DUEL WITHOUT END

DUEL WITHOUT END

Mankind's Battle with Microbes

STIG S. FRØLAND

Translated by John Irons

REAKTION BOOKS

Published by
REAKTION BOOKS LTD
Unit 32, Waterside
44–48 Wharf Road
London N1 7UX, UK
www.reaktionbooks.co.uk

First published in English 2022
Copyright © Stig Sophus Frøland 2022
First published in Norwegian as *Kampen mellom mennesket
og mikrobene*, © Stig Sophus Frøland 2020

This translation has been published with
the financial support of NORLA

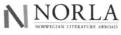

NORLA
NORWEGIAN LITERATURE ABROAD

Printed and bound in India by Replika Press Pvt. Ltd

A catalogue record for this book is available from the British Library

ISBN 978 1 78914 505 2

Contents

Foreword

THROUGHOUT HUMAN HISTORY a duel has been fought between man and microbes. This has not only led to countless infectious diseases and an inconceivable number of deaths but has had far-reaching consequences for culture and society.

For several years after the Second World War there was a widespread belief that the era of infectious diseases as a serious threat was over. This turned out to be a formidable miscalculation. Not only have many of the well-known infectious diseases held their own in many parts of the world, but over the past decades we have also encountered a large number of previously unknown microbes that have caused life-threatening disease problems and, to a certain extent, major epidemics. The HIV, Ebola, SARS and COVID-19 viruses are just a few characters in the sinister cast of microbes that have appeared on the scene. The mass media constantly come up with announcements of new infectious diseases and epidemic threats.

We now know that the duel between man and microbes is an ongoing affair – and that it will continue for as long as humanity exists on this earth. But we also know far more about the factors that influence the outcome of this eternal duel, including the consequences of the ever-increasing, man-made changes to nature around us. The new knowledge gleaned about the connection between infection and ecology is important for our duel against microbes in the future.

The new insight into the interaction between man and the world of microbes has shown itself to be useful in trying to understand the history of human infection through the ages. In recent years we have also seen an increased understanding of the importance of infectious diseases and epidemics for the course of history.

This book provides an updated presentation of the eternal duel between man and microbes and the many factors that influence its outcome. I describe the major transitions in the history of human infection from the time when the first representatives of *Homo sapiens* roamed the African savannahs. I also deal with a number of the large epidemics that have affected humanity through history, of which the Black Death is just one of many examples. One chapter is devoted to the significance that many of these epidemics may have had for the downfall of civilizations and empires. Some of the new infectious diseases that were discovered from the second half of the twentieth century onwards are dealt with in separate chapters.

The book also deals with how man has fought back against microbes via vaccines and antibiotics. Here I describe a number of the microbial threats we will probably have to face in the future, and how we can combat them. This includes the constant threat from new epidemics and pandemics. From the beginning of 2020 the world has been confronting a new pandemic involving a formerly unknown coronavirus: SARS-CoV-2. We have been shown once again the considerable consequences a pandemic has for both the individual and society – an echo from the pandemics of the past that have repeatedly shaken humanity. In the book I emphasize that the question is not *whether* we will encounter new pandemics in the future but *when* – and which particular microbe from the multifarious world of microbes will be involved.

The history of human infectious diseases is dramatic and colourful. But it is also extremely comprehensive and complex. My project may thus appear to be highly ambitious. I have decided to write this book in spite of this for two main underlying reasons.

First, as a doctor I have spent practically all of my working life dealing with infectious diseases and the immune response to microbes, partly as a researcher, and partly as a clinician and doctor with patients. For a number of years I have also worked at many levels on one of the largest pandemics of recent times: the AIDS pandemic. I have been involved in much teaching and have given countless lectures on these subjects. Second, since my childhood I have had a burning interest in history, one that has not diminished over the years. With this dual background I succumbed to the temptation to combine my medicinal and historical interests.

The result is this book. It is not an academic thesis intended for specialists. The primary target group is interested readers without previous specialized knowledge. Even so, I have included a number of references for those who might wish to see something of the background of the material I am presenting.

If I am able to convey just a fraction of the fascination I myself have for this topic, I will be content.

Prologue: The Invisible Enemy

Homo sapiens – our own species of the human race – originally came from Africa. The first fossil finds of human types that manifestly looked like present-day humans were made in Africa and are more than 200,000, perhaps closer to 300,000, years old.

About 60,000 years ago some of our ancestors left Africa and gradually spread out over all the earth's continents, with the exception of Antarctica. This, until now, has been the prevailing view,[1] but new research finds can be argued to imply that this migration started somewhat earlier, perhaps more than 100,000 years ago.[2]

The first humans doubtless faced many threats and challenges. Considerable changes in climate conditions put their adaptability to the test – from tropical conditions on African savannahs to much cooler climates in temperate zones. Predatory animals of many kinds threatened our ancestors, including fearsome species that have long since become extinct, such as the sabre-toothed tiger and huge types of cave bear. Even so, human beings managed to develop strategies to survive these visible threats, although many lives must unquestionably have been lost in the struggle.

From the outset, however, our ancestors were exposed to other threats, at least as dangerous, about which they were unaware: attacks from invisible enemies, microorganisms that can cause infectious diseases. Bacteria, viruses, fungi and other microorganisms have been the cause of acute and chronic, deadly and more harmless infections.[3]

Throughout our entire history of development, a duel has been taking place between man and microorganisms – a never-ending duel that is still being fought and will continue to be so for as long as humans exist on the planet. This duel has had enormous consequences for *Homo sapiens*, not only from a medical point of view but on our history, culture and society.

To understand the history of human infections through the ages it is not sufficient just to look at the two duellists – man and the microbes – and their attributes. It has gradually become apparent that the outcome of the duel is very often decided by ecological and environmental relations.

This book deals with this interaction between man, microbes and ecological factors throughout the thousands of years of man's history of infection.

ONE

The Duellists

T he fact that microorganisms such as bacteria and viruses can cause infectious diseases is now common knowledge, a natural part of what we learn as children. The same applies to an understanding of which diseases can be passed on from one person to another. Even so, not all that many years have passed since such views made their breakthrough via a number of epoch-making research finds in the second half of the nineteenth century. For several hundreds of thousands of years prior to this insight, *Homo sapiens* has constantly been the victim of a large number of infectious diseases both acute and chronic, fatal and banal.

What ideas did our ancestors have about the cause of such diseases, which quite often took a dramatic course as epidemics, with great consequences for society? An important characteristic of our species, one that distinguishes us from other animal species, is the wish to understand the surrounding world and what goes on around us. For that reason, humans have doubtless thought a great deal about the causes of the many diseases that we now know are infections. These early theories about disease were naturally shaped by the prevailing conceptions about the world and the place of humanity within it.

Apollo's Arrows or Miasmas?

It seems highly probable that religious ideas – the belief in supernatural forces in nature, and subsequently in various types of god that could intervene in human life – arose during an early stage of human development. The earliest conceptions of the causes of infectious diseases, naturally enough, were that they were a result of the intervention of gods or demons.[1]

In the ancient civilizations of Sumer and Babylon in Mesopotamia, and also in China, we find over a period of thousands of years widespread popular belief in demons as the cause of infectious diseases.[2] One important Mesopotamian deity was Nergal, the ruler of the underworld, who was worshipped as the god of fever, plague and war. Similar concepts were also found in ancient Chinese civilization.

In the Old Testament we find accounts of how Yahweh punished Israel's foes with plagues.[3] The Philistines were punished in this way when they stole the Ark of the Covenant from the temple in Jerusalem, and the Assyrians were struck down by a plague when they threatened to conquer Jerusalem. In the New Testament demons play an important role in diseases, including infections.[4]

In ancient Greece religious concepts of the causes of disease were important, particularly in the event of epidemics. Here the god Apollo was a central figure, both as a bringer and curer of disease.[5] He could

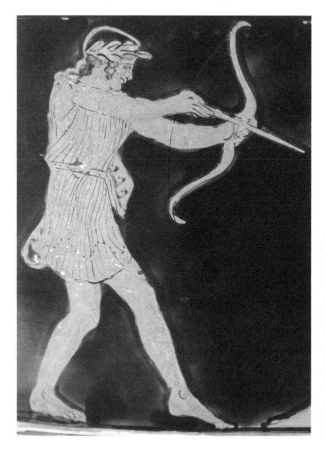

Apollo with his bow. Apollo – son of the god of heaven, Zeus – was one of the most popular gods of ancient Greece. One of his many tasks was to be the god of healing and diseases. But he could also bring about epidemics by shooting plague arrows with his bow when he wished to punish humanity.

cause epidemics by taking his bow and shooting plague arrows at people. In the very first book of the *Iliad*, Homer describes how Apollo sent a plague sweeping through the Greek armies because Agamemnon, the Greek commander, had offended the priest of Apollo:

> The arrows clanged at his back as the god quaked with rage,
> the god himself on the march and down he came like night.
> Over against the ships he dropped to a knee, let fly a shaft
> and a terrifying clash rang out from the great silver bow.
> First he went for the mules and circling dogs but then,
> launching a piercing shaft at the men themselves,
> he cut them down in droves –
> and the corpse-fires burned on, night and day, no end in sight.[6]

In the *Iliad* the plague does not cease until Apollo has been pacified. In the tragedy *Oedipus the King* by Sophocles, the city of Thebes is ravaged by a plague epidemic. The oracle of Delphi announces that this is the punishment of the gods because the present ruler of the city, Oedipus, has killed the former king, who was his father. It is the patricide that here represents the offence against divine law.[7]

The views of Homer and Sophocles were without a doubt in accordance with the people's conceptions of the divine causes of epidemics. These concepts were retained among most people throughout antiquity and the Middle Ages. In Rome there were no fewer than three temples dedicated to the goddess Febris, who controlled fevers, the most common of which was probably malaria. Even in our own time we occasionally come across such attitudes in certain religious environments. When the AIDS epidemic broke out in the early 1980s, certain Christian preachers announced that this was the Lord's punishment for ungodly sexual behaviour.

From antiquity until the present day, in many cultures there have also existed ideas that diseases, including infectious diseases, can be caused by black magic carried out by witches and magicians who are in contact with evil, supernatural powers. This has contributed to witch hunts down the ages and still occurs in certain African societies.

Sagas from the Norse period in Iceland and Greenland reveal that people also assumed there were supernatural causes of epidemics. There

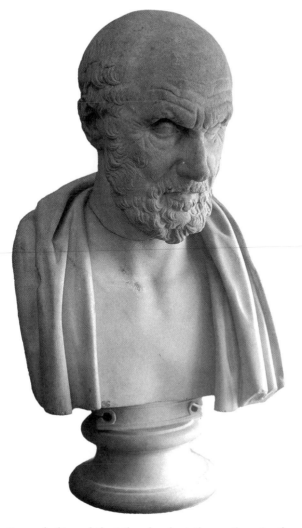

Hippocrates of Kos is the most famous physician of all time. He lived and practised in Athens in the 5th century BC, at the same time as Plato and Socrates.

it was believed that the dead, at the outbreak of an epidemic, sought to drag the living along with them into death.[8]

Ancient Greece has strongly influenced Western civilization in a great many areas. We have mentioned the religious explanations of the causes of infectious diseases in ancient Greek culture. At the same time, there were early alternative ways of thinking that attempted to under-stand nature and the place of humanity in it without resorting to religious explanations. The beginnings of natural science arose with the Greek philosophers of nature in the sixth and seventh centuries BC.[9] A recurrent idea found in their works was that the universe consisted of a small number of basic elements that are normally in a state of balance. The same laws that apply to the macrocosm – the world around us – must also apply to the human body, they believed. Some of these philosophers claimed that illness resulted from the balance between the elements or components of the body being disturbed in some way or other. These basic ideas were developed by the semi-mythical doctor Hippocrates of Kos and his many successors.

Despite the fact that Hippocrates is indubitably the most famous physician of all time, we know very little about him. He lived and practised in Athens in the fifth century BC, at roughly the same time as Socrates and Plato, the latter of whom refers to him in a number of his writings as being an excellent physician. The medical teaching ascribed to Hippocrates and his pupils is to be found in the so-called Hippocratic Collection (*Corpus hippocraticum*). We do not know which of these, if any, Hippocrates wrote himself. Among other things, they include a discussion of fevers and epidemics as well as their causes.[10] The basis of the views of diseases in the collection, highly simplified, is that illness results from a disturbance of the balance in the body between the most important body fluids: blood, yellow gall, phlegm (mucus) and black gall. Pandemics are caused by the influence of harmful vapours – miasmas – in the air. The Greek word *miasma* means pollution.[11] Such pathogenic miasmas can come from stagnant water and ponds, unhealthy sumps or the rotting corpses of animals or humans. Miasmas are typically accompanied by a foul stench. There is emphasis on the fact that both the seasons of the year and meteorological factors are significant in epidemics, and that a role is played by the positions of the planets and the stars. People also display individual differences in how susceptible they are to miasmas.

The views of diseases expressed in the Hippocratic Collection, and its teaching on miasmas, were developed by Galen, who, alongside Hippocrates, is the most famous physician of antiquity.[12] He was Greek, born in Pergamon in Asia Minor, but practised in Rome in the mid-second century AD, and was employed by the philosopher-emperor Marcus Aurelius as his personal physician. Galen was to have an enormous influence on European medicine for the next 1,500 years. The teachings of Hippocrates and Galen about diseases were also translated into Arabic in the eighth and ninth centuries and came to have a profound influence on medicine in the Muslim world.

The concept that miasmas caused disease survived well into the nineteenth century, even though the old Hippocratic theories about disease being the result of an imbalance between bodily fluids had gradually been abandoned. From the Enlightenment onwards, there was an increasing belief in the positive influence of hygiene and good sanitary conditions. The ideas that miasmas were a cause of epidemic diseases was one of the driving forces behind the many measures during the nineteenth century intended to improve the sometimes dreadful sanitary conditions that characterized the rapid growth of cities during industrialization.

The Pioneers of Germ Theory

Religious conceptions regarding the causes of what we now consider to be infectious diseases had a firm hold on people's minds from the beginnings of history, while non-religious explanations such as the belief in miasmas gradually also came to influence human thought, particularly in the upper echelons of society. These differing conceptions seem to have existed alongside each other.

Many infectious diseases are also extremely contagious, yet it is surprising that the existence of contagion was not recognized early on. If we return to the Hippocratic Collection, we find detailed descriptions of symptoms and the course of infectious diseases, but there is no evidence anywhere that the author took into account the spread of infection from one person to another. This also applies to learned physicians, it should be noted, in the centuries after Hippocrates and Galen. Were ordinary people unable to observe contagion in their everyday lives during epidemics? Did people blindly accept the scholars' theories? No; opinions are sometimes expressed supporting the theory that there was some knowledge of contagion being passed from one person to another in infections, and that this characterized people's behaviour during epidemics.

The first basis for this can be found in the Greek historian Thucydides.[13] In his comprehensive account of the epidemic that ravaged Athens in the fifth century BC, it seems as if he reckoned on the disease being passed from one person to another. And, just as interesting, one gains the impression that he also believed this to be a quite common view among Athenians.

We must move forwards more than 1,700 years before we find further evidence that person-to-person contagion was a widely held concept, one that even had political consequences. One of the most famous epidemics of all time, the Black Death, was then ravaging the world. In its wake, an increasing number of European cities, based on the model used for Italian cities, introduced measures that were clearly aimed at preventing the spread of infection.[14] These included the introduction of quarantine: sailors from newly arrived ships were kept on board, isolated from the population, for forty days, to see whether or not they fell ill. The word quarantine comes from the Italian *quaranti giorni*, which means forty days in a Venetian dialect. When syphilis exploded as an epidemic in Europe at the beginning of the sixteenth century, it was also abundantly obvious to most people that this disease was transmitted from person to person.

Although the idea of contagion was clearly accepted in sections of the population, at any rate as far as certain diseases were involved, the classic teaching of miasmas still prevailed among learned physicians, who held on to the legacy of Hippocrates. And even though some of them accepted the idea of contagion with regard to certain diseases, there was, naturally enough, no clear understanding of why and how this occurred.

There was, however, one man who diverged greatly from the conventional views of his colleagues. This was the Italian Girolamo Fracastoro, or, as he called himself in his Latin writings, Hieronymus Fracastorius. Fracastoro wrote during the first half of the sixteenth century. In many ways he was a typical Renaissance figure who excelled at both science and art.[15] He was a physician, indeed the pope's private physician, a professor of logic at the university of Padua, an astronomer and a poet who wrote in elegant Latin. Two of Fracastoro's works give him a place in the history of medicine: his poem on syphilis (*Syphilis sive morbus gallicus*, 1530) and his later work *De contagione et contagiosis morbis et eorum curatione* (On Contagion and Contagious Diseases and Their Cure, 1546).[16]

Fracastoro's poem on syphilis is not some sort of dirty limerick but an epic in no fewer than three volumes, in which he gives a thorough account of the disease – its symptoms, origins and treatment – and employs the term 'syphilis' for the first time. He also deals with the

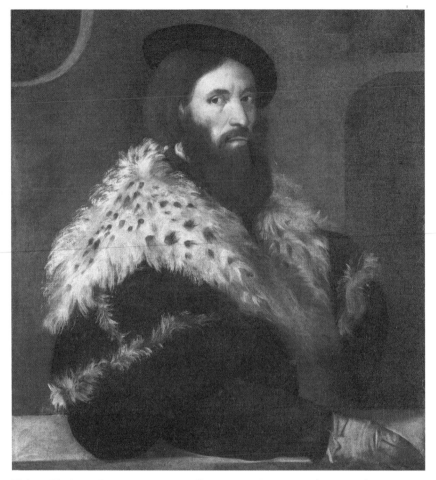

Titian, *Girolamo Fracastoro*, *c.* 1528, oil on canvas. Fracastoro (1478–1553) was a physician, and a typical Renaissance figure who engaged in medicine, poetry, philosophy and astronomy. He is best known for a work on syphilis and for one in which he presents a comprehensive theory about contagion and contagious diseases.

mechanisms of infection, but does not present his final theories on germs until several years later in the second work, in which he claims that infection is caused by the transmission of extremely small, invisible particles, which he calls *seminaria*. These can be transmitted directly from person to person, via objects such as clothing or through the air. This accords well with our present-day conceptions, and Fracastoro has been praised to the skies in our own age as a visionary pioneer. Others have more soberly pointed out that one cannot know for sure what Fracastoro meant by his *seminaria*, and that he did not, at any rate, regard them as living organisms.

It has also been claimed that Fracastoro was not completely original, since it has been discovered that certain antique writers before him mentioned that disease can be caused by minute creatures, or *animalcula*, as they are called in Latin. At certain points in Galen's comprehensive writings he also talks about 'plague seeds', without explaining the basis for this or developing the theme further, to the great frustration of modern Galen scholars.

Despite these objections, Fracastoro's theories are interesting. They gave rise to a certain amount of interest in some decades to follow, but were then consigned to oblivion until they were rediscovered with enthusiasm in the twentieth century, when he was almost declared to be the father of modern infection medicine.[17]

Just over a century after Fracastoro's death in 1553, the Dutch amateur researcher Anton van Leeuwenhoek came up with some epoch-making discoveries that, seen in retrospect, ought to have brought Fracastoro to the fore once more and accelerated scientific development towards our present-day view of microbes and infection.[18] Van Leeuwenhoek, who was born in 1632, was a respected draper from Delft. He had no real formal education, but he had a hobby that engrossed him: the use of the microscope for studying nature. He taught himself to make microscope lenses in a new way and the microscopes he created, of which he had around two hundred, were considerably better than the somewhat primitive instruments known until then. One day in 1674 he placed a drop of water from a pond under the microscope and, to his amazement, could see a great many minute creatures that were invisible to the naked eye. What he probably saw were a number of single-cell organisms, which today are called protozoa. Two years later, when he had further improved his microscope, he took a sample from his own gums and placed it under the microscope. He emphasizes in his account how meticulous he was with his own oral hygiene. Despite this, he was amazed to see a great number of minute organisms, of which he made very precise drawings. There can be no doubt whatsoever that this is history's first description of bacteria, which are even smaller than the protozoa he had seen earlier.

Van Leeuwenhoek published his findings and became famous for his discoveries using a microscope. Prominent people from all over Europe wished to look through his microscope, including Tsar Peter the Great of Russia and Queen Mary II of England and Scotland, who were given microscopes as gifts.

Van Leeuwenhoek never understood that the small organisms he had discovered could be the cause of disease: he spoke and wrote only Dutch and was unfamiliar with Fracastoro's germ theories. Surprisingly enough, no medical scholars linked these newly discovered bacteria to Fracastoro and infectious diseases. The time was not yet ripe, and Van Leeuwenhoek's small creatures were regarded as an amusing curiosity.

The Breakthrough – and the Preceding Struggle

Let us move forwards to the first half of the nineteenth century. Was the world now ready for more modern theories about the transmission of infection by germs? Not at all. Admittedly, people realized in practice that a number of the common infectious diseases such as syphilis, gonorrhoea, smallpox and measles were transmitted from person to person, but this was not linked to the idea of live pathogens. In some countries the authorities had long since established various quarantine measures to prevent the spreading of epidemics, mainly the 'big three': the plague, yellow fever and cholera. But this did not mean that there was any sort of agreement that they were infectious diseases, in the modern sense of the term. People explained the possible effect of quarantine measures by rather ingenious interpretations of the miasma theory.

It was not only reactionary and anti-scientific sticks-in-the-mud who were opposed to germ theory. Many of the antagonists were excellent scientists who fought against what they considered to be outdated theories and traditions from earlier times – and they were in a fairly strong position. Even though the belief in contagion had been widespread for centuries, no one had been able to explain how it could actually take place. And the experiences gained from quarantine measures for the major epidemics such as the plague, yellow fever and cholera did not point unequivocally towards person-to-person infection. Today, we know why. When it comes to the plague and yellow fever, infection with the microbe is normally not from person to person but via a bite from infection-carrying insects. In the case of cholera, it is usually waterborne. This means that one will often encounter cases where the infected person has not been in contact with patients who are already ill. This was why the classic quarantine measures used from as early as the medieval period did not always work. This was taken to be evidence against person-to-person infection. And it meant that the miasma theory, in updated versions with the emphasis on the importance of comprehensive sanitary measures, seemed considerably more plausible to many people. The miasma theory had gradually been modified to such an extent that it was now thought that the pathogenic 'miasma contaminants' were not only airborne but could also be transmitted via clothing and objects.

Prominent researchers knew about the existence of the micro-organisms already demonstrated by Van Leeuwenhoek, but no one had yet convincingly documented that such microbes cause disease in human beings. Furthermore, it had been demonstrated that bacteria could exist in the bodies of completely healthy individuals. Through the somewhat primitive microscopes of the time, all bacteria also looked more or less the same, and it was thought to be hardly probable that there were many different types of bacteria with completely different capacities to cause disease.

There were also other factors in the mid-nineteenth century that consolidated the resistance to the theories of contagion by germs.[19] An influential middle class had emerged that was highly involved in inter-national trade and supported economic liberalism without too much intervention from the authorities. All the old quarantine regulations that were still enforced in many places were regarded as being damag-ing to trade, because they could lead to considerable financial loss and, as we have seen, were not even always effective. The opponents of such measures saw themselves as men of the future who were fighting for the freedom of the individual and trade against reactionary and despotic regimes. Their ingrained resistance led to the abolition of a number of quarantine measures in several European countries.

Even though political and economic considerations certainly played a role in this debate, there is no doubt that the opponents of germ theory were completely convinced they were right. For that reason, some of them fearlessly carried out experiments by exposing themselves to all kinds of infectious material from patients with diseases such as yellow fever and the plague. Surprisingly enough, no infection resulted in most instances. In certain cases, however, things went badly wrong: one experimenter, for example, died of self-inflicted yellow fever after having survived an attempt to give himself the plague. Often, though, the negative results of these fearless experiments fitted the theory, with people concluding that contagion did not play any role.

A final factor that contributed to the polarization between supporters and opponents of germ theory was the dispute about spontaneous generation, a concept that is alien to us now that Charles Darwin and the theory of evolution are part of our schoolday knowledge.[20] The theory of spontaneous generation – the belief that life can come into being out of dead matter – has its roots in antiquity and originally had many supporters.[21] It was believed, for example, that small animals such as mice and frogs could come into being spontaneously from dead, rotting matter. The dispute about spontaneous generation became important because it also reflected the feud between the Church and critics of religion, who had become increasingly vociferous from the time of the Enlightenment in the latter half of the eighteenth century.

While Christians held that the idea of spontaneous generation was blasphemy, since only God could create new life, a number of the thinkers of the Enlightenment and their successors supported the theory. In the nineteenth century there were still many who were convinced that microorganisms such as bacteria could spontaneously come into being, for example in rotting matter. Representatives of the two camps were carrying out experiments of varying quality as early as the eighteenth century to find means of justifying their points of view, without this leading to any unequivocal conclusion.

Why was the theory of spontaneous generation of importance for the dispute about germ theory? It was because those people who thought that bacteria could arise out of nothing claimed that this could also take place within the human body, without it having to do with an infection from outside. This idea, which we now know is wrong, was held by highly respected scientists who rejected the theories of contagion and the ability of bacteria to cause disease.

Around 1850 the outcome of the hard-fought and at times emotional dispute between opponents and supporters of germ theory and the role of bacteria was still completely undecided.[22] The supporters, however, were not just twiddling their thumbs during this period. A number of new findings were made, based partly on real experiments and partly on meticulous and intelligent observations, that gradually caused those opposing germ theory to beat a retreat, laying the basis for what we can call the bacteriological revolution. Several of these discoveries were made by relatively unknown researchers and doctors, which meant that initially they did not get much publicity. In certain cases they were also the subject of strong criticism. Let us take a look at some of them with fresh eyes.

One famous story is that of the British surgeon John Snow and cholera.[23] Europe was still being ravaged by cholera epidemics. Snow had studied the details of a number of these epidemics and had become convinced that the disease must be caused by some infectious substance present in the patients' faeces, which infected new individuals via drinking water. During an epidemic in the London district of Soho in 1854, he observed that cholera particularly afflicted those people who fetched water from a particular public water pump in Broad Street, and he became convinced that this must be infected by the contaminant. He persuaded the local authorities to remove the pump handle, which led to a dramatic fall in new cases of cholera. It must be admitted, however, that by then the epidemic was already very much on the decline.

Snow did not content himself with this. London's water supply was provided by various private firms that sourced it from the Thames at different points. Snow was able to show that districts supplied by companies that fetched water *upstream* of London – water that had not been polluted by sewage from the city – suffered far fewer cases of cholera than those where the water was drawn from the Thames *inside* London – water that was highly polluted by the then quite primitive refuse and sewage systems.

Initially Snow met with considerable resistance to his germ theory and was unable to have his reports printed in the most recognized periodicals. Gradually, however, his message got home and had practical consequences for the organization of London's water supply. Although Snow could not himself demonstrate the infectious agent that caused cholera, he deserves a place in the history of medicine. His views on cholera infection were admittedly not completely original, but he made an impressive effort to get them confirmed in practice. He has also had a pub named after him in what is now Broadwick Street, even though he was teetotal for most of his life.

Far more tragic is the story of the Hungarian obstetrician Ignaz Semmelweis. In the mid-nineteenth century infections raged in surgical

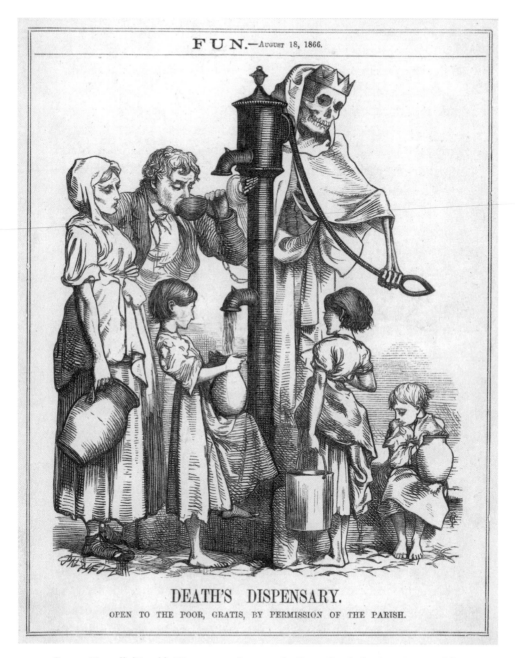

DEATH'S DISPENSARY.

OPEN TO THE POOR, GRATIS, BY PERMISSION OF THE PARISH.

George Pinwell, 'Death's Dispensary: Open to the Poor, Gratis, by Permission of the Parish', *Fun*, 18 August 1866. This satirical drawing shows the water pump in Broad Street in London's Soho district that spread the deadly cholera infection.

wards in European hospitals.[24] There was an extremely high mortality rate from bacterial infections after operations. One surgeon stated that a patient hospitalized for an operation had a greater risk of dying than a British soldier on the battlefield at Waterloo in 1815. This was also the case in most of the maternity wards, where the risk of childbed fever, which is caused by bacteria, was considerable and led to a high mortality rate.

Semmelweis worked in the maternity ward of one of the largest hospitals in Vienna, where he was shocked to observe the high incidence of childbed fever. This maternity ward was divided into two, one where student midwives assisted at the births and one where medical students were responsible. Semmelweis meticulously recorded the occurrence of childbed fever in the two sub-wards and was able to show unequivocally that this complication followed the medical students, not the midwives. What could be the reason for this? He discovered that the medical students very often came from maternity-ward autopsies. He concluded that the students' hands were probably contaminated with what he called 'corpse particles', which were then brought into contact with the women's genitals. It was these 'corpse particles' that Semmelweis believed were the cause of childbed fever. He was unaware that these were living microorganisms, but he ordered the students to wash their hands thoroughly in chlorinated water before taking part in births from then on. This led to a dramatic fall in childbed fever at the hospital.

An important part of the classic story about Semmelweis is the amount of resistance he encountered from the medical authorities, who doubted his theories, and his tragic end in a mental hospital, where he was physically maltreated. He died in 1865, probably as the result of a wound infection caused by the very same bacterium he had fought against.

To a great many people, Semmelweis has gone down in history as a martyr for new scientific truths, but a great deal of this is myth. He actually won over many supporters who gradually spread his message across Europe. That he also met with some resistance from sections of the medical elite in Vienna is probably correct, but it is not really all that surprising. It calls for a certain amount of personal and social talent to 'sell' completely new and revolutionary truths in science. Semmelweis was probably devoid of such a talent. He was a difficult man who gradually developed major personality disturbances with paranoid characteristics that estranged friends and supporters. Nor was the political climate in Vienna at the time favourable, with considerable antagonism between Austrians and Hungarians, which was hardly an advantage for the Hungarian Semmelweis.

Although Semmelweis may not have realized it, one doctor before him had also arrived at the conclusion that childbed fever was caused by an infectious substance. The Scottish doctor Alexander Gordon came to this conclusion around 1790, but was greatly thwarted by his colleagues and ended up a broken man on his brother's farm.[25]

A now-little-known pioneer who made discoveries that paved the way for later breakthroughs in germ theory and the role of bacteria was the French physician Casimir-Joseph Davaine. In the 1860s Davaine carried out a series of elegant studies of the bacterial disease anthrax, which raged, with serious economic consequences, among various kinds of livestock, even occasionally causing death among human beings. He was able to detect the bacteria in the blood of sick animals and show that blood containing the bacteria transmitted the disease to healthy animals. Initially he met with considerable resistance from the medical profession, and was later completely overshadowed by the giant figures Louis Pasteur and Robert Koch, who became dominant in the bacteriological revolution in the second half of the nineteenth century.

Davaine, however, was not the only one to make important discoveries that led to major breakthroughs in the understanding of the role of bacteria in diseases. Norway, which in the nineteenth century must be said to have been quite marginalized in European intellectual life, was able to make a considerable contribution within this area. In 1873 the Norwegian doctor Armauer Hansen, who worked at a leprosy hospital in Bergen, made an important discovery.[26] He was profoundly interested in the disease of leprosy, which at the time people assumed was either hereditary or caused by miasmas.[27] Hansen, however, was able to detect under the microscope small rod-like bodies inside cells from sick tissue, and concluded that these must be the cause of leprosy. This was the first identification of the leprosy bacterium. A German researcher, Albert Neisser, attempted to steal the honour of the discovery, but today Hansen has gained his rightful place in the history of leprosy, and

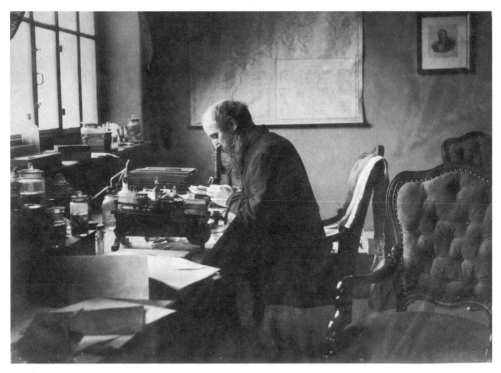

In 1873 the doctor Armauer Hansen, who worked at one of the three leprosy hospitals in Bergen, was the first person to detect leprosy bacteria in tissue from a leprosy patient. Leprosy is often referred to as 'Hansen's disease'.

internationally leprosy is often referred to as 'Hansen's disease'. It must, however, be admitted that Hansen's sense of ethics was not quite at the same level as his talent for research: he attempted to transfer the bacteria into a woman's eye. She already had leprosy, but Hansen wanted to see if she now contracted the same type of leprosy as the patient from whom the bacteria had come. He was given a relatively mild sentence, but lost his position at the leprosy hospital in Bergen.

The Toreadors Enter the Arena

A great many important observations had been made that spoke in favour of transmitted bacteria being of crucial importance for a number of diseases, but as yet there was no irrefutable evidence. The situation in the germ theory dispute in the mid-nineteenth century is reminiscent of a bullfight. During the first rounds of a *corrida*, as it is called in Spanish, the bull is weakened in various ways by riders with lances, known as picadors, without being defeated. Then comes the climax as the toreador enters the arena. If all now goes well, the bull is killed by an elegant thrust from the toreador's sword, to thunderous applause and music from the tribune. This is called 'the moment of truth'. The researchers whom I have named so far have, in a sense, the role of picadors preparing this 'moment of truth' in the history of germ theory. The ecstatically acclaimed toreadors in the story normally told about

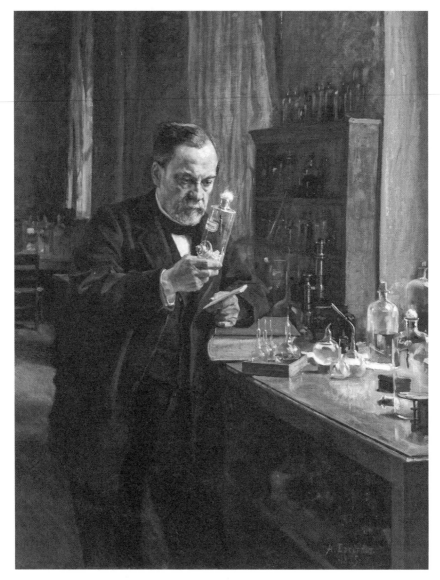

Albert Edelfelt, *Louis Pasteur*, 1885, oil on canvas.

the bacteriological revolution are the Frenchman Louis Pasteur and the German Robert Koch.

Louis Pasteur was born in 1822, the son of a tanner who had previously fought bravely in Napoleon's army. Louis studied chemistry and eventually became a professor in the subject, in which he made interesting and original finds.[28] Partly as a result of coincidences, he became interested in the mechanisms of fermentation processes, which the authorities claimed were caused exclusively by chemical reactions. Pasteur, however, was able to show that the various forms of fermentation were completely dependent on living microorganisms: yeast fungi and bacteria. He proved that different bacteria produced different results of the fermentation. In his laboratory he managed to cultivate the various bacteria and fungi he was studying. He also demonstrated that certain bacteria caused harmful fermentation in, for example, the brewing of beer, and that one can prevent this by heat treatment, which kills the microorganisms responsible. This is the basis of what later became known as pasteurization, of milk for example, where the treatment deactivates the bacteria that spoil the milk.

Pasteur then threw himself into the dispute about spontaneous generation that was still taking place. As his point of departure, he did not believe that spontaneous generation was possible. This phenomenon was also incompatible with his religious beliefs. In a series of elegant experiments he definitively crushed this centuries-old idea.[29]

Once again via a number of coincidences, Pasteur started to investigate the possible cause of various diseases that destroyed the silkworms that were vital for the economically important silk industry in France. After a considerable number of experiments he managed to demonstrate that the diseases that affected the silkworms were caused by microorganisms. So it was a case of infection!

Pasteur's results were also to be of great consequence for French wine production. This, it goes without saying, brought him great popularity, since according to the current president of the republic, Emmanuel Macron, wine 'represents the soul of France'.

From then on, Pasteur became increasingly interested in microbes as the cause of disease, also in humans, and he devoted the rest of his life to attempts to prove this. He studied infections in animal experiments and also followed up on Davaine's studies of anthrax bacteria. His results also convincingly confirmed the recently published finds by the young Robert Koch, to whom we will return. Pasteur's most important contribution during these years, however, is his epoch-making studies of vaccines for human beings, which in many ways laid the foundation of the triumphs of modern vaccination medicine. We will return later to that part of his contribution, which was just as significant as his fundamental studies of bacteria.

Pasteur's historic discoveries of the role of bacteria gained a great deal of attention, both in France and abroad. A young British surgeon, Joseph Lister, was among those fascinated by Pasteur's finds.[30] Like other surgeons of the time, he was greatly interested in the post-operative infection of wounds, which was a major problem as it led to a high mortality rate.

Lister had the idea that wound infections were quite simply caused by surrounding bacteria that got into the wounds, leading to harmful processes of the same type as Pasteur had proved took place in fermentation. He believed that it must be sensible to treat such infections with germicidal substances and chose the chemical substance phenol, which he applied directly to wounds from operations and also used as a spray in the air around the patient. His results showed convincingly that phenol had an effect.

Lister's methods were very soon adopted on the continent, first in Germany, then in France. In Britain and the USA, on the other hand, he initially met with considerable scepticism. Among other things, this was because of a certain distrust of the theories of bacteria and germs in general in the world of medicine. Gradually, however, Lister gained full recognition as a pioneer, and he was given the title Baron Lister by Queen Victoria in 1897. The dedicated work carried out by him and other surgeons in combatting wound infections has been of enormous importance for the development of surgery over the past 150 years.

We now come to Pasteur's great rival, the other true giant of the bacteriological revolution, Robert Koch.[31] Early in his medical career be became fascinated by infectious diseases, including cholera, with which he became familiar during an epidemic, as well as the wound infections that he experienced as an army doctor during the Franco-Prussian War of 1870–71. As a practising local doctor in the small town of Wöllstein (now Wolsztyn in Poland), he became interested in the

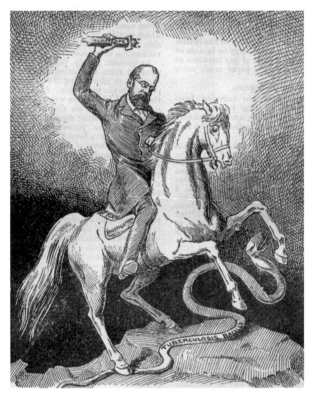

Robert Koch depicted as St George fighting the dragon tuberculosis. Koch's weapon is the microscope.

disease anthrax, which at the time was ravaging flocks of sheep and also causing a number of human fatalities.

Koch's wife gave him a microscope as a present on his 29th birthday. He set up a somewhat primitive improvised laboratory separated from his doctor's surgery by a curtain, and, with hardly any contact with other research environments, made a number of fundamental discoveries showing that anthrax was caused by a bacterium. Like Davaine before him, Koch found the bacterium in the blood of sick animals. He managed to cultivate it and was able to transmit the disease to experimental animals via the bacteria. He further discovered that the bacterium could mutate into spores, a kind of dormant state that was extremely hardy and capable of surviving for a long time in nature before they once more converted to fatal bacteria, which could infect both animals and humans.

Koch published his anthrax finds in 1876. This must be regarded as one of the great breakthroughs in the history of infection medicine, since it was the first time that anyone had been able to show that bacteria cause disease in humans. The discovery caused quite a stir, although some people doubted the findings. As mentioned, Pasteur was able to definitively confirm them somewhat later.

Koch followed this up with a number of new discoveries that laid much of the foundations of modern bacteriology.[32] He launched a series of new cultivation methods for bacteria and devised staining methods that could easily demonstrate them. He also contributed to technical improvements to microscopes, which proved very important for the further study of bacteria.

Today, it may seem strange that several prominent researchers at the time claimed that there was only one type of bacterium that could mutate into other bacteria. With his extremely thorough studies of, among other things, various kinds of wound infection, Koch was able to completely refute such assertions: a large number of different bacteria exist, and dissimilar bacteria cause different types of infection. This also agreed with Pasteur's findings concerning the role of different bacteria in fermentation.

Then came perhaps Koch's finest hour, his discovery of the bacterium that causes tuberculosis. Anthrax was a relatively uncommon infection in human beings and mainly played a role in agriculture. Tuberculosis, on the other hand, was an extremely widespread disease, responsible at the time for one death in every seven in Europe. The theory that it might be an infectious disease was not completely new.[33] A French army doctor, Jean Villemin, had shown as early as 1865, through epoch-making experiments, that he could transmit tuberculosis by injecting rabbits with diseased tissue from tuberculosis patients. But he was unable to prove the existence of any bacterium, and so his findings were treated with scepticism. Koch was convinced that there had to be a tuberculosis bacterium in the diseased tissue from patients, one that was not visible using his usual dyeing methods for bacteria. Via meticulous trial-and-error methods he managed to create a completely new dyeing method, which convincingly demonstrated the existence of bacteria in tissue from both humans and experimental animals with tuberculous infection.

After further laborious experiments, Koch also managed to cultivate these tuberculosis bacteria. He subsequently showed that experimental animals he infected with the bacteria developed typical signs of tuberculosis.

In March 1882 Robert Koch presented his tuberculosis finds at a scientific gathering in Berlin. His audience, which counted several celebrities from the research world, was almost speechless with admiration. A later Nobel Prize-winner who was present, Paul Ehrlich, stated that this 'was the most important experience of my life as a scientist'. In the course of a couple of months, Koch had become internationally famous.

Shortly after this success with tuberculosis, however, Koch took up a new challenge: cholera.[34] Cholera still gave rise to serious epidemics with high mortality and had now descended on Egypt. After a request from the Egyptian government, research teams from Germany, led by Koch, and from France, under one of Pasteur's men, travelled to Egypt. Koch and his assistants managed to detect the cholera bacterium in a patient's intestinal system in 1883. He also managed to cultivate the bacterium and show that in all probability it was transmitted via polluted drinking water. When the epidemic had peaked in Egypt and the number of patients was on the decrease, Koch and his team continued their studies of cholera in India.

On their return home to Germany, they were celebrated as heroes. The French group, however, was completely unsuccessful and had to return home crestfallen after one of their team had died – of cholera. This was a new humiliation for France after its defeat in the Franco-Prussian War.

Despite Koch's extremely thorough studies of cholera, many still doubted his finds, partly because no one was initially able to infect experimental animals with the cholera bacterium. One prominent critic was the influential German scientist Max von Pettenkofer.[35] He had developed a highly complex variant of the miasma theory as an explanation of cholera and was not prepared to accept that the bacterium could cause the disease on its own. He requested a bacterium sample from Koch, which he then drank. He did not contract cholera. Despite this negative result, which von Pettenkofer exploited to the maximum, it became increasingly clear over the next few years that Koch was right. After years of worsening depression, von Pettenkofer shot himself in 1901.

After several years of important administrative work as a professor, Koch returned to his study of tuberculosis. This time he worked on developing a ground-breaking treatment for the disease. After one year's intense work in the laboratory, he announced at a research convention in August 1890 that he had found a bactericidal substance that halted tuberculosis in animal experiments. He did not initially reveal that this was tuberculin, an extract of tubercle bacteria in glycerol that was injected into the subcutis. The reason he kept the tuberculin 'recipe' secret was that he wished to earn money from selling it and did not want any competition from other researchers. Koch gave this tuberculin to a number of patients with tuberculosis and claimed, on the flimsy basis of rather unsystematic experiments, that the treatment had a dramatic effect.

This 'cure' commanded enormous international attention, and Koch was once more acclaimed – at least at first.[36] The announcement of the new tuberculosis treatment led to tremendous enthusiasm. In one of Germany's most prestigious medical journals Koch was compared with St George, who slayed the dragon. The illustration depicted Koch on his horse, named 'Science', attacking the tuberculosis bacterium with his sword – the microscope.

Thousands of tuberculosis patients flocked to Berlin to be treated, with the hotel capacity of the city almost at bursting point. Koch persuaded the government to set up a new institute for infectious diseases, with himself as head. He gradually formed a large team of excellent colleagues who over the next few years made a great many discoveries in the field of bacteria, including identifying the bacteria that cause such major infections as typhoid fever, diphtheria, tetanus, pneumonia and meningitis. Koch and his team also inspired many other researchers to seek bacterial causes for diseases. The thirty years that followed Koch's discovery of the anthrax bacterium could well be called the golden age of the history of bacteriology.[37]

Koch's launch of tuberculin as a treatment for tuberculosis, however, proved to be a disaster – for both him and for his patients.[38] By the end of 1890 it began to be clear that Koch's acclaimed treatment had no convincing effect. Tuberculin caused fever in the patients and occasionally marked allergic reactions that could be serious, but did not lead to a cure. It is surprising that Koch's usual critical sense deserted him during this period, and we do not have any convincing explanation as to why this occurred. Was this a modern version of what the ancient Greeks called hubris, overweening pride that was punished by the gods? When enthusiasm for the tuberculosis treatment dwindled,

Koch's prestige also faded and his marriage collapsed. But he rose again after the tuberculin fiasco and made further important research contributions, especially in the field of tropical infections. His reputation was re-established and he was awarded a well-deserved Nobel Prize in 1905.

A Retrospective Look at the Bacteriological Revolution

The breakthrough in modern germ theory, linked to the convincing demonstration of bacteria as the cause of infectious diseases, was a milestone in the history of medicine, a revolutionary development that was to have tremendous consequences for the prevention and treatment of such diseases. It also overthrew 2,500 years of quite literally airy miasma thinking. If one is to be pedantic, the term 'revolution' is not quite accurate, since this radical change in the traditional view of illness, as we have seen, took many decades.

When one speaks of revolutions, certain key figures are often emphasized in the historical presentation. The Russian Revolution has its Lenin and Trotsky, the French its Robespierre and Danton. One often forgets all the others who also contributed to the breakthrough of the revolution.

In the most conventional historical presentation of the bacteriological revolution, it is quite clear that Pasteur and Koch are considered giants, while all the others who contributed and tilled the soil for the breakthrough are consigned to the shadows and partly forgotten. I have earlier compared them to the picadors at a bullfight, which culminates with the *coup de grâce* – the moment of truth – from the toreadors Pasteur and Koch. Naturally, it is unjust to ignore all these other proficient and partly visionary researchers, who often have been given only walk-on status in the historical narrative. I have mentioned some, but could well have mentioned many more.

There is further good reason not to ignore the many people who contributed to the feats of the giants. Popular representations of science generally have a tendency to focus exclusively on the efforts of a few key individual figures resulting from ostensibly genius-like inspiration. This is well illustrated by the anecdotes about Archimedes leaping triumphantly out of his bath after having realized the law of the upward buoyant force of a body immersed in water, and Isaac Newton, who recognized the law of gravity after seeing an apple fall to the ground. The truth is that all researchers, even the most brilliant ones, base their findings on earlier work; research is a laborious task placing one stone on top of another. This also applies to a high degree to the intellectual contributions that led to the bacteriological revolution.

Even so, there can be no doubt that both Pasteur and Koch deserve their towering position in the history of infection medicine. They were truly impressive researchers with vision, iron-hard discipline and, not least, an enormous capacity for work. It is said that when Pasteur was working late in the laboratory, as usual, some of his young assistants would hear the Master muttering a particular sentence time and time again. To find out if this was the magic formula for success, one of them concealed himself behind a curtain and learned by heart the magic words that Pasteur constantly repeated: 'Il faut travailler, il faut travailler' (Work must be done, work must be done). Pasteur in particular has been granted hero status, to such an extent that people have spoken of the 'pasteurization' of France.[39]

Both Pasteur and Koch also possessed another quality that is useful for success in research: the ability to market one's discoveries and oneself, and to stay on good terms with the leading politicians. Both of them were tough polemicists with their opponents: Pasteur was once even challenged to a duel by an infuriated old surgeon he had provoked.

It is hardly surprising that a lifelong hostility existed between the two stars in the firmament of infection medicine. This was probably due partly to subject-related rivalry between two highly ambitious researchers, a not uncommon phenomenon in science. But it was also caused by the highly tense relationship between France and Germany both before and after the Franco-Prussian War, which ended in French humiliation. Pasteur furiously returned a gold medal he had formerly received from the university in Bonn.

What we can call the golden age of the bacteriological revolution laid the foundation for a comprehensive international research process which gradually broadened the field with the discovery of new microbes as well as bacteria: viruses, protozoa, fungi and prions. This we will return to later.

Accounts of the bacteriological revolution often concentrate on the consequences for modern infection medicine and the treatment of patients. This, in a sense, is scarcely surprising, for the consequences within these areas have been tremendous. Even though this book concentrates on the purely medical aspects of the never-ending duel between humanity and the world of microbes, it is nevertheless important to remember that active research in this field over the past 150 years has increased our total sum of knowledge about the world far beyond the field of infection medicine. Studies of bacteria in particular have given us new and valuable knowledge about the life processes of all living cells. We have gained insight into the vital importance of microbes for the maintenance of all life on the planet – animal as well as plant. Furthermore, we have learned to make use of bacteria in the production of new medication. It is also probable that bacteria and viruses will be able to be used in completely new forms of treatment for a number of diseases, including various forms of cancer. Viruses, in particular, are included in many forms of gene therapy that are showing great promise for the treatment of a series of diseases.

The Multitudinous World of Microbes

It is first and foremost the duel between man and microbes that is our theme. The term 'microbe', or 'microorganism', means an organism that is not visible with the naked eye, only with a microscope. But *Homo sapiens* and other living creatures can also be subject to infection by organisms that are clearly visible without a microscope: various forms of parasitic worm. For this reason I use the term 'microbes' in a broader sense, one that also includes these parasitic worms, which are the cause of many common and serious diseases.

Before presenting the various forms of microbes known as pathogens, which are of interest as causes of infection and disease, let us start at the beginning with the origins of life.

The 'primeval soup' and the beginning of life

The formation of our planet is estimated to have taken place somewhere between 4.5 and 5 billion years ago.[40] For the first billion years, no life existed: the earth was almost an inferno. The temperature was extremely high, the atmosphere lacked oxygen and probably consisted of such gases as carbon dioxide (CO_2), nitrogen, hydrogen and methane. There were violent volcanic eruptions, electric storms with lightning strikes and bombardment by meteorites. There was no protective ozone layer in the atmosphere, which meant that the earth's surface was continuously exposed to ultraviolet and cosmic radiation. Despite these highly inhospitable conditions, something happened to the warm seas after a billion years when the planet had cooled to a certain extent, with the water no longer existing as vapour: a form of life arose that marked the beginning of everything subsequently alive on our planet. There are many more or less well-founded theories as to how this took place, but these lie outside the scope of this book. The prevalent theory during the past eighty years has been that the first bacteria arose in the seas of that time, also known as the 'primeval soup', about 3.5 to 4 billion years ago.

For the next 3 billion years, bacteria were the only form of life on earth. They made good use of their time. Numerous new forms developed according to the eternal laws of evolution, and the extremely hardy bacteria gradually conquered every nook and cranny of the planet.

As mentioned, the atmosphere lacked oxygen for the first billions of years. But about 2 billion years ago the concentration of oxygen began to increase considerably. This was because bacteria had now emerged that could use energy from sunlight to convert water and hydrogen into chemical energy in the process we now know in plants, photosynthesis, resulting in the production of oxygen. Gradually, some of the bacteria learned how to use oxygen in the production of energy, and this proved to be far more efficient than earlier forms of energy production. The foundation had now been laid for the next major event in the history of life on the planet: the development of what are called eukaryotic cells about 1.5 billion years ago.[41] This form of cell is the basis for all life forms other than bacteria, which are known as prokaryotic cells. The new eukaryotic cells were definitely derived from the bacteria, but they broke away from the bacterial world and developed further – with *Homo sapiens* as the final result so far.

There are fundamental differences between the prokaryotic bacterial cells and the eukaryotic cells we find in all plants and animals, including humans. Bacterial cells are smaller and much more primitive than eukaryotic cells, which have a cell nucleus that contains the genetic material – DNA – made up of a number of chromosomes. Bacteria lack a cell nucleus and have their hereditary material (also DNA) on a single, circular chromosome that swims freely in the cytoplasm, the cell fluid that is surrounded by the cell membrane. While bacteria nearly always have their own cell wall outside the cell membrane, the former is lacking in eukaryotic cells. There are also a great number of other basic differences, including propagation and metabolic processes, between the two types of cell.

After a billion years, the eukaryotic cells began to combine for their mutual benefit, and the next great leap occurred in the development of life – multicellular organisms in which the individual cells gradually began to specialize in various directions and to form various organs. And, as the saying goes, the rest is history, even though there are still a great many blank pages in this history book.

Bacteria: the first inhabitants of the planet

Bacteria, then, are single-cell organisms that can only be seen under a microscope, since their size varies between 0.2 and 10 μm. Today there are around 12,000 species of named bacteria.[42] Despite this, there is no doubt that the number of bacterial species is far greater; they have just not been discovered and studied as yet. Bacteria are found everywhere on the earth, even under the harshest conditions: in sources of boiling water, deep under the polar ice, in extremely saline or extremely acid lakes and on the seabed, as well as deep down in the earth under the pressure of many atmospheres. Among all these many types of bacteria, only a few – around 1,400 perhaps – cause disease in human beings.

There is enormous variety in the world of bacteria as regards their characteristics and their role in nature. One property, however, they all have in common: a virtuoso capacity to adapt themselves. For billions of years this adaptability has been a unique survival factor for bacteria, but it also makes pathogenic bacteria dangerous opponents of humanity.

This great capacity for adaptation has to do with the way bacteria reproduce and deal with genetic material (genes).[43] Bacteria reproduce by the cell dividing once it has doubled in size, resulting in two daughter cells with identical chromosomes. Cell division takes place quite frequently in most bacteria: every thirteen minutes in the case of cholera, for example. Not infrequently, mutations (or changes) take place in the DNA molecules. This changes the genetic information and sometimes the characteristics of the bacterium.

The genetic information (hereditary material) of the bacteria, however, is not only linked to DNA on the single chromosome. Many bacteria, in addition to their one chromosome, also have single, circular DNA molecules (plasmids) with extra genetic information that can be useful to the bacterium. This plasmid-borne genetic information can be exchanged between single bacteria by plasmids being transmitted to an adjacent bacterium via the formation of a pipe-shaped channel between them. In this way the recipient acquires new genes.

Bacteria can also freely pick up DNA from dead bacteria in their surroundings. Finally, a bacterial cell can have new hereditary material transmitted to it if it is attacked by special types of virus known as bacteriophages, something we will return to later.

So bacteria have a number of different ways to quickly change their DNA, that is their genetic material. This makes them particularly well suited to the evolutionary process and contributes to a major problems in today's infection medicine: the constantly increasing number of bacteria that are resistant to present-day antibiotics.

Viruses: small but dynamic players in the life processes

Already in the golden age of bacteriology, when constantly new pathogenic bacteria were being discovered, people were well aware that bacteria could not be detected in a number of diseases that were clearly clearly infections.[44] For some of these suspected infectious diseases – measles, smallpox, influenza, mumps – it was possible to show that a contagious agent was present in material from patients after filtering that removed bacteria. These agents, therefore, had to be extremely small particles, much smaller than bacteria. They were given the name 'viruses'. A virus, with just a small number of exceptions, is far smaller than a bacterium and cannot be seen using an ordinary light microscope. Virus particles only became visible with the arrival of the electron microscope in 1932.

Viruses are probably the most numerous of all microorganisms on our planet. They are far simpler in their construction than bacteria. The hereditary material (the genes) consists of either DNA or RNA. It is surrounded by a kind of capsule (capsid) of proteins. Many viruses also have an outer membrane, the viral envelope.

Are viruses living organisms? People disagree about this, but the answer depends to a great extent on how life is defined. If the ability to reproduce is a sign of life, viruses must be said to be living. If, on the other hand, one believes that a living organism must be able to reproduce completely on its own, then viruses are non-living. A characteristic all viruses share is that they can only reproduce within living cells. This happens when viral particles penetrate cells after having latched onto specific molecules on the surface of the cell that act as 'door openers' so the virus can enter the cell. After this, it takes over control of the cell and forces it to start to produce numerous new virus particles, specified according to the virus's own genetic material. The newly produced virus particles leave the cell and can infect new cells. Very frequently, the host cell dies during this process, which one could describe as the microbe world's version of hijacking.

The special lifestyle of the viruses accounts for their cardinal importance for all living beings on the planet. A virus can infect all forms of life: bacteria, plants and animals. Virus genes are very often absorbed into the genetic material of many forms of life after a former 'visit'. One could say that it has left behind its calling card as DNA in the cell. This may have had a great influence on the processes of evolution. With their ability to destroy and break down infected cells, viruses also contribute to the never-ending and absolutely necessary cycle of nutrients in nature.

Only a few representatives of the vast world of viruses, until now at any rate, have caused diseases in humans. On the other hand, many of the pathogenic viruses cause some of the most serious infectious diseases. Some viruses are among the classic causes of widespread epidemics with a high infection rate, such as the smallpox, measles and influenza viruses.

The origin of viruses is mysterious. Are they a form of degenerate bacteria that have lost the ability to manage completely on their own? Or do they come from plasmids, the small, ring-shaped DNA structures that are often found in bacteria? Nobody knows for sure.

Protozoa: 'the first animals'

Protozoa (Greek for 'the first animals') are unicellular organisms which, unlike bacteria, are eukaryotic, as is the rest of the animal and plant world.[45] Among other things, this means that unlike bacteria they have their own cell nucleus and a more complex metabolism. Certain protozoa are about the same size as bacteria, while others are somewhat larger. There are more than 200,000 different species of protozoa, but only a few cause disease in humans. However, these diseases are often widespread and serious, such as malaria, amoebic dysentery and African sleeping sickness. As disease-causing microbes, protozoa are extremely effective. It is difficult for our immune response to combat them. They are also more difficult to treat with drugs than bacteria. This is because their metabolism is more similar to that of humans than that of bacteria is.

Most pathogenic protozoa are to be found in tropical regions. The increase of international travel has increased the incidence of these infections in Western countries. The constant increase in patients with a reduced immune response has also contributed to this, as we shall see.

Fungi: the cause of both banal and life-threatening infections

Fungi are unicellular or multicellular organisms that, like human cells, are eukaryotic.[46] They differ from human cells in that they have a solid capsule outside the cell membrane. Of the 250,000 species that exist, only a few cause disease in humans. Some fungal infections cause quite trivial skin problems, such as ringworm or athlete's foot, while others are some of the most serious infections we know in medicine, with a mortality in patients of almost 100 per cent.[47] It is mainly patients with a reduced immune response that are struck down by these life-threatening infections.

Parasitic worms: large and small causes of infection

Parasitic worms are one of the commonest causes of human infection.[48] Such infections are extremely common in tropical regions, but we also have a few forms in other parts of the world, quite harmless ones on the whole. Parasitic worms are multicellular organisms which, unlike the other organisms that cause infectious disease in humans, are visible to the naked eye. They are between 1 centimetre and 10 metres in length.

Many of them have quite a complex life cycle, with the human being as merely the intermediate stage between various species of animal that the worm can infect.

Infectious diseases caused by parasitic worms vary from relatively harmless, often chronic intestinal infections to life-threatening diseases in inner organs such as the liver and the brain. Examples of serious infections are trichinosis, which one can get from eating infected pork, schistosomiasis, which one can get from contact with infected water, and tapeworm, with which one can be infected by eggs in animal faeces.

Prions: deadly protein molecules

Prions represent the smallest and most primitive cause of infectious disease and were not discovered until a few decades ago.[49] They can hardly be called living organisms, since they probably only consist of a single protein molecule, do not have their own genetic material and cannot reproduce without a host organism. The prion protein has the

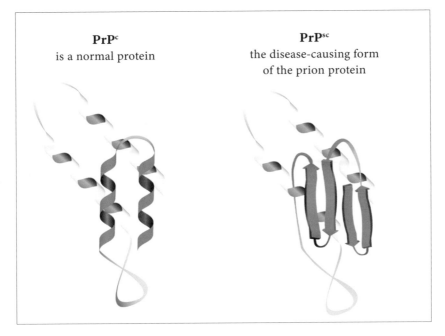

PrP^c
is a normal protein

PrP^sc
the disease-causing form
of the prion protein

The simplest form of infectious agent known is prions, which consist solely of protein molecules. They are almost identical with normal molecules in the brain of the species of animal they attack, but the prion molecule is folded in a different way. When the prion molecules come into contact with corresponding normal molecules, the latter are transformed into new prion molecules. After a time, this results in brain disease.

forbidding characteristic that it attacks an almost identical molecule that is normally found in the central nervous system and converts it into a new prion molecule where the amino-acid sequence is the same, but the three-dimensional structure is abnormal. This gradually leads to the destruction of nerve cells via a kind of 'domino effect', with an increasing number of normal protein molecules being transformed.

In both animals and humans, prions give rise to some quite rare and as yet incurable diseases that particularly attack the brain and spinal cord. So-called mad cow disease (bovine spongiform encephalopathy or BSE) is one example. Another is chronic wasting disease (CWD) in the deer family, including reindeer and elks in North America and Scandinavia. Prion diseases are infectious, but can also be hereditary.

Evolution and microbial invasion

From the time the first bacteria – the very first inhabitants of the planet – appeared, they displayed an impressive adaptability and occupied every conceivable place of residence.[50] Then new forms of life emerged: protozoa, multicellular organisms and, in particular, viruses. The bacteria doubtless quickly saw new possibilities to develop in the new forms of life, which they invaded with great success using their adaptive powers. Viruses also greedily fed on the other fauna, so that there is scarcely any form of life on earth that is not infected by viruses, very often with ruinous consequences for the host cells. The world of plants has not managed to avoid the virtuoso invasive capacity of microbes.

The result of the invasion of other forms of life by microbes was sometimes peaceful coexistence to the benefit of both parties, and sometimes disease and damage for the host. This is also the situation for the interaction between bacteria and *Homo sapiens*, and probably also for our relation to the other microbes that invade us: viruses, fungi and protozoa.

From the very beginning of time, then, a constant interaction has existed between the forms of life, in which the various players, subject to the laws of evolution, have constantly faced challenges from their opponents via new adaptations, which in turn lead to countermeasures. Humanity was inexorably drawn into this ancient process.

Microbes and Humankind

The entire series of developments of multicellular organisms that has resulted in *Homo sapiens* has, over hundreds of millions of years, been invaded by microbes. We initially inherited a microbe repertoire from our immediate ancestors, apemen. Subsequently our challenges from the world of microbes have constantly changed, partly through the evolutionary adaptations that have governed the interaction between microbes and host organisms, and partly through ecological and environmental relations that, to a great extent, control this interaction.

Microbes as allies

Our main theme is the ability of the world of microbes to cause infectious diseases. Even so, it is necessary to emphasize that the invasion by microbes does not necessarily cause disease, but can on the contrary be useful – even vitally necessary. Our knowledge about this is the result of quite intensive research into what is called the microbiota, the total microbial mass that at all times exists in a healthy human body in the digestive channel (particularly the intestines), on the skin, in the air passages and in the birth canal in women.[51] The microbiota consists of bacteria, viruses, protozoa and fungi, but until now it is the bacteria that have been studied most intensively. We reckon on there being more than one bacterium for each of our own body cells. In total, we each carry more than a kilogram of bacteria around with us.

In our intestines alone, which have been studied most – since one finds by far the most bacteria there – it is estimated that there are about 1,000 different species of bacteria. As each species of bacteria has about 2,000 genes, we thus have far more bacterial genes than the 23,000 human genes in our bodies. This gene mass is called the microbiome.

These genes find expression via the generation of a great many bacterial products in the intestines. The microbiome has important functions in the human body. It protects it against alien pathogenic microbes, contributes to our digestive processes and produces inflammation-suppressing substances.[52] The bacteria in the intestines also produce important nutrients such as vitamins and amino acids.

New and fascinating research has also shown that the microbiome in the intestines, via its metabolism products, can influence other areas

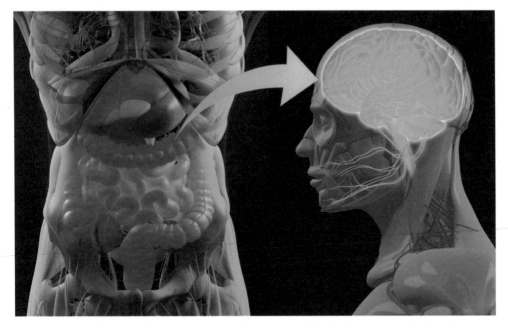

The microbiome in the intestines can affect areas outside the intestines, including the function of the brain, and can be of great importance for its normal development.

of the body, including the function of the brain.[53] Conversely, the brain, via its nerve paths and own hormones, can affect the intestines and the microbes there: the microbiota. Animal experiments have also shown that the microbiome seems to be of great importance for the normal development of both the brain and the immune system. We must assume that this also applies to humans.

The exploration of the role of the microbiome is still only in its infancy, but the results so far are extremely promising for an understanding of both the normal function of the human body and the development of various diseases connected to disruptions in the microbiota, such as diabetes and obesity, and the possibility of new methods of treatment in the future, based on manipulation of the microbiota.

Microbes and disease

Even though microbes do not always cause disease when they invade us, and even though the great majority of microbes are not the cause of infections, it is a fact that some microbes within all the main groups – bacteria, viruses, protozoa, fungi and prions – do cause infections in humans. Some of these infections have been with our ancestors ever since they took their first step out of the African rainforest and onto the savannah. Others arose later, in connection with changed life conditions for humanity. And many of them have had great consequences for the human race, not just in the medical field but for the historical, cultural and psychological development of man. They have also influenced the development of the human race more directly by affecting our genetic material.

How can microbes exert such a strong influence? Let us first examine the mechanisms microbes make use of to invade the human organism, for this is of course the first necessary step in developing an infection. In other words, how does infection occur?

The paths of microbial infection

The impressive adaptability of microbes is shown by their often fantastic ability to find ways of entering the human body.[54] Most microbes have specialized within individual paths of infection, but we also have plenty of examples of a microbe using various alternative ways.

The first obvious question to ask is where the invading microbes come from. Where are they before invading a victim? Here there are various possibilities. Microbes that cause infection can come from other people who transmit the microbe involved. Such a source of infection need not be a sick person, but might be a healthy carrier. Healthy disease carriers play an important role in many epidemics. There is often a far greater number of healthy disease carriers in society than those who become ill because of the microbe in question. An example of this is the Pneumococcus bacterium, which can cause inflammation of the lungs and membranes of the brain.

But the source of infection does not have to be other human beings; animals can also carry microbes that affect humans and cause infection. This applies to common and serious infections such as yellow fever, Ebola and the classic plague. In these cases, the microbe causes infection in the species of animal concerned where the animals are reservoirs for the microbe, and we speak of zoonoses – animal infections. Zoonoses have played a very important role in the history of human infection and are still extremely topical.[55] We now know that many of the most important microbes that have caused infection problems throughout history originally come from animals.

Certain pathogenic microbes can also live freely in nature and only cause infection if humans are unlucky enough to come into contact with them. One example of this is the bacterium that causes tetanus, which is found in soil. Another is the bacterium that causes legionnaires' disease, which is found in water.

Microbes can gain entry into our body via various paths of infection as the first stage in the infection process.[56] Let us briefly take a look at the most important of these paths, since the many evolution-related environmental factors that are crucial in infection medicine often act by influencing the infection paths of microbes.

Many microbes infect via direct contact between human beings. This can be via intimate (such as sexual) contact or via what is known as droplet infection, when an infected person coughs or sneezes, so that small droplets containing microbes are flung out into the surrounding air and inhaled by the person exposed. Direct infection can also take place if pathogenic bacteria in the soil or in water come into contact with open wounds, as in the case of tetanus, and via bites by infected animals, as in the case of rabies. Children can also be directly infected by the mother during pregnancy or via breast milk. HIV infection is an important example of both types.

Many microbes can transmit infection through the air, over greater distances than droplet infection, which can only operate within a radius of about 1 metre. Small particles that contain microbes, either extremely small droplets or very finely divided aerosol dust particles, are breathed in by the person exposed. Such small particles can remain in the air for quite a long time and be spread over considerable distances. Tuberculosis and measles are examples of this. Particles containing microbes that cause airborne infection can also come from skin rashes with particles of dried scabs, such as chickenpox and smallpox.

Infection via the mouth or intestines from polluted food or water is also of great importance. This is the usual form of infection for microbes that cause intestinal infections, from banal diarrhoea to such life-threatening infections as cholera. Since infection is via the intake of food or drink polluted by faeces, one often talks about faecal-oral infection. This is how another serious viral infection, polio, often occurs.

Infection can also take place through the transmission of microbes via various objects, such as polluted toys, clothing, bed linen and medical instruments. In a medical context this can take place via blood transfusions and blood products. This has occurred before with the HIV virus and viruses that cause inflammation of the liver – hepatitis B and hepatitis C. The same can happen with drug abuse through the sharing of infected syringes.

The last of the important paths of infection is transmission via stinging or biting insects that transport microbes from infection-carrying humans or animals to the next victim. The great classic example of this in human history is the plague, whose bacteria were passed on through fleas. Malaria and yellow fever are today more important examples of insect-transmitted infectious diseases than the plague. In both instances species of mosquito transmit the microbe.

Our Immune System: An Exceedingly Sophisticated Defence System

For millions of years, all the various forms of life on the planet were threatened by invasion from microbes in a never-ending struggle of all against all. In many instances, the invasion ended in peaceful coexistence, but the possibility of harm and death resulting from infection has always been there. So it is not surprising that even in the most primitive of life forms we find early defence mechanisms against infection. During the process of evolution, we see that multicellular organisms gradually develop an increasingly complex immune system based on specialized cells and molecules. Let us be confident enough to say that the human immune system represents the high point of this process.

The investigation of the human immune system began with a number of basic discoveries at roughly the same time as the bacteriological revolution. Many of the pioneers belonged to the circles around Pasteur and Koch or were influenced by the revolutionary discoveries made by these giant figures and their colleagues and pupils. Over the past 130 years, knowledge of the immune system – immunology – has gradually increased and acquired major importance, particularly in medicine.

The medical use of immunological discoveries got rapidly underway in the second half of the twentieth century.[57] Today, immunology is an important complementary subject within many disciplines of medicine, particularly that of infection. We know much about the role of the immune system in the defence against infection as well as the consequences of our immune system or important parts of it failing to function. Although we still lack a great deal of knowledge of this unusually complex system, we know a great deal more than we did only a few decades ago, thanks to intensive research.

From cradle to grave, at every second of the day and night, we are in constant contact with a great number of different microbes in the air, in what we eat and drink, and on many of the objects with which we are in contact. And we have large quantities of microbes as permanent guests on our mucous membranes and skin. Even though the vast majority of these are harmless and never cause infection, we regularly encounter some that can be pathogenic if the conditions are right. Despite this, not even these microbes are always able to get the better of otherwise healthy individuals. Most of us in Western countries manage to get through life with only a few of the more serious infectious diseases, mainly because of our immune system. This system consists of various types of highly specialized cell – white blood cells – and a great many molecules that to a significant extent are produced by the cells of the immune system and are utterly vital for their proper functioning.[58]

The different types of white blood cell in the immune system have various tasks in the defence against the microbes we face as an infection threat. The key to the success of the immune system in the human defence against infection is an intimate cooperation between the various cell types. This takes place partly via direct cell-to-cell contact, and partly by the cells releasing various kinds of signal molecule that can take a 'message' from one cell type to another and alter the function of the recipient cell. Cytokines are a large and important group of these signal molecules. Some of them can stimulate other immune cells, while others can inhibit them. Certain cytokines can also influence other cells in the body outside the immune system itself.

The cells of the immune system are distributed among most tissues and organs of the body, including the blood. They are to a great extent localized in lymph tissue, where lymph nodes, spleen and thymus are important, as well as the lymph tissue in the mucous membranes of the intestinal canal.

For the sake of simplicity, we can divide the immune system into two main parts on the basis of tasks and function: one part that is responsible for so-called natural or innate immune response, and one that mediates so-called acquired immune response. The two parts do not, however, operate separately: they cooperate closely. Both parts of the immune system have the capacity to react to certain substances that are foreign to the body and that are found on microbes which can invade the body. This ability to distinguish between our own and foreign molecules is crucial for the proper function of the immune system. It is particularly well developed in cells that mediate acquired immunity.

Natural immune response is the first line of defence against invading microbes, and it is rapid in its response. This part of the immune system is extremely old (at least 2 billion years) and we see the first signs of it in extremely simple cellular forms of life. The cells here, the advance guard in the battle, attack the microorganisms in various ways and often manage to overcome and kill them. The battle can then be called off. A key cell among these frontline soldiers is the macrophage (Greek: large eater), which has the ability to 'swallow' many microbes and subsequently kill them. Another important cell type is the neutrophil granulocyte.

Also important to this line of defence against viruses are NK-lymphocytes, a type of white blood cell, which also have a role in combatting cancer cells that arise in the body. I must confess that these cells have a particular nostalgic appeal for me. As a laboratory researcher in the early 1970s, I took part in the detection of this type of cell, which were then called K-lymphocytes (an abbreviation of killer-lymphocytes), and sometimes 'the third type of lymphocyte', since they have characteristics that distinguish them from both B and T lymphocytes, which are white blood cells vital to the acquired immune response.[59]

If the microbes cannot be defeated quickly, and the infection shows signs of spreading, the acquired immune response – the heavily armed main troops – is activated. This takes place via direct contact with the cells of the frontline defence as well as via signals communicated by the cytokine molecules that are released by these cells. In the further combatting of the microbe, the natural and acquired immune responses continue to cooperate.

The acquired immune response is much younger than the natural response, being 'only' 500 million years old. It is found in all higher species of animal. This immune response comes several days after initial contact with a microbe, but becomes increasingly strong as new cells are constantly mobilized and join the fray. In this part of the immune system, one type of white blood cell in particular is vital: lymphocytes. There are two main types, B lymphocytes and T lymphocytes, each with different tasks. These cells have a highly specialized ability to recognize and react to molecules that are foreign to the body – antigens – which are found on microbes and elsewhere. Every single B and T lymphocyte is highly specialized to react only to one antigen with a distinctive molecular structure. Because of the large number of lymphocytes, the immune system is nevertheless capable of reacting against a large number of foreign antigens.

When the individual B or T lymphocyte meets its corresponding antigen, it reacts and starts active cell division that forms an increasing number of lymphocytes to attack this particular microbe. In a great many cases this will lead to effective combatting of the infection and the neutralizing and elimination of the invading microbe.

How do the B and T lymphocytes neutralize infections so effectively? The essential weapon of the B lymphocytes is their ability to produce antibodies, the important type of molecule known as immunoglobulins (formerly often called gamma globulins). When the B lymphocyte has reacted against an antigen, it is converted into a plasma cell that specializes in the production of immunoglobulins. This is a specially constructed protein molecule that has the ability to bind itself to precisely the same antigen on the microbe that the mother B lymphocyte recognizes. The role of the antibodies in the combatting of infection is partly to deactivate and damage the microbe after binding itself to it, and partly to react with and neutralize any possible dangerous substances – toxins – which are released by the microbe and are important for the development of infection and disease.

The T lymphocytes have different, more varied tasks in combatting infection. This is a larger family of cells, with various subgroups that have different functions. The most important of these are the so-called $CD4^+$ T lymphocytes. These can be said to be the most central cell type of our entire immune system. They coordinate the various parts of the immune defence in fighting against the microbial invasion, and can be compared to the conductor of a symphony orchestra, where the members of the orchestra are the various types of cell and the signal

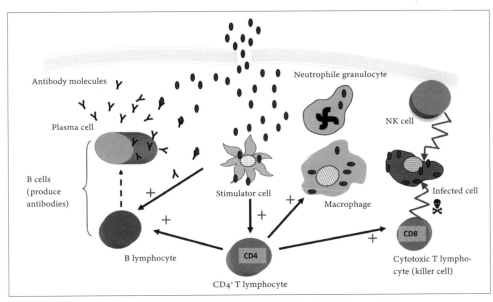

The most important types of cell in the immunological defence against infection. When the microbes get into the body via mucous membranes or skin, they are met by the various cells of the immune system that efficiently cooperate in combatting infection. The CD4+ T cell is the 'general' in the defence, coordinating, controlling and activating the other types of cell. The 'stimulator' cells, which are related to the macrophages, are the first to make contact with the microbes and activate the immune system.

molecules, which in harmonious interaction can effectively fight the infection. Among other things, the CD4+ T lymphocytes stimulate the B lymphocytes to increase their production of antibodies. The rest of the T cell types have other functions, including the ability to actually kill virus-infected cells. Yet other T lymphocytes can slow down immune responses that get too strong and can be harmful. Such regulating mechanisms are important to prevent an immune response from 'over-killing' and causing damage.

An essential characteristic of the B and T lymphocytes in the immune system is their capacity for immunological memory.[60] After these cells have encountered microbial antigens just once, for example in an earlier infection, the memory of this is stored in special 'memory cells' that are retained in the body for years, sometimes for the rest of the person's life. If the immune system is once more exposed to the same microbe, the memory cells have the ability to react quickly and ensure a much swifter immune response than during the first contact with the microbe. In a great many cases this will completely prevent re-infection, or possibly ensure that the infection is much weaker than the first time. It is this immunological memory that we can thank for having many infectious diseases only once. We have become immune to the microbe involved. Measles and chickenpox are examples of this. The memory of the immune system is the key to an understanding of the principle underlying vaccination against infectious diseases.

Why Does Infection Lead to Disease?

Certain premodern cultures believed that serious infectious diseases were caused by the influence of supernatural beings and evil demons. The fact that we know since the bacteriological revolution that microbes play a central role as a cause of disease naturally does not mean that we ascribe to microbes any wish to harm the human organism. Microbes invade our body and possibly cause disease as a result because of just one prime aim, which matches that of all other organisms throughout the often bloody history of evolution: to acquire food, reproduce and spread their genetic material further via descendants.[61] This can harm the host organism (the human involved), but from the microbe's point of view it is an unintended side-effect.

What exactly do we mean by 'infection'? We normally carry a large number of microbes on our mucous membranes and skin. They are our permanent companions, do not usually harm us, and are often useful at the same time. We use the term 'infection' when a microbe that normally is not one of these companions – our microbiota – settles either on or inside our body. This visit is often short-lived and does not create any disease problem. Only by laboratory testing can we see if the presence of the microbe has been discovered by our immune system. Sometimes a recently infected person can carry the microbe around for a while and infect others. Such bearers of infection often play an important role in the spread of infections, for example in epidemics.

Microbial weaponry

Some microbes have the characteristic of relatively often causing disease when infecting people with a normal immune system. These microbes have a strong capacity to establish themselves in our body, to seize necessary nutrients, actively reproduce and use efficient methods of leaving the body, so spreading to new victims.[62] Compared with many other microbes that do not normally cause disease, these microbes, known as pathogens, have a formidable arsenal of attributes that cause greatly varying effects.[63] Such harmful genetic products of the microbe are given the name 'virulence factors'. These help the microbe during the various stages of the infection process. Certain factors ensure that the microbe latches onto the mucous membrane cells as the first stage of invasion and infection. Others, found in many bacteria, are enzymes that break down barriers in the tissues, allowing the bacteria to penetrate further into the body.

It is crucial to the success of the microbe to ensure that it is not neutralized quickly by the patient's immune system. Its microbial weaponry includes a number of virulence factors that can ingeniously hamper the various components of the immune response. Let us look at a small selection of the mechanisms that microbes have developed thanks to their impressive capacity to adapt themselves in their duel with a human opponent.

Certain bacteria, pneumococci for example, which are a common cause of pneumonia, and meningococci, which cause meningitis, have an extra-thick capsule that prevents the bacteria from being swallowed by macrophages – the 'great eaters' – in the natural immune response. Other bacteria, such as those that cause tuberculosis and leprosy, happily allow themselves to be swallowed, but have developed tricks that ensure they survive inside the macrophages and continue to infect without being killed, as more harmless bacteria would be. Many common bacteria and certain protozoa produce toxic substances (toxins) that kill the cells in the natural immune response.

Some bacterial toxins play a role by helping newly produced bacteria to leave the body and thereby ensure a further spread of the microbe. We find this in a number of diarrhoea-producing bacteria, where abundant, thin evacuations of the bowels spread them effectively to the surroundings, so that new individuals become infected. The most dramatic example here is the cholera bacterium, which causes violent diarrhoea that can lead to a swift dehydration of the patient and death after only a few hours.

Certain bacteria produce toxins that have a particularly harmful effect on the patient. This applies, for example, to tetanus bacteria, which with its highly poisonous toxin causes tetanus (lockjaw) by means of its effect on the patient's nervous system. This toxin leads to violent convulsions that can create life-threatening breathing difficulties by affecting the muscles used for breathing. Even more poisonous is the botulin toxin, produced by the bacterium *Clostridium botulinum*, which leads to widespread paralysis of the nervous system. One milligram of this toxin is sufficient to kill hundreds of thousands of humans. In such cases, the use-value of the toxins for the microbe is somewhat unclear.

Pathogenic viruses also have a considerable repertoire of mechanisms that help the microbe and cause harm in patients. Viruses always have to invade cells if they are to survive and reproduce. Various viruses have specialized in different cells and organs in the host's body. Certain viruses, for example, attack liver cells and cause hepatitis (inflammation of the liver); others invade brain cells and cause various diseases of the brain, such as poliomyelitis. When a virus invades cells and takes control, this often leads to the death of the cell, resulting in the release of newly produced virus particles that are then able to attack new cells.

Many viruses also use tricks to hamper the host's immune response. The EBV virus, which causes mononucleosis (glandular fever), produces a molecule that inhibits the production of important cytokines in the response. Other viruses weaken the response by attacking and infecting the immune cells themselves. This applies to the measles virus and, most dramatically, the HIV virus, which causes life-threatening collapse of the immune system (AIDS) by destroying the most central cell of our immune system, the CD4+ T lymphocyte.[64]

A refined way of 'fooling' the immune system is the microbes' ability to change their antigens, the molecular characteristics of the microbe that the immune system recognizes as being foreign and therefore reacts against.[65] A dramatic example of this is the protozoon *Trypanosoma brucei*, which is the cause of African sleeping sickness, an extremely serious infection where the patient is subject to brain disease that includes sleep disturbances. During the infection, which always lasts a long time, this microbe alters its surface coat as soon as the immune system has started to react against the coat antigens in order to combat the microbe. The immune system then has to start all over again and build up a new, powerful immune response against the new antigens. This happens time after time, so that the immune defence system never manages to combat the microbes effectively. In this way, infection is maintained. This can really be called trimming one's sails to every wind! The ability to alter antigens is also seen in a number of viruses, such as HIV and influenza, where it greatly contributes to the problems encountered. In the case of influenza, this means having to have a new vaccine every year, since the virus has changed its antigens from the previous season.

The immune system as a cause of disease

Part of the explanation of why patients with infections fall ill is not actually the microbe itself but the patient's reaction to it. This can be in the form of inflammation or as so-called autoimmune reactions.

The combined effect of the virulence factors and the propagation of the microbes in the tissues releases, via the natural immune response, the phenomena everyone recognizes as inflammation when seen in the skin and mucous membranes: redness, heat, swelling, pain. Inflammation is the body's basic reaction to every form of injury, even if triggered by a microbe. It is useful in infection because it facilitates the afflux of the cells and molecules of the immune system in the local battle against the microbial invasion. Unfortunately, the inflammation in itself will, in many instances, aggravate the disease when it involves important organs and tissues in the body, for example in the brain, heart and liver.

The acquired immune response, which makes its attack if the natural response does not succeed in effectively combatting the microbe, can also contribute to the problems caused by the disease through the inflammation mechanisms. In certain infections, a considerable part of the disease is actually caused by the attempts of the B and T lymphocytes to clear up after the attack.

An example of this is chronic inflammation of the kidneys, which can be the result of immunoglobulin antibodies reacting against microbe antigens and forming so-called immune complexes that circulate in the blood and damage the kidneys. This occurs, for example, in malaria and after throat diseases involving streptococcus bacteria. In the case of chronic hepatitis B, such immune complexes in the blood can occasionally cause extensive, life-threatening damage to the walls of the blood vessels in important organs such as the kidneys.

Similarly, a type of T lymphocyte (killer cell), which act by killing virus-infected host cells, can cause serious illness when too many such cells are killed in important organs. Those infected by the hepatitis B virus are an example of this: virus-carrying liver cells are killed by T lymphocytes that react against the virus antigens.

Finally, some parts of the pathological picture in infections are a result of the fact that certain microbes can cause what is called an autoimmune disease.[66] The cells of the immune system are normally able to distinguish clearly between the body's own antigen molecules and foreign ones, first and foremost the microbe antigens. This is vital for the proper functioning of the immune system. Sometimes, however, the immune system is no longer able to make this clear distinction. In that case, the B and T lymphocytes start attacking their own cells and this gives rise to autoimmune reactions. This can result in serious disease via the mechanism we have just discussed, including T lymphocytes and harmful immune complexes.

There are several possible causes of autoimmune reactions and disease as a consequence of infection. One happens in infections where the microbe, in nature's unpredictable way, carries molecules that are extremely like antigens on some of the patient's own cells, making it difficult for the immune cells to distinguish between them. Inflammation of the heart valves, which can be observed in rheumatic fever (a possible complication when infected by certain streptococcus bacteria), is an example of this. There is also evidence to suggest that the EBV virus that causes mononucleosis can trigger serious rheumatic diseases via autoimmune reactions.

There is enormous variation in the pathological pictures caused by different microbes, and in no way do we have complete knowledge of all the important disease mechanisms possible. For the sake of completeness, we cannot refrain from mentioning that certain viruses can actually cause cancer.[67] Once again, the mononucleosis virus (the EBV virus), which can trigger various types of lymphoma, is the first example of this to have been discovered. Other examples are the hepatitis B virus, which can cause liver cancer, and the HPV virus, which can cause various kinds of cancer, including cervical cancer and cancer of the oral cavity. The bacterium *Helicobacter pylori*, which usually causes stomach ulcers, can also trigger stomach cancer. And chronic infections with certain parasitic worms can also cause cancers.

The fragile balance of power between man and microbe

Microbes have a thousand ingenious methods of surviving in our body and overcoming the resistance of our well-developed, efficient immune system. There are several possible results of an acute infection. It can completely gain the upper hand and lead to the patient's death, but much more often the infection is effectively neutralized by the immune system and the patient recovers completely. In certain cases, the infection is dealt with relatively effectively but not completely, so the microbe still manages by various ways to stay in the body. In such cases the microbe can be 'encapsulated' without causing any further damage, as we often see with tuberculosis. With viral infections such as chickenpox and herpes, the virus, after the acute illness, enters an inactive and symptom-free phase, but does not disappear from the body. Later in life, these dormant viruses can 'wake up' and cause new signs of disease.

Alternatively, a microbe that remains in the body after the acute phase of an infection can quietly be active and cause chronic damage, until finally the disease becomes overt once more, possibly resulting in death. A dramatic example of this is untreated patients with an HIV infection; in most cases this ends with AIDS, which is fatal.

Which result is actually in the microbe's own interest? Or, to put it another way: which result is desirable from the microbe's point of view, according to the laws of evolution?

A pathogenic microbe that is well adapted from an evolutionary point of view has one aim: to reproduce and pass on its genetic material via descendants as effectively as possible. Obviously it is not in the microbe's interest to cause such a violent acute infection that the patient dies rapidly. This will drastically reduce the possibility of the microbe being spread by the patient infecting others. Nor is it always in the microbe's interest for the patient to fall so ill as to be bed-ridden and immobile; this depends on the infection mechanism of the disease in question. Effective droplet infection via the air passages and the transmission of sexual diseases are dependent on the patient being able to move around and infect others, so a well-adapted microbe does not want to cause symptoms of disease that are too serious. Conversely, this will not play so important a role in diseases that are transmitted via biting insects, such as malaria, or in infections where large quantities of microbes are released by violent diarrhoea, as with cholera. Here the spreading of the microbes can often be extremely effective even when the patient is passive, possibly bed-ridden.

Moreover, the tendency of certain microbes to cause chronic infections that are often symptom-free for years on end can, from an evolutionary point of view, be useful in cases where further infection is not spread as effectively as via air-passage infections and diarrhoea diseases. This applies, for example, to infections with the hepatitis B and C viruses, while the hepatitis A virus, which infects much more easily, via faeces, never causes chronic infection.

But does this mode of thought fit with what we can observe in extremely serious infectious diseases such as rabies, where mortality is very high even when treated? Yes, such infections fit this evolutionary way of thinking. When these microbes infect a human, it is not an essential part of their lifestyle, more a chance affair. The rabies virus normally infects a number of wild animal species, where the microbe is well adapted without causing disease problems that are too serious. That the infection is fatal in humans is thus irrelevant for the survival of the microbe and its dissemination in nature.

It is in the interest of a microbe for there to be a certain balance of strength between patient and microbe, a sort of parallel to the balance of power during the Cold War. The disturbing thing about this was that the balance of power was extremely fragile – and the same applies to the balance between humans and pathogenic microbes. For it is not the case that the microbes' arsenal of virulence factors and general ability to create disease problems have been determined once and for all. It is precisely the tremendous adaptability of the microbes that has ensured their success on our planet from the beginning of time. Their ability to cause infection and disease is central to their history of evolution: their struggle to survive and spread. This means that changes to surrounding conditions will rapidly lead to change in the microbes' characteristics and their ability to cause disease. A relatively well-behaved microbe can suddenly change and become much more aggressive. Conversely, the pathogenic capacity of a microbe can decrease if it is in the microbe's interest.

Formerly, it was almost an established fact that a microbe will gradually produce milder infections. Research undertaken in recent years has shown that this is not necessarily the case. Changes to a microbe's pathogenic ability can go in both directions, mainly depending on the ecological and environmental challenges to which the microbe is exposed. Many of these factors affect the characteristics of the microbes by intervening in their possibilities for infection and thereby their ability to spread and survive, which is the microbes' primary aim.

Genetics and Defence Against Infection in *Homo sapiens*

The cause of the vast adaptability of microbes throughout the history of evolution, which has made them formidable opponents of *Homo sapiens*, is the rapidity with which they can change their genetic characteristics.[68] Bacteria reproduce by dividing. This division takes place very quickly, for example right down to 20 seconds for staphylococci. When dividing, the DNA of the bacteria – the carrier molecules of the genes – can be changed by mutations. Furthermore, the bacteria can easily acquire new genes by the exchange of plasmids and bacteriophages. Many viruses also have the ability to rapidly change genetically, partly via frequent mutations, as for example the HIV virus, and partly via the exchange of parts of their genetic material with other viral variants, as we see in the influenza virus.

When it comes to rapid change of the genetic material, microbes have an enormous competitive advantage compared to *Homo sapiens*, where an individual takes on average between twenty and thirty years to reproduce. One would then expect that we could be vastly inferior in the duel with the microbes and that we ought to have been eradicated from the surface of the planet long since after constant pathogenic attacks for hundreds of thousands of years. That this has not happened is basically due to our sophisticated immune system.

Homo sapiens has also been under the influence of the laws of evolution in the interaction with the world of microbes. Physicians of former times believed that the characteristics of the individual patient – the balance between the key body fluids – were of crucial importance for the outcome of infectious diseases.[69] This view was held from the time of Hippocrates until the bacteriological revolution.

With the new insight into the seminal role of microbes as the cause of disease, interest diminished in individual differences in the powers of resistance in the event of microbial attack. A key pioneer such as Robert Koch has posthumously been criticized for a far-too-one-sided focus on the role of the microbe and a correspondingly small interest in individual differences in the patients' potential for resistance.[70] As new bacteriological methods gradually started to be used for an increasing number of infectious diseases, it became clear that the outcome of infection by one and the same microbe varied a great deal from patient to patient, as regards both mortality and the general course of the disease. Had the physicians of former times perhaps been right about something? Are there differences from one individual to the next in their susceptibility to infections? I am here ignoring the difference between immune and non-immune individuals.

With the advanced methods that have been developed in recent years for genetic studies of human beings, it has become clear that in every population group there are distinct differences in the genes of each individual, which, to a greater or a lesser extent, affect their susceptibility to infection by various microbes.[71] This has probably been the case since the infancy of the human race. Studies of the total genetic material of the single individual – the genome – have also shown that the duel between man and microbes during the past hundreds and thousands of years has left distinct traces in our genes. Infectious diseases that throughout history have followed an extremely serious course, with high mortality, or chronic illnesses that have led to increased mortality, bad health and reduced ability to reproduce, have via the process of natural selection led either to an increase in the frequency of genes that provide an increased resistance or to a loss of genes that increase susceptibility to the microbe involved. The process of evolution has weeded out genes that are unfavourable for survival and protected genes that are favourable. We are talking here of negative or positive selection of such genes.

Such genetic investigations have been carried out by comparing population groups from various parts of the world. When our ancestors spread out from Africa to other continents between 60,000 and 100,000 years ago, they were exposed to new microbes that varied from region to region. This has influenced human beings' genetic equipment in different ways in various climes. If occurrences of genes are compared today with what we know about the frequency of the individual important infectious diseases in the same geographical area, the results are interesting. Even though much is still unclear, certain finds are worth mentioning.

Most often, it is not a single gene among the 23,000 genes a human has that exerts a decisive influence on an individual's powers of resistance to a microbe. In most instances, it is a series of genes that together influence the result of an infection, even though single genes can have a greater influence than the others. This is probably the case with tuberculosis, where the accumulation of disease in certain families has been known for a long time. Before the microbial cause of this infection was discovered by Robert Koch, many people believed that tuberculosis was hereditary.

Studies in Bangladesh, where cholera is a considerable threat, have shown that certain genes apparently have a protective effect against this life-threatening infection and that their occurrence in the population has therefore increased. At the same time, the population has the world's lowest occurrence of blood group O, which is connected to an increased susceptibility to cholera.

There are also some examples of single genes that offer considerable protection against particular microbes. An example from Africa and Asia is a gene that encodes for a special blood type (in the so-called Duffy system). A mutation variant of this gene is strikingly frequent in West and Central Africa, compared with other parts of the continent. In the same regions, the special malaria parasite *Plasmodium vivax* is lacking, a parasite that is the most widespread malaria type in other regions of Africa. So it is natural to assume that individuals with this gene have had a competitive advantage in the population. And we know the explanation: the normal molecule variant of the blood type in question on the surface of the red blood cells is necessary for the malaria parasites (the plasmodia) to be able to penetrate the cell, whereas the mutated form does not work in the same way. Since so many in the population bear this gene, *Plasmodium vivax* malaria is rare in these regions. As a new example of the arms race between the microbe and humans it must be added that new variants of *Plasmodium vivax* have emerged that can also infect individuals with this gene mutation. And in the case of a formerly feared disease such as leprosy, there are finds indicating that single genes have a protective effect. Such a gene is present in no less than 70 per cent of the European population, where leprosy has been virtually eradicated over the past centuries. The occurrence of this gene is only 2 per cent in China and 9 per cent in India, where leprosy is still a considerable health problem.

Let us take a look at the HIV virus, which, until the events of 2020, has given rise to the largest pandemic – a worldwide epidemic – in recent times.[72] Here too we find that genetics influences the susceptibility to infection. The clearest example is the CCR5-Delta32 gene, a mutation variant of a gene that controls the production of a molecule on the surface of the CD4⁺ T lymphocyte. The normal variant of this gene is necessary for the HIV virus to be able to penetrate into the cell and cause infection. An individual who has a double dose of the mutated gene (from both mother and father) cannot be infected with the HIV virus. This special gene has a distinctly higher occurrence in Northern Europe than in the rest of the world. Suggestions have been made that it is because the gene also offered protection against the extensive plague epidemic that ravaged Europe in the fourteenth century and also later, but there is considerable disagreement about this. Many other genes, when acting together, have a certain effect on the course of HIV infection, though none so dramatic as the CCR5-Delta32 gene.

The pressure exerted by microbes on human genetic material has occasionally had surprising consequences. We know of a number of serious diseases that are hereditary and are due to a single gene. In terms of evolution, such genes ought to be unfavourable for the survival of the carriers. In a few of these diseases the gene responsible, possibly as a result of mere chance, has a protective effect against certain infectious diseases. This has led to the gene being preserved in population groups where the microbe in question exerts a particularly large infection pressure. The gene has, then, given a survival advantage to the carriers, one that counterbalances its harmful effect.[73]

The classic example of this 'use value' of certain hereditary diseases is the so-called sickle-cell gene in certain parts of Africa. This gene gives rise to a variant of the iron-binding haemoglobin in red blood cells which cause anaemia, a reduction in the number of red blood cells. At the same time, the gene offers effective resistance to serious forms of malaria, and it therefore occurs far more frequently in regions where serious malaria is extremely common than elsewhere.

Another example is the serious hereditary disease cystic fibrosis. This disease is due to a number of possible mutations of the so-called CFTR gene. These mutations, and thereby the disease, are much more common in ethnic Europeans than in Africans. The responsible gene actually also provides a high level of protection against cholera, an infection that has a high mortality rate. The high frequency of gene mutations in Europeans is thought to be a result of the major cholera epidemics that struck this part of the world in the nineteenth century, in which the carriers of the mutations had a survival advantage, making this an example of positive genetic selection.

A third example is the rare but serious hereditary metabolism illness Tay-Sachs disease, which is far more frequent among Jewish people with a background from East and Central Europe than other population groups.[74] The disease arises when an individual has the relevant gene from both father and mother, and it leads to a gradual destruction of the nerve cells in the brain and spinal cord, which normally starts in the first year of life and leads to death after just a few years. Individuals who have the Tay-Sachs gene from only one parent are healthy. Surprisingly enough, the gene probably has a protective effect against tuberculosis, which was formerly very common among Jews in crowded ghettoes in Eastern Europe. Descendants who carry the gene actually have a lower frequency of tuberculosis than other population groups in the same area. The gene has therefore been retained in the population.

What is the mechanism behind the influence of the genes on powers of resistance and susceptibility to infections? As far as many genes are concerned, we still do not know. Many of the genes involved control genetic products that are important in our immune system. This probably applies to many genes relevant to infection.

Work on mapping the importance of our genes for the defence against infections is still in its infancy. All the examples provided show that throughout the history of *Homo sapiens* the world of microbes has to a great extent left its imprint on our hereditary material, the genome, and affected its development. The genetic profile of humanity today is not the same as when our ancestors left the African rainforests and moved out onto the savannahs.[75] Subtle differences in the genome then developed between the various branches of *Homo sapiens* after they migrated to different parts of our planet, since the microbes they encountered differed. These genetic differences are conceivably not only important for the variation in our susceptibility to infectious diseases but for the occurrence of other diseases in which genetic factors play a role.

TWO

The Third Factor:
Ecology and the Environment

Until now we have concentrated on the two duellists – man and microbes – and seen how the fight takes place once they are at close quarters when infection has occurred. We have seen how evolution has influenced the fighting capacity of the duellists via genetic adaptations, and how *Homo sapiens* is definitely a slow learner compared with the microbes. But the prerequisite for this interaction between microbe and man is that the players come into contact with each other in such a way that infection is the outcome. And here we meet the third factor that has always played a key role in the duel between man and microbes. It comprises both relations linked to the physical nature that surrounds humans, and human behaviour in the broadest sense down through the ages. It is only in recent years that research has become aware of the enormous significance of these factors, both for an understanding of the history of infection from earliest times and the present and future challenges we face from the world of microbes.

Many of the important ecological and environment-related factors often exert their influence at the same time, and many of them overlap to a certain extent. For that reason, there are several ways of subdividing them that are equally valid. As far as a number of the factors are concerned, human activity and intervention in nature are of crucial importance. These human-related factors have acquired ever-increasing importance in the period leading up to our own time, a period that is now beginning to be called the Anthropocene, because human intervention in nature has had such stark consequences.

Trading, Travel and Migration

As *Homo sapiens* spread out from Africa to other areas of the planet, various cultures and civilizations arose which for thousands of years remained separate from each other. Such factors as differences in geography and climate as well as the local panorama of microbes led, over the course of time, to considerable dissimilarities in the threats that came from microbes and the predominant infections in various parts of the world.[1]

About 2,500 years ago, the various civilizations in Asia, Europe and Africa began to come into contact with each other. This was mainly the result of the development of trade. Since then, international trade has in various ways been a lasting and important factor in changes to the picture of infections around the world.

The most famous of all trade routes down through the ages is the Silk Road, which went westwards from northwestern China, north of the Himalayas, through Central Asia to the Middle East and Europe.[2] There were other important trade routes, including one from India, across the Indian Ocean to the Middle East and Africa. As the name 'Silk

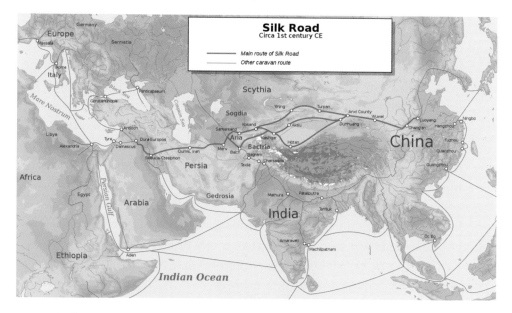

The famous Silk Road between China and the eastern part of the Mediterranean. This route was already central to trading, war and the transference of microbes several centuries before the birth of Christ.

Road' implies, silk was an important commodity transported along this and other trade routes. But less congenial commodities were also transported. The transportation of microbes along the trade routes is regarded as explaining some of the great epidemics that ravaged Europe, Asia and Africa from antiquity until far into the Middle Ages. One example of this is the plague bacterium that repeatedly savaged Europe and the Middle East, including the Black Death of the fourteenth century. It is assumed that this plague epidemic started in China and then moved westwards along the trade routes, first and foremost the Silk Road.

The cholera bacterium has resulted in a number of worldwide pandemics since the beginning of the nineteenth century.[3] Since time immemorial, this bacterium has lived in brackish water at the mouth of the Ganges in India, where it normally lives in peaceful coexistence with plankton and small shellfish. But it also flourishes in human intestines if given the chance. The spread of the cholera bacterium the rest of the world as an epidemic to has taken place partly via trade routes and partly via shipping, where the bacterium has stowed away in water taken on board as ballast.[4] This bacterium is not the only organism transported by shipping around the world. More than 3,000 species of plants and animals have been shown to exist in ballast water and are imported to new parts of the globe, sometimes with serious consequences, not only for humans but for the local fauna and flora in the country of arrival.

The extensive global trade in various food commodities can also lead to infection problems.[5] The import of microbe-polluted fresh vegetables, fruit and berries from developing countries where hygiene levels are poor has led to outbreaks of a spectrum of different infections, including acute inflammation of the liver by the hepatitis A virus and various diarrhoea-related diseases.

There is also widespread trade in various species of animals, both as pets, such as birds and reptiles of various kinds, and as experimental animals for medicinal purposes. Here there is ample opportunity for undesired microbes to be present, including microbes that can cause serious infectious diseases in both humans and tame or wild animal species in the recipient country. A present-day example is the importation of street dogs for adoption, which can be carriers of many microbes that can cause diseases in humans as well.[6]

A more macabre commodity – slaves – played an important role for about three hundred years from the sixteenth century onwards in the spread of dangerous microbes between continents. Malaria, which was unknown in the New World, was imported to the American continent by slaves from West Africa in the eighteenth century.[7] The viral infection yellow fever was transported along with African slaves to the New World in the seventeenth century.[8] The same ships brought with them a variety of mosquito, *Aedes aegypti*, which has specialized in the transference of yellow fever between human beings. Both malaria and yellow fever hit indigenous Americans as well as the European settlers hard. African slaves got off more lightly because of their immunity and probably also a certain genetic resistance built up via contact with these microbes over a long period of time.

The exchange of microbes between parts of the world has, then, been going on for more than two thousand years, as contact between these various areas increased. Today, global trading is far greater than in previous ages, and various forms of travel have mushroomed during the last few decades, running parallel with the expansion of international flight connections and ever shorter travelling times. Today one can reach the most distant destinations in the space of a few hours (even though much of this time is spent travelling to and from airports and waiting). Similar journeys by ship used to take weeks or months.

It is estimated that normally 10 million people fly every day, and a great many of these flights are international.[9] Obviously, the potential for the international transportation of microbes is dangerously large. This is particularly important when it comes to the spread of infections that are transmitted via direct contact, such as airborne droplets or sexual contact. Infection can be spread by everyday tourism or commercial travel activity. Sex tourism has played a great role, particularly in the spread of the HIV virus to all the inhabited continents in the space of a few years.

Groups of people have always set out on journeys for various reasons and forms of migration are important for the spread of microbes. A special example of this is the *hajj*, the annual Muslim pilgrimage to Mecca from all parts of the globe.[10] Tens of thousands of pilgrims come into close contact with each other, and the conditions for the spread of infectious diseases are very much in evidence. This has given rise to many serious epidemics. In 1987 pilgrims from Asia brought with them a special meningococcus bacterium that causes inflammation of the membrane of the brain (meningitis). This led to an epidemic with almost 2,000 cases in Saudi Arabia alone, and more cases in the pilgrims' home countries after their return. Down through the ages, pilgrims have also been hit by a number of cholera epidemics. In both 1821 and 1865 thousands of pilgrims died in connection with the *hajj*.

In today's world, both economic migrants and refugees from parts of the world where sanitary and medical conditions are below Western standards because of war and poverty lead to a high risk of infection.[11] This applies, for example, to diseases such as tuberculosis, HIV and, in the wake of the war in Syria, the viral disease poliomyelitis, which has been eradicated from Western countries.

It is not only human transporters of infections that are important for global dissemination. Many important infectious diseases are transmitted via stinging insects. Such insects also participate in comprehensive international travel, contributing to the spread of microbes.[12] This particularly applies to mosquitoes. Certain types of mosquito prefer transport by ship, which definitely contributed to the spread of malaria and yellow fever to the New World. The Asian tiger mosquito (*Aedes albopictus*), which can transmit several viral infections, was recently introduced to North America via the import of used car tyres from Asia. This variety of mosquito has actively contributed to the spread to the North American continent of the Zika virus and the virus that causes dengue fever, and possibly also the West Nile fever virus (WNV). Other varieties prefer air travel and are able to survive quite low temperatures in aircraft cargo compartments. This applies, for example, to the *Anopheles* mosquito. This is the underlying cause of the many cases of so-called airport malaria that have been found at airports in Paris, Brussels and London, all of which regularly receive aircraft from malaria-ridden areas. The WNV virus first appeared in the Western hemisphere in New York in 1999, probably because of plane-borne *Culex* mosquitoes.

During the major plague epidemics, to which we will return later, the black rat (*Rattus rattus*) was a key player in the spread of the plague as a passenger on ships. Today, a special problem with infection is connected to the extensive tourism on board huge cruise liners.[13] They can accommodate more than 3,000 passengers, who may come from various locations and are transported from port to port during the cruise. These 'floating cities' can contribute to the global spread of microbes. The ships have also been the setting of their own small epidemics with various microbes. A great many of the passengers are elderly people, often with various chronic diseases that weaken their immune systems and result in more serious periods of illness. Intestinal infections that cause diarrhoea are common, often caused by either viruses or *Salmonella* bacteria. Respiratory-tract infections are also often found among cruise passengers, frequently accompanied by the influenza virus. The SARS-CoV-2 virus has also recently hit cruise ships.

The Key Role of Animal Infections Over Thousands of Years

Homo sapiens is of course not the only species of animal to which the world of microbes has taken a fancy. For millions of years before our ape-like ancestors came onto the scene, microbes were well adapted to the extremely varied fauna and flora that existed on the earth. And today all existing species of animals also have their own special microbe partners, some of which live in peaceful coexistence with their hosts and some of which cause disease. The 'rules of the game' are more or less the same as they are for humans. Given this fact, it is perhaps not surprising that human beings, as one of the most recently arrived animal species on the earth, have taken over a great many microbes from the animal world, where they were already well established. Of the more than 1,400 microbes one can at present identify as causes of infectious diseases in human beings, more than 60 per cent also cause animal infections.[14] In many instances, animals are the most important reservoir for the microbe, and often the microbe does not cause disease in its preferred animal species, but does so in humans.[15] These infectious diseases in humans are called zoonoses. Knowledge of these infections is absolutely crucial for an understanding of the history of human infections, present-day infection problems and the challenges regarding infections we will face in the future.

The most important source of pathogenic microbes in human beings throughout our history of development has been the animal world. The vast majority of infections were initially zoonoses.[16] Animal microbes have, whenever contact between humans and animals has made this possible, attempted with varying degrees of success to infect humans. These microbes have probably often been unsuccessful because they have not been adapted to the conditions of the human body. Evolution and the vast adaptability of the microbes have in many instances led to the microbe using the human being as a host and partner exclusively, often with disease as the result. In this last phase of development, the microbe must have developed mechanisms for effective transmission of infection from one human being to another to be able to survive. We must assume that this has gradually taken place. At the first 'leap' from an animal species to a human being, the microbe has probably not managed to pass infection on to other human beings, but further adaptation has made this possible, with ever greater efficiency.

If we look at present-day zoonoses, we can see illustrated the various stages of development in the adaptation of animal microbes to human beings. They vary from one microbe to another. We have earlier mentioned the rabies virus as the cause of often fatal canine madness. This virus has its animal reservoir, from which it is effectively transmitted, but the virus cannot pass from one human being to another. Other examples are the bacterium that causes anthrax, which Robert Koch studied with such success, and the *Borrelia* bacterium (Lyme disease), which gets much attention from the media during tick season. None of these bacteria can be transmitted from one human to another.

An example of a microbe that has reached the next stage – human-to-human infection – although not particularly effectively, is the dreaded Ebola virus. In such cases, the epidemics tend to burn out relatively quickly, although we are perhaps witnessing an increase in the infectiousness of the Ebola virus.

Examples of the next stage of adaptation – even more efficiently spreading from one human to another, although still an important animal infection – are yellow fever, African sleeping sickness and the influenza virus. Well-known examples of microbes that have reached the final stage in the obstacle race of evolution – that is, they only cause infection in human beings – are the viruses that cause measles, mumps and smallpox, the protozoon that causes the most dangerous form of malaria (*Plasmodium falciparum*), the bacterium that causes syphilis (*Treponema pallidum*) and, last but not least, the HIV virus.

Do we know the animal origin of the microbes that now only cause infection in human beings? As far as a number of these microbes are concerned, we believe we can locate their original in the animal world, even though we lack the final proof.[17] Most people believe that the measles virus has developed from the related cattle plague virus. This virus has now been eradicated worldwide. And the smallpox virus may also come from a related virus in cattle, although recent research would actually suggest that it comes from the camel. The whooping cough bacterium is thought to have come either from the dog or the pig. As far as all these microbes are concerned, the assumed origin is domesticated animals. In other words, the transition from animal to human must have taken place after *Homo sapiens* started to keep animals, approximately 10,000 years ago. It was probably around the same time that humans acquired the most dangerous malaria microbe – *Plasmodium falciparum* – from birds. And we know that the HIV virus comes from African apes after having adapted itself to human beings in the twentieth century.

We cannot leave the topic of zoonoses without mentioning that we also have examples of microbes that normally infect humans exclusively sometimes also attacking animals. We have a number of examples of the great apes, both chimpanzees and gorillas, being infected by the human tuberculosis bacterium.[18] This has also happened to apes in the wild in connection with so-called eco-tourism.

Man-made Changes to the Natural Landscape

From the time that *Homo sapiens* settled and started to cultivate the land, about 11,000 years ago, our ancestors have constantly changed the natural landscape. The felling of forests to create more agricultural land and residential areas, the building of roads through deserted areas and the construction of dams have led to drastic changes in the ecological balance between various species of animals and plants.[19] Deforestation has escalated in our age and acquired alarming proportions. In the decade between 2000 and 2010 alone, it is estimated that 13 million hectares of forestland was lost, an area the size of Alaska.

The ecological consequences of man-made changes to the natural landscape are often unpredictable. Certain animal species will disappear; others will increase in number. A possible result of this is that people will for the first time encounter unknown microbes from species of animals that have now acquired more favourable life conditions and are therefore more plentiful in number. This particularly applies to various kinds of rodent that are carriers of pathogenic microbes. Whether or not such a microbe will manage to start an epidemic with transmittance of infection from human to human will depend on a number of adaptations that we looked at earlier.

In certain cases a microbe has already established itself as a cause of disease in humans, but only in remote, isolated population groups such as in jungle areas. If the group's isolation is broken, for example by building new roads, this can lead to the spread of the microbe, and only then does one realize that one is facing a new microbe. This may have been the case with the epidemics involving both the HIV and Ebola viruses, which existed as animal infections in the African jungle before adapting to humans. For years there may have been only a few infections caused by these viruses in isolated tribes before the possibility of further spreading arose.

There are a number of well-documented examples where the destruction of wilderness areas through the expansion of agriculture has led to formerly unknown microbes causing infections in humans following increased contact with a microbe-carrying animal species. Three such examples with exotic names originated from South America in the mid-twentieth century.[20]

The Junin virus was discovered to be the cause of serious infection in humans in Argentina after sections of the natural pampas were converted to maize cultivation. A special kind of mouse greatly appreciated this and its population increased rapidly. Unfortunately, this species of mouse was a reservoir for the Junin virus, which caused an epidemic of the so-called Argentine haemorrhagic fever (AHF).

Haemorrhagic fever is a life-threatening pathological condition in which the walls of small blood vessels burst, so that blood seeps from the skin and bodily apertures, while comprehensive internal bleeding also occurs. At roughly the same time as the outbreak in Argentina, there were a number of instances of a similar serious infection in Bolivia. This Bolivian haemorrhagic fever involved a formerly unknown virus that was given the name Machupo virus; one-seventh of the local population died. Here too the cause was wooded land that had been converted

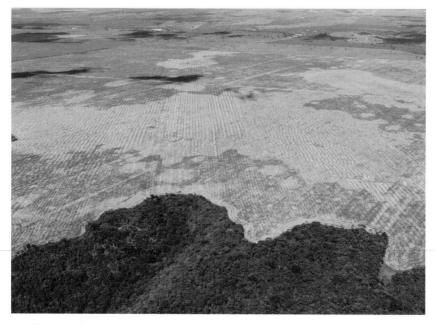

The felling of rainforest areas in the Amazon region. Deforestation often has major ecological consequences that can lead to new infectious diseases.

to agricultural use, which led to the increase in a species of mouse that carried the virus. Later, yet another new virus was discovered in Venezuela, the Guanarito virus, which also causes haemorrhagic fever and is found in small rodents on agricultural land.

Dam installations built to improve irrigation conditions in drought-ridden regions of the world also lead to ecological changes. This can have serious infection-related consequences for humans in the areas concerned.[21] One example is infections with the intestinal worm *Schistosoma*, which is widespread in Africa and Asia. The worm has a complex life cycle with various intermediate stages that develop outside human beings. One of these stages is dependent on a small freshwater snail. After maturing in the snail, small free-swimming worms are released that can infect human beings on contact via the skin. There are three species of this intestinal worm that can cause disease, particularly in the intestines and urinary bladder, but also in other organs such as the liver and the brain.

We know that this *Schistosoma* infection was already widespread in ancient civilizations such as Egypt and China, where artificial irrigation was an important component of agriculture, offering fine conditions for the intestinal worms. Both the building of the enormous Aswan dam in Egypt and other major dam projects in West Africa in our age have led to a marked increase in schistosomiasis in the populations close to the dams and the irrigation systems linked to them.

Species of mosquitoes are also completely dependent on water for their propagation. The building of dams will therefore possibly lead to an upsurge in their numbers, including those that transfer pathogenic microbes such as malaria. This has undoubtedly occurred many times throughout history. We have a modern example in Ethiopia, where a number of so-called micro-dams were built for agricultural irrigation in Tigray province, leading to a considerable increase in malaria in the local population. The same has been seen in Asia, including Sri Lanka.

Even though man-made changes to physical nature have been going on for centuries, constantly giving rise to new problems with infectious diseases, this is nowadays taking place at a more rapid tempo than ever before. There can be no doubt that there are still countless as yet undiscovered microbes in animal species that up to now have had little contact with human beings. Many of these microbes will perhaps not be able to infect humans, but some are certain to cause new infections in the years to come. During the past decades new pathogenic microbes have constantly been discovered, most of them coming from the animal world.[22] Such infections have greatly contributed to our increased awareness of the role of ecological changes in the interaction between man and microbes.

Human Behaviour: Sex and Syringes

As the world's dominant species, *Homo sapiens* also contributes to the ecological processes of the planet via its behaviour. We have already mentioned many examples of this from nature. But human behaviour at the more private and social level, which we can refer to as human ecology, also plays an important role in interaction with the world of microbes and the possibilities for infectious diseases.[23]

Sexual contact is an important means of infection for many microbes, and not only for those that cause what are commonly regarded as sexually transmitted diseases. Human sexual behaviour has undergone major changes down through history and social norms for acceptable behaviour have varied. A continuous characteristic, at least since the first human settlements were established about 11,000 years ago, has been that society has been based on the family, and that sexuality has been linked to propagation and the production of offspring. This has led to various restrictions as regards sexual practice. As a rule, this has especially affected women, since many societies have allowed men greater sexual freedom, with a certain acceptance of sexual activity outside the family, including the use of sex workers. The view of homosexuality has also varied through history. Since the introduction of Christianity, homosexuality has not been accepted until quite recently. The same applies to traditional Islamic societies. Corresponding to these shifting cultural and social conditions, microbes spread via sexual contact have had changing circumstances. In a great many cultures sex work has played a key role in the spread of sexually transmissible infections.

A dramatic change occurred in most Western societies from the 1960s onwards. The reasons for this sexual revolution are many. Former religion-based norms of sexual behaviour gradually lost their hold, particularly among younger people. The fear of pregnancy disappeared with the advent of the Pill. Irrespective of the causes, this led to a number of changes in heterosexual behaviour. The age of first sexual activity became lower. The number of sexual partners increased, particularly among young people. Casual sex, 'one-night stands', became more common. Forms of sexual practice also changed, with more frequent enjoyment of anal and oral sex in addition to 'conventional' sex. An increased use of various narcotic substances contributed to the decline of sexual inhibitions.

The sexual revolution was just as dramatic among male homosexuals, leading to a 'gay revolution'. While homosexuality had traditionally been a taboo phenomenon and homosexual practice a shady activity that was criminalized in most countries, there now came an increased acceptance of this form of sexuality. Gradually, homosexual practice was decriminalized in Western countries. Flourishing homosexual subcultures came into being with their own saunas and meeting places, where sexuality was given free rein. In some of these subcultures it was not unusual for some to exceed a thousand sexual partners. Here, too, it was increasingly common to use drugs and other substances such as so-called poppers to release people from their inhibitions. Many homosexual men were also frequent sex tourists to international meeting places, both big cities and holiday destinations such as Haiti.

All these changes to both heterosexual and homosexual environments sowed the seeds for an upsurge in infections through sexually transmissible microbes. With the introduction of penicillin, syphilis had declined in the years following the Second World War, only to flare up again from the 1960s onwards, both among heterosexuals and, especially, homosexual men. Cases of other 'classic' sexual diseases such as gonorrhoea and chlamydia increased dramatically, particularly because condoms were used much less by heterosexuals after the advent of the Pill. Condoms offer good protection against a number of sexually transmissible infections. The human papilloma virus (HPV), which is transmitted sexually, became more widespread and has led to a steady increase in cancer of the cervix in women and of the anal orifice and oral cavity in both women and homosexual men.

Last but not least, the sexual revolution provided a breeding ground for the largest infection catastrophe of our age – the HIV pandemic. The far higher level of sexual activity among homosexual men, with an increased number of partners, highly varying use of condoms and high level of travel and sex tourism, greatly contributed to the rapid spread of the HIV virus. Particular forms of sexual practice, such as fisting, where the partner's fist or lower arm are inserted into the rectum, also led to wounds and rents in the mucous membrane, which increased the risk of infection. The same applied to the use of an artificial penis (dildo).

Heterosexuals were also hit by the HIV epidemic, but during the early years they were less affected in Western countries than homosexuals. In Africa, on the other hand, various factors led to the virus spreading violently among heterosexuals.

It was not only infections that are usually perceived as being sexually transmitted that increased strongly in the years after the sexual revolution. This was also true of infections such as hepatitis, particularly the hepatitis B virus, which increased particularly among homosexual men.

In the second half of the twentieth century Western societies also faced another societal problem that had serious consequences as regards infectious diseases. Widespread abuse of drugs, first and foremost various forms of intravenous abuse through sharing contaminated syringes, offered many microbes new possibilities of infection. This applied to the hepatitis viruses HBV and HCV and, most dramatically, the HIV virus, which in many countries exploded among drug abusers. In Norway, for example, it proved possible to restrict this development with greater success than in many other countries, partly by action to distribute clean syringes to intravenous drug users. In many countries, however, this was forbidden. Bacteria can also cause life-threatening infections in people who inject drugs, with bacteria being injected directly into the bloodstream via contaminated syringes, leading, among other things, to inflammation of the heart valves (endocarditis). Access to clean syringes can also prevent this. In countries such as Italy and Spain, those who injected drugs were the group hardest hit by the HIV epidemic.

Cities: An El Dorado for Pathogenic Microbes

After *Homo sapiens* had settled to a life based on agriculture and animal husbandry, population densities gradually increased, leading to the formation of towns. These were established as early as between 3000 and 2000 BC in Egypt, Mesopotamia, the Indus Valley and China, as well as in Central America.

As we have already touched on, the transition to agriculture and animal husbandry led to comprehensive changes in the history of human infection as well as of medicinal issues in general. This tendency was in many ways intensified by the increasing urbanization. It is a historical fact that right up to modern times, microbes have presented a serious threat to towns and cities – and to a great extent continue to do so. Various factors have contributed to this.[24]

Urban environments, which involve close contact between those living there, have naturally always afforded optimum possibilities for microbes that transmit infection directly from one human being to another. For that reason, they are prone to epidemics and infectious diseases in general. The increased social stratification that gradually developed led to there being, from the earliest times, a large, poor lower class that lived in cramped, wretched dwellings, where conditions were particularly favourable for direct infection from person to person. Malnutrition, often connected to poverty, increased vulnerability to serious infections. The accumulation of rubbish and excrement attracted rats and insects that were often carriers of pathogenic microbes.

Even the more prosperous strata of urban society were, until modern times, exposed to infections because of poor sanitary conditions in towns and cities, with lamentable water and sewage conditions that were ideal for the spread of waterborne infections and epidemics such as cholera, typhoid fever and poliomyelitis. Some historians believe that entire urban civilizations may have perished because of serious waterborne epidemics. A possible example is the so-called Harappa culture, which flourished in the Indus Valley between about 3000 and 2000 BC.[25]

Ancient Rome was less affected by waterborne disease because of its system of aqueducts to transport relatively clean water from distant country districts, and, as a legacy from the Etruscans, its well-constructed sewage system; parts of this are still in use. This superior sanitary system disintegrated after the fall of the Roman empire and was eventually consigned to oblivion. The Roman drainage system, however,

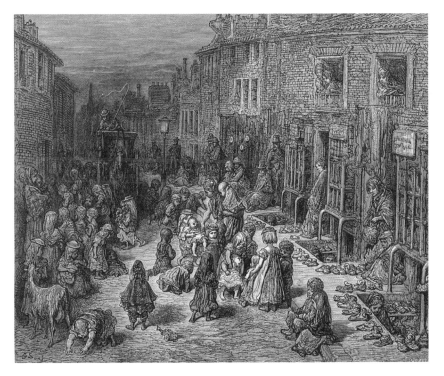

Slum district in London during the Industrial Revolution in the 19th century. Drawing by Gustave Doré, published in Gustave Doré and Blanchard Jerrold, *London: A Pilgrimage* (1872).

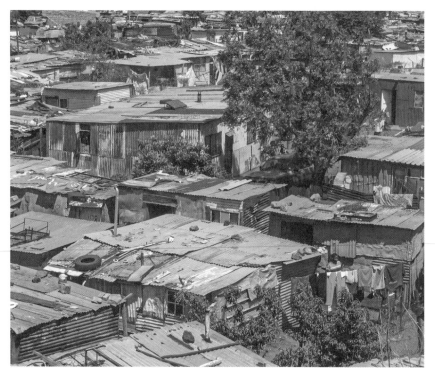

Shanty town in South Africa. These are urban districts with a high population density, simple dwellings made of gathered scrap materials, primitive sanitary and sewage conditions and an unsatisfactory water supply. At least 50 per cent of the population of Africa live in shanty towns.

also had serious defects since most of the private dwellings were not connected to the sewage system and unhygienic solutions were often adopted to get rid of excrement and other forms of waste, which were occasionally simply thrown out onto the street or on rubbish tips.[26]

Medieval towns and cities had far more primitive sanitary conditions than the Rome of antiquity. Human and animal excrement was often left lying in the streets, and the potential for microbial pollution of wells was always present. It was not until the first half of the nineteenth century that real improvements took place within this area in Western countries.

Urban problems with infectious diseases were undoubtedly aggravated by the fact that personal hygiene and cleanliness were extremely deficient throughout the Middle Ages and well into the eighteenth century. This did not apply only to the lowest social classes. Bathing and washing one's body were regarded as hazardous to health, since they could disturb the normal balance between body fluids or humours, on which Hippocrates and Galen had placed so much emphasis. The few public baths that existed in the early Middle Ages, as a memory of ancient Rome, were gradually regarded with great scepticism as being centres for immorality and crime. Cities have also been centres for sex work, very frequently connected to poverty, which has been a fertile source of sexually transmissible diseases.[27]

All in all, cities have always represented a health threat. Until about a century ago, mortality, especially among children, was so high that cities were completely dependent on immigration from the rural districts to maintain their population levels.[28] Infectious diseases contributed greatly to this high mortality rate.

The urbanization of the world's population took place at an accelerating tempo through the twentieth century. Today, more than 50 per cent of all humans on the earth live in towns and cities, and it is estimated that 65 per cent will do so by 2025.[29] In the poorer parts of the world, this urbanization has taken place so swiftly that in many places there are megacities where health conditions are in many ways just as bad as they were in the cities of the past. This is particularly the case in certain big cities in Africa, such as Lagos in Nigeria and Kinshasa in the Congo, which have widespread slums or 'shanty towns' whose inhabitants are exposed to well-known pathogenic factors such as poor access to clean water, wretched sewage conditions, poverty, malnutrition, sex work and drug abuse. These cities are in actual fact undetonated bombs of infection for new, serious epidemics. The explosive development of the HIV epidemic in Africa took place to a great extent in such urban environments.

War and Infection: an Ancient Alliance

As civilizations gradually arose, armed conflicts between individual civilizations as well as civil wars became a recurrent phenomenon. Unfortunately this is still the case.

Early written accounts from various civilizations show that humans have always been aware that war and epidemics are inextricably linked to each other. We earlier quoted Homer's description of the plague that ravaged the Greek army during the siege of Troy. Although the plague is ascribed to Apollo's wrath, the account faithfully reflects the fact that the Bronze Age Greeks were already aware of the connection between war and epidemics.

In the famous vision of the Four Horsemen of the Apocalypse in the Book of Revelation, there is a dramatic description of the plague as war's henchman, while Death forms the rear guard. This is not the only place where this theme is named in the Bible. At various places it is stated that the angel of the Lord struck down the army of the king of the Assyrians, Sennacherib, after he invaded Israel in 701 BC and besieged Jerusalem, where the prophet Isaiah also happened to be living. During a single night, 185,000 Assyrian soldiers are said to have died, and Sennacherib had to beat a retreat.

The account by the Greek historian Herodotus of the Persian Wars between Greeks and Persians – the first major east–west conflict – states that the invading Persian army lost thousands of its men because of epidemic diseases (and I have already mentioned the epidemic that ravaged Athens during the war with Sparta).

The connection between war and infectious diseases that we see throughout most of human history over thousands of years raises three important questions.[30] What is the cause of this connection? Who is affected? What consequences has the connection between war and infection had throughout history?

Let us first consider the causes. There are a number of these and some are complex. Army recruits came from various parts of the country, from both urban and rural districts, and these to a certain extent have very different histories of infection. The recruits encountered microbes they have never been exposed to before and therefore have no immunity against. The barracks and camps for the soldiers were often quite primitive, with even worse sanitary conditions than in the rest of society. In addition to such cramped quarters, conditions were ideal for pathogenic microbes that are transmitted via direct contact, such as influenza, smallpox and measles. Bad sanitation meant that parasitic infections transmitted via food and water, such as dysentery, typhoid fever and cholera, were common. Severe wound infections from battle injuries were common and, before the bacteriological revolution led to more modern treatment of wounds, there was little that could be done as war surgery was primitive, with brutal amputations.

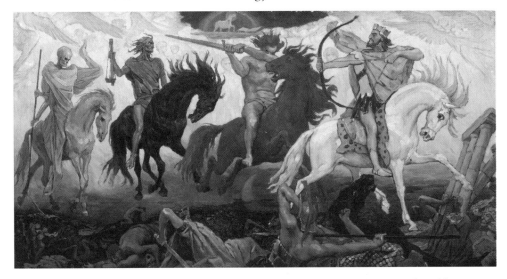

The Four Horsemen of the Apocalypse in St John's Book of Revelation in the Bible, painted by Viktor Vasnetsov, 1887. Here the four gruesome knights have been given the power 'to kill with the sword and with famine and with plague'. In the picture we see Death – 'the pale knight' – at the rear of the retinue.

In addition to all these factors, there were new medical problems with infection when military forces moved into distant climes with microbial flora that the soldiers had never met in their own country. This is a situation that armed forces from Western countries have encountered down through history.

Napoleon's forces during his campaign in Egypt encountered classic plague, which had long since disappeared from Europe. This probably contributed to his decision to abandon his campaign against the Ottoman Turks who ruled in the area. With his highly developed flair for public relations, he later took care to be painted by Antoine-Jean Gros as fearlessly visiting his plague-stricken soldiers at the plague hospital he had established in the city of Jaffa.[31]

Right up to the present age, malaria and yellow fever have created considerable problems for military operations in hot climates. During the Second World War, for example, the allied forces in Southeast Asia were troubled by malaria. In addition, British and American soldiers were hard hit by a particular bacterial disease, 'scrub typhus', which is transmitted from birds and small rodents via bites from mites. The case fatality rate was between 10 and 15 per cent. During the Vietnam War, classic plague appeared once more, mainly among the civilian population. As a conclusion to this cavalcade of exotic infections suffered by Western soldiers in distant climes, it should be mentioned that there has recently been a considerable number of cases of the protozoan parasite disease Leishmaniasis in American personnel in Afghanistan.

Until now we have not mentioned a type of infectious disease that has always flourished in military contexts: sexually transmitted diseases. It is fairly self-evident that such infections are likely to occur when large numbers of young men are gathered together, often far from their home country, not infrequently under stressful war conditions that often lead to casual, uncritical sex. Sex workers often have a lucrative business close to military divisions, which in former times would often have brought their own women along with them.

A dramatic example of the connection between war and sexually transmitted diseases is syphilis, which entered Europe during the long war between France and Spain in the 1490s. The French, who had brought a large number of sex workers with them from home, besieged Naples. The fall of the city in 1495 unleashed violent excesses against the civilian population as the victors celebrated. During these, a formerly unknown disease broke out, the sexually transmitted infection that our earlier acquaintance Girolamo Fracastoro christened syphilis. In the years that followed, syphilis was efficiently transported around Europe by soldiers and sex workers from the dissolved French army.

The list of examples of extensive and serious outbreaks of infectious diseases in military personnel is a long one. Let us instead take a look at examples of the consequences that these diseases have had for warfare – and so how they have influenced history.

We have seen that in the Old Testament there is an account of how Sennacherib had to withdraw the Assyrian army from Israel on account of the plague, apparently because the epidemic reduced the striking power of the army. This is not the only example of epidemics greatly curtailing military operations, with crucial consequences for the course of wars. We can clearly see this from the statistics known for the causes of death in armies of former times.

It is perhaps surprising that until the beginning of the twentieth century it was more common for soldiers to die from diseases (mostly infections) during campaigns than from the sword, bullets and bombs.[32] During the Napoleonic Wars, seven times as many British soldiers died from disease than from war wounds, particularly from typhus (also known as spotted fever) and dysentery, which are caused by bacteria. During the Crimean War (1853–6) almost four times as many allied soldiers died from disease than from injuries sustained on the battlefield. Even during the Second Boer War (1899–1902), twice as many British soldiers died of disease, particularly typhoid fever, as from war wounds.

It was not until the Russo-Japanese War (1904–5) and the First World War (1914–18) that more soldiers died on the battlefield than from disease in the field hospitals. Unfortunately, this is only partly because of improvements in the prevention and treatment of infections. The increased effectiveness of the weaponry doubtless also played a part.

Let us return to the endless war between France and Spain in Italy during the sixteenth century and to a later French siege of the Spanish-held city of Naples. Once again, a serious epidemic disease now made its first appearance on the European stage, typhus, caused by the bacterium *Rickettsia prowazekii*. The bacterium is transmitted from person to person via the faeces of lice. As Naples was about to fall in 1528, a violent epidemic of typhus broke out among the besieging French army: in the space of a month, half of the army was dead, the siege had to be broken off, and the rest of the army was swiftly dissolved. This had major political consequences, since Spain now became the dominant power in Italy, with the pope on its side. The Spanish Habsburg king, Charles V, confirmed his right to be Holy Roman Emperor in 1530 when he was crowned by the pope 'by courtesy of typhus', as it has been said.

We have already touched on the Napoleonic Wars. Napoleon's tragic and humiliating retreat from Moscow in 1812 is another example of an epidemic ravaging an army. The Russian winter, for which the Frenchmen were unprepared, combined with guerrilla attacks by the Cossacks, weakened Napoleon's army, but there is no doubt that the impact of typhus was even harder, well assisted by dysentery.

The American Civil War (1861–5) was an extremely bloody affair. This was the last major military conflict prior to the bacteriological revolution and the modern concept of microbes as a cause of disease. It is estimated that 660,000 soldiers perished during this war, but no less than two-thirds of these deaths were due to infectious diseases, mainly typhoid fever, dysentery, pneumonia and malaria. On a number

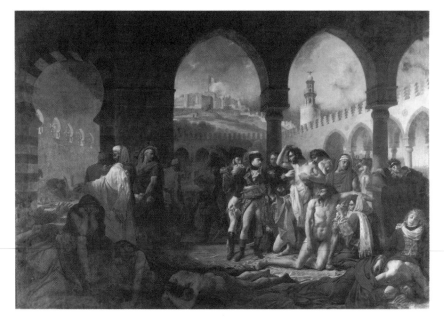

Napoleon at the plague hospital in Jaffa during his Egyptian campaign of 1798–1801, painted by Antoine-Jean Gros in 1804. Plague broke out in the army, leading to a fear of infection and weakened morale. Napoleon attempted to turn this around by visiting the hospital, where he also helped to carry a plague patient.

of occasions these epidemics prevented important military operations from taking place. Military historians have established that this probably lengthened the civil war by two years.[33]

But it was not only the soldiers who were affected by the preference of infectious diseases for war as their arena. Civilian populations have to a high degree paid the price for this linkage.[34] There are a whole series of examples of infectious diseases that have broken out in sections of the army and then spread to the civilians, starting large-scale epidemics. This is the natural explanation of the vision of the Four Horsemen of the Apocalypse in the Book of Revelation, where War is one of the riders.

There are many reasons why civilian populations are subject to infectious diseases in wartime.[35] Transmission from military personnel can take place during warfare, but it can also become widespread when the soldiers are demobilized and return home. Civilians are often forced to flee their homes during wars and can end up in geographical areas with microbes they are not immune to. Refugees are often housed in more or less improvised camps where conditions are highly favourable for outbreaks of infectious diseases, with cramped quarters, bad sanitary conditions and frequently undernourishment as well. During war conditions, the normal medical infrastructure in society can fail, with vaccination and medical treatment no longer taking place. The German concentration camps during the Second World War are a particularly shocking example of humanity's ground zero. Here infectious diseases such as typhus raged, resulting in a horrendous number of deaths.

We have already seen how the syphilis epidemic of the sixteenth century began among French soldiers in Naples. From there it spread out across all of Europe and affected all levels of the civilian population. During the bloody Austro-Prussian war of 1866, which was won by the Prussian forces, a smallpox epidemic broke out that also spread to the civilian population and led to 165,000 deaths in Austria alone. The smallpox virus struck again during the Franco-Prussian War of 1870–71, causing the death of 300,000 French and German citizens. A century after the Russian Revolution, which resulted in many deaths, we should not forget that in the wake of the revolution and the ensuing civil war there was a typhus epidemic that caused 2.5 million deaths.[36]

The most extensive epidemic known to have been linked to a war is the Spanish influenza epidemic (Spanish Flu), which broke out towards the end of the First World War and spread in the months that followed. This developed into a pandemic, with death figures variously estimated at between 50 and 100 million people. Both armies in the conflict were also badly affected.

From the German side, it has even been claimed that the influenza epidemic led to the failure of the German offensive of July 1918, which could otherwise have led to a German victory. This infection-related variant of the 'stab-in-the-back' conspiracy theories about the causes of the German defeat is not all that realistic, but it is certain that influenza had a significant effect on the military operations.[37]

The linkage between war and epidemics is not just a thing of the past. We have a relatively fresh example of a special epidemic in the wake of the long-lasting state of war in South Sudan.[38] Exacerbated by starvation and undernourishment, a large-scale epidemic broke out of the serious protozoon disease *kala azar* (visceral Leishmaniasis), which, if not treated, has a very high mortality rate. Given the wretched conditions in which the population lived during the war in South Sudan, the death figures were also horribly high.

There are even more recent examples in modern media. Polio has broken out during the war in Syria, even though the disease was formerly well under control in the country, with widespread vaccination.[39] As a consequence of the war in Yemen, a cholera epidemic has been taking place and a measles epidemic has recently broken out after the vaccination routine ceased to function because of the warfare.

These examples of the unhappy alliance between war and infections across the millennia illustrate yet again how microbes, with their virtuoso adaptability, exploit every possible change in human behaviour. The countless tragedies this has led to show that the unknown author of Revelation, with its apocalyptic vision, was not without a realistic insight into the misery of this world.

Technological Advances : A Double-edged Sword

In the struggle to survive, *Homo sapiens* has had one decisive advantage: its brain capacity and its ability to construct tools, from the first primitive flint knives to sophisticated space probes that can be sent to distant planets. Modern technology has changed the world and everyday human life in a thousand different ways, compared to our ancestors not only on the African savannahs but of just a hundred years ago.

Despite this, there has been no lack of critics of the rapid technological development. Even though some of this criticism may be exaggerated and based on unrealistic and nostalgic dreams about the past, we must not be blind to the fact that some of the advances we now regard as self-evident, and are also quite proud of, have their drawbacks. As far as our leitmotif is concerned – microbes' adaptation to human behaviour – there are a number of key examples of infection-related medical consequences of modern technology that should be taken into account.

At all times, polluted food has played a role as a mode of transmission for microbes. Formerly epidemics were triggered in this way at a quite local scale, since practically all food production was carried out privately. This has changed in Western countries, where over the past fifty years private households have become highly dependent on industrially produced foodstuffs.[40] The raw materials are processed, and the final products packaged industrially on a large scale and dispatched far and wide. If the raw materials used are polluted with microbes as a result of a failure in quality control, the foundation may be laid for a widespread epidemic. We have seen many examples of this in recent years.

Industrial production of chickens and eggs has often led to epidemics with bacteria that cause intestinal infections, in particular *Salmonella* and *Campylobacter*. Meat products from both small and large livestock have also caused infections via special pathogenic species of the bacterium *Escherichia coli*, which can cause life-threatening disease, especially among young children and old people. Such infections have also created problems for fast-food chains that sometimes serve inadequately cooked hamburgers.

Modern cooling technology and globalization have also led to large-scale international trade in foodstuffs. Imports of food to Western countries from developing countries with bad hygienic control of their food production have led to epidemics with various types of microbes. In the USA, for example, importing raspberries from Guatemala led to an epidemic with the protozoon *Cyclospora*, which causes intestinal infection. Even the cholera bacterium was imported in a consignment of frozen coconut milk from Thailand, which resulted in a small epidemic.[41]

Another example of the exploitation by microbes of modern technology is infection with the *Legionella* bacterium.[42] This is often found in water and usually does not cause any disease problems. In cooling towers connected to modern air-conditioning plants the bacterium can find favourable growth conditions and be emitted in water vapour in the form of aerosol clouds that have led to epidemics in the vicinity. Increased growth of the bacteria in water heaters has also led to infection via showerheads.

Since the Second World War, swift advances have been made in medical treatment and technology that have produced impressive results within a wide range of diseases.[43] A striking example of this is modern transplantation medicine. The transplantation of the heart, liver, kidney, pancreas and bone marrow has saved countless lives. A precondition for successful transplantation is that the patient takes immuno-suppressive medication, which reduces the immune system's reaction to the 'foreign' transplanted tissue, for the rest of his or her life. Similar medicines are also used on a large scale for many other illnesses that result from the harmful effects of immunological reactions; this applies, for example, to rheumatological diseases.

The price we pay for these major advances achieved by the use of immuno-suppressive medicines is that we have created a steadily increasing group of patients with more or less serious immune deficiency. Once again, the world of microbes has watched out for a chance to strike. A large number of microbes that are unable to cause infection and disease in humans with a normal immune system can now cause serious, sometimes even fatal, infection in these patients. Such microbes, known as opportunists since they exploit the patients' weakened immune system, have given rise to a completely new and steadily expanding field of infection medicine.

Medical technology has also celebrated triumphs within modern emergency medical treatment. In the intensive-care units at hospitals patients are kept alive using advanced technological forms of treatment with needles and tubes in natural and non-natural apertures. This too presents new opportunities for microbial invasion, sometimes with very special microbes. The prevention and treatment of infections are thus an important part of medical activity in such wards.

All these examples show how human activities, even those which start out by being extremely rational, constantly shift the balance in the duel between man and microbes.

Climate and Infections: A Highly Complex Interaction

It is beyond doubt that climate in many ways plays an important role in the interaction between man and the world of microbes. This has consequences for the occurrence of infectious diseases, which vary in frequency and significance according to the climatic conditions. The factors of import here are temperature, rainfall (precipitation), wind and sunshine.[44]

The connection between climate and infectious diseases is particularly complex and our knowledge of it is still incomplete. This is not limited to various climatic factors. In the interaction between man and microbes there are a large number of factors and players that are affected by the climate: the microbes, infection-carrying insects, animals that are hosts for the microbes in the event of zoonoses – and, in particular, humans who can change their behaviour and powers of resistance to infections in the wake of large-scale climate change.[45]

94

First, the microbes themselves can be influenced by climatic factors, including temperature. This is the case with malaria. The maturing of the malaria parasites (*Plasmodium* species) cannot take place at less than 16°C or over 33°C. Malaria infection comes from a bite by the *Anopheles* mosquito. The development of the mosquito is optimal at temperatures between 28°C and 32°C. The mosquitoes also bite more frequently at higher temperatures. These conditions explain why cooler, higher areas in Africa are malaria-free in regions where malaria otherwise is widespread. The mosquito that transmits yellow fever and dengue virus, like the malaria mosquito, cannot tolerate temperatures above 34°C and therefore disappears from areas when the temperature is in excess of this.

At higher temperatures, the propagation of cholera bacteria in water and *Salmonella* in foodstuffs increases, and this can lead to epidemics. The resurgence of the cholera bacterium is even stronger in the event of strong sunshine. The water bacterium *Vibrio vulnuficus*, a relation of the cholera bacterium, can increase sharply if the seawater is strongly warmed and cause wound infections in bathers, especially in the event of open wounds and reduced immunity against infection. We also see this in northern latitudes during periods of hot weather.

Changes in rainfall can influence both microbes and infection-carrying insects. Floods after long periods of heavy rain are often, especially in developing countries, accompanied by epidemics of parasitic infections because drinking water has become polluted. Such epidemics can also occur in developed parts of the world after long periods of drought, when the pathogenic microbes have gained a stronger concentration in sources of drinking water and the capacity to purify the water is exceeded.

The amount of rainfall can also affect infection-carrying insects.[46] The malaria mosquito, for example, thrives with increased rainfall, since dryness reduces the potential for the maturation of larvae, which takes place in water. But, as an illustration of the unpredictability of the connection between climate and infectious diseases, periods of drought in usually humid areas can also provide more breeding grounds of stagnant water for the mosquito. Heavy rain can also be catastrophic for the insects, since it washes them away from their breeding grounds.

Wind also plays a role in the spread of airborne diseases through viruses, fungi and bacteria, where dust particles containing microbes can be spread over large distances in the event of strong winds. Some people believe, for example, that the influenza virus can be transported from Asia all the way to the American continent in this way.

Then there are zoonoses, infections where the main hosts for the microbes are animals, but where infection can also affect humans. As mentioned, zoonoses have played a major role in the history of human infection, and the majority of newly discovered microbes over the past few decades also belong to this group. Rodents of various kinds are important with regard to many of these infections. Climate changes strongly influence the rodent population, which in turn can affect the occurrence of infections with microbes that rodents carry. Periods of extreme drought will often reduce the number of rodents, which can explode when rainfall returns. Humans will then come into contact with infected animals to a greater extent than usual. This happened for example with an epidemic of a previously unknown virus that was given the name *Sin Nombre* ('Nameless') in the southeastern part of the USA in 1993. Recent research findings indicate that climate causes can be involved in the outbreak of plague epidemics through the influence exerted on the rodent population in the areas concerned.

Lastly, major climate changes – both acute disasters and more chronic changes – will lead to altered human behaviour resulting in migration, poverty, undernourishment and the collapse of already poor health services, which in themselves make people more susceptible to infectious diseases.

The examples mentioned reveal how complex the interaction is between climatic factors and infectious diseases. Intensive research has been carried out within this field in recent years, mainly triggered by the ongoing debate about climate development and the risk of serious global warming and its consequences. Many claim that these include an increased risk of the spread of infectious diseases from tropical and subtropical areas to temperate zones such as Europe and North America. The time has not yet come for making any sweeping conclusions within this field.

In discussing climate and infections, we ought to distinguish between possible consequences of long-lasting climate changes, first and foremost global warming, and more acute, extreme climate occurrences. What can we learn from history? We have written accounts of major epidemics from as far back as almost 4,000 years ago, but the oldest say little about possible connections to climatic conditions.[47]

If we consult the imperial Chinese archives, which provide information about major epidemics in all the provinces, we find there were 881 such epidemics between 1300 and 1850. If we analyse a possible connection with warmer and cooler periods, we find that there was a 35 to 40 per cent greater probability of large epidemics in cold periods than in warm ones. However, it is impossible today to determine what kinds of epidemic were involved.

The connection between variations in climate and epidemics is highly complex since so many factors are often involved. Many historical accounts tell of epidemics in the wake of extreme climatic conditions that led to a failure in agricultural production, famine and undernourishment. Very frequently these climatic crises were also accompanied by social unrest and war, which has a clear link to outbreaks of epidemics. The period around the Thirty Years War (1618–48) illustrates this

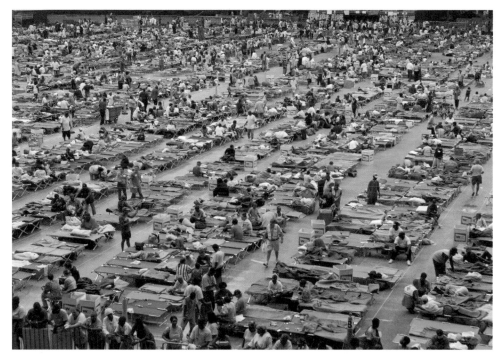

Thousands of refugees during Hurricane Katrina, which ravaged New Orleans and Louisiana in 2005, were collected together by the Red Cross in improvised centres, as here at the Houston Astrodome. Almost 900 acute infectious diseases followed in the wake of the hurricane.

dramatically, with plague and typhus epidemics constantly following in the footsteps of the armies involved.

We also have a number of clear examples from our own age of the link between extreme, acute climatic occurrences and the outbreak of infectious diseases.[48] Hurricane Katrina in 2005 led to almost nine hundred acute infectious diseases, mainly intestinal and respiratory infections as well as skin and wound infections.

In summer 2010 Pakistan was hit by extensive flooding after violent monsoon rains. In addition to the considerable material destruction, the disaster led to 37 million acute infections, particularly intestinal and respiratory tract infections, skin infections and malaria.

In recent years there has been an upsurge in interest in the importance of the so-called El Niño phenomenon.[49] This is a complex, linked change in the temperature of the sea and the atmosphere that has major climatic consequences, particularly in the southern hemisphere. El Niño occurs at intervals of between two and seven years. Storms and hurricanes, heavy rainfall, regional drought and higher-than-normal temperatures are then common. Several malaria epidemics have been seen in connection with El Niño. The epidemic caused by the *Sin Nombre* virus in the southeastern USA in 1993 followed rainfall after many years of pronounced drought in the wake of El Niño. Some researchers claim that the El Niño disturbances will become more intense in connection with the feared global warming in the years to come. It would, however, hardly be justified to assert on the basis of the El Niño effects described here that lasting global warming will lead to more chronic consequences.

In conclusion, we can state, all things considered, that climatic conditions will doubtless be of great importance for the spread and frequency of a whole series of infectious diseases, and also for major epidemics. A great many factors are significant, as regards both the climate and the interaction between man, microbes and environment.[50] The future situation is thus extremely complex and difficult to predict.

The trinity: microbes, man and the environment

In the never-ending duel between microbes and men, the outcome will to a great extent be decided by ecological and environmental factors, and here we are including humans' own behaviour in the ecological picture. These are the factors that actually determine if the duellists will confront each other in a trial of strength. At the same time, one of the duellists, *Homo sapiens*, greatly influences many of the environmental and ecological factors, partly consciously, but in the vast majority of cases unconsciously. This process has been going on for several thousand years, but has rapidly accelerated in recent times.

The consequences resulting from human behaviour and our relationship to the world of microbes constitute just one example demonstrating the ever-increasing influence *Homo sapiens* has acquired over nature. Human activities now make a vast impact on the physical and biological state of the planet, notably climate change with global warming as a result of greenhouse gas emissions, pollution of the earth, sea and sky, the loss of species diversity, deforestation and fallout from radioactive isotopes. This is why many people have proposed the introduction of a new term, 'Anthropocene', to describe the geological epoch in which we now find ourselves (*anthropos* is the Greek for man/human) and which until now has been called the Holocene, starting about 12,000 years ago.[51]

There is disagreement as to when the new epoch started, although the majority of a committee set up to deal with this question are in favour of placing the starting point in the mid-twentieth century.[52] It is nevertheless obvious that this is a somewhat random choice. That particularly also applies for our theme: the consequences of human behaviour for the microbial world and the history of infectious diseases. This process has been going on for thousands of years, long before what we refer to as historical time.

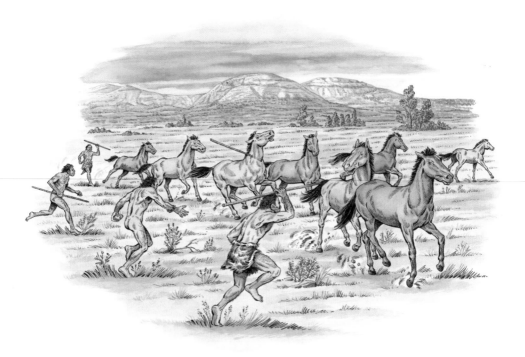

Homo sapiens roamed around as hunters and gatherers in small groups until c. 8500–9000 BC, when the first epidemiological transition came. This led to people having fixed dwellings with animal husbandry and agriculture.

THREE

A Bird's-eye View of the History of Human Infection

*H*omo sapiens – modern man – is the only survivor of several species of the human race. Our history stretches back at least 300,000 years. Naturally enough, our knowledge about most of this history is somewhat imperfect. Even so, via contributions from various sciences over a century we have gained an impression of the living conditions experienced by *Homo sapiens* during the various periods leading up to today, and especially of the role of infectious diseases in human history.

As we have seen, it is not sufficient to simply focus on humanity and the microbes in order to understand how infectious diseases arise and eventually spread. After we became aware of the importance of the third factor (ecological conditions and the environment) as the result of contemporary research, we have acquired a different understanding of the history of human infection down the ages.

A widespread modern conception is that the development of human history has taken place fairly gradually and with a constant improvement of living conditions, although interrupted by crises and disasters of various kinds. This is probably incorrect, particularly with regard to the history of human infection. Instead of an even development with constant progress, it is now believed that the development has been characterized by a great many comprehensive adjustments – so-called epidemiological transitions – when the relationship between man and microbes and infectious diseases has changed quite drastically, running parallel with other major changes in human life conditions.

The reason for the large-scale alterations in the panorama of infections in relation to these transitions is precisely the major changes in the ecological factors that are so important in the interaction between man and microbes. Even though most present-day researchers within the field now believe in the existence of such major and epoch-making transitions in the history of human infection, there is not complete agreement about what merits the term 'epidemiological transition', or about the number of such transitions. Most researchers in this field are not medically qualified and probably place less emphasis on purely medical factors than I as a medical doctor find natural. Based on the knowledge we have today, I feel it is reasonable to talk of five different transitions in the history of infection from the time when the first members of the species *Homo sapiens* roamed the African savannahs. Let us take a look at the timeline of our history of infection and at the various transitions that convincingly illustrate the interaction between man, microbes, and ecological and environmental factors.

Man as Hunter and Gatherer

The forefathers of *Homo sapiens* had already moved out of the African rainforests, where high temperatures and humidity result in a particularly rich microbial life, and where numerous insects and various species of animals can all pose a threat of infection. For tens of thousands of years *Homo sapiens* roamed the African savannahs as hunters and gatherers, without any fixed dwellings.

What sort of life did the humans have, living in small groups of perhaps thirty to fifty individuals? Did they lead such a frightful existence that the seventeenth-century philosopher Thomas Hobbes was right when he described the life of primitive man as 'solitary, poor, nasty, brutish and short'? Or was the eighteenth-century Jean-Jacques Rousseau right when he enthusiastically wrote about 'the noble savage' who lived in 'celestial and majestic simplicity'? The truth probably lies somewhere in between.

How can we possibly know anything about these people who lived thousands of years ago? Our conception is based on two types of knowledge, comparing in-depth studies of the few surviving hunter-gatherer communities in recent times with archaeological finds, particularly skeletal remains.[1] On this basis, it is reasonable to assume that humans of this period led a demanding life. They had considerably shorter lives than present-day people in the richer parts of the world, although not much shorter than what we now find in the poorer parts, or indeed in Europe a few centuries ago. In periods when there was little game, the hunter-gatherer communities probably had problems with their calorie intake. Despite this, they had a quite varied diet consisting of meat from various types of game, plants, roots and berries. Their skeletons display no convincing signs of malnutrition or lack of vitamins. This is why certain modern romantics have praised what they refer to as the 'stone-age diet'.

What infectious diseases were these people plagued by? There is reason to believe they actually had a smaller infection load than people at a later stage of development. One of the reasons for this is precisely that a nomadic existence involves a regular change of place and relocation of dwelling. In this way they could avoid the dangers of piling up excrement and polluting drinking water, two things that can lead to the spread of microbes that cause intestinal infections: bacteria, intestinal worms and protozoa.

We also believe that the individuals of these small groups were only to a very limited extent afflicted by microbes that cause acute infectious diseases, either killing the patient or being passed on, leaving the patient with permanent immunity.[2] Once all the individuals have been infected, immunity acquired by the survivors will lead to the disappearance of the microbe. We have seen examples of this in isolated hunter-gatherer groups in the present day. Infections such as measles, smallpox, mumps and whooping cough therefore did not exist at that time. These microbes did not develop as important threats until much later, when people lived in permanent larger communities.

Despite this, these early humans also contracted infections. The two most important types were probably zoonoses (infections from animals) and chronic infections that are transmitted at close quarters. The risk of zoonoses from wild animals was probably considerably greater for the hunter-gatherers than for later humans, since contact with wild animals during hunting was far more frequent. Many of these infections were also transferred from animals to humans via stinging insects. Examples of such diseases are malaria, yellow fever and African sleeping sickness. Hunters could also risk contracting anthrax from various kinds of wild animal. Microbes that live in the soil, such as the tetanus bacterium and certain fungi, could also result in serious infections. But neither such infections nor many of the zoonoses were passed on from human to human, and for that reason there were only isolated cases in a group that was not itself wiped out by the microbes. On the other hand, it was often the adults who were affected, and that could have serious consequences for a small, vulnerable group where all the adults were important for the group's survival.

The chronic infections that were probably important were mainly fairly mild diseases that were transferred via close bodily contact, droplet infection or food. An example of the first may have been the disease yaws, which is caused by a microbe closely related to the syphilis bacterium (*Treponema pallidum*) and possibly a precursor of this infection. Yaws produces chronic wounds of the skin and still exists in Africa. There are reasons to believe that leprosy also occurred at this early stage. The leprosy bacterium is, as mentioned earlier, a close relative of the tuberculosis bacterium (they are both mycobacteria). Did tuberculosis, which is also a chronic disease, occur among the small hunter-gatherer groups? We have no certain information about this, but we know that the bacterium that causes tuberculosis in humans, *Mycobacterium tuberculosis*, is extremely old, at least as old as *Homo sapiens* and possibly older.

Chronic infections by viruses from the herpes group very likely existed, probably both chickenpox and infections with *Herpes simplex*. These viruses remain in a latent form in the body after the acute infection and can flare up again and cause infection later in life. The chickenpox virus, for example, is able, after existing in a dormant state for many decades, to reappear in older people as shingles, which is infectious to all who have not had chickenpox earlier in life.

Wound infections naturally existed among the hunter-gatherers, partly via bacteria from the soil and partly via bacteria that are normally a part of human microbiota. Staphylococci are a possible example of this, since these bacteria are normally found in the nose and on the skin.

After roaming the African savannahs for a couple of hundred thousand years, *Homo sapiens* gradually moved beyond Africa and, over time, populated all other continents except Antarctica. The encounter with new environments with different fauna as regards both microbes and animals, including insects, doubtless led to a change in the panorama of infections.[3] People took with them the chronic infections already mentioned that are transmitted from human to human, but the pattern of the actual zoonoses changed, since many of the earlier types of animals and insects transmitting microbes remained in tropical Africa. However, *Homo sapiens* now met new species of animals that had their own infections, including new zoonoses. Lower temperatures in the new climes led to hides and skins increasingly being worn, offering ideal conditions for such parasites as lice and fleas that could pass on infections. Generally speaking, there are nevertheless reasons to believe that the total infection load was somewhat less for humans in temperate habitats than in tropical Africa, where the variation in all forms of fauna is particularly large.

On the whole, then, we can conclude that the first humans' state of health in their hunter and gatherer existence was not all that bad. In many ways their state of nutrition was probably better than that which has characterized the majority of people in subsequent history until recent times. The same applies to their infection problems. Even now, one still finds large groups of people in the so-called developing world who live in poverty and who in many ways are worse off than our first ancestors were, both as regards nutrition and infection load.

But the situation was to change drastically with the first transition in the history of human development: the transition to agriculture and animal husbandry.

The First Transition: Agriculture and Animal Husbandry

About 11,000 years ago the first clear signs that *Homo sapiens* had changed its means of living appeared. From having been small groups of vagrant hunters and gatherers, many people now settled in a permanent location and begin to farm and keep animals.[4] This dramatic transition occured at various places in the world, but it started about 8500 BC in the Middle East, in the area known as the Fertile Crescent, centred on the land between the Euphrates and the Tigris and extending to present-day Israel, Lebanon, Jordan and the southern part of Turkey. Egypt is often also included. A similar development took place, although not at precisely the same time or in exactly the same way, in both North and South America, parts of Africa and regions of Asia. All in all, it probably occurred in nine areas, independently of each other. The new mode of living then gradually spread out beyond these original areas.

There is an ongoing debate about the causes of this dramatic shift in human existence, one that involved major changes of social organization,

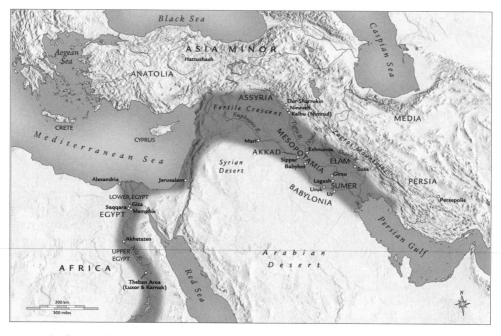

The first epidemiological transition – when humans began to settle permanently and engage in agriculture and animal husbandry – took place *c*. 8500–9000 BC in the Middle East.

behaviour and, in particular, state of health – including the infection load.[5] Many people emphasize that the climatic conditions had become more favourable for agriculture, since the last Ice Age was then on the wane, accompanied by higher temperatures.

This led on the one hand to a greater variation in wild, edible plants that were suitable for cultivation. On the other hand, the increase in temperature led to drought in some areas, resulting in fewer edible wild plants. The amount of large game also gradually diminished considerably. At the same time, the population of the hunter-gatherer communities had already started to increase and it is possible that the increased need for more food contributed to the great transition, which cannot have been a sudden change. Over a long period of time, there were probably settled communities alongside the hunter-gatherer groups, which gradually decreased in number.

As a point of departure, many will probably view the dramatic transition as a major step forwards in the development of the human race. And in many ways this was undeniably the case. The new living conditions provided the basis for comprehensive social, political and cultural development. This also led to material advantages: the production of food increased and enabled a considerable increase in population to take place. Dwellings that were more solid and permanent provided better shelter in unfavourable weather conditions.

But there was also a reverse side to the coin.[6] The workload was probably greater than for those in the hunter-gatherer communities and, in terms of health, this new form of existence actually represented a considerable step backwards, despite the undeniable material advantages. Life expectancy decreased, and so did people's average height. This was due to various factors.

In terms of nutrition, it actually seems as if people were now worse off than before. Their diet became too one-sided, being mainly based on grain products. The population also became more vulnerable to undernourishment if the harvest failed or the stores of grain were stolen by hostile groups. Vitamin deficiency probably also became more common. All of this would have weakened the immunological defence against infection in such a way that the first permanent settlers became easier prey to infectious diseases than their nomadic forefathers. This had serious consequences, since both agriculture and animal husbandry drastically changed people's relation to the world of microbes and infectious diseases. There were many reasons for this.

In their previous existence as vagrant hunters and gatherers people moved to a different place to live from time to time. As we have seen, their excrement and other forms of waste did not get the chance to pile up and pollute the sources of drinking water.[7] And so people at this stage were not seriously troubled by acute and chronic intestinal infections caused by contact with faeces, which, via food or water, may lead to so-called faecal-oral infection. Nor did various forms of intestinal worms that need an intermediary stage outside the body in order to mature get a chance to do so, since people frequently changed dwelling places. For settlers the situation was completely different. For that reason, the frequency of many such intestinal infections increased considerably after the first transition. Infection often took place during childhood and resulted in chronic illness and diarrhoea, which also weakened their nutritional state, as we can still see in poor countries around the world. The spread of intestinal infections in these communities further increased as human excrement was used as manure in the fields. Piles of manure and excrement doubtless attracted swarms of insects and small rodents, who were very frequently carriers of microbes, some of them dangerous, such as plague and various types of virus that can cause haemorrhagic fever.

An important factor in the problems causing new infections was the introduction of agriculture.[8] The natural environment surrounding *Homo sapiens* now seriously started to change, along with the natural ecological conditions. Such changes to the eco-balance could cause new infection problems because humans came into contact with microbes that formerly never or only rarely created them. This occurred partly because of increased contact with animals, most often small rodents, which were carriers of a pathogenic microbe, or by infection-carrying insects changing their behaviour towards humans. An example of the latter is malaria, which clearly became a far greater problem after the first transition than it had previously been. The clearing of agricultural land and the introduction of irrigation often created new dams and dykes that were ideal breeding grounds for malaria mosquitoes, which increasingly developed a taste for human blood, and this was far more accessible than before in the new, permanent settlements. In the same way, the yellow fever virus also became a greater threat.

Intestinal worms that cause the chronic infection schistosomiasis also became a real problem in agricultural societies where large-scale irrigation systems were used. The snail that is an intermediary host for the intestinal worm thrives in water under such conditions, and humans become infected by wading in infected water. This became a serious problem early on in both Egypt and Asia, where the paddy fields are under water. Agriculture also increased the risk of becoming infected by microbes that exist in the soil, including the bacterium that causes tetanus. This bacterium thrives in the intestines of horses and livestock and, via the animals' excrement, gets spread over the pastureland on which they graze.

All these factors increased the human infection load and contributed to the larger health problems that the hunter-gatherer peoples had to put up with. In spite of this, the major transition in human existence led to a sharp increase in the population, which has continued up to the present day. Precisely this development provided the basis for a completely new situation as regards threats from the world of microbes:

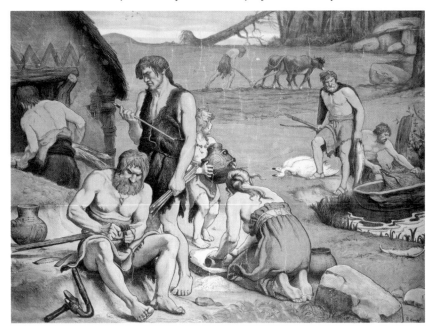

With the first epidemiological transition, *c.* 8500–9000 BC, people began to settle permanently and engage in agriculture and animal husbandry, as seen in this painting by Arthur Kampf, *c.* 1900.

acute, epidemic infections now entered the turbulent history of human infection, as we shall see.

For settled farmers, hunting wild animals no longer played the central role that it had previously done. This meant that people suffered far less exposure to the zoonoses that wild animals could pass on than had the hunter-gatherer communities. On the other hand, people came into far more intimate contact with all the animal species that had now been tamed, and very often humans lived alongside many of them, such as pigs, dogs and cows. These tame animals also had their own infectious diseases, and the basis was therefore established for new zoonoses. This was to have major consequences for humanity's later development.

A number of the commonest pathogenic microbes in humans were thus originally passed on from domestic animals at the stage when humans started to settle and engage in agriculture and animal husbandry. The most important of these microbes are those that typically cause acute infections which are either short-lived and confer immunity or are fatal, often after new individuals have been infected. This created the basis for an epidemic. It is these infections that are often referred to as 'infectious childhood diseases', such as measles, mumps, German measles and whooping cough. The smallpox virus, which has now been eradicated, followed this pattern. In order to survive, these microbes constantly have to infect new victims, so they are utterly dependent on there being a large number of individuals available who can be infected. In small population groups exposed to the microbe, everyone will either become immune or succumb to the infection. The microbe will then disappear from that group. For that reason, such infections were not a serious threat among the small hunter-gatherer communities. These diseases are called 'crowd infections'.

The situation changed, however, with the large population increase resulting from the transition to agriculture and animal husbandry. After several thousand years, urban communities sprang up where sheer numbers made it possible for the microbes involved to stay in the population, partly because new, non-immune, children capable of being infected were constantly being born, and partly because of an influx of formerly uninfected individuals from the distant peripheries of the community who had not been in contact with the microbe concerned.

The microbes causing such 'crowd infections' appeared as epidemics according to a certain time-pattern. At certain intervals, when a sufficient proportion of the population had acquired immunity, the epidemic abated. The population had then reached so-called herd immunity. But the microbe was still present in the population. Everything was quiet until the next epidemic with the same microbe broke out. How many people are needed for this situation to be able to arise? This has especially been studied concerning the measles virus, where both theoretical calculations and practical experience show that the population must be at least 300,000 to 500,000 strong for the virus not to disappear but to continue to exist in the community and give rise to repeated epidemics. This result has partly been arrived at via mathematical calculations and partly by observing measles epidemics in smaller, isolated communities: in the latter circumstances the virus disappears from the population group because there are no more individuals left who are susceptible to infection.

The common conception today is that most of the microbes causing such epidemics derive from closely related microbes in many of our domestic animals.[9] These can cause corresponding animal epidemics. At a certain point in time, the animal microbe involved has 'jumped' to humans, where, probably after many unsuccessful attempts over a lengthy period of time, it has managed to gain a foothold and cause infection. Through increasingly improved adaptation to human hosts it has learned how to pass on infection from one human to another.

The measles virus has many quite close relatives among several animal species. Most people believe that the virus originated from the related rinderpest (cattle plague) virus, but it may also have come from a different, related virus in dogs.[10]

The smallpox virus has relatives in many animal species. It has been claimed that the human virus, which cannot infect other animal species, derives from cattle. Recent research, however, seems to indicate that 'our' virus comes from a closely related virus in the camel, which has 'jumped' to humans and then further adapted.[11] This kind of research is not only of theoretical interest. Today, the smallpox virus is considered to have been eradicated from our planet. Is it possible for a new smallpox virus to reappear, introduced from the camel or other animal species? Another related virus in monkeys – monkey pox – can actually cause serious illness in humans, but it is not particularly infectious. Could this virus adapt itself to human beings and become just as infectious as the 'classic' smallpox virus?

Let us pause for a moment and ask an important question. Did this development of 'new' infectious diseases with microbes from domestic animals take place in all parts of the world where the great transition to settlers engaging in agriculture and animal husbandry occurred? The answer, perhaps surprisingly, is no, because here we have to make a sharp distinction between the development in Europe and Asia, where the transition first started, and that in the Americas, where the first transition also took place in several centres in North, Central and South America. In the Americas no corresponding development of major epidemic diseases such as measles and smallpox took place. What was the reason for this? Were the conditions on the American continent basically different from those in Europe and Asia?

The American biologist Jared Diamond believes that the explanation for this is that a great number of large mammal species had died out on the American continent at the end of the last Ice Age, about

13,000 years ago.[12] Among these were cattle, the horse and the camel. Although this may partially have been the result of climate changes, it is probable that intensive hunting by the first humans in America was the main cause.

The general conception is that *Homo sapiens* immigrated to North America from Siberia across the Bering Strait during the last Ice Age or some time earlier, about 20,000–30,000 years ago, when there was probably a land bridge between Asia and North America. When the first epidemiological transition came to the American continents, several thousand years after Europe and Asia, there were far fewer large animals suitable for animal husbandry: the llama and the related alpaca were the most important exceptions. We do not, however, know of any microbe that has 'jumped' to humans from these animals, which existed only in a fairly small area in the western regions of the Andes. Nor do they live as domestic animals in such close contact with humans, as was the case with domestic animals in the Old World. Zoonoses from domestic animals were therefore a far less serious problem in the Americas.

To a certain extent, people were far more fortunate in Europe and Asia, where there were many large animals well suited to animal husbandry, such as cattle, pigs, sheep and goats. But this came at a price: 'new' epidemic diseases. No matter the cause, people in the Americas initially avoided such raging epidemics. Diseases such as measles and smallpox were unknown until Europeans arrived. This was to have tragic consequences.

Before we conclude this discussion of zoonoses and the transfer of microbes by domestic animals to humans, we must take a look at tuberculosis, which has played such an important role in the history of human infection and is still a very great health problem in parts of the world. How does the tuberculosis bacterium (*Mycobacterium tuberculosis*) fit into the picture we have drawn?

The prevailing conception until recently was that the human tuberculosis bacterium was a further development of a related bacterium, *Mycobacterium bovis*, in cattle. This bacterium is able to infect humans partly via milk and then further mutate, as we have observed with so many other microbes. New research, using sophisticated molecular-biological methods, has now shown that this conception can hardly be correct, for the human bacterium seems to be much older than its related bacterium in cattle. Either they must have developed in parallel with each other from a common 'ancestor', or the cattle bacterium is a descendant of 'our' bacterium after humans infected cattle.

When we look back at the many changes to humanity's way of life in the wake of the transition to agriculture and animal husbandry, it is not difficult to accept that this really was a dramatic transition for *Homo sapiens* – for better or for worse. We have seen that human health in many ways deteriorated compared to that of their nomadic ancestors. This applied both to the nutritional situation and the infection load. If one focuses on these negative aspects of the first transition, one can be tempted to say, as some have done, that the transition from hunters and gatherers to settlers is one of the biggest mistakes of humanity. Such an extreme claim, however, naturally ignores the fact that the first transition laid the necessary foundation for formidable progress within a large number of fields.

During the first millennia after humans became settlers, the constant increase in population as well as political and social developments led to more densely populated societies and the development of cities, city states and empires. For thousands of years, the main civilizations – in China, India, the Middle East and eventually Europe – were quite isolated from each other. We must assume that each of them, to a great extent, developed its own pattern of infections, including regular epidemics.[13] In addition to people developing immunity towards the microbes that caused epidemics at intervals – crowd infections – we must also assume that certain genetic changes gradually took place in the defence against the local microbes. This would have increased the ability to combat such microbes and contributed to differences in the genetic material, the genome, which we now see in various parts of the world.

Sooner or later, however, increased contact between the formerly isolated civilizations was inevitable, and it was to have consequences for the threats from the microbial world. Now the foundation was laid for an exchange of microbes between the civilizations of Europe and Asia. The American historian William H. McNeill in particular has spotlighted this in his classic book *Plagues and Peoples* (1976).

During the last centuries BC, the conditions were right for a considerable increase in trade between the Asian civilizations and European societies, particularly the Roman empire. This partly took place over land, especially along the famous Silk Road, and partly by boat across the Indian Ocean. And on board were stowaways from the world of microbes, which now gained access to completely new populations that had not developed either immunological or genetic defence against them. The results did not fail to materialize.

The exchange of pathogenic microbes that ensued made such a vast medicinal and political impact that it is tempting to call this the second epidemiological transition in the history of human infection. Some scholars have done so. My reasons for choosing not to follow suit are these: first, we have very little firm knowledge about the microbes that evolved at the time of the exchange between Asia and Europe, even though there are many theories and suggestions; second, this exchange of microbes took place over quite a long period of time and in a somewhat complex fashion. The final result was a considerable levelling out of the differences in the major epidemic infectious diseases such as smallpox and measles. This process, however, took several centuries. And there remained large geographical differences in the infection load for many other pathogenic microbes, corresponding to permanent local differences in the panorama of microbes, fauna, climate and ecological conditions in general.

The first meeting with alien microbes, however, was a violent affair. We can best see this in Europe, where we have two dramatic examples from the Roman empire: the Antonine plague (AD 165–80) and the plague of Cyprian (AD 249–62). Both these epidemics severely taxed the Roman empire and probably had lasting consequences for its stability. We do not know for certain which microbes were involved, but we will later examine these epidemics in more detail.

The Second Transition: The Exchange of Microbes between the Old and the New World

The same development of acute epidemic infectious diseases did not take place on the American continent as in Europe and Asia. This naturally meant that people there had not encountered these microbes; nor had they developed any immunological or genetic defence against them. This was unimportant as long as the Americas were isolated from the rest of the world, but an abrupt end came to this with the arrival of

Europeans in 1492 and the 'discovery' of America. Here I am ignoring the sporadic visits of Norsemen, which apparently did not alter the infection situation in North America. Their stays were relatively short and comprised only a few visitors who had practically no contact with the indigenous population.

A very different microbial drama was enacted, however, in the wake of the Spanish conquerors, the conquistadors, who in a very short space of time invaded and suppressed the large civilizations they encountered in Central and South America.[14] They did so with forces that were quite small. Although the conquistadors had many unattractive characteristics, no one can doubt their courage and willpower. But that in itself would have been insufficient to ensure their formidable success as conquerors. How could Hernán Cortés, along with a few hundred men, conquer the mighty Aztec empire in Mexico in such a short space of time? Well, he brought with him – admittedly without realizing it – a decisive weapon: the smallpox virus. This virus had developed in the Old World and did not exist in the Americas, so the indigenous population had no defence of any kind against it. The violent epidemic that broke out thus had catastrophic consequences for the military and psychological resistance of the Aztecs.

Another of the famous conquistadors, Francisco Pizarro, who conquered the flourishing Inca empire in Peru, was also greatly assisted by the smallpox virus, which had rapidly spread from Mexico to South America.

It has been calculated that the first smallpox epidemics that followed the conquistadors took the lives of a third of the indigenous population.[15] In the years following the arrival of the Europeans, the virus spread further to other parts of the continent, with equally tragic consequences.

It was not only the smallpox virus that was new to the American population. Hard on its heels came the measles virus, which also led to epidemics with a high mortality rate, just as we have seen elsewhere when this virus is introduced into a population that has not developed immunity against it after former contact. The Europeans also had with them the viruses that cause mumps and German measles, as well as those that give rise to whooping cough (pertussis) and diphtheria. It is further possible that the typhus bacterium (*Rickettsia prowazekii*) was imported, but this is not known for sure. Other epidemics also raged, the causes of which we do not know with any certainty, but they may well have been caused by microbes that the conquistadors had brought with them.

Between 1545 and 1548 Mexico was ravaged by an epidemic that may have taken the lives of almost 15 million people (about 80 per cent of the indigenous population), according to Mexican researchers.[16] The pathological picture was new to the doctors, with high fever, bleeding from nose and mouth, and jaundice. The Aztecs called the epidemic 'cocoliztli' in their language, Nahuatl. A new outbreak of the same disease occurred in 1576–8, leading to the deaths of 2 million people. The cause of these epidemics is unclear. It is interesting that a period of extreme drought hit Mexico just before the outbreaks. Mexican researchers have therefore claimed that cocoliztli may have been some sort of haemorrhagic fever caused by a virus from rodents where the population has been influenced by climatic disturbances. They doubt whether the microbe in question came from the Old World.

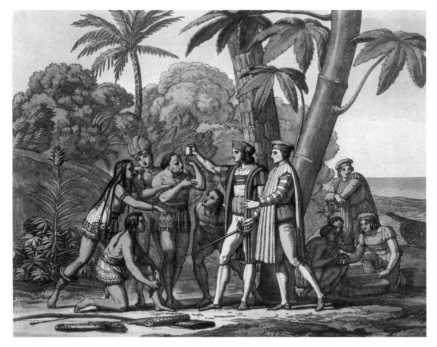

The 'Columbian exchange' is the term used for the exchange between the Old and the New World of, among other things, plants, types of food, animals, population groups and infectious diseases that took place after the arrival of Christopher Columbus in 1492, an event seen here in an illustration by Pelagio Palagi, from Giulio Ferrario, *L'Amerique*, vol. 1 (1820), part of *Le Costume ancien et moderne*.

Very recent finds, using advanced molecular-biological methods, have now indicated that the possible cause may have been a member of the large *Salmonella* family of bacteria, more precisely a bacterium that is called *Salmonella paratyphi C*.[17] This bacterium can give rise to paratyphus, an intestinal infection that is often serious. Was this bacterium a gift from the Old World? Even though this cannot be affirmed with certainty, there is much that implies it could be the case. The same bacterium that hit the Aztecs in 1545 has been found in the thirteenth-century skeleton of a young woman from Trondheim in Norway. So it already existed in Europe three hundred years before Columbus came to America. The pathological picture of cocoliztli, however, was not what we normally associate with paratyphus. We do not yet know the answer to the mystery of cocoliztli.

In the course of the following century, yellow fever and malaria were introduced to the American continent via the slave trade. Did miseries from the world of microbes only pass as one-way traffic between the Old World and the New? Were no 'new' infectious diseases brought to Europe from America? There is actually one possible example of this, syphilis, which, as we have seen, broke out as a malignant epidemic connected with the French siege of Naples in 1494, shortly after Columbus had returned from his first journey. Did he bring the syphilis bacterium home with him? Or was it already established in Europe? This issue has been discussed for years by researchers and as yet no definitive answer has been found.

One can at any rate claim that this second transition led to a transatlantic levelling of microbial threats in the history of human infection, one that runs parallel with the exchange of microbes between Europe and Asia about 1,000 years earlier. The same occurred, although on a smaller scale, later in connection with the Europeans' arrival in Australia and the Pacific area. The aborigines of Australia, for example, were decimated by smallpox epidemics.

The Third Transition: The Industrial Revolution

From the time of the emergence of the first cities, some four to five thousand years ago, humanity has undergone rapid development both historically and culturally. Urbanization has constantly increased, with more than half the world's population now living in cities. And the growth of cities has been astonishingly rapid in developing countries during the second half of the twentieth century.

The human health situation in general, and the infection load in particular, remained unaltered in cities on the whole up until the end of the medieval period. The explosive growth of population after the transition to agriculture and animal husbandry often led, despite the increase in food production, to poor nutrition in the lowest levels of the population resulting from the increase in social stratification.[18] The birth rate was always high, but the mortality rate, especially the infant mortality rate, was too. For that reason, the average life expectancy for thousands of years was only between twenty and thirty years. To a great extent this has been the result of infectious diseases and malnutrition. Naturally enough, the poor lower classes were most affected, although the wealthy and well-fed upper classes could not avoid infectious diseases.

The total number of humans on the planet at the time of the first transition ten thousand years ago was around 10 million. By 1830 it had swelled to around a billion, after which it increased fourfold by 1975. Today, global population is estimated to be around 7 billion. What is striking is that the increase in population really got underway around three hundred years ago, since when it has simply accelerated.

Historians have examined what exists in the way of official birth and death figures, which are often quite deficient in most countries. Even so, the conclusion would seem to be clear: the birth rate has on the whole remained unaltered, with a slight tendency to decrease, while the mortality rate from infectious diseases has gradually fallen, particularly when it comes to infant mortality. For that reason, life expectancy has increased steadily over the past three hundred years. It is this period that is referred to as the third epidemiological transition. What lay behind this? Can medical science take all the credit for it?

The bacteriological revolution did not take place until the end of the nineteenth century. Knowledge about the role of microbes in infectious diseases and the development of antibiotics and the vast majority of vaccines thus came long after the mortality rate from infectious diseases had started to fall. No matter how proud physicians may be, and rightly so, about the advance of medical science over the past 150 years, they have nevertheless been obliged to admit that there must have been other explanations (up until the nineteenth century at least) for this than just the medical treatment of patients. One researcher in particular, the social scientist and doctor Thomas McKeown, is responsible for this conception of what is viewed as the third transition in the history of human infection.[19] This transition partly coincides with the Industrial Revolution from the end of the eighteenth century.

If active prevention and medical treatment of infectious diseases, based on medical science, are not the explanation of the increase in life expectancy and the decrease in infant mortality, what is responsible for the third transition? What is McKeown's explanation?

Human living conditions, particularly among the poor, were virtually unchanged until the Industrial Revolution. The material situation of the lower classes with regard to cramped living quarters and wretched sanitary conditions, which had been important for the infection load since the first transition, now deteriorated rather than improved in the slum-like workers' districts of the dreary industrial cities at the beginning of the nineteenth century. McKeown dismisses improvements to these areas as being the explanation for the decrease in the mortality rate from infections. His great idea, known as the McKeown thesis, is that the entire explanation lies in a gradual improvement of nutrition over the past three hundred years. He believes that it has to do with increased food production in this period, resulting from a number of improvements in agriculture in Western countries.

It is a well-known fact that both undernourishment and malnutrition increase one's susceptibility to many infectious diseases and worsen the course they may take. This admittedly does not apply to the same degree for all infectious diseases, but it is obviously an important factor when it comes to such diseases as tuberculosis and measles.

McKeown's explanatory model, which is mainly based on the improvement in nutrition being the key to an understanding of the third transition, has been animatedly discussed and criticized. A number of objections can be raised against it.

First, it cannot be documented from historical sources that human nutrition improved greatly during this period. This is a fact that McKeown readily concedes. Furthermore, he is probably mistaken in ignoring the significance of the large improvements in the sanitary conditions and standard of hygiene in the cities that took place in both England and other countries from the mid-nineteenth century onwards. The driving force here came from supporters of the miasma theory. The belief in the influence of miasmas meant that they regarded it as absolutely necessary to improve the cities' horrible sewage and waste situation, to ensure a water supply, to improve personal hygiene and clear the worst of the slum areas. Even though their point of departure, based on the miasma theory, was wrong, their comprehensive measures were effective in practice in preventing many infectious diseases. There is no doubt that they contributed to the reduction in the mortality rate for such infections as tuberculosis and cholera, which ravaged cities in the mid-nineteenth century. Within the hospital system this so-called sanitary movement was also influential. It is interesting that the nurses' great idol Florence Nightingale was also a supporter of the miasma theory. Her major contribution was made during the Crimean War of 1853–6, when she reformed sanitary conditions and hygiene in the military hospitals, resulting in a marked drop in the mortality rate. It goes without saying that most of the measures introduced by the miasma supporters were also shared by the growing numbers of supporters of the idea of a bacteriological revolution.

In my opinion, McKeown also goes too far when he dismisses medical science as having any kind of influence on the role of infectious diseases right up until 1935, fifty years after the bacteriological revolution. Vaccination against smallpox, which started at the end of the eighteenth century, undoubtedly played a considerable role in the fall of the mortality rate, as did other vaccines developed after the breakthrough of bacteriology. The new insight into microbes and conditions of infection also rapidly made an impact on surgery and childbirth medicine, leading to a reduction in post-operative infections and deaths in childbirth, forming the basis of many practical measures to prevent infectious diseases, including tuberculosis. And the belief in the role of bacteria has certainly strengthened the belief in measures to improve hygiene and sanitary conditions.

The gradual improvement of the human infection load over the past centuries in Western countries has a wide range of different causes. Other factors than scientifically based infection medicine have certainly been of vital importance for the development throughout most of the period we refer to as the third transition, up until the beginning of the twentieth century, but from then on the results of the bacteriological revolution and modern infection theories begin to assert themselves.

Before leaving the important third transition, it is important to emphasize that the presentation I have given applies to the situation in Western industrialized countries. The poorer developing countries lag many years behind and major changes did not really get underway until after the Second World War. It is also uncertain whether it will continue in the right direction, for there are many obstacles, such as war, civil war, poverty and overpopulation. In major cities that expanded rapidly there are often slum areas where sanitary conditions, nutrition and infection load are comparable to those of earlier times in the industrialized world. And one can fear that developments from now on will not be the same as in the West, since the non-infectious lifestyle diseases that now characterize rich countries have already started to get a foothold in developing countries.

The Fourth Transition: The Bacteriological Revolution

Most researchers within the field of the history of infectious diseases operate with defined transitions in their description of developments, although their definitions do not always completely coincide. In my opinion, it is surprising that what I have called the bacteriological revolution at the end of the nineteenth century is not normally considered to be such an important transition. The major discoveries made by Pasteur and Koch, as well as their precursors and successors, totally changed the conception of the causes of infectious diseases and have also been highly important for their prevention. Furthermore, this insight gradually led to the epoch-making breakthrough in diagnostics and the treatment of these diseases. Sulpha drugs began to be used in the mid-1930s, a few years after penicillin and a range of other antibiotics. The basis for new vaccines that have saved millions of lives was also established at the end of the nineteenth century.

An important reason for what I regard as a downgrading of the significance of these advances is possibly the strong influence of Thomas McKeown. He was undoubtedly right in saying that the gradual improvement in the infectious disease situation that led to reduced mortality over a long period of time was to a considerable extent due to other factors than the contributions of medical science. But the consequences of the new ground won by the bacteriological revolution, in my opinion, became noticeable several years before McKeown is prepared to admit, and this has undoubtedly had a greater effect on the mortality rate of infectious diseases throughout the twentieth century than he asserts.

Perhaps it is significant that most researchers who nimbly vault over the bacteriological revolution when talking about the major epidemiological transitions are not medically qualified, but are anthropologists and historians. (Thomas McKeown, with his medical background, is the exception.) When one has worked with infectious diseases for a lifetime, as I have, one is in no doubt that the time around the bacteriological revolution must be regarded as an important transition in the history of human infection, on a par with the other transitions named. I will later return to the many gains resulting from the transition, which has greatly tipped the odds in favour of *Homo sapiens* in the duel with the world of microbes.

The Fifth Transition: The Global Village

During the first decades after the Second World War there was a widespread view among both politicians and populations in Western countries that infectious diseases were beginning to lose their importance as a cause of illness and death.[20] There were now other groups of illnesses that to an increasing extent were being considered important, including cardiovascular diseases, arthritis and cancer. A significant reason for this change of attitude was the discovery of penicillin and a string of other antibiotics that came from the research laboratories. More and more vaccines were also developed. All of this led to a downgrading of the role of infectious diseases. The ancient Greeks would probably have called this an expression of hubris, an overweening confidence by humans that would inevitably lead to punishment from the gods.

Punishment was not long in coming: from the mid-1950s an increasing number of unknown microbes announced their arrival and caused serious disease problems, including epidemics. Something was clearly on the move on the infection front. Many people who had not understood the writing on the wall before now did so – at any rate when the AIDS epidemic exploded in the early 1980s.

What was the reason for the emergence of ever-new threats from the world of microbes? Many factors were involved. The short version is that this world has demonstrated its impressive ability to adapt and exploit changes in the environment, including changes in human behaviour. The leitmotif in the history underlying all threats of infection is that they are very frequently a consequence of human behaviour and comprehensive intervention in nature. Increased human interference with the workings of nature on our planet in recent times has led to the concept of Anthropocene becoming relevant, an addition to the traditional terms of various geological periods in the earth's history.[21]

An important aspect of the Anthropocene is precisely changes of balance in the struggle between *Homo sapiens* and the world of microbes that have led to many new, or at any rate newly discovered, microbes and infectious diseases which we will consider later. Significant examples of these are HIV, Ebola and the SARS viruses as well as the *Legionella* bacterium, which causes legionnaires' disease.

There are many mechanisms behind this development that give cause for serious concern. In fact, one could say that all the environment- and ecology-related factors we have already discussed are involved in this fifth epidemiological transition in the history of human infection.

Let us consider one single factor that fundamentally separates our age from earlier periods in human history. In former times microbes and epidemics could not move faster than a horse or camel. Sailing ships spent up to a year making the journey from England to Australia in the eighteenth century. The fast clipper ships still took three months to do so at the beginning of the nineteenth century, while steamships in the first half of the twentieth needed 58 days.[22] That is why the French writer Jules Verne caused a furore in 1873 with his fantastic book *Around the World in Eighty Days*, a travelling time which would have been an amazing feat. Modern air traffic has completely changed this. Today a trip to Australia, and possibly around the world, can be managed in just a few hours. Normally, more than 1.5 billion people fly every year, half of them on international flights. This means that infected humans, animals and pathogenic insects can move between continents in the space of a few hours and start an epidemic on arrival.[23]

The many aspects of globalization are now an extremely important topic in many areas of the social debate. When it comes to our relationship to the world of microbes, I am afraid that there is an important downside to 'the global village', a term often used by globalization enthusiasts. The possibility of passing on an infection in today's globalized society is in fact just as large as it was in the villages of former times. The consequences, in the form of potential intercontinental epidemics, known as pandemics, are simply so much more devastating. Convincing examples are HIV/AIDS and influenza epidemics during the twentieth century and, very recently, the rapid development of the COVID-19 pandemic.

The development in the field of infectious diseases during the last of the five transitions in the history of human infection has led to the launching of the new concept 'emerging infectious diseases', meaning new infections with previously unknown microbes or infections with known microbes which have recently increased rapidly in incidence or geographic range.[24] I prefer to call these 'new infections', even though the microbes themselves existed earlier. These infections have gained considerable publicity and, understandably enough, caused great concern. But when one knows about the history of human infection and the never-ending duel between *Homo sapiens* and the world of microbes, it ought not to come as a surprise that the microbes, with their impressive ability to adapt and mutate, have once again exploited the quite drastic changes in ecological and environmental factors for which we have been responsible over the past hundred years. These are issues we must take far more into account than previously when preparing ourselves for combatting the new threats from the world of microbes that will undoubtedly come in the future.

FOUR

Major Epidemics and Pandemics: Examples from History

For hundreds of thousands of years, the duel between man and microbes has swayed back and forth. For shorter or longer periods, the duellists have at any rate apparently kept each other in check, without any obvious drama. But then the microbes more or less suddenly gained the upper hand, resulting in epidemics. An epidemic is a considerable increase of an infectious disease in a population over a relatively short time. Epidemics can only develop in fairly large population groups, where the microbe is able to infect a considerable number of individuals. That is why we do not see epidemics until after the first transition in *Homo sapiens*' history of infection, after people began to settle and engage in agriculture and animal husbandry. There is little agreement about how many instances of disease are needed in order to speak of an epidemic, or how rapidly it has to develop. If an epidemic strikes a whole continent or several continents, we use the term 'pandemic'.

Many infectious diseases such as measles, mumps and smallpox follow a quite typical course, rapidly spreading to a large number of individuals who are not immune, after which they disappear for a while when there are no longer any receptive individuals in the population. These are examples of classic epidemics, with microbes that cause what I call 'crowd infections'. But we also use the terms 'epidemic' and 'pandemic' about a number of non-acute infections that spread much more slowly and do not necessarily retreat after a certain period of time. Examples of such infections are tuberculosis, leprosy, malaria and HIV. These epidemics also change their profile over time, return to previously afflicted regions and then spread further.

In former times, when microbes were not known to be a cause of disease, we naturally had no clear conception of the causes of epidemics and pandemics. And it was not until the last few decades that we clarified the many mechanisms – the ecological and environment-related factors – that have a crucial influence on the interaction between man and microbes. Extremely often, it is significant changes in these factors that underlie the many epidemics we know from history. A number of factors are frequently in operation at the same time.

But we also have examples of changes to the pathogenic qualities of the microbes that have been crucial: microbes use many methods to alter their genetic characteristics when this is favourable for adapting to their surroundings. Changes in human behaviour, which we can refer to as human ecology, also often play an important role in epidemics, whereas the process involved for humans to change genetic characteristics is far more cumbersome than that of microbes.

With all this recently acquired knowledge, we can now look back at history and try to analyse the background of the many epidemics of which we have accounts, and which have definitely had major consequences for humanity within many areas. The insight we can gain from such studies can also prove extremely valuable for our future duel with microbes.

How can we state anything with any degree of certainty, however, about the epidemics and infections of the past, since knowledge of microbes only came at the end of the nineteenth century? How can we be sure that the epidemics of earlier ages were caused by microbes? These are perfectly natural questions to which we are actually able to provide good answers. Before dealing with some important examples of epidemics and pandemics, we should therefore take a look at the basis of what, to a great extent, is historical detective work using what in criminology are called 'cold trails'.

How can one follow the cold trails of history?

For as long as we have had written accounts, about the past 4,000–5,000 years, we have also had accounts of major epidemics. These descriptions are of course important sources for studying the epidemics of former times. Many of those that struck humanity, however, are not mentioned in ancient writings. Some descriptions may also have been lost. In surviving accounts there may also be additional interpretative problems that make the work more difficult. Often the writers of chronicles are not representatives of the physicians of the time, but are historians or monks, so they are not necessarily familiar with the specialized concepts of medicine in their own time. Translation thus often involves considerable problems, since one is at a loss to know what the authors mean by the medical concepts they use to describe the disease in question. Furthermore, the conceptual apparatus of former medicine differs from that of the present day. One example of this is the description of rashes, which are an important sign of a number of epidemic diseases and may provide the key to a diagnosis. Ecclesiastical writers often concentrate on religious considerations in theories about the causes of diseases and are less inclined to give a sober description of possibly more prosaic aspects.

Even so, we do have some excellent examples of thorough analysis of epidemics in the past. A classic example we have already touched on is the description by Thucydides of the Athenian plague during the war between Athens and Sparta in 431–404 BC.[1] This description has been studied closely down through the centuries and often influences descriptions of epidemics by later writers, since they use the same vocabulary in their accounts and interpretation of disease as Thucydides.

Despite the many problems involved in translating and interpreting the ancient accounts of epidemics, they are nevertheless invaluable for our understanding of both the geographical occurrences and spread of the epidemics, and tell us a great deal about pathological pictures and mortality.

A valuable supplement to the ancient chronicles are other written sources such as wills, contracts of employment, sales contracts and other non-literary registers and records. These sources are probably not gripping reading for the layman, but for historians they can provide invaluable information about the course, spread and consequences of major epidemics. This source material has also been the subject of intensive studies.

Although this historical approach can often give us a good picture of many of the epidemics of the past and their probable microbial causes, it can of course seldom provide a completely sure basis for analysis on its own. With many epidemics the various sources on which historians build do not enable any definite conclusions to be made. A number of famous epidemics from the past belong to this group. We will later look at a few of these enigmatic epidemics, including the Athenian plague already mentioned.

In the studies of infections of past ages, historians have been helped by archaeologists.[2] Archaeological excavations often uncover human remains from various epochs in the development of *Homo sapiens*. Normally, there are only skeletal remains, since the soft parts (skin, muscles, inner organs) usually decay quickly as a result of bacteria. Under special circumstances, such as desiccation, low temperature, lack of oxygen or chemical influence, this decaying process may be prevented, resulting in what we call mummification. In that case the soft parts may be quite well preserved, which means that the tissues and organs of the body can be studied using ordinary microscopic methods as used in present-day medicine, for example when carrying out autopsies. Such mummification is most frequently man-made. It is primarily the several thousand-year-old burial customs of the ancient Egyptians that have given us the term 'mummy'. Certain other cultures, however, have also embalmed their dead. Under special climatic conditions such mummification can also take place spontaneously. A famous example of this is the 5,000-year-old 'Ötzi the Iceman', who was found frozen in the Alps. In such instances, the content of the intestines can also provide valuable information, for example about chronic infection due to parasites. This was the case with Ötzi.

The mummification of human remains is unfortunately the exception. In most cases only the remains of skeletons are found. With various processes of chronic diseases, however, changes take place in the skeleton that can provide valuable information about the state of health of former humans.[3] This applies, for example, to tuberculosis and syphilis, which can cause characteristic changes. The great majority of the microbes that have caused widespread epidemics, however, attack only the soft parts of the body, not the skeleton. For that reason, examining the skeletons will not tell us anything about the occurrence of these infections.

Fortunately, modern science has come to the rescue of historians and archaeologists. The major breakthroughs in molecular biology after James Watson and Francis Crick's discovery of the structure and role of the DNA molecule in 1953 have also revolutionized research within the history of infection and epidemics. DNA molecules are carriers of the genetic information of all living creatures (with the exception of certain viruses that have RNA instead, and prions – if they are to be counted as living). Modern molecular-biological methods can be used to detect microbe DNA in remains from humans and animals from thousands of years ago that show signs of infection. These new methods can also be used to study the DNA from humans and animals, leading to sensational new data that also provide information about the process of evolution.

There is first and foremost one method, PCR (polymerase chain reaction), which has been used when examining ancient DNA. Using this method, which has revolutionized diagnostics within many areas of medicine, one can detect extremely small amounts of DNA and increase the original amount to such an extent that one has enough material for further studies using other methods.[4]

Although the new methodology for detecting old DNA has been an important breakthrough, such studies are extremely demanding with a number of sources of error. Ancient DNA can be damaged to varying degrees, depending to a great extent on outer, climatic conditions. DNA is best preserved under dry, cool conditions. Unfortunately, these conditions do not exist in many of the most important areas where human remains from major epidemics are found, such as the Mediterranean. DNA, however, is often well preserved after mummification, so it is no coincidence that some of the first successful detections of old microbial DNA were of the tuberculosis bacteria (*Mycobacterium tuberculosis*) in mummies from Egypt and Peru. This took place in the 1990s. Later, it proved possible to identify DNA from a number of other microbes, including the leprosy bacterium, *Mycobacterium leprae*, and the plague bacterium, *Yersinia pestis*. The finds of the plague bacterium in human remains from various ages have given us probable answers to previously unanswered questions concerning the major plague epidemics.

DNA studies using the PCR method are very susceptible to sources of error because of pollution from other irrelevant DNA, such as from naturally occurring microbes at the site of the find or in the laboratory when the investigation is being carried out. For this reason, particular demands are made of these laboratories.

The methods used to examine ancient DNA have become increasingly sophisticated over the years. In addition, we now have methods that can detect proteins in archaeological material. Such methods will probably be of considerable use, since protein molecules, under favourable conditions, can stay unchanged for hundreds of thousands of years, whereas DNA has a limited 'shelf-life'. However, neither of these methods can be used exclusively when studying infection problems of the past. The finds must always be combined with solid archaeological assessments, including the dating of the remains in question, along with other conditions at the site.

It is highly likely that the rapid development of modern molecular biology will also come up with other methods that can be used when studying epidemics from former ages and old microbial material. The methods we already have, however, are only in their infancy and a great many interesting archaeological finds have yet to be investigated using modern DNA methods.

The Plague Epidemics

In everyday speech few words are as negatively charged as 'plague'. The word is often used to characterize a phenomenon or a person as quite horrible. The term is also used when one is faced by a choice between two equally frightful alternatives: in Germanic and Romance languages, choosing between the Devil and the deep blue sea, or between Scylla and Charybdis, can be called 'a choice between plague and cholera'. This use of the word is derived from the memory of terrifying historical epidemics. In purely medicinal usage, the word 'plague' is solely the term for infection caused by the bacterium *Yersinia pestis*, not for epidemics with other microbes. However, 'plague' has often also been applied less precisely to other epidemics.

The best-known plague epidemic, one that most people have heard about while still at school, is the Black Death, which raged in the mid-fourteenth century.[5] In the history of infection, we also include two other comprehensive plague epidemics.[6] All three of them deserve the term 'pandemics'.[7] The first of these, the Plague of Justinian, broke out in the mid-sixth century AD, followed by the Black Death in the mid-fourteenth century and the third pandemic at the end of the nineteenth. In addition to these pandemics, several centuries saw a number of smaller epidemics in the wake of the first two. Outbreaks of the plague still occur in certain parts of the world: most recently there have been outbreaks in Madagascar and the Congo.

A large majority of physicians and historians now feel it is beyond all doubt that all these epidemics are due to the bacterium *Yersinia pestis*. Yet agreement is not unanimous.[8] For several decades there has been a lively debate on the subject that has sometimes become heated. There is also disagreement about a number of other facets of the various plague epidemics, to which we will return in due course. Let us first look at the great plague epidemics of history before we discuss the underlying mechanisms behind them, the special characteristics of the plague bacterium and how the duel between *Homo sapiens* and *Yersinia pestis* was enacted under the influence of the ecological and environmental factors we discussed earlier. The plague epidemics of history are excellent examples of the significance of these factors.

The Plague of Justinian: the first plague pandemic

In the year AD 542 the Byzantine emperor was Justinian, residing in his magnificent capital, Constantinople, the largest city in the world at the time.[9] Justinian had good reason to be content with his career up to that point. The son of poor peasants in the Balkans, he had risen through the ranks thanks to his own capability and the help of his uncle Justinus I, who had also overcome a humble background to become emperor. Justinian succeeded Justinus in 527. As his empress, Justinian had the beautiful, strong-willed Theodora, one of the most talked-about female figures of history, with an extremely varied and rather dubious past, according to certain contemporary historians, particularly Procopius. In addition to his official historical works, in which he praised the deeds of Justinian, Procopius wrote another, anonymous, work, *The Secret History* ('Anecdota' in Greek), which contains a sharp attack on the imperial couple.[10] He writes about Theodora that she was the daughter of a bear-keeper at the Hippodrome circus in Constantinople, that she became a famous actress, notorious for her highly indecent performances, and early on had become a sex worker. She then caught Justinian's attention and he married her despite her dubious reputation. Soon afterwards he ascended the imperial throne, and the daughter of the bear-keeper became empress.

The Roman empire was admittedly not the same as it once had been. The western parts of the empire had gradually fallen away and been conquered by various Germanic tribes. The year 476 is often cited

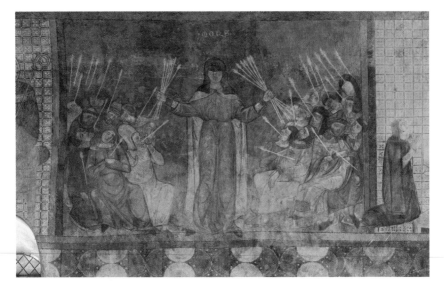

The Plague of Justinian broke out in the Byzantine empire in the year AD 541, under Emperor Justinian. It was undoubtedly a burden on the kingdom, but there is a certain amount of disagreement among historians about its extent. Seen here is a rare and early personification of the plague, possibly the only depiction of the Plague of Justinian, 1315, fresco, Saint-André Abbey in Lavaudieu.

as the date of the fall of the Roman empire. Emperor Justinian's great plan was to re-establish the empire in its former greatness and extent, and he was well on the way to succeeding, partly as a result of the help of capable generals. The foremost of these was Belisarius, who is ranked by military historians as a strategist on a par with Alexander the Great, Julius Caesar and Napoleon. By 542 Justinian's generals had recaptured areas that included parts of North Africa, Italy and Spain.

The incredibly industrious Justinian had also ensured the preparation of a comprehensive legal code that was to have an impact on European law for centuries. In addition, he had taken the initiative for the erection of a number of wonderful buildings. The most impressive of these was the enormous cathedral of Hagia Sophia (the Church of Holy Wisdom), which can still be admired in what is now Istanbul. At the solemn consecration, the emperor exclaimed, with a reference to the magnificent temple of King Solomon, 'Solomon, I have surpassed you!'

Had Justinian's many successes now caused him to display what the Greeks called hubris, which usually led to the wrath and punishment of the gods? Some perhaps thought so, particularly because they still believed in the ancient gods that the emperor was now seeking to eradicate with fire and sword. In that case, they probably felt that this punishment of the gods really came in dramatic fashion in 541–2.

An epidemic with an extremely high mortality rate broke out in 541 at the small Egyptian port of Pelusium in the eastern part of the Nile delta.[11] This spread rapidly, both northwards to Palestine, Syria and Persia, and westwards to the nearby city of Alexandria, one of the largest ports in the Mediterranean. From Alexandria the epidemic spread via maritime traffic to the rest of the Mediterranean, and in spring 542 it struck Constantinople with full force. We have comprehensive written accounts, both by the most prominent historian of the age, Procopius, and from ecclesiastical chroniclers.[12] One of them, John of Ephesus, had with his own eyes seen how the epidemic ravaged Egypt and the neighbouring countries to the north, with deserted villages and uncultivated fields. Procopius gives harrowing accounts of the consequences of the epidemic in Constantinople, where between five and ten thousand people died daily. The ecclesiastical historian Evagrius Scholasticus writes that the epidemic claimed 300,000 lives in Constantinople alone, a terrible figure considering that the population was probably less than 600,000. Even though these figures are uncertain, mortality was unquestionably very high. Gradually people had to abandon the usual burial

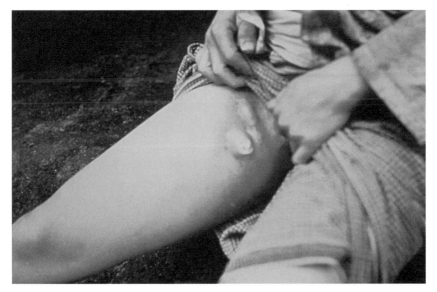

In the classic form of bubonic plague one finds large, pus-filled lymph nodes (buboes) on the neck, in the armpits and in the groin, as in this photograph from 1993.

routines and make use of mass graves; in Constantinople it was also necessary to dispose of bodies at sea.

The written accounts also provide details of the usual pathological pictures of epidemics. Those attacked were suddenly seized by a fever. Quite rapidly most of them started to develop large swellings in the groin and armpits and on the neck. We now know that these were infected lymph nodes that developed into abscesses. Such a swelling is called a bubo and it is a characteristic feature of infection by the bacterium *Yersinia pestis*. For that reason the infection is also known as bubonic plague.

Typical of the pathological picture was also that the patients quickly became muddled, often with hallucinations, before going into a coma and dying. Some nevertheless recovered. The disease could develop extremely quickly. Both in Constantinople and Alexandria, it was common for people, when leaving the house in the morning, to wear a tag with their name and district on a string round their necks, so that their relatives could be contacted if they collapsed in the street. Procopius states that the emperor himself was struck down by the disease, but survived.

The plague raged on until 543. By then it had spread to the rest of the Mediterranean countries, Germany, England and Ireland as well as to most of today's Middle East and to Central Asia.[13] Between fifteen and seventeen new plague epidemics followed over the next two hundred years or so, at intervals of five to seven years.[14] Sometimes the Plague of Justinian is also used as an umbrella term for all these epidemics, while other scholars simply use the term for the first major epidemic in 541–3. Certain scholars have claimed that some of the later epidemics also reached Scandinavia, but the documentation for this assertion is not very reliable.

After the year 750, Europe and the neighbouring areas were, for unknown reasons, spared plague epidemics until the second great plague pandemic, the Black Death, struck in the mid-fourteenth century.

What did people think about the cause of the epidemic at the time of Justinian? Among physicians, the theories of disease of Hippocrates and Galen were naturally strongly represented.[15] What we have in the way of written accounts from the sixth century suggests, nevertheless, that there was a widespread view that the plague had been sent by God as a punishment for people's sins, their godlessness and worldliness. Several ecclesiastical chroniclers, including John of Ephesus, place great emphasis on this. But even those who claimed that the plague was divine punishment believed that it must be allowable to seek to flee from it, since they also believed that miasmas played a role. And many people did flee from the cities that were hardest hit.

Procopius, on the other hand, has a different view of the causes of the plague: in his *Secret History* he describes the emperor as an evil, almost demonic figure. According to Procopius, the plague is God's punishment for the emperor's misdeeds.[16]

Many who had continued to believe in secret in the ancient gods had their own thoughts about the origin of the plague. It is also said that some Christians began to worship the ancient gods once more, since they felt that the Christian God had deserted them.

While the epidemic apparently started in Pelusium, the general view at the time of Justinian was that the plague had actually begun far further south, in Ethiopia, and from there had been brought downstream to Egypt. Some scholars hold the controversial opinion that the ancient view is correct, and that the Plague of Justinian came from Africa, possibly by ship through what was probably a canal linking the Gulf of Suez and the Nile. Others reject this theory outright, claiming that the plague came to the Mediterranean region via trading routes from Central Asia.

There are also other issues related to the Plague of Justinian that have given risen to lively debate among historians, for example what consequences the epidemic had for the late Roman empire and for subsequent development in the Mediterranean countries.[17] Can anyone doubt that the plague had major societal consequences when all the historians and chroniclers at the time and in all the countries concerned affirm with one voice the enormous mortality in the urban and rural areas, and how the machinery of society almost ground to a halt during the epidemic? Some contemporary researchers have their doubts about the accounts, claiming that for various reasons they strongly exaggerate the effects of the plague epidemic.[18] These critics believe that archaeological finds do not confirm the dramatic narratives of the contemporary writers concerning the high mortality rate during the plague. All things considered, however, there seems to be a broad perception among historians that the Eastern Roman empire, which gradually became called the Byzantine empire, was hit extremely hard both by the first plague pandemic of 541–3 and by the later waves of plague up until the eighth century.[19]

Justinian and his successors on the imperial throne repeatedly had to wage war on various fronts, which involved considerable expenditure from the imperial coffers. Much of the state's income came from the taxation of landowners, but this source of income dried up as the plague ravaged the rural areas, with a resulting loss of labour. Recruitment to the army, which to a great degree was based on the peasantry, was severely affected. Even though a number of successful campaigns were conducted after the first wave of the epidemic, many historians believe that the military clout of the Byzantine empire was permanently reduced because of the plague, and that this prepared the ground for both the conquests made by the Islamic armies of Byzantine territory – Syria, Palestine and North Africa – and the invasion of the Balkans by the Slavs, from the seventh century onwards. Despite this, the Byzantine empire managed to survive for seven hundred years after the last plague epidemic.

In Spain, waves of the plague might have weakened the resistance of the Visigoths to the Islamic invasion of the eighth century. It has even been claimed that the spread of Anglo-Saxon control of England in the seventh century was easier because Romano-British society had been weakened by the plague.

Plague epidemics raged for two hundred years and disappeared around 750. It seems quite certain that the plague must have had serious consequences for the political, social and cultural development of the countries involved, probably most dramatically in those of the Mediterranean area. But the historical conditions during the period concerned are extremely complex, and it would be naive to give the bacterium *Yersinia pestis* the main responsibility for the historical and cultural development during these years.

A great many contemporary witnesses in the Byzantine empire were convinced that the Plague of Justinian was God's punishment for people's sins. It is interesting that a similar way of thinking was employed in various places to explain why the plague finally disappeared.[20] In the year 750 the ruling Muslim Ummayyad dynasty in Damascus was overturned. The new victorious dynasty, the Abbasids, claimed that Allah stopped the epidemic because the evil Ummayyads were overthrown.

Similarly, the end of the plague epidemic in France was explained by the fact that the new Carolingian dynasty had defeated the former ruling family, the Merovingians, which traced their line of kings back to the heathen gods.

The Black Death: the second plague pandemic

The second great pandemic involving the plague bacterium broke out in the mid-fourteenth century, six hundred years after the last plague epidemic in Europe.[21] It has become known as 'The Black Death', but this name was introduced later. The first record we have of the term is from a Swedish text that dates from 1555. It was originally known by other names, such as 'The great Pestilence', 'The great Death of Man' or simply 'The Plague'. Most researchers today reckon that this epidemic was also caused by the *Yersinia pestis* bacterium, but apart from that there is much that is unclear. This applies, among other things, to the infection mechanisms and the spread of the epidemic.[22]

Its place of origin is uncertain. China has been proposed by a number of historians. The first well-documented cases of the plague appeared in Mongol-controlled territory between the Black and Caspian seas, which was no coincidence, as we shall later see. The 'official' start of the European epidemic is near the city of Kaffa (now Feodosia) in the Crimea in 1346. This city, which was established by Genoese traders, was then under siege by Mongol troops led by Jani Beg Khan. The siege was not a success, particularly because after two years a plague epidemic broke out among the Mongols. This had a high rate of mortality and 85,000 soldiers died in the course of a few weeks. Jani Beg, in an act later described as the first attempt at bacteriological warfare, decided to sling plague-infected bodies into the city by catapult, so that its defenders would also be struck down by the plague. This strategy was a considerable success and the plague now broke out violently inside the city as well. A number of Genoese then chose to flee by sea, which was still open to them. But the Genoese galleys had a dangerous cargo on board: the plague bacterium. This became clear after a few days at sea when the first deaths from the plague began.

The Genoese galleys sailed through the Bosphorus, taking the plague with them to Constantinople, where the emperor himself, John VI Kantakouzenos, describes the epidemic extremely precisely:

In most cases plague spots broke out over the entire body. All those who fell ill, felt depressed when the first signs came, then they lost all hope of recovery, and gave themselves up for lost as well. This hopelessness meant that they were even more susceptible to the disease, and it precipitated death. Amazingly enough, some of those who fell ill were able to recover, and of these none was later attacked once more. The disease was highly contagious by nature: those who cared for the sick fell ill themselves. In many families all of their members died.

From Constantinople the ships spread out, taking the plague with them to most of the ports in both the eastern and western Mediterranean. An important hub of the spread to the European continent and North African harbours was the port of Messina in Sicily, where twelve Genoese galleys arrived from Kaffa in October 1347. When the inhabitants saw the first cases of the plague, all the ships were chased out to sea and they now spread the disease as far north as Paris and to ports in southern England. In the course of the following year all of England, Ireland and parts of the Netherlands and Germany were affected. The pattern was the same all over Europe: first the plague came by ship to the ports. Then it spread inland along the trade routes.

Schoolchildren in Norway were always taught that the Black Death arrived in Bergen in September 1349 on board an Icelandic ship from London. Recent research, however, would seem to indicate that the plague had already reached Oslo by that time, on board an English ship in the summer of 1348.[23] It then spread out along the trade routes. From Oslo and Bergen the plague spread to the rest of the country and to Sweden and the North German and Baltic ports. From there it spread further east to Russia, arriving in Moscow in summer 1353. By then it had burned out in most of the rest of Europe. At each location the plague would normally rage for five to six months, generally in spring, summer and early autumn.

The Black Death raged for a total of seven years, and most of Europe was affected. The Middle East and Northern Africa were also heavily hit. Iceland and Finland avoided the plague this time round.

A frightful pathological picture

We have a large number of eyewitness reports of the pathological picture of the plague. According to these accounts, in most cases large, painful swellings quickly developed in the groin, armpits and on the neck, the so-called buboes that had been described during the Plague of Justinian. These were infected and inflamed lymph nodes. Patients developed a high fever and became muddled. After a few days the buboes burst and the pus inside them emptied out. Often the skin of the patient had by then developed blue-black spots. This is a classic form of what is called bubonic plague. The mortality was high, but just how high it really was during the Black Death is uncertain. Some people survived and probably became immune to the *Yersinia pestis* bacterium, which meant that they could be in contact with patients later without falling ill once more.

In addition to this pathological picture of bubonic plague, there were two other possible courses. Some patients developed a life-threatening form of pneumonia, pneumonic plague, which led to the patient coughing up bloody sputum and having breathing difficulties. Practically all such patients died quickly. A third form, which led to death in the course of a day or two, had neither buboes nor pneumonic plague. Instead black spots developed and the skin started to bleed. This was probably what we now call septicaemia, where bacteria spread through the bloodstream, leading to a fall in blood pressure, and causing shock and the failure of most organs.

What is obvious from most of the eyewitness accounts of the pathological picture of the plague is that it gave rise to fear and disgust to a degree one does not often see with other diseases. A contemporary account says that 'all the secretions from their bodies had an intolerable stench. Sweat, faeces, sputum and breathing all had a vile smell.'

Let us pause and consider the term 'Black Death' and the reason for it. At the time itself, this term was not used; as we have seen, it was first used in Scandinavia in the second half of the sixteenth century. It is hardly correct, as many people have believed, that the term reflects the physical appearance of the patients prior to death. In Latin the plague was called *atra pestis*. Because *atra* can mean both 'great' and 'black', it is probable that *atra pestis* originally meant 'the Great Death', and that at a later date *atra* was mistakenly translated as 'black'.[24]

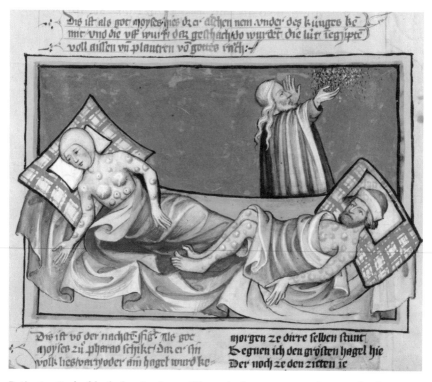

Patients attacked by bubonic plague. The artist has exaggerated somewhat by placing buboes over the entire body, not only in the groin, armpits and on the neck, which is where they usually appeared. Miniature from the Toggenburg Bible (Switzerland), 1411.

Although we do not know for sure what percentage of the individual victims died, we do know that a large part of the population in the areas involved were attacked. The percentage of the population that died of the plague has been assessed by various historians as being from 30 per cent upwards. The Norwegian historian Ole Jørgen Benedictow, who is internationally recognized for his comprehensive studies of the Black Death in Europe and Scandinavia, estimates that no less than 60 per cent of the European population died of the plague.[25] If the population of Europe is estimated to have been 75–80 million, this means that almost 50 million people may have lost their lives.

The general pattern for the spread of the plague was that it followed the sea and land trade routes. However, there were considerable geographical differences in the ferocity of the plague; certain areas got off surprisingly lightly without there being any good explanation as to why. In northern Italy, cities such as Florence, Pisa and Venice were very hard hit, while Milan, also an important commercial city, escaped. Inside individual cities one could also observe large differences from one precinct to another.

All classes of the population were struck down by the plague, but the main impression is that the poor succumbed most. The reason for this is probably that the rich, unlike the poor, had the opportunity to flee from the plague, the only measure that could have a certain effect. This was also the background of one of the most famous depictions of the Black Death in world literature, Giovanni Boccaccio's *The Decameron*, even if it has admittedly been read throughout history more for its erotic portrayals than its information about the plague.[26] The background for the action is that seven rich, upper-class women with their servants flee from the plague in Florence to an idyllic, isolated country estate along with some young men. They while away the time by telling each other erotic stories as they wait for the plague epidemic to lose its grip.

Boccaccio gives the reader a dramatic depiction of the plague in Florence, both the pathological picture and people's reactions to the plague. About the actual disease, he says:

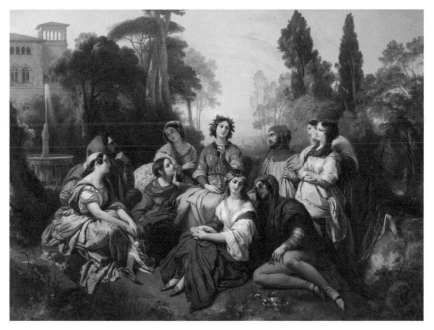

The plague in Florence is the background of the Florentine Giovanni Boccaccio's work *The Decameron*. Franz Xaver Winterhalter, *The Decameron*, 1837, oil on canvas.

it began both in men and women with certain swellings in the groin or under the armpit. They grew to the size of a small apple or an egg, more or less, and were vulgarly called tumours. In a short space of time these tumours spread from the two parts named all over the body. Soon after this the symptoms changed and black or purple spots appeared on the arms or thighs or any other part of the body, sometimes a few large ones, sometimes many little ones. These spots were a certain sign of death, just as the original tumour had been and still remained. No doctor's advice, no medicine could overcome or alleviate this disease.

Boccaccio was apparently surprised at the rapid spread of the plague:

And this epidemic increased in strength because it spread from the sick to the healthy when they had intercourse with each other, in the same way that fire spreads over dry and inflammable materials. Yes, so dangerous was this disease that merely to talk with and have intercourse with the sick gave those who were healthy the disease and sent them to their deaths. But to touch

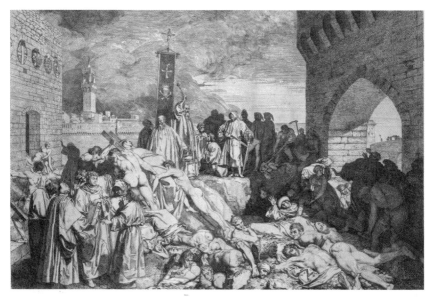

The plague in Florence in 1348, depicted here in an etching by Luigi Sabatelli, c. 1801, based on the description in Boccaccio's *Decameron*. According to Boccaccio, 100,000 people died, but recent research estimates the figure to have been approximately 70,000.

A plague doctor in full work attire, with cloak, gloves and headwear with its characteristic beak, from an 18th-century manuscript by Giovanni Grewembroch. The staff the plague physician always wore was used to keep people at a distance and to examine patients with. This attire was particularly common in Italy and France in the 17th and 18th centuries.

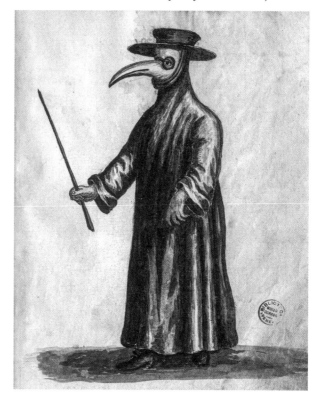

clothing or other objects the sick person had been in the vicinity of was also sufficient to transmit the disease.

According to Boccaccio, 100,000 Florentines died of the plague. Modern calculations indicate that the real figure was about 70,000.

What could the physicians of the time do when faced with the plague? Precious little.[27] Medical science still swore by the principles of classical medicine from Hippocrates and Galen. Many doctors thought that the plague was a consequence of a strong imbalance between the body fluids. For that reason, blood-letting was used, and not infrequently buboes were opened and the pus let out. As we have heard, some patients with bubonic plague survived, and their recovery tended to be ascribed to the treatment.

The best-known physician of the time, Guy de Chauliac, physician-in-ordinary to the pope, studied the plague and the various forms of treatment used, which he found to be ineffective. He advised Pope Clement VI to isolate himself in the papal palace in Avignon and placed

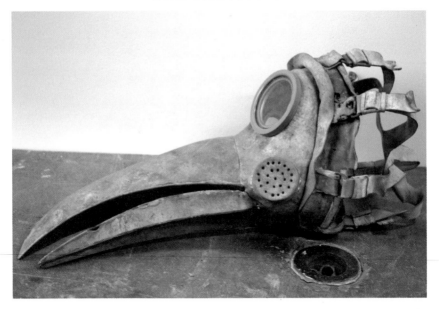

Plague doctor beak. It contained a mixture of aromatic herbs which it was believed would cleanse the air of plague-causing miasmas.

him between two flaming open fires in the belief that this would keep the miasma at a distance.[28] The pope survived, even if he was probably somewhat overheated. Some people have suggested that the reason for this could have been that the plague-carrying fleas could not stand the great heat.

The prevailing conception of the plague and the reactions to it

From both Boccaccio and many other writers we know quite a bit about people's view of the Black Death at the time. As in former ages, there was a widespread belief that the plague was God's punishment for the people's sins. This was also stated in a papal bull. The university in Paris, however, produced a long and learned statement that concluded by saying that the plague was due to an unfortunate constellation of the heavenly bodies. Most people doubtless shared the pope's view, and many energetically went in for acts of penance and a pious life.

Boccaccio had a highly balanced view of the causes of the plague:

Some people say that it struck down the human race because of the influence of the heavenly bodies, others that it was a punishment which showed God's just anger at our shameless way of life.

144

But no matter the cause, it had started some years earlier in the East, where it had taken countless lives before it unfortunately spread westwards.[29]

Religious reactions to the plague ended quite often in hysterical phenomena. One of the most dramatic was the flagellant movement.[30] This consisted of groups of people who travelled around, particularly in Germany, and whipped themselves at public mass meetings until the blood came in order to do penance for their sins. The flagellants often regarded themselves as a kind of holy army that sometimes had supernatural powers. They gradually started to challenge the power of the Church, both verbally and at times even physically, by interrupting Mass. This led to the pope and the Catholic Church successfully retaliating against the excesses of the flagellants.

Although the flagellants were probably able to stimulate a kind of religious revival in some places, the movement also clearly had negative aspects, including its encouragement of one of the most tragic outcomes of the plague: persecution of the Jews.[31] Throughout history, a common psychological reaction to major catastrophes has been to search for scapegoats. During the Black Death it was in particular Jewish people

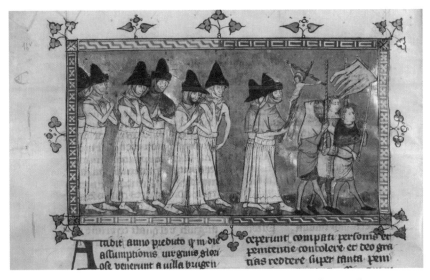

A procession of flagellants from the Netherlands, illumination from Gilles Li Muisis, *Antiquitates Flandriae*, *c.* 1350. In the belief that the Black Death was God's punishment for man's sins, they whipped themselves until they bled in order to do penance.

who were assigned this role. They were suspected of having caused the plague by poisoning wells, and this led to a series of horrible massacres in a number of European countries, even though most monarchs and especially Pope Clement VI attempted to stop them. Tens of thousands of Jews lost their lives during these massacres, which led to large numbers emigrating to Eastern Europe, where they established their own communities that lasted until the Second World War.

Certain other groups, although to a lesser extent, were also singled out as scapegoats. This especially applied to lepers, who were suspected of colluding with the Jews. A quite astonishing phenomenon that makes one think of pre-Christian times, and is said to have taken place in Scandinavia, is the occurrence of human sacrifice – of apparently completely innocent individuals – in order to appease the forces behind the plague epidemic.

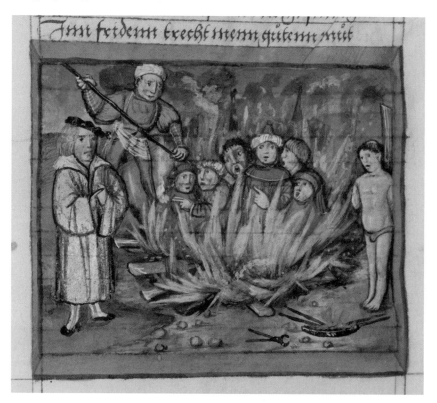

Jews were burned at the stake during the Black Death, accused of having caused the plague, as seen in this illumination from Nikolaus Marschalk, *Mecklenburgische Reimchronik*, 1521–3. Leprosy victims were also burned, suspected of having colluded with the Jews.

The many consequences of the Black Death

It would be extremely surprising if such a disaster as the Black Death, during which perhaps 60 per cent of the European population perished, did not have great consequences within a number of areas. The literature on this field is also comprehensive. Nevertheless, this is one of the many topics where there is still considerable disagreement among historians.

Some claim the Black Death had decisive importance for the subsequent history of Europe, acting as a watershed between the Middle Ages and modernity. Others have a far more belittling view of the long-term effects of this pandemic. Without going into detail, we will attempt here to find the conclusions that seem most plausible.

There can hardly be any doubt that the Black Death had a considerable impact within the economic and social spheres, particularly in rural districts.[32] When more than half the population dies, as was the case in many countries, it cannot help but have serious consequences.[33] Before the pandemic, considerable areas of cultivable land were worked by leaseholders and lessees, who were obliged to provide services to the wealthy landowners. Paid farm labourers were also beginning to become common. The Black Death led to a marked reduction in the labour force, which created serious problems for the operation of the landowners' farms, both because of this lack of labour and because demand for, and thus prices of, agricultural products fell. The farm labourers managed to push up wages, while the leaseholders exploited their bargaining power to secure better conditions. In many places this led to marked social unrest, since the authorities attempted via legislation to support the demands of the landowners. This eventually led to a number of violent peasant revolts. One of the largest of these hit England in 1381. Despite this, the Black Death eventually led to a certain social levelling in the rural districts.

In Norway, the consequences for agriculture were extremely serious. A large number of farms lay deserted and unused, particularly inland. Agricultural production of grain and meat plummeted to about a third of earlier output. This led to a strong decrease in the Crown's income, which in turn had a negative effect on the administration of the kingdom. But in particular, the plague hit the major landowners of the upper class, who lost a great deal of their income and were often 'degraded' to large farmers. The fact that the Norwegian upper class, which played an important role in governing the country, was so hard hit by the Black Death certainly contributed to the weakened country entering into the later union with Denmark. The lack of labour after the plague also led to major technological advances, with the development of labour-saving innovations, such as water-driven sawmills.

The increase in religiosity that the Black Death inspired in many people did not necessarily mean increased support for the established Church. On the contrary, it is probable that the Black Death seriously weakened the Church's prestige and spiritual authority.[34] Even though many of the clergy performed their duties well during the time of the plague, there were far too many examples of priests who did not, fleeing from the plague-ravaged areas for which they were responsible, or immodestly hiking up prices for burials and other church rituals. Things went so far that the pope himself had to chastise his clergy for their greed. During and after the Black Death, many empty positions in the Church had to be filled by men who were less educated than those who

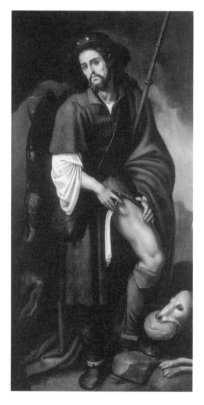

St Roch is the patron saint of the plague. He is normally shown with a distinct bubo – a swollen, pus-filled lymph node – in his groin. Francisco Ribalta, *St Roch*, c. 1610, oil on canvas.

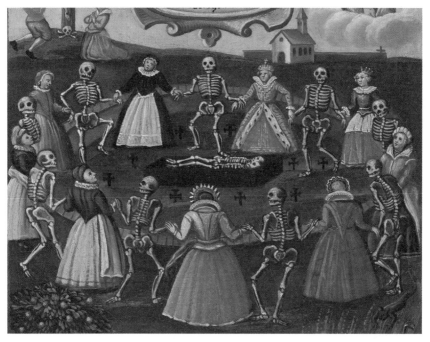

Few ages have been so preoccupied with death as the one when the Black Death raged. It also became the basis for a highly popular motif in art: the dance of Death and humans – the so-called *danse macabre*. Here, Death is depicted as a smiling dancer who invites everyone to dance. Franciszek Lekszycki or his circle (attrib.), detail from *The Dance of Death*, late 17th century, oil on canvas.

had been lost. This did not enhance the reputation of the Church either. All in all, it is not unreasonable to assume that the increased scepticism towards the Catholic Church caused by the Black Death prepared the ground for the Reformation of the sixteenth century.

Although in many people's eyes the Church had lost a great deal of its authority after the Black Death, there were, paradoxically enough, also many who wished to support it at a time of menacing upheaval in society. This particularly applied to the rich bourgeoisie, who now gave large donations to the Church, endowing the construction throughout Europe of many new churches, both large and small. The most famous of these, perhaps, is Milan Cathedral.

Many people claim to have detected a clear change in visual art after the Black Death. After the plague, the motifs in religious art became much more sombre, with an emphasis on suffering, death and punishment. The common motif of the *danse macabre*, with Death leading the dance, was regarded by many as being an echo of the Black Death.

The motif is still familiar, appearing in the final scene of Ingmar Bergman's film *The Seventh Seal* (1957), which provides a gripping depiction of the psychological atmosphere during a medieval plague epidemic.

There is a clear difference in architecture created before and after the Black Death, possibly because the relatively limited number of qualified stonemasons had been decimated by the plague.[35] Simpler styles than the classic Gothic now became common.

Throughout the Middle Ages, and up until quite recent times, Latin was the language of the learned as well as the main language within the Catholic Church. After the Black Death there was an increase in the use of the vernacular languages, which might have been partially due to the considerable decrease in university teachers proficient in Latin. A number of universities were even closed down during the time of the Black Death.

Considerable disagreement remains about the extent of the long-term effects of the Black Death. A number of historians have pointed out that some of the changes attributed to the plague were actually under-way before the epidemic and would possibly have developed further

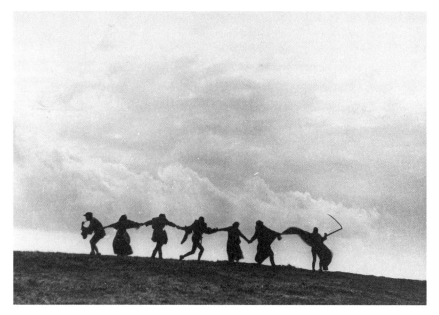

The final scene of Ingmar Bergman's film *The Seventh Seal* (1957) – with plague in the Middle Ages as its theme – is a representation of the classic *danse macabre* motif, with Death leading the main characters of the film in a dance along a ridge.

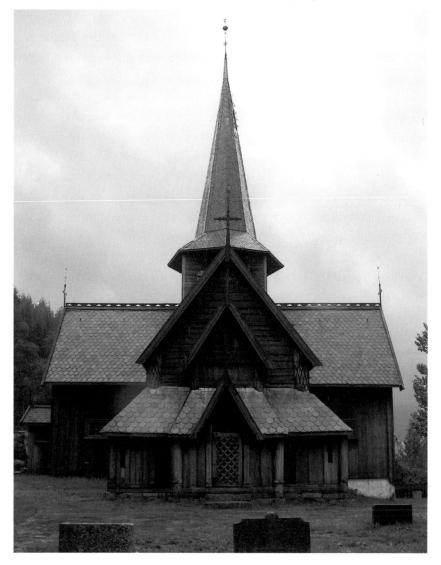

Hedalen stave church in the Norwegian mountain valley of Hedalen, Valdres, built in 1163. According to legend, the church was forgotten when Hedalen was depopulated during the Black Death, but rediscovered by huntsmen after many years. At the altar the huntsmen found a bear, which they shot. A bearskin, dating from the time of the Black Death, hangs in the vestry.

without it. Even so, it is reasonable to assume that such a huge disaster as the Black Death did at least speed up many of the changes that have been mentioned.

The epidemic had an enormous psychological impact on its own and subsequent ages, reflected in the many legends containing this motif that exist around Europe. It also very much applies to Norway, where most parts of the country have local accounts of the plague and its consequences. One of the best known comes from Sogn in Western Norway and deals with the Jostedal grouse. The legend states that a number of farmers in the Sogn area decided to flee from the plague to the remote valley of Jostedal, where they attempted to isolate themselves. But the plague caught up with them and all of them died, except for a young girl. She was later found in a semi-wild state, like a shy grouse, and was known as the Jostedal grouse. The legend states that she later became the first ancestress of a long line, the grouse family. This may well be a migratory legend, since similar stories are also found elsewhere in Europe where the plague had depopulated large rural areas.

Just as well known is the legend of the famous stave church in the Norwegian mountain valley of Hedalen in Valdres. This was built before the time of the Black Death and is first recorded in 1327. Hedalen was apparently almost completely depopulated by the ravages of the plague, and both the church and the farms in the valley were forgotten. The

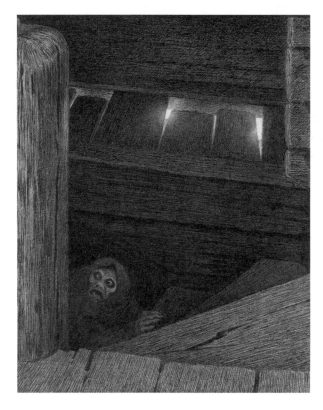

Theodor Kittelsen, *The Plague*, 1894–6. Kittelsen builds on the popular traditional view of the plague as an old, pale grey woman who went from farm to farm with broom and rake. Where she used the broom, nobody survived. Where she used the rake, some survived.

The Plague comes to a farm in Theodor Kittelsen's representation, published in Kittelsen's *Svartedauen* (1900).

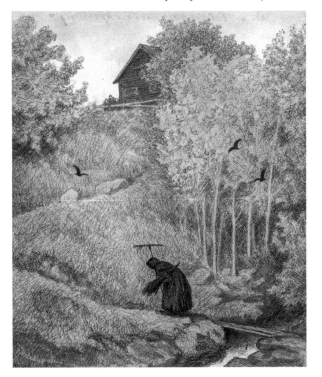

legend says that a huntsman from outside the area shot an arrow at a bird while hunting capercaillie. He missed, but instead could hear a sound like that of a bell where the arrow had fallen. It had struck the bell of the stave church, which in this way was rediscovered. The legend also states that a bear had lain down at the altar. The huntsman killed the bear and flayed it. The bearskin still hangs in a glass case on the wall in the vestry.

What is the reality behind this legend? A few years ago it was demonstrated that the bearskin, which is now in a rather poor state, is from the period between 1290 and 1370, indicating that it fits well with the period of the Black Death. So there may be some truth behind this fascinating tale, even though the presentation of the original events may have changed somewhat through having been retold countless times and possibly influenced by similar tales from the time of the Black Death.

Norwegians' ideas of the Black Death have without a doubt been strongly influenced by the popular artist Theodor Kittelsen's brilliant pictures of motifs from the plague: depopulated, scary farms with skeletons in beds and plague corpses lying at the roadside. Of particular note are his depictions of the plague as an evil old woman, which was how she was often seen in popular belief. Everywhere the plague came with her broom and rake, she left behind death and misery.

Later plague epidemics

The term 'Black Death' is normally used about the pandemic in the period 1346–53, but Europe was by no means finished with the plague. During the next few centuries, Europe was hit at intervals of just ten to fifteen years by new plague epidemics, some smaller, some larger, although none had the same scope as the pandemic. The last major epidemic in northern Europe, and one of the best known, was that which struck London in 1665–6, which has gained its place in world literature partly because of Daniel Defoe's *A Journal of the Plague Year* (1722), in which he gives vivid depictions of the fear and sufferings of those living in London (even though Defoe himself was only five at the time of the epidemic).[36]

'Death now began not, as we may say, to hover over every one's head only, but to look into their houses and chambers and stare in their faces', Defoe writes. 'People sickened so fast and died so soon, that it

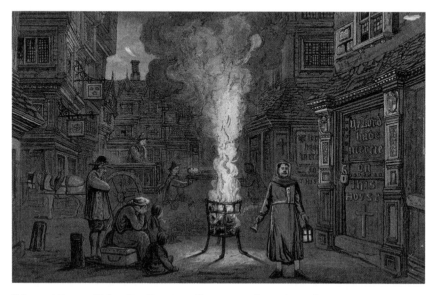

Edmund Evans, 'Bring Out Your Dead', c. 1864, coloured wood engraving. During the last major epidemic of *Yersinia pestis* in northern Europe, in 1665–6, the hearses in London drove through the streets after nightfall to collect the day's victims.

The contents of a hearse are emptied into a mass grave during the plague epidemic in London in 1665–6. Engraving by Samuel Davenport, 1835, after George Cruikshank.

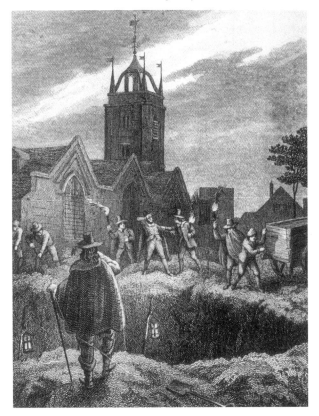

was impossible, and indeed to no purpose, to go about to inquire who was sick and who was well.' According to Defoe, the disease developed so fast that 'we see men alive and well to outward appearance one hour, and dead the next'. Today it is estimated that 75,000–100,000 died out of a population of 460,000 in London.

Gradually the plague disappeared from Europe. The last major epidemic in Western Europe hit Marseilles in 1720–21. In Eastern Europe, however, there were still outbreaks, the last major occurrence being in Moscow in 1771. In Egypt and the Middle East, there were outbreaks until well into the nineteenth century.[37]

Gradually both the population and the authorities learned to live with the threat of plague. Most European countries introduced various protective measures, including quarantine regulations that were in force until well into the nineteenth century.

Many researchers believe that the constantly recurring plague epidemics contributed to keeping down the European population

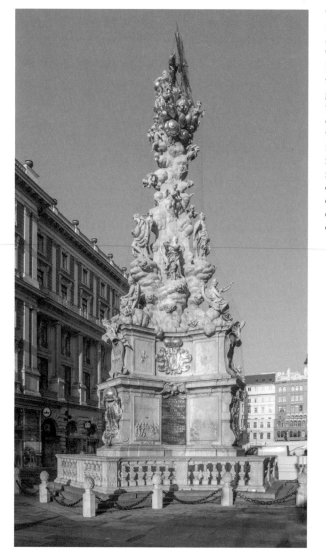

The plague column in Graben in the centre of Vienna. This impressive Baroque column was raised in gratitude when the major plague epidemic came to an end in 1679. It was the inspiration for many similar columns in other parts of the Habsburg empire.

figures until we see the beginnings of an increase from the eighteenth century onwards that has continued ever since.

The third plague pandemic: the pieces fall into place – or do they?

There were still plague outbreaks outside Europe until well into the nineteenth century, but on the whole these were quite local epidemics. Then came the third pandemic – and it was not until this point that people came to realize the cause of bubonic and other forms of plague that earlier eyewitnesses had described: the bacterium *Yersinia pestis*.

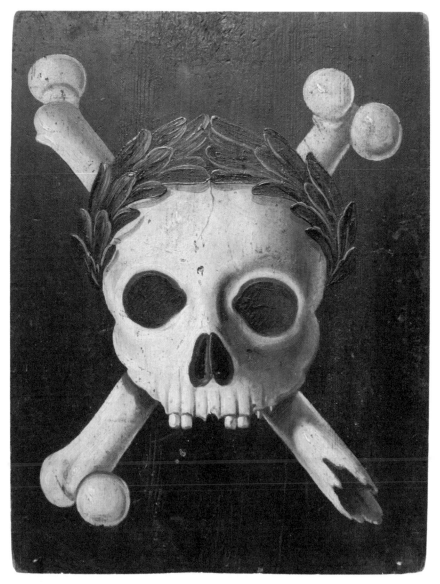

Plague panel with the triumph of death, 17th century. Panels of this kind were placed on the walls of houses to warn against the plague. A plague epidemic raged in Augsburg between 1607 and 1636.

This third plague pandemic, which left its mark on several continents, probably began as early as the 1770s in the Chinese province of Yunnan and gradually spread to other parts of China.[38] It flared up strongly in the 1850s, when the country experienced considerable social unrest, including the bloody Taiping rebellion. This civil war involved constant troop movements and large floods of refugees, which without a doubt contributed to spreading the plague effectively. In 1894 the plague reached the two major ports of Canton and Hong Kong, in each of which it is estimated that between 50,000 and 100,000 inhabitants died. These ports now became the starting point of a global spread of the disease over the next few years via shipping. Modern steamships enabled the plague to spread much more rapidly and over far greater distances than it had during the Black Death. Important ports in all inhabited parts of the world were now hit by the plague: Bombay and Calcutta in 1896, and such distant ports as San Francisco and Buenos Aires in North and South America, Sydney in Australia and Glasgow in Europe in 1900. It arrived in Cape Town in 1901. In most of these cities it proved possible to limit the spread of the disease via, among other things, active quarantine measures. The tragic exception was India, where probably 12 million people

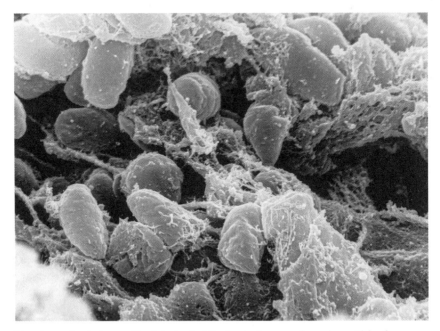

The plague bacterium – *Yersinia pestis*. The bacteria are rods with a width of 0.5–0.8 μm and a length of 1–3 μm.

lost their lives in the 25 years after the arrival of the plague. It is estimated that a total of around 13 million people died during the third pandemic, which considerably declined after 1914.

But even if it was possible to combat the plague in most cases, *Yersinia pestis* did manage to retain a foothold on several continents as a lasting threat.

The moment of truth

The disease picture of the victims of this third pandemic was in principle the same as with the other great historical plague epidemics and many later ones until well into the nineteenth century.[39] The physicians of that period were thus familiar with the forms the disease could take. As we have seen, people had for centuries suspected that the plague was contagious in one way or another, although they had explained this by variants of the miasma theory. In 1894, however, the bacteriological revolution was in full swing. The bacteria that caused anthrax, tuberculosis and cholera had been discovered, to great fanfare. Many researchers were now convinced that the plague was also caused by a bacterium.

The two main research teams competing with each other during the first years of the bacteriological revolution were the groups around Robert Koch in Berlin and Louis Pasteur in Paris. Koch's group had won the race to detect the cholera bacterium. Now there came a repeat performance of the rivalry between the two most prestigious bacteriological research teams in the world.

In June 1894 the imperial Japanese government sent the bacteriologist Shibasaburo Kitasato to British-governed Hong Kong to investigate the cause of the plague.[40] Kitasato had worked as a member of Koch's group for a number of years. He was received most kindly by the British, who did everything to facilitate his work, granting him free access to plague corpses for his research. A short time afterwards the young Swiss physician Alexandre Yersin arrived in Hong Kong, also to carry out plague research. Yersin had studied as a bacteriologist under Pasteur and had now been sent out by the French colonial secretary.

For obscure reasons, Yersin was given a rather unfriendly reception and was denied access to hospital laboratories and plague corpses, which were important for his research. He had to set up his own laboratory in a somewhat ramshackle shed outside the mission hospital in the city, and acquire corpses under cover of darkness by bribing the seamen whose task it was to bury them. By injecting rats with extracts of tissue from the swellings of these corpses, Yersin managed to detect the plague bacterium, which he called *Bacterium pestis*. Later it was called *Pasteurella pestis* in honour of the famous head of the Pasteur Institute, but in 1944 it was given the name *Yersinia pestis*, a belated posthumous tribute to its enterprising discoverer. As early as September 1894 Yersin published his discovery of the bacterium that caused the plague. In the race for the plague bacterium, therefore, Pasteur's laboratory avenged its defeat in the hunt for the cholera bacterium.

Meanwhile Kitasato had also detected a bacterium in the plague corpses, but hung back from publishing his findings.[41] When he did so, his description of the bacterium was imprecise, so there is still doubt as to whether Kitasato actually had detected the 'true' plague bacterium.

Fleas and rats leap onto the stage

Yersin's findings were convincing, and it now became generally accepted that the plague was due to infection with *Yersinia pestis*. Both Yersin and many other researchers were also convinced that the former plague epidemics of history, including the Black Death, were caused by this bacterium.

But how did humans get infected with *Yersinia pestis*? This question Yersin had not answered. Quite early on in the epidemic in India, both Yersin and other physicians suspected that rats played an important role in this respect. The predominant species of rat in India was the black rat (*Rattus rattus*). Prior to most outbreaks of the plague it was observed that there was a comprehensive spike in deaths among the rat population.[42] Their corpses floated around the gutters and streams, and were found in houses' nooks and crannies. A number of researchers therefore believed that the rats had also been smitten with the plague. The question then was how the bacterium was transmitted from rat to human being.

In 1898 Paul-Louis Simond, who also had a background at the Pasteur Institute in Paris, published an answer: the plague bacterium was transmitted from rats to human beings via the oriental rat flea with the fine-sounding name *Xenopsylla cheopis*. Infected rats contain a lot of bacteria in their blood, and the blood-sucking fleas transmit the

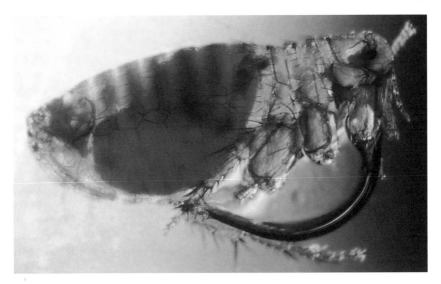

The oriental rat flea – *Xenopsylla cheopis* – infected with *Yersinia pestis* bacteria. Its intestines are blocked with blood and bacteria that the flea regurgitates when attempting to suck blood from a human being, and thereby it transmits the plague infection.

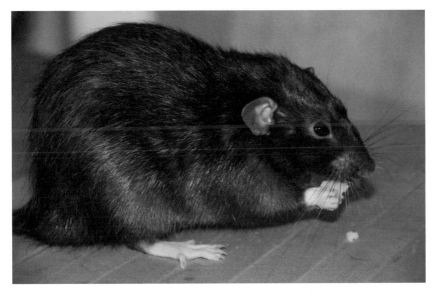

The black rat – *Rattus rattus* – which has played a key role as a carrier of *Yersinia pestis* in plague epidemics. In large parts of Europe it has been ousted by the brown rat, *Rattus norvegicus*.

bacteria from animal to animal. When the rats die, the fleas have to find new hosts, including humans. In all fairness, it must be said that the Japanese physician Ogata Masanori had already shown the previous year that rat fleas contained plague bacteria.[43]

Later research has shown that the rat flea is particularly well suited to the transmission of *Yersinia pestis* since the bacterium has the ability to create a blockage in the flea's digestive tract. This blockage means that the blood cannot be absorbed as nutrition by the flea, which therefore spews the blood into the bite wound at the next attempt to suck blood, and thus the bacterium is transmitted to the human being. The fleas gradually became wild with hunger and extra-active as blood-suckers, before dying after a few days.[44]

In the course of the following years, it became generally accepted that the mechanism involved in plague infection is that the rat flea transmits *Yersinia pestis* from rats to humans, so we are dealing with a zoonosis. Plague bacteria that are transmitted via flea bite are transported to the nearest lymph nodes, where inflammation leads to the classic bubo (plague swelling), often in the groin or armpits. The bacteria then spread out further, via the blood, and serious complications arise, including an intense activation of the coagulation mechanisms and the immune system. Untreated, the patient dies after four or five days. With some patients who have classic bubonic plague the bacteria also get into the lungs and cause what is known as pneumonic plague. In a few patients the bacteria get into the blood very rapidly after infection, which accelerates the process, so that death takes place in the space of a couple of days, without plague swellings necessarily being formed.

The usual view has long been that people sick with the plague most often do not infect each other directly. Only if the patient has pneumonic plague is droplet infection a possibility. The person who is infected can then either develop pneumonic plague or the usual bubonic plague. It is thought that this kind of infection has been the exception rather than the rule in most epidemics. Droplet infection does not extend very far and is therefore not normally all that effective.

Even so, we know that there have been epidemic outbreaks of the plague where droplet infection has been predominant. In 1910, during the third pandemic, a local plague epidemic broke out in Manchuria in which droplet infection with pneumonic plague was the most important transmission mechanism.[45] This is particularly likely in a relatively cold climate where people live close to each other, as was the case in Manchuria.

Until well into the twentieth century the infection theory based on the three-leafed clover of rat–flea–human being was the only one used to explain plague infections, and was also applied to the earlier pandemics. In recent decades, however, many researchers have begun to question this explanation as the only possible mechanism for plague epidemics. It definitely applied to the outbreak of the third pandemic, but was it also the mechanism for the Plague of Justinian, the Black Death and many others? It has gradually been understood that humans can probably be infected in more ways than we have already discussed. But let us first take a look at the role ecological factors can play in plague epidemics, since interesting research discoveries have been made in this area.

The hiding places of plague bacteria

It became obvious early on that rats were not the only mammals playing a role in the spread of plague. We now know that *Yersinia pestis* can infect a large number of mammals. Many rodents are particularly important and more than two hundred species of rodent can be infected by this bacterium.[46] In certain parts of the world we now have so-called plague reservoirs, areas where wild rodents (and their fleas) are constant carriers of the bacterium. Some species of rodent live more or less in peaceful coexistence with it and do not necessarily die, so the bacterium remains in this environment. Many of these rodents live in underground burrows, where it is also possible for the plague bacteria to live freely in the soil for months or years – and then re-infect the rodent inhabitants.[47]

Such plague reservoirs exist on several continents. The largest of these areas covers large parts of Central Asia, including Kazakhstan, and was probably formed several thousand years ago. Another plague reservoir is found in the western states of the USA, where it is gradually spreading eastwards. Less comprehensive plague areas are found in South America, Africa and parts of Asia. Such areas form the basis of new outbreaks of plague around the world. No such reservoirs have been detected in Europe or Australia. We will return later to the controversial issue of whether there have ever been such in Europe.

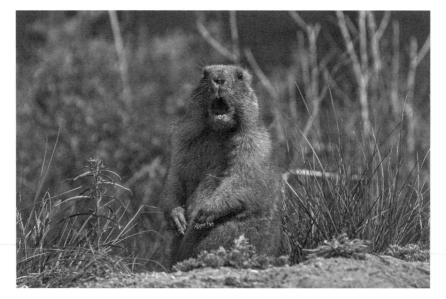

Marmot, also known as prairie dog. This relation of the squirrel, which lives in colonies in underground passage systems, is one of the many species of rodent that are carriers of the plague bacterium – *Yersinia pestis* – in such areas as Central Asia and North America.

Isolated cases of plague in humans or small-scale epidemics are most frequently caused by direct contact with infected wild rodents from a plague reservoir.[48] But infection from such a reservoir can also spread to other animals that live close to humans, not only rats but cats, which are susceptible to *Yersinia pestis* infection. The transmission to humans can then occur via the fleas on the animal or, when cats are involved, even with droplet infection from animals with pneumonic plague. Dogs are far less likely as sources of infection. Both animals and humans can also be infected from eating infected animal meat, including camel. It is also possible for predatory birds to spread the bacterium over quite large areas.

Major plague epidemics can be a consequence of an infected rodent population in a reservoir temporarily having violently expanded, resulting in a mass death of the animals. Fleas that carry the plague bacterium will then leave dead animals and jump onto other animals (rats in particular) and pass on infection to humans. The number of infected fleas will also be able to increase rapidly as a result of certain climate changes. We will later look more closely at the influence of climatic factors on plague epidemics.

Attempts to dethrone Yersinia pestis *as the cause of the plague*

The history of plague epidemics continued to fascinate many scholars during the twentieth century. Several of those who studied the historical accounts of the first two pandemics in detail and compared them with the facts related to the third found that there was something that did not tally. From about 1970 some researchers raised objections to the prevailing theories of plague infection, as presented in schoolbooks, for example, and now openly claimed that *Yersinia pestis* could not possibly be the cause of the plague epidemics of former times. This unleashed a tremendous debate, one that has lasted for several decades and, to a certain extent, is ongoing.

Why did those we can call plague-deniers wish to dethrone *Yersinia pestis*? Well, because they believed that both the first and the second pandemics were completely different in nature from the most recent pandemic, where nobody has doubted the key role played by *Yersinia pestis*.[49]

The earlier epidemics, such as the Black Death, definitely spread far more rapidly than the third pandemic, as seen for example in India. Mortality was also far greater than in modern times. As we have seen, rats played a key role in the third pandemic, and large numbers of dead rats were a sure sign that an outbreak of the plague was on the way. The critics claimed, however, that there is no mention of large numbers of dead rats anywhere in accounts from the Black Death or the Plague of Justinian. Furthermore, they argued, rats were in short supply in northern Europe during the earlier pandemics. Nor was the oriental rat flea *Xenopsylla cheopis* to be found in the northern parts of Europe where the plague ravaged so severely. Some historians also claimed that the descriptions of the disease from the time of the Black Death do not fit the plague cases of recent times. The plague-deniers assert that the so-called plague epidemics of former times must have been caused by other microbes than *Yersinia pestis*. Both the anthrax bacterium and Ebola types of virus have been proposed, but without any documentation.

How weighty and real are these objections? Can the differences claimed between plague in our times and the historical epidemics be explained without discarding *Yersinia pestis* as the cause of disease? I am absolutely sure that this is possible, and to cut a long story short, I believe we can maintain that the role of *Yersinia pestis* as a cause of plague in the two earlier pandemics is viable. Modern molecular biology has come to the rescue. As we have touched on earlier, in the last few years we have acquired methods of detecting extremely small amounts of DNA, mainly using the so-called PCR technique.

Since the 1990s researchers have successfully detected the DNA from *Yersinia pestis* in excavations from the time of the Plague of Justinian, from that of the Black Death and from later plague epidemics.[50] Admittedly, such finds have until now mostly been made in the Mediterranean countries, and in continental and eastern Europe. However, we can now say that *Yersinia pestis* was the probable cause of all three great pandemics and of lesser epidemics in their wake.

But what about the plague-deniers' other assertions about profound differences between modern and historical plague epidemics? Could the explanation be that there were very different variants of the plague bacterium that were responsible for the various pandemics, variants that behave differently when it comes to infection and mortality? There is no basis for this assertion; nor is it likely, based on the molecular biological studies that have been carried out on the DNA of bacteria from the various pandemics.

To be able to cut through the long-lasting plague debate we must probably look once more at the century-old teaching that the trinity of *Yersinia pestis*, rats and rat fleas supplied the only, or at any rate the dominant, mechanism for the major plague epidemics. We now know that not only the oriental rat flea can transmit plague bacteria, but so can other species of fleas, including the human flea, *Pulex irritans*, which jumps from person to person.[51] During plague epidemics the bacterium *Yersinia pestis* has also been detected in body lice. So is it not likely that the bacterium can *also* be transmitted directly from person to person via these 'human-loving' insects? In the start-up phase of epidemics, rats and rat fleas quite probably play a role as a bridge between infected wild rodents from plague reservoirs to humans, but later the epidemic can perhaps be self-driven via human-to-human infection. In this way, the plague could spread considerably faster than the classic rat model allows. Recently an international group of researchers has shown, via mathematical calculations, that infection with human fleas or body lice corresponds better with the rate of infection spread in the Black Death than the classic rat model.[52]

That the role of the rats may have been more modest than previously assumed can also explain why Norwegian researchers have not been able to detect archaeological remains of rats from the time of the Black Death far inland in Norway, where the plague raged.[53] Could it be that the pest bacterium during the Black Death there was transmitted from human to human via fleas and lice? This theory is also strongly opposed. Ole Jørgen Benedictow, in particular, is convinced that the 'classic' rat–flea–human model that was mapped during the third pandemic also applied during the Black Death in Norway.[54] Nor can one completely ignore the fact that pneumonic plague with direct droplet infection may have played a role in a cool country like Norway, as it did during the epidemic in Manchuria in 1910.

There is still a great deal we do not know about the earlier plague epidemics. As yet we have not found the final answers to the original cradles of the great pandemics and their initial spread. What was it that actually triggered these pandemics? What can explain the fact that the plague, having raged after both the Plague of Justinian and the Black Death, disappeared from Europe (apart from Eastern Europe)? And where was *Yersinia pestis* between the individual epidemics? Some of the answers to these questions we can probably get from climate research.

The interaction between climate and the plague

Studies in Central Asia and North America have shown that the risk of a plague outbreak is considerable when the rodent population in a plague reservoir increases strongly over several years with good nutritional conditions, then decreases with mass deaths when the conditions change.[55] This cycle is a result of climate changes that first favour vegetation rich in nutrition, then become less favourable. Could similar mechanisms explain the recurring epidemics in Europe that broke out time after time at intervals of ten to fifteen years after both the first and the second pandemic? The problem here is that we do not have any basis for the establishment of any permanent plague reservoir in Europe, as is the case in several other continents. Even so, we cannot completely exclude the possibility that such reservoirs in the rodent population also existed in this part of the world.

A new theory has recently been launched to explain the constant recurrence of plague epidemics in Europe after the Black Death.[56] A group of international researchers under Norwegian leadership found that outbreaks of new plague in ports in the Mediterranean area came fifteen years after marked climate changes in Central Asia that might have activated plague reservoirs. Their theory is that the plague bacterium followed the caravan routes to the Mediterranean – something that would take many years – and was then spread further on ships by rats, fleas or humans. That the plague bacterium has repeatedly been re-imported into Europe from Asia in this way does not exclude the possibility that it also remained in the local population of black rats between new plague outbreaks. In recent times, however, the black rat has to a great extent been replaced by the brown rat in large parts of Europe. There are also recent findings suggesting that infection during the earlier plague epidemics was mainly from human to human via fleas and lice, as mentioned earlier.

It is beyond doubt that climate changes play a considerable role in plague epidemics. That the explanation of the constantly recurring plague epidemics in Europe over several hundred years is the constant re-importation of bacteria as a result of Asian climate fluctuations must nevertheless be considered to be only one of several possible explanations of the epidemic patterns.

Several observations suggest that patients who survived the Black Death developed lifelong immunity. If the *Yersinia pestis* bacterium should in some way or other have managed to retain a hold between epidemics, a possible explanation of the recurrence of new epidemics could be that they struck when a sufficiently large percentage of the population had grown up that was not immune to the bacterium. Further research will perhaps be able to answer these questions.

Yersinia pestis: *an unusually adaptive opponent for* Homo sapiens

Microbes, in their never-ending duel with man, have a quite extraordinary capacity to adapt to new life conditions. In many ways *Yersinia pestis* is a shining example of this, so let us take a look at the plague bacterium's CV.

The plague bacterium comes from a fairly modest family of bacteria.[57] Its closest relative today is the bacterium *Yersinia pseudotuberculosis*, which gives rise to only quite harmless intestinal infections in humans. The two bacteria share the same progenitor and they separated some

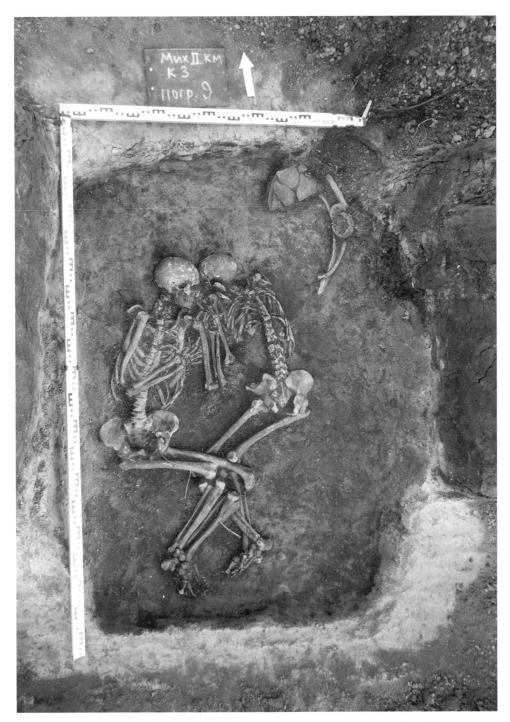

Two skeletons from 1800 BC, found in the Samara region in Russia, are the oldest finds of humans infected with the plague bacterium *Yersinia pestis*.

thousands of years ago. From then on, the one destined to become the dreaded plague bacterium gradually changed in character, partly by deactivating some of its genes, partly by assimilating new genes from its surroundings in the form of two plasmids that we have previously mentioned as an important part of the genetic equipment of many bacteria. With these new genes, the bacterium now acquired the ability also to cause life-threatening infections elsewhere in the body than the intestines. The genetic changes led, among other things, to the bacterium becoming able to combat the victim's immune response and trigger dramatic disturbances in the coagulation and immune system.[58] Even so, the bacterium was still not particularly effective in its transmission mechanism from human to human. Finally, genetic changes came about that made it possible for the bacterium to utilize fleas as a medium of transportation from rodents to human victims and possibly from human to human – a considerable advance, seen from the bacterium's point of view.

We cannot determine for sure when the fully developed plague bacterium entered the arena. Researchers have recently demonstrated that infections with the bacterium were common among people in southeast Asia as early as 3000 BC and that this bacterium had apparently acquired the ability to spread via fleas.[59] Other researchers, however, are of the opinion that this ability did not develop in the bacterium until about AD 1000.[60]

During our account of the plague epidemics through history we have seen that the plague bacterium, with great virtuosity, has exploited a number of the ecological and environmental factors that influence the interaction between microbe and man. The bacterium has started to use blood-sucking insects to infect new individuals. It has the ability to remain in wild rodents and in the soil for considerable periods of time. It spreads via trade routes, as is clear from all three major historical pandemics. It also often flares up in war situations with influxes of refugees. This was seen at the beginning of the Black Death in Crimea, during the Thirty Years War in Europe, during Carl XII of Sweden's campaign in Russia in the early eighteenth century, and in China in the mid-nineteenth century during the Taiping rebellion.

Let us conclude our account of *Yersinia pestis* by pointing out that there are still new incidences of the plague as an after-shock of the third pandemic. This epidemic led to the establishment of plague reservoirs, both in and outside Asia. According to the World Health Organization (WHO), 3,248 cases of the plague were recorded between 2010 and 2015, with 584 deaths. And *Yersinia pestis* can cause major problems because of its great adaptability: plague bacteria have already been detected that have developed considerable resistance to the common antibiotics used to save the lives of plague patients. The future therefore gives us cause for a certain anxiety.

Smallpox: 'the most terrible of all the ministers of death'

In 1980 the WHO was able to proclaim that smallpox had been eradicated from our planet after the last naturally occurring case had been seen in a young Somali in 1977.[61] This was the result of an intense campaign lasting twelve years, a key element of which was targeted vaccination. Victory over the smallpox virus is one of the greatest triumphs *Homo sapiens* has achieved so far in its battle against microbes, for smallpox is probably the infectious disease that has claimed most lives through the history of humanity. It was fully justified when, with Victorian pathos, one of England's greatest historians, Thomas Babington Macaulay, described smallpox as 'the most terrible of all the ministers of death'.[62] In the twentieth century alone, the smallpox virus claimed 300 million lives, three times as many as all those who died fighting in wars. It is estimated that over the past thousand years it has been responsible for 10 per cent of all deaths in the world, a quite incredible figure.

Smallpox is an acute infectious disease that is caused by a virus.[63] This virus only infects humans and is not found in any species of animal, even though it has many relatives in the animal world. It is thus not a zoonosis. The fact that it does not have an animal reservoir is one of the reasons it was possible to eradicate it.

When one becomes infected by the smallpox virus, the course of the disease is fairly predictable.[64] The incubation time is ten to twelve days on average. The patient then has a high fever, back pains, a headache and often vomits. Then the rash breaks out, first in the oral cavity, then all over the body. It takes the form of small red spots that develop into blisters, which initially contain a clear liquid and then pus. After seven to ten days the sores start to dry out and become scabs, which gradually fall off. After around three weeks all these scabs have normally fallen off.

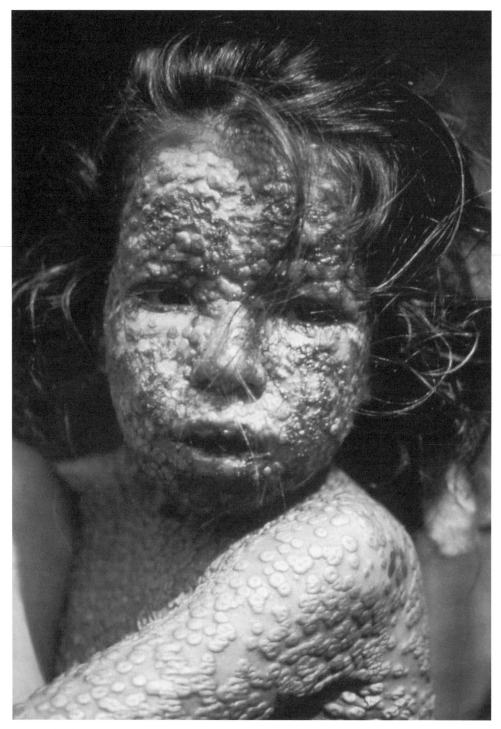

Child with smallpox, Bangladesh, 1973.

The case fatality rate of this commonest form is about 30 per cent. In a few such cases the rash develops differently, possibly with extreme skin bleeding, in which case perhaps 97 per cent of patients will die. Most of the deaths from smallpox are from this form of the disease, one of the features being that the patient's coagulation system is knocked out, which results in bleeding complications.

In addition to the high mortality rate, smallpox was also feared because many people had permanent damage from the infection. Conspicuous scars, particularly on the face, were extremely common. The eyes were also attacked, resulting in up to 30 per cent of the victims going blind.[65]

During the nineteenth century a considerably milder form of the disease, known as alastrim, appeared in Africa and Central America, the fatality rate of which was only 1–2 per cent and with far fewer lasting complications.[66] The variant responsible for the serious form of smallpox is called *variola major*, while the form that causes alastrim is called *variola minor*. Both forms normally lead to lifelong immunity against both types of virus.

The commonest form of transmission is droplet infection, which particularly takes place during the first week after a rash appears.[67] That means the disease is not normally extremely infectious. Infection can also take place via direct contact with skin scabs or with objects, especially fabrics such as clothing and bed linen, that contain the virus. The virus in its desiccated form can survive for a very long time outside the body, and thus it is also possible for airborne infection to take place through tiny aerosol particles.

Camels, goddesses and mummies

Smallpox is a typical example of what we earlier referred to as 'crowd infections', which require a large population for the microbe to be able to survive after an epidemic. For this reason, the smallpox virus must have arisen quite a long while after people began to settle around 10,000 years ago. The virus has many relatives within the animal kingdom, and we must assume that they originate from a related virus in animals. It is probable that they originally come from rodents. The animal virus that is most closely related to the smallpox virus, however, according to new finds, is found in the camel.[68] This virus could possibly be the source of the smallpox virus. Either way, smallpox was probably originally a zoonosis until it adapted itself completely to the human race and lost contact with its original animal host.

Exactly where the first smallpox epidemics occurred is lost in the obscurity of history, although there are many fascinating pieces of information in the ancient Indian and Chinese accounts that have been emphasized in various ways down the centuries. The most likely areas of origin are Southwest Asia, Egypt and Mesopotamia, although others favour India.[69] Sanskrit accounts from several centuries BC mention epidemics in India that may have been smallpox, but the descriptions of the diseases are not unequivocal. For centuries Hindus have worshipped a special goddess of smallpox, Shitala, which indicates the significance of this infection in their society. The goddess was feared, and worship of her was widespread.

Smallpox probably made its way into China from the north, imported by nomadic horsemen around 250 BC, not long before the Great Wall of China was built to prevent invasions. The Chinese also had their own goddess of smallpox, who was worshipped in special temples all over China and prayed to for protection against infection and for cures. The smallpox virus spread from China in the eighth century AD to Japan, which was ravaged by several large epidemics during that period.

Egypt is also of interest when discussing the origins of the smallpox virus, as there is some evidence of smallpox in several mummies from the second millennium BC. The best known is the mummy of the pharaoh Rameses V, who died in 1157 BC.[70] He had the impressive title 'Mighty bull. Victor of millions. Golden Horus. King of Upper and Lower Egypt. Lord of the Two Lands'. His elevated position possibly did not protect him against the smallpox virus, for the mummy has clear signs of a smallpox-like rash on the face, neck, stomach and lower belly. It is not, however, a completely certain diagnosis, since the Egyptian authorities have not allowed molecular-biological investigations of the pharaoh's rash to be carried out.

The Egyptians were frequently at war with the powerful Hittite kingdom in Asia Minor. Hittite clay tablets tell of a terrible epidemic that struck them down, allegedly transmitted by Egyptian prisoners of war in the mid-thirteenth century BC. This may have been smallpox.

Russian researchers have recently found evidence suggesting that the smallpox virus might have originated in Somalia, in the Horn of

The Hindu goddess of smallpox – Shitala – has been worshipped for at least 2,000 years. She is extremely popular and has temples all over India – four in Benares alone, which is Hinduism's holiest city. Shitala is often portrayed in red clothes.

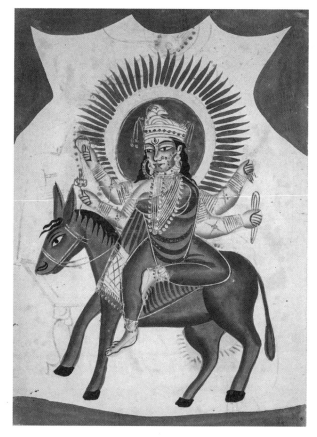

Africa, which in antiquity was called Punt.[71] In ancient times there were trade links between this part of Africa and Egypt, and the virus could therefore have been imported to Egypt from there. The virus could also have followed the trade routes or been spread eastwards by sea to India.

As we have seen, an exchange of microbes took place between the civilizations in Europe and Asia in the first centuries AD.[72] We must assume that this also applied to the smallpox virus, but we do not know exactly when the virus arrived in Europe. Most researchers now doubt that smallpox existed in the classical Greek world.[73] If it did, it would be extremely surprising as the Hippocratic writings do not contain any references to a fever that is reminiscent of smallpox. The Antonine plague during the reign of Marcus Aurelius in the second century AD may possibly have been smallpox, but this remains uncertain.

In all probability, the smallpox virus had established itself to a certain extent in the Christian part of the Mediterranean world in the

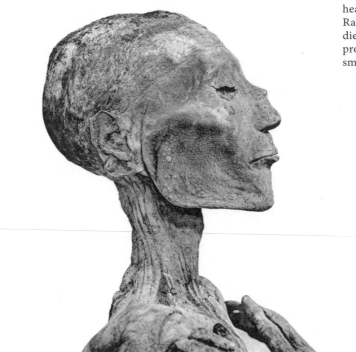

The mummified head of pharaoh Rameses V, who died in 1157 BC, probably of smallpox.

middle of the first millennium AD, but hardly to the same extent as in the Arab world.[74] It has been a common view that the first unequivocal account of smallpox was written by the Persian physician Abu Bakr Muhammad ibn Zakariya al-Razi, known in Europe as Rhazes, who worked in Baghdad at the end of the ninth century AD. He was also the first person to make a clear distinction between smallpox and measles, which has been a problem for physicians, even much later in history. It has gradually become known that a Chinese alchemist, Ko Hung, had made a quite exact description of smallpox as early as the fourth century AD. We do not know if Rhazes was familiar with this.

There are reasons to believe that the conquering Islamic armies during and after Muhammad in the seventh century brought the smallpox virus with them. This could possibly explain part of their success in lands around the Mediterranean that were formerly Christian, since their opponents, unlike the Muslim conquerors, had hardly any immunity against the virus. During the succeeding centuries there was a series of examples of the smallpox virus having a decisive influence on campaigns and military conflicts.

As early as the tenth century smallpox had arrived in northern Europe, including Scandinavia.[75] Norway possibly received the virus from Denmark, while in turn Norwegian ships took smallpox with them to Iceland, which was hit by a series of epidemics. From the late eleventh century returning crusaders brought home with them new supplies of the smallpox virus.

The virus became one of the many players from the world of microbes influencing human life in Europe during the Middle Ages and up to around 1500. Yet smallpox was not feared in the same way as the plague, and up to that point had not had the same influence on mortality across the population. As we shall see, however, all this changed during the seventeenth century.

The smallpox virus crosses the oceans

With the arrival of Europeans to the Americas in 1492, led by Christopher Columbus, we come to the second epidemiological transition in the history of human infection. This led to an exchange of microbes between the Old and the New World.[76] There can, however, be no doubt whatsoever that the 'trade balance' was in Europe's favour. More microbes were transferred to America than vice versa, and this led to great tragedies for the indigenous American population.

The both fascinating and gruesome account of how the Spanish conquistador Hernán Cortés conquered the mighty Aztec kingdom in Mexico is one of the best-known examples of the influence of the smallpox virus on the path of history.[77] In 1519 Cortés sailed from Cuba to Mexico with a modest force of four hundred foot soldiers, sixteen cavalrymen and fourteen cannons. In order to demonstrate that retreat was inconceivable to him, he burned his boats on arrival, an act that has entered the language as a sign of uncompromising commitment. He then marched towards the magnificent capital, Tenochtitlan, along with allied indigenous warriors who were hostile to the ruling Aztecs. The emperor of the Aztecs, Moctezuma (earlier often called Montezuma), and his counsellors were seized with fear because these white-skinned intruders were said to have supernatural, perhaps divine qualities: there were legends that the god Quetzalcoatl, who had once been driven into exile, would one day return from the east. The Aztecs were scared stiff by the Spaniards' horses, their metal armour and the thundering firing weapons, which they had never seen before. Could it be Quetzalcoatl, who according to legend had a light-coloured skin and beard, who had now returned? For this reason, the Spaniards were not initially attacked by the Aztecs, who had tens of thousands of well-trained soldiers, but were received as honoured guests in the capital, which lay out in the middle of a lake, joined to the land by a number of bridges. After a few months, however, much of the awe of the Aztecs had disappeared because of the Spaniards' violent behaviour and somewhat ungodly appetite for gold. This culminated in a rebellion against the Spaniards, which led to them having to flee the city.

This flight from Tenochtitlan was a terrible experience for the Spaniards and their indigenous allies. In popular Spanish tradition it has been given the name *La noche triste* ('the night of sorrow'). Since the Aztecs had destroyed sections of the bridges to the mainland, the Spaniards had made a mobile wooden bridge intended to help them across such gaps. This went well for a while, but then they started to have problems positioning the wooden bridge and became stranded on the remaining sections of the bridge, caught in a life-and-death struggle and attacked both by Aztec warriors from the city and those who surrounded them in canoes. Many Spaniards fell while others were dragged out into the water. The Spaniards, however, filled the gaps in the bridge with cannons, chests of booty, and the corpses of men and horses, and many of them managed to get across. Throughout, the war drums of the Aztecs could be heard. Those who managed to escape had to see their captured comrades hauled up to the top of the highest temple in the city, that of the god of war, Huitzilopochtli, to be sacrificed in Aztec manner by the sacrificial priests ripping the heart out of the living body.

Cortés lost half his men and the survivors sought refuge with indigenous allies. Why were they not caught up with and slaughtered by Aztec warriors before reaching safety? This is where the smallpox virus comes in as perhaps the most important of all allies. As the historian William McNeill has emphasized, smallpox broke out on the same night as the Spaniards fled.[78] The powerful new Aztec leader after Moctezuma's death in Spanish captivity, his brother Cuitlahuac, was also struck down with smallpox, as were large swathes of his warriors and the population in general, perhaps 50,000 of the 300,000 who lived in Tenochtitlan. This paralysed the Aztecs and probably explains why they did not follow up their success after driving Cortés and his men from Tenochtitlan and crushing them with their well-trained army. When, after several months, Cortés and his men returned and managed to gain control of the city, they found it full of dead and dying Aztec victims of smallpox. One of the Spaniards who took part in the fighting in the city, Bernal Diaz, wrote later: 'We could not go anywhere without treading on heads and bodies of dead Indians. There were piles of corpses lying on the ground.' In addition to smallpox, famine had now also descended on those defending the city.

The smallpox virus had come from Cuba to Mexico the same year with Spanish forces that joined up with Cortés. And now smallpox

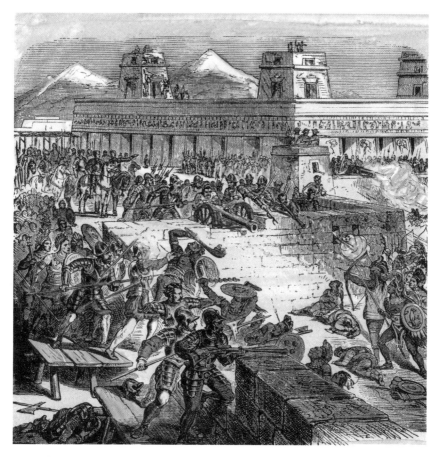

La noche triste – the night of sorrow – was a harrowing experience for Hernán Cortés and his men during their conquest of Mexico. During the night of 1 July 1520 the Spaniards attempted to leave the Aztec capital, Tenochtitlan, over one of the bridges while under heavy attack from Aztec warriors from both land and water. Cortés lost half his men, who were sacrificed to the Aztec god of war, Huitzilopochtli.

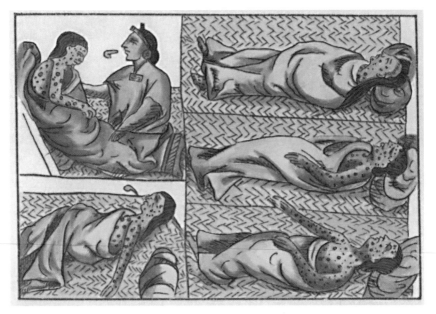

Dying Aztecs infected with smallpox, illustration by an Aztec artist from the
Codex Florentinus (book xii), written by the Franciscan monk Bernardino
de Sahagun in 1575–7.

spread through the Aztecs and other indigenous peoples like wildfire
through dry grass. The smallpox virus was a newcomer in the New
World. The native population had acquired no immunity whatsoever
against the virus, and it is also possible that genetically they were not
optimally equipped to tackle it.

The Spaniards, on the other hand, had centuries of experience with
smallpox, and the great majority of them had had smallpox as a childhood disease and were now immune. The Aztecs gazed with awe and
fear at the white conquerors who were unaffected by the terrible disease
while they were sorely afflicted, and regarded this as a sign that it was the
will of the gods that the Spaniards should gain supremacy. This demor-
alized them. Furthermore, the Spaniards interpreted the preference of
the smallpox virus for the Aztecs as God's will, as an eyewitness wrote:
'When the Christians were exhausted from war, God sent smallpox to
the Indians.'

It is estimated that at least half of all the Aztecs who contracted
smallpox died. The death figures are not completely reliable, but we are
talking of many millions in the space of just a few months. New smallpox
epidemics broke out in the succeeding years, and the native population

of Mexico was further afflicted by other epidemics involving microbes brought from the Old World.

The smallpox virus was also extremely useful for the conquest by the Spanish conquistadors of the other great civilization of the New World: the Inca kingdom in the western part of South America. The Spaniards had heard rumours of a land rich in gold further south, and this drew the attention of another conquistador, Francisco Pizarro.[79] He started his

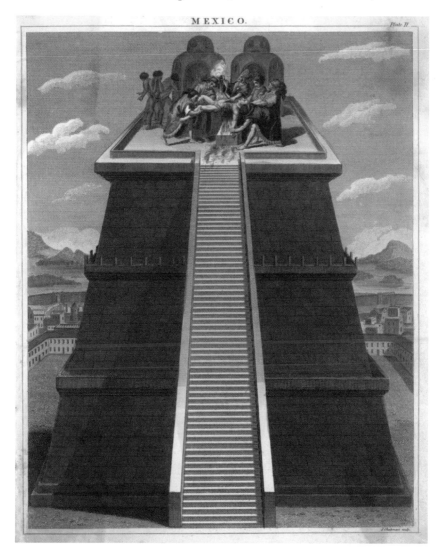

MEXICO.

Plate II

Countless people were sacrificed by the Aztecs on the top of the pyramid-shaped temple to the god of war, Huitzilopochtli, in the capital, Tenochtitlan, as seen in this engraving by J. Chapman for *Encyclopaedia Londinensis*, vol. xv (1817).

campaign in 1531 with only 180 men, 37 horses and a couple of cannons. The kingdom he attacked, however, had already been ravaged by two disasters: civil war and smallpox, which had swiftly spread southwards from Mexico. The smallpox virus attacked the kingdom as early as 1525, with fatal consequences for all strata of society, leaving a high mortality in its path. The timeline between the attack by the virus and the arrival of the conquistadors, however, differed from Mexico.

As with the Aztecs, the Incas had no natural immunity against the virus: at least 200,000 died during this first epidemic. The smallpox virus gave Pizarro and his men invaluable assistance in their conquest of the Inca kingdom. The mighty ruler Huayna Capac was among those who succumbed to the disease. After bidding farewell to his family and friends, he announced that his father, the sun, was calling him back to him. He then had himself immured in his palace, so that no one should witness his death throes. After his appointed successor died at roughly the same time, another son was nominated king by the Incas, but was challenged by an illegitimate son of Huayna Capac. This led to a devastating civil

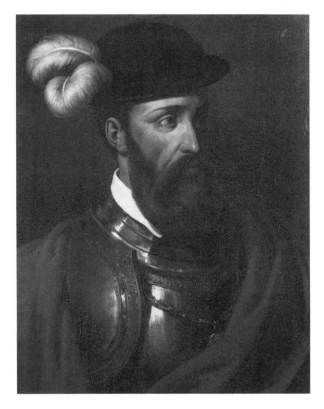

The Spaniard Francisco Pizarro, seen here in a painting by Amable-Paul Coutan from 1835, conquered the Inca kingdom in 1532–3 with a very small army. The smallpox virus had preceded the Spaniards and laid the foundation for the conquest.

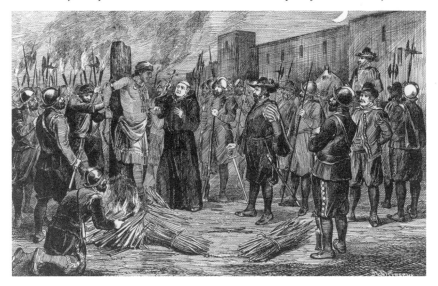

The execution by the Spaniards of the last ruling Inca, Atahualpa, engraving by
A. B. Greene, *c.* 1891.

war that lasted five years and paved the way for Pizarro and his men when they arrived in 1532. The reigning Inca, Atahualpa, who had won the civil war, was tricked by the Spaniards, taken prisoner and murdered. Two new smallpox epidemics then broke out in quick succession. In less than two years, Pizarro and his men, with ruthless brutality, had conquered the kingdom and the Spaniards were able to march in triumph into the Inca capital, Cuzco, in 1533, their path cleared by the smallpox virus.

During the sixteenth century the smallpox virus spread over large regions of Central and South America.[80] It was brought to the coastal areas of Brazil by the Portuguese, and then spread inland across the continent, wiping out entire tribes of native peoples. Some of this infection took place at Jesuit mission stations, where tens of thousands of indigenous people had gathered to receive the blessings of religion and civilization, seeking protection against the predation of Portuguese slave traders. The mission stations, however, were nothing less than factories for infection.

South and Central America received regular new influxes of the smallpox virus as a result of the increasing slave trade from West Africa in the following centuries. The numerous slave caravans that crossed the African continent contributed greatly to the spread of the virus. Smallpox seems to have been present on the east coast of Africa as far back as the tenth century, probably brought there by ship from Arabia, Egypt or India. About the same time, the countries south of the Sahara probably received the virus from caravans passing through the desert from North Africa.[81] It was present on the west coast as early as the sixteenth century. As in India and China, a West African tribe, the Yoruba, had its own god of smallpox, Shapona, who was feared to such an extent that people did not even dare utter his name. It was not until the nineteenth century that the smallpox virus started to lose its grip in South America, for three reasons: vaccination was gradually introduced; the import of African slaves ceased and thereby so so did the constant re-importation of the smallpox virus to South and Central America; and finally, the 'mild' variant *variola minor* replaced the more deadly form, against which it also provided immunity.

In North America the spread of the smallpox virus was delayed for a hundred years compared to the situation in the south, but the result after its arrival in the north at the beginning of the seventeenth century was the same: regular new epidemics with a high mortality in the native population.[82] The first epidemics came on the east coast and then spread inland. Here too the native population was highly prone to infection, partly because of a lack of immunity, and partly because cramped living quarters and constant nomadic roaming increase the possibilities of infection. One often saw the most serious forms of smallpox infection, with a particularly high mortality rate. Since various tribes were affected to a different extent, this led to considerable shifts in the power relations between the various indigenous nations on the North American continent.

European immigrants in the British and French colonies in North America did not escape smallpox either, since they had less immunity than the Spaniards in the south, but they were much less affected than the indigenous people. In the seventeenth and eighteenth centuries there were repeated smallpox epidemics at intervals of several years among the white immigrants, but the smallpox virus did not rage as violently as in Europe during the same period.

Smallpox came to Australia in the 1780s via British ships. The result was a repetition of the tragic scenario we have seen when the virus is introduced to a 'virgin' population that lacks immunity: the aborigines of Australia were hit very hard.

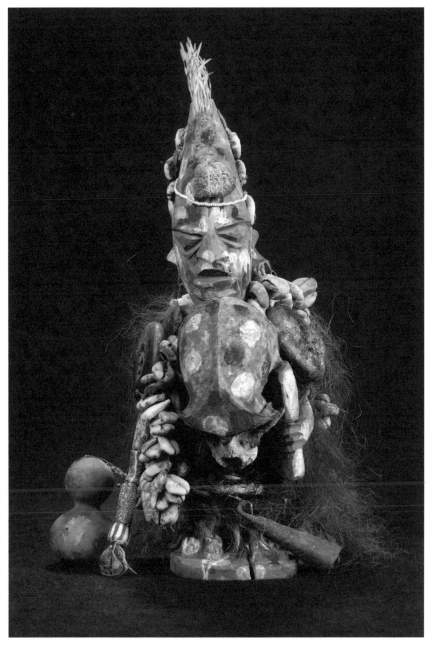

A special god for smallpox – Shapona – was worshipped by the Yoruba people in
present-day Nigeria and Benin in West Africa. Shapona, who was lord of the earth
and could punish humanity with smallpox, was greatly feared. He had his own
temples and priests. As late as the 1970s, there was strong resistance to smallpox
vaccination among Shapona worshippers.

The heir to the plague in Europe

The smallpox virus unquestionably contributed to much illness and death in Europe throughout both the Middle Ages and the Renaissance.[83] Even so, the virus was overshadowed during these periods by *Yersinia pestis* as a cause of epidemics with high mortality. This, however, began to change during the seventeenth century, as the plague began to lose its grip on the population of Europe until the last epidemics in the early eighteenth century.

Smallpox now overtook the position of the main cause of death among the most important epidemics – plague, typhus and dysentery – all of which flourished in the wake of the warfare that ravaged Europe, particularly the Thirty Years War.[84] There is a German saying that 'Few people escape falling in love and smallpox.'

It is unclear why smallpox epidemics and possibly also the intensity of the disease increased from the end of the sixteenth century and during the seventeenth. One theory is that the virus increased in virulence, its ability to cause illness. So far it has not proved possible to document this using modern methods. Molecular-biological examinations of a child mummy from Lithuania from around 1650 suggest that during the past two to three hundred years genetic changes in the virus have taken place, but we do not know if it has become more aggressive in this period than earlier in history.[85]

The smallpox virus was always present in large cities, but major epidemics also started to recur at shorter or longer intervals.[86] In the mid-eighteenth century more than 400,000 people died every year from smallpox in Europe (excluding Russia). A great many were attacked by the virus during childhood, but there were also many adult victims, especially young people. In Sweden every tenth baby died from small-pox, in Russia every seventh. The disease was also the cause of a third of all cases of blindness during this period.[87]

Perhaps half of Europe's population was characterized by early smallpox with disfiguring facial scarring that often must have led to considerable psychological problems. Such scars particularly influenced the chances of young women on the marriage market. The historian Macaulay, cited earlier, gives a vivid account of the ravages of smallpox:

The smallpox was always present, filling the churchyards with corpses, tormenting with constant fears all whom it had not yet stricken, leaving on those whose lives it spared the hideous traces of its power, turning the babe into a changeling at which the mother shuddered, and making the eyes and cheeks of the betrothed maiden objects of horror to the lover.

Beggars and emperors

As we touched on earlier, the first epidemiological transition, when humans settled and practised agriculture and animal husbandry, inevitably led to social stratification, with a wealthy elite and a large, poor lower class. The living conditions were of course utterly different in the various strata, especially when it came to the state of nutrition and housing conditions that influence the liability to infection. As far as some infectious diseases were concerned, this probably led to a greater liability among the under-privileged section of the population. But since the microbial causes and infection mechanisms of such diseases were unknown, the social elite did not necessarily get off scot-free.

What is extremely striking, as far as smallpox is concerned, is that it was more 'democratic' than most of the other common causes of epidemics in former ages. All levels of society were affected, from beggars to emperors. When smallpox was introduced to Iceland in 1240, the epidemic was given the name *farkonusótt* (beggar-woman's disease) since it was believed that it was spread by itinerant beggar-women.[88] But it was not only beggars who were stricken with the disease, but members of European royal families and other prominent figures from the sixteenth century onwards, particularly the eighteenth. This is of special interest because it often had historical consequences. Let us take a look at some of the royal victims.[89]

The most famous sixteenth-century smallpox victim was the young Elizabeth I of England, the Virgin Queen. After only four years on the throne, she contracted smallpox in 1562. She managed, however, to survive without any disfiguring facial scars, a topic she wrote about, with a slightly triumphant tone, to her beautiful rival Mary Stuart. Nor did she lose her hair, as has been claimed. Two of her ladies-in-waiting were not so lucky: one died and the other was so facially disfigured that she wore a mask at court for the rest of her life. Nor was one of the queen's rejected suitors any more fortunate. François, Duke of Alençon and Anjou, was the youngest son of the French king Henry II, who had already lost one son to smallpox, while another became blind in one eye. The duke was so badly pockmarked that Elizabeth used this as a (probably welcome) excuse for turning down his proposal.

After the childless Elizabeth I, the throne passed to the Scottish royal house, the Stuarts.[90] Queen Mary II died of smallpox in 1694. We know something of the course of the disease and the treatment she received as her physicians published the details in order to defend themselves against accusations that they had caused her death. Her sister, who was to become Queen Anne, had a mild attack of smallpox when aged twelve in 1677. Her death in 1714 marked the end of the House of Stuart, since the heir to the throne, the eleven-year-old William Henry, Duke of Gloucester, had died of smallpox in 1700. The German royal house of Hanover, which then took over the throne, can therefore thank smallpox for this.

King Louis XIV of France, the Sun King, was struck down with small-pox as a boy but survived, apparently without ill effects.[91] Later, two of his daughters were victims of smallpox but survived, unlike one of his sons-in-law. The order of succession was very much influenced by the smallpox virus, as Louis' son and grandson died of the disease. Only his young great-grandson, later Louis XV, survived, probably because his governess hastily removed him from Versailles. But the smallpox virus had not forgotten Louis XV: the virus's last, dramatic attack on the French royal house took place when he died horribly in 1774, his body first swelling up and then almost disintegrating. The stench from the sickbed was apparently so intense that the servants fainted. The heir apparent, later Louis XVI, who was the king's grandson, was denied access to the sickbed for fear of infection. This demonstrates, as we have touched on earlier, that the concept of person-to-person transmission of infection was very much in circulation long before the bacteriological revolution.

A few historians have claimed that Louis XV's death may have precipitated the French Revolution, but so-called counterfactual thinking of this type is of course highly uncertain and seldom fruitful. It is less uncertain to propose that the dramatic death of Louis XV from smallpox possibly accelerated the first form of smallpox vaccination, so-called inoculation, in France.

The Habsburg dynasty, one of the most powerful European royal houses across more than six hundred years, was also hard hit.[92] In 1711, in the midst of the War of the Spanish Succession, the gifted, liberal Holy Roman Emperor Joseph I died of smallpox. This led to the grandson of his opponent, Louis XIV, gaining the throne of Spain, which the Habsburg dynasty now lost. Joseph's talentless brother Karl became emperor, but on his death his daughter Maria Theresa, who ascended the throne, only received the title Archduchess of Austria, since as a woman she was barred from election to emperor. From here she was to influence European politics for several decades, but her environment was very much affected by the smallpox virus.

Having lost her future husband when young as a result of smallpox, she married his brother. They had sixteen children: two sons and a daughter, as well as two daughters-in-law, died of smallpox. Two daughters survived, but were so disfigured that they remained unmarried and ended their days as abbesses in nunneries. Her daughter Maria Antonia (Marie Antoinette), who later became queen of France, survived the infection without after-effects. It was to be the guillotine and not the smallpox virus that ended her life and that of her husband in 1793.

The list of members of ruling royal houses that became victims of the smallpox virus is much longer. The sixteen-year-old King Luis I of Spain died in 1724, after only eight months on the throne. His queen, Louise Elisabeth d'Orléans, who had faithfully nursed her husband while the rest of the court fled, became infected, but survived.

In Russia, the grandson of Peter the Great, thirteen-year-old Tsar Peter II, died of smallpox in 1729. He was the last of the male line of the Romanov dynasty. A few historians believe that he would probably have reversed many of the progressive reforms introduced by Peter the Great. His later successor Tsar Peter III survived smallpox, but was so greatly disfigured that it is believed it had serious psychological consequences for him. He entered into a highly unhappy marriage with his second cousin Sophia of Anhalt-Zerbst: it is uncertain what role she, now Tsarina Catherine, later called the Great, played in his assassination.

In Sweden the childless queen Ulrika Eleonora, who briefly succeeded her brother Carl XII after his death in battle before abdicating in favour of her husband, died of smallpox in 1741.

The smallpox virus also affected the succession in many other dynasties around the world, but we have less detailed information about this than for Europe.

The last phase of the battle

There are a number of reasons why historians have been so interested in the ravages of the smallpox virus in European royal houses. The prominent status of the royal victims meant that very often there was considerable publicity relating to the course of their illnesses, which can tell us quite a lot about the prevailing conceptions of disease and forms of treatment. In addition, the royal houses of former times had far more influence on politics than present-day monarchs. For that reason, their illnesses often made a considerable impact on politics both nationally and internationally, as we have already seen.

There are also reasons to believe that the dramatic inroads made by the smallpox virus in European royal houses gave the infection much publicity and led to greater efforts to speed up the development of effective medicinal measures against it. It is this struggle that has characterized the history of the smallpox virus over the past three hundred years – a long-drawn-out phase including dramatic events and medical breakthroughs. During this period, the battle between man and the smallpox virus has swayed back and forth until the virus was finally defeated and eradicated during the 1970s.[93]

A key element throughout this long period has been the gradual introduction of various forms of vaccination against the smallpox virus, starting with what is called inoculation (vaccination with ordinary smallpox virus), and then the more modern vaccination with a related but considerably 'milder' virus. We will return later to this history, one that comprises major advances, obstacles and setbacks, when dealing with vaccination in general.

Typhus: Napoleon's Nemesis

While such concepts as plague and cholera live on in people's consciousness – at any rate in the language – the infectious disease typhus has unquestionably been forgotten. This is really rather surprising, for during the past five hundred years typhus has given rise to epidemics large and small that have cost millions of human lives, including in Europe, where the infection still created serious problems during the Second World War.

Typhus, often referred to as epidemic or louse-borne typhus, is caused by the bacterium *Rickettsia prowazekii*. To understand why this bacterium has given rise to such major problems over the centuries, and why it has struck in particular situations, we have to take a closer look at the special infection mechanisms the disease employs. The history of typhus also illustrates many of the basic characteristics of the interaction between man, microbe and the environment.

Filth, lice and hunger – a deadly trio

Rickettsia prowazekii belongs to the rickettsia subgroup of bacteria, which has a series of special characteristics, notably that they are smaller than bacteria usually are and, like viruses, can reproduce only within living cells.[94]

The typhus bacterium is transmitted from human to human via lice, *Homo sapiens'* faithful companion since time immemorial. This is the key to understanding how infection occurs and why typhus epidemics arise. The connection was first discovered at the beginning of the twentieth century. When people live in close proximity to each other under conditions marked by a high level of filth, and most of them are plagued by lice, conditions are ideal for *Rickettsia prowazekii*. Malnourishment is very often part of the overall picture. The typhus bacterium has specialized in human beings and does not infect other species of animals, with one exception: flying squirrels in North America.

Before taking a closer look at the typhus bacterium and its henchmen – lice – we will consider the disease typhus itself, which can be extremely dramatic. One to two weeks after being infected, the victim, after feeling ill for a couple of days, suffers acutely painful headaches, and muscular and back pains. After four to five days there is a rash of red spots that often develop into small bleeding sores. The face, hands and soles of the feet are normally spared. At the same time the patient often becomes muddled and may lose consciousness or suffer attacks of cramp. The name of the disease comes from the Greek word *typhos*, which means misty or unclear.[95] There are often signs of pneumonia. Patients can also develop gangrene of the fingers, toes and other parts of the body, resulting in necrosis of the tissue and even in fingers and toes falling off. Without modern treatment, the case fatality rate is almost 60 per cent. Patients who recover are not free of the bacteria, which remain dormant in the body. Years later, they can become active once more and cause new disease.

A newcomer among epidemics

The typhus bacterium is nowhere near as old as a cause of epidemics in humans as, for example, the plague bacterium *Yersinia pestis*. It is possibly only about one thousand years old. The first epidemic of what we can be fairly certain was typhus occurred in Spain in 1489.[96] Christian Spain's reconquest – *La Reconquista* – of the southern part of the country after seven centuries of rule by the Moors from North Africa was then entering its concluding, furious phase with the capture of Granada, the Moors' last foothold. In the intoxication of victory, Queen Isabella and King Ferdinand decided to finance plans for a certain Christopher Columbus that were to have major consequences.

The recapture of Granada, however, did not take place without complications. The Christian army was attacked by a dangerous epidemic that was previously unknown: 17,000 soldiers died from the disease, whereas only 3,000 fell to Moorish weapons. Spanish chroniclers believed that the disease had been introduced by mercenaries from Cyprus, where they had contracted the disease from the Turks. Perhaps the typhus bacterium came from the East.

No matter its origins, the typhus bacterium spread during the next few years to all of Spain and Portugal. As early as the beginning of the sixteenth century it reached Italy, probably transported there by Spanish soldiers taking part in the endless war between Spain and France, where Italy was an important theatre of war. The French were thus obliged to break off from their promising siege of Naples in 1528 because their army was attacked by typhus.[97] Half of the soldiers died and the weakened survivors fell easy prey to guerrilla troops and murderous peasants as they retreated, in addition to the effects of typhus. The major political consequences of this led to Spain becoming the dominant power in Italy, with the pope as an obedient ally of Emperor Charles v. Indirectly, this also came to influence British history. For fear of offending the victorious and mighty emperor, the pope refused to approve the application for divorce made by the English king Henry VIII when he wished to divorce his Spanish queen, Catherine of Aragon, who was the emperor's aunt. This led to Henry declaring the English Church independent of the pope and starting the Reformation in England. He was now also free to approve a series of new queens for himself.

The new disease established itself in Europe during the sixteenth century.[98] We earlier met Girolamo Fracastoro, the universal talent from the Italian Renaissance, who wrote both a long poem about syphilis and a book in which he put forward his theory about infection. *De contagione et contagiosis morbis et eorum curatione*, which appeared in 1546, provides an excellent description of the pathological picture of typhus, with keen observations about the spread of epidemics.

Even as typhus gradually spread northwards in Europe, the typhus epidemics' centre of gravity was in Eastern Europe. For centuries Christian Europe fought against the Turks, who were still a potent threat. Twice the Turks stood outside the walls of Vienna – in 1529 and 1683 – and both times they were repulsed. The fighting against the Turks took place especially in Hungary and the Balkans. On several occasions German armies were attacked by serious epidemics that were probably typhus. Their Hungarian allies and Turkish opponents got off more lightly. This could indicate that they had developed immunity from earlier contact with the typhus bacterium. Hungary was called 'the Germans' grave' and for a time typhus was called 'the Hungarian disease'. When the German armies returned to the western parts of Europe, they brought typhus with them and started new epidemics. These continued in Europe until the nineteenth century.

We saw earlier how the plague bacterium raged during the Thirty Years War. Typhus, however, was just as great a problem, accompanied by dysentery, a bacterial intestinal infection. All the major wars that haunted Europe in the seventeenth and eighteenth centuries were accompanied by typhus epidemics, but one example is worthy of special mention: Napoleon's disastrous Russian campaign in 1812.

Cold, Cossacks and catastrophe

In 1812 Napoleon was at the pinnacle of his power. He was master of virtually the entire European mainland, and the tsar of Russia had been his ally for several years. The friendship between Napoleon and Tsar

Alexander, however, had cooled after the tsar had permitted himself to go against Napoleon's major political objectives. Napoleon decided to teach the tsar a lesson and to attack Russia. He gathered together an enormous army, which marched through Poland and East Prussia towards Russia in the summer of 1812. The *Grande Armée*, as it was known, comprised more than 600,000 men, of whom one-third were French, while the rest came from various allied countries. In addition, they were accompanied by many civilians, as was usual during military operations in earlier times.[99]

Napoleon's army, with banners waving and music playing, crossed the border at the River Niemen and entered Russia on 23 June. The summer, however, was unusually hot and dry, and the lack of water made it harder for the soldiers to wash and bathe. The local Polish and Russian population were unusually dirty and lice-ridden. On the march the soldiers commandeered the locals' simple shacks for over-night accommodation and naturally became infested with lice. These were areas where the typhus bacterium had exerted a firm grip for centuries, so it did not take long before the first instances of typhus were reported, with a steadily increasing number of deaths. Supply problems to the vast army also led to food shortages among the soldiers, who became increasingly undernourished. Polluted drinking water added waterborne infections such as dysentery, which contributed greatly to the ill-health of the soldiers, making them unfit for warfare. Despite this, the army thrust deeper and deeper into Russia, with regular skirmishes against the Russian army, which retreated using scorched-earth tactics until the armies finally clashed at Borodino. This battle was regarded as the bloodiest in recent history until the Battle of the Somme during the First World War.

On 15 September Napoleon was able to enter Moscow with a considerably reduced army of about 90,000 men, but the Russians quickly set the city on fire. All the while typhus continued to rage. The conquest of Moscow did not, however, lead to the end of the war, as Napoleon had counted on, and on 19 October he left the city with his troops and began to withdraw westwards. He had to leave several thousand typhus patients behind, nearly all of whom died. Throughout the retreat the French army was constantly harried, partly by regular Russian forces, partly by hordes of Cossacks on horseback, who struck fast and unexpectedly and then disappeared once more.

The Russian winter set in early that year, with low temperatures for which Napoleon's soldiers were neither clothed nor prepared. Snowfalls and bitter cold led to increasing numbers of soldiers freezing to death, and famine was rife. At night the soldiers were forced to huddle together to keep warm and for safety. What had once been a proud army was now characterized by filth and lice. Even the emperor was attacked by lice, which clearly still believed in the French Revolution principles of *egalité* and *fraternité*, which the emperor had apparently forgotten. Everything was perfectly set up for typhus, which raged among the soldiers as they staggered on until they often ended up lying by the roadside. Stragglers and those left behind by the main column were nearly always taken prisoner by Cossacks and infuriated peasants: at best they were robbed and left naked in the snow, but often they were beaten to death after horrible torture.[100]

We have accounts of the inconceivable suffering from a number of eyewitnesses, both ordinary soldiers and higher-ranking officers. Dramatic descriptions of this phase of the war are also to be found in one of world literature's great works, Leo Tolstoy's *War and Peace*. Despite the enormous suffering, which also afflicted the Russians, particularly the common people, the war of 1812 was unquestionably a Russian triumph, reflected in the music of Tchaikovsky's *1812 Overture*, which was commissioned for celebrations of the seventieth anniversary.

It is now estimated that around 400,000 soldiers from the *Grande Armée* lost their lives during the Russian campaign. Less than a quarter of them died in battle. A large proportion had been victims of typhus. Tens of thousands of civilians who had followed the army were also dead, partially because of typhus. It should be added that the Russian army pursuing the French also lost more than 60,000 men, most of them to typhus.[101]

The accounts of this catastrophe and description of the epidemic mean that we cannot be in any doubt that typhus was the disease in question. Here, however, we also have an example of how modern molecular biology can help provide a definitive diagnosis. In 2005 French researchers who had also worked on the plague detected DNA from *Rickettsia prowazekii* in corpses from a mass grave of French soldiers at Vilnius in present-day Lithuania.[102] This city had been a temporary reception area for the countless sick soldiers from the *Grande Armée* during the retreat, and a great many ended up in mass graves there.

French soldiers who returned home from Russia across parts of Central Europe brought with them the typhus bacterium, leaving behind numerous new cases. The hospitals where the badly wounded soldiers had been housed were very hard hit indeed. But 'General Typhus' was not yet finished with Napoleon: the new troops he had managed to assemble in his heroic but unsuccessful attempt to survive were also hard hit by the disease.[103]

The result of Napoleon's Russian campaign was to have considerable political consequences and marked the beginning of the end of his short-lived but glorious empire. His almost supernatural aura of invincibility began to fade and his many opponents, both nations and individuals, gained new courage to continue the fight. Despite heroic efforts and a number of military triumphs, Napoleon had to admit defeat after a further three years and begin his exile on St Helena.

We now know that the small, innocuous-looking bacterium *Rickettsia prowazekii* played an important role in Napoleon's downfall. One of Napoleon's top generals, Field Marshal Ney, called 'the bravest of the brave' after his heroic contribution during the retreat from Moscow, wrote to his wife: 'General Famine and General Winter, not Russian bullets, have defeated the *Grand Armée*.'[104] He forgot to mention 'General Typhus'.

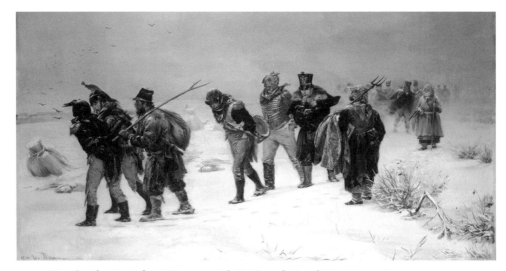

Napoleon's retreat from Moscow with *La Grande Armée* in autumn 1812 was one of the great disasters of military history, as seen in this painting by Illarion Pryanishnikov from 1874. The French soldiers suffered from the biting cold, they were constantly under attack from Russian forces, and typhus raged in the French army.

Death sentence for both judge and jury

Until well into the nineteenth century conditions in prisons were generally so wretched, with tightly crammed cells, filth, lice and bad food, that they were ideal for typhus. This became so common that it was often called 'jail fever'.[105] As such, prisons often served as the starting point of serious typhus epidemics that also came to affect those employed in the justice system. We have dramatic examples of this at the so-called Black Assizes in England from the end of the sixteenth century until 1750. At these court sittings, the judges and members of the jury, as well as many of those attending the sessions, became infected with typhus from sick prisoners. At one such trial in Oxford in 1577, the accused came directly from a prison where a number of inmates had just died from typhus while in chains. More than five hundred people died in connection with the court case. The accused, who was sentenced to have his ears nailed to the local pillory for blasphemy, survived.

Typhus also often raged on board ships, since the conditions were ideal for *Rickettsia prowazekii* and its henchmen: lice. 'Ship's fever' was therefore another frequent name for typhus.

We have previously noted famine and undernourishment as an important factor with relation to typhus epidemics. The importance of famine is dramatically illustrated by the great famine that afflicted Ireland between 1845 and 1851 after a fungal disease resulted in the failure of the potato harvests.[106] Ireland was one of the most densely populated countries in Europe, and social conditions were already bad in large sections of the population. Hand in hand with the famine, a typhus epidemic broke out, with terrible consequences. Naturally, filth and lice also played an important role here. A surprisingly large proportion of those in the upper echelons of society were also hit, especially those who, in the course of their work, came into close contact with typhus patients from the lower classes. Many doctors became victims of the disease. This may have been due to the fact that typhus is able in certain situations to infect without any assistance from lice.

The typhus epidemic in Ireland was accompanied by recurrent fever, an infection caused by another bacterium transmitted by lice, *Borelia recurrentis*. Modern historians estimate that at least half a million people died of these two infections, most of them probably of typhus.

The consequences of the Irish famine epidemic were considerable. It led to enormous emigration, particularly to North America. After the epidemic economic and social conditions improved for the poorest section of the population, as we also saw in the wake of the Black Death.[107] But the disaster also led to great and lasting bitterness towards England, since people felt that the British government had not done nearly enough to help the Irish people. Some even claimed that assistance was held back so as to reduce the size of the population.

Bolshevism, lice and world wars

From the mid-nineteenth century onwards typhus epidemics ebbed away in Western Europe, where *Rickettsia prowazekii* was no longer a serious problem, but the bacterium was still active in Eastern Europe and the Balkans. Then the it got its big chance: the first of the two bloody world wars, which was triggered by Austria declaring war on Serbia in July 1914 after the Austrian heir to the throne, Franz Ferdinand, was assassinated by Serbian terrorists.

The typhus bacterium struck first in the Balkans, as early as autumn 1914 in Serbia.[108] Then the epidemic exploded in camps holding thousands of Austrian prisoners of war, where the hygienic conditions were appalling. It spread with tremendous speed via the transportation of prisoners and troops. Practically all of Serbia's nearly four hundred doctors became infected and up to half of the 60,000 Austrian prisoners of war died. Military historians believe that at this point Serbia would have been helpless if Austria had mounted a full-scale attack. But this did not happen, because Austria feared the typhus epidemic. Thus Austria and its allies probably lost valuable time that might have had a decisive influence on the outcome of the war. Once again, General Typhus had crucially intervened in the course of a war.

To the east, the Austrians' German allies were fighting against Russia. The German troops here managed to keep typhus in check via effective hygienic and medical measures, but conditions on the Russian side were considerably worse. After the Russian government sued for peace in 1918, one of the largest of all typhus epidemics broke out across the country. At the same time, the civil war that followed the Bolshevik Revolution of 1917 brought about the only too well-known pattern of famine, social chaos and floods of refugees that provides optimal conditions for typhus among both soldiers and civilians. It is estimated that around 25 million people were infected with typhus between 1916 and 1921, and that 3 million died. A third of the doctors in the Red Army were infected, and a fifth of them died. The situation was so serious that Lenin is said to have remarked: 'Either socialism will defeat the louse, or the louse will defeat socialism.' On this occasion socialism won, and the typhus epidemic ebbed away.

During the Second World War both sides put in place fairly effective measures for combatting typhus among the soldiers, but a number of typhus epidemics broke out among the civilian population in war-torn areas, such as the Balkans, North Africa and the Far East.[109] Appalling tragedies took place in the German concentration camps, where tens of thousands died of typhus as a result of undernourishment and terrible hygienic conditions. In principle, it was in the interests of the camp commandants to fight typhus in order to ensure there were enough prisoners capable of providing labour, but the measures adopted were sometimes barbaric and contrary to all forms of medical ethics.[110] If an accommodation block was attacked by typhus, the rule was that all the prisoners in the block, both those with and without the disease, were to be killed. Individual patients with typhus were quite frequently killed after admission to the camp hospital. The ss doctors also carried out experiments on prisoners by injecting them with contaminated blood in order to see how long they remained infectious; they were subsequently killed. The German-Dutch girl Anne Frank, famous for her gripping diary, died of typhus at the age of fifteen in the Bergen-Belsen concentration camp.[111]

A macabre aspect of the war against typhus is that the gas Zyklon-B, used in the mass-killing of Jews and other prisoners at extermination camps such as Auschwitz, was originally manufactured as a disinfectant by German chemists in 1923, when it was believed to mark an advance in combatting lice – and thereby also typhus.[112]

Typhus has played an extremely minor role in Europe over the last few decades, but it is still active in other parts of the world, particularly Africa and Central and South America.[113] A comprehensive epidemic that broke out in connection with the civil war in Burundi in the 1990s is known to have caused more than 45,000 cases, of which 15 per cent of the patients died.

Of lice and men: the evolutionary history of the typhus bacterium

The special group of bacteria (*Rickettsia*) to which the typhus bacterium belongs possibly began their career in the distant past by infecting various kinds of insect. Some of these gradually developed the capacity to support themselves as blood-suckers of higher species of animals, particularly many types of rodents. The accompanying bacteria, like the insects, adapted themselves in turn to the animals, which led to infection. After hundreds of thousands of years' adaptation, the bacteria have attained a kind of peaceful coexistence with both the insects and rodents they infect, and neither insects nor rodents fall ill. Unfortunately, developments did not stop there. Some of the blood-sucking insects that took part in this interaction found it occasionally necessary to fetch their blood-meal from humans. And if the insect in question was a carrier of the bacteria, this could result in infection and illness.

This sequence of development is not simply an armchair theory. We now know that *Rickettsia typhi*, a bacterium closely related to that which causes typhus, is found in rats.[114] Occasionally, humans are infected by being bitten by the oriental rat flea, *Xenopsylla cheopis*, which we met earlier in connection with the plague. This results in an infection that resembles ordinary typhus, but it is considerably milder and has a much lower mortality rate. It is reasonable to believe that 'our' bacterium – the typhus bacterium – has developed further from this relative. The great breakthrough probably came when the bacterium learned how to infect human lice. It then acquired the ability to bring about human-to-human infection. Once again, we see an example of the microbes' impressive ability to adapt via evolution.

Since lice play a key role in typhus and a number of other infectious diseases, the species actually deserves a closer look. It is first and foremost the human body louse, with the full name *Pediculus humanus corporis*, that is central to typhus.[115] It spends its life in human clothing, interrupted only by meals of blood, which it sucks from its host four or five times a day. Louse eggs are also laid in clothing. When a louse sucks blood from a typhus victim, it too becomes infected since the bacteria are found in the blood. The bacteria penetrate the cells in the louse's intestines and are excreted in the faeces, which are fine-grained, like powder. When an infected louse bites another healthy human, infection does not occur from the sucking of blood. It takes place because louse excrement containing bacteria is rubbed into the skin when the bite starts to itch and the human scratches it. Infection can also take place if the powdery louse excrement is inhaled. The bacteria can survive in the louse excrement for several months.

It is first and foremost the adaptation by the bacterium to lice that has made possible the major typhus epidemics down through history. To be completely fair, it should be said that the infected louse pays with its life after about three weeks. Often its intestines burst, turning the louse blood-red.

It was Charles Nicolle, who worked in North Africa after a time at the Pasteur Institute in Paris, who discovered the significance of lice for typhus and realized that they had to be carriers of the microbe transmitting the disease.[116] This was a considerable breakthrough, one that enabled effective means of fighting the disease; Nicolle's award of the Nobel Prize in 1928 was well deserved. The person who discovered the actual bacterium in lice from typhus patients was Stanislaus von Prowazek, who in the course of his researches with Henrique da Rocha Lima became infected and died, but his memory lives on in the name given to the bacterium, *Rickettsia prowazekii*. The fatal nature of the *Rickettsia* bacteria is further illustrated by the fact that Howard Taylor Ricketts, who identified the first bacterium in this group, of which typhus is a member, also lost his life to the disease.

When we look at the cultural history of the louse, we also realize that a fertile soil for typhus epidemics has existed for almost the whole of human history. Lice have followed *Homo sapiens* from the very outset, as a legacy from our more hirsute ancestors. Lice have been found on Egyptian mummies, and throughout the Middle Ages they were widespread, especially because cleanliness had such a low status. As late as the seventeenth century lice were widespread in all social classes. Courts had their own rules of etiquette as to how one's own and other people's lice could be dealt with in an elegant manner.

It is not only the typhus bacterium that makes use of the louse as a Trojan horse for infection. This also applies to *Bartonella quintana*, a relation of *Rickettsia prowazekii*, which causes a condition known as 'trench foot' that plagued soldiers in the trenches on the Western front during the First World War. As has been mentioned earlier, lice have recently become a focus of attention when seeking to explain the infection mechanism of the Black Death, where previously the main role had been assigned to fleas.

Do we know all the secrets of the typhus bacterium?

For a long time it went almost without saying that *Rickettsia prowazekii* differed from all its relatives by exclusively infecting humans and having no reservoirs in the animal world, such as we see with zoonoses. In 1975, however, it was discovered that the typhus bacterium also infects a special type of rodent on the eastern seaboard of the USA, the southern flying squirrel.[117] Occasionally the bacterium can be transmitted from squirrel to human via a flea bite. In Europe there is no known corresponding animal reservoir – but have we looked closely enough?

Can the typhus bacterium remain in the population without infected lice or any animal reservoir? Yes: it turns out that the bacterium does not completely let go of its victim even if the patient becomes completely healthy and free of symptoms. Somewhere or other in the body (we have no idea where) the bacterium goes into hiding. After many years during which the host is completely without symptoms, the bacterium can once more become active and produce signs of illness like those of common typhus, although they are often less severe. We do not know for certain what 'wakes up' the bacterium, but a weakening of the immune system for some reason or other is the probable explanation. Lice do not have anything to do with this, but if this 'resurrection' of the bacterium takes place in an environment where lice are widespread, the spread of infection can occur in the usual manner.

I began this section by stating that typhus, despite its highly sinister history of millions of human lives on its conscience, has disappeared from the common consciousness. But the bacterium has not disappeared from the surface of the earth, as the smallpox virus has done. It can still cause big problems if the conditions are right – or, as the German-American researcher Hans Zinsser writes in his book *Rats, Lice and History* (1934): 'Typhus is not dead. It will live on for centuries, and it will continue to break into the open whenever human stupidity and brutality give it a chance, as most likely they occasionally will.'

Cholera: The Violet Death

Like the plague, cholera has also entered many languages as an expression for a choice between two evils – plague and cholera. In English this corresponds to a choice between the Devil and the deep blue sea. This saying is probably an echo of the great fear created by the cholera epidemics of the nineteenth century, for cholera was and is a truly dramatic and frightening disease.

Cholera is caused by the small, comma-shaped bacterium *Vibrio cholerae*, which provokes an acute and often violent intestinal infection. Its manner of appearance down through history is a highly illustrative example of many aspects of the duel between man and microbe, showing its virtuoso ability to adapt to external circumstances, particularly climatic factors. Cholera epidemics have had considerable political and cultural consequences and had an important role in the development of medicine and the health services during the nineteenth century.

The cholera bacterium was detected by Robert Koch in 1883 and he gave it the name *Vibrio cholerae*. Since then it has become clear that it was in fact an obscure Italian anatomist, Filippo Pacini, who discovered the bacterium as early as 1854 and deduced that it was the cause of cholera. This passed unnoticed in Italy, where the miasma theories were still

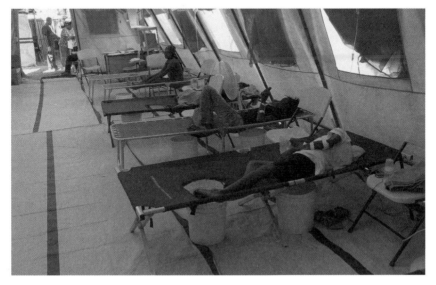

Improvised ward for cholera patients, with special 'cholera beds' including drains for fluid, during the epidemic in Haiti in 2016.

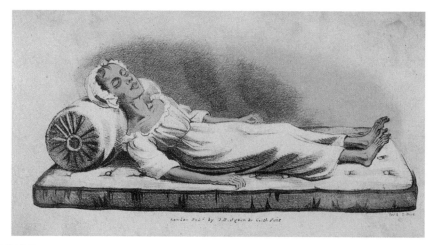

A dead cholera victim, with the characteristic violet skin colour that gave the disease the epithet 'the violet death'.

strongly believed at the time. He died the same year Koch published his discovery. It was not until 1965 that Pacini received greatly belated recognition of his discovery, when the cholera bacterium was renamed *Vibrio cholerae pacini*.[118]

The cholera bacterium does not infect any species of animal other than humans. It is first and foremost connected with water. Infection takes place when water or food that contains bacteria is ingested, most often by the water being polluted with bacterial excrement. Between less than a day and five days after infection the patient experiences nausea and violent diarrhoea, with up to a litre of liquid being excreted per hour. This enormous loss of liquid leads to severe dehydration. Because of the large quantities of liquid that patients excrete, special 'cholera beds' are used where the diarrhoea liquid is collected in special containers. In the space of a few hours, the patient becomes a shrunken caricature of him- or herself and gradually acquires a blue-violet skin colour, which has led to the term 'the violet death'. Finally, the blood pressure falls and the patient dies, sometimes after only a few hours. If untreated, most people die within the first 24 hours of the disease.[119]

It is uncertain where the term 'cholera' comes from. It was used by Hippocrates and other writers of antiquity about isolated cases of heavy diarrhoea. The name 'cholera' is probably derived from the ancient Greek term for drainpipes from gutters, reflecting the violent, watery diarrhoea.[120] The cases that Hippocrates described were not infections

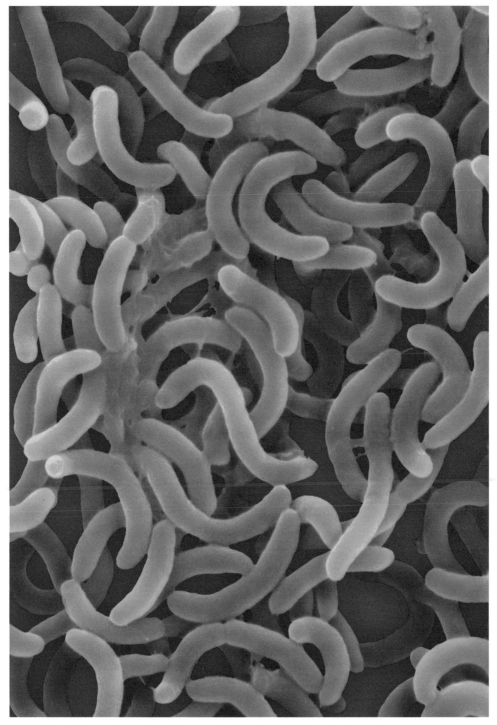

The typical comma-shaped cholera bacterium – *Vibrio cholerae*.

caused by the cholera bacterium, since in all probability it did not exist in Europe at that time.

The detection of the bacterium in 1883 was one of Robert Koch's major triumphs, but it turned out that this did not solve all the problems. *Vibrio cholerae* still had many secrets up its sleeve. And almost 150 years after Koch's discovery, it still gives rise to great suffering in a number of places in the world.

The threat from the East

Where does the cholera bacterium come from? Once again, as in the case of the plague and typhus, we have to turn our gaze to the East. The present prevailing view is that cholera originated in India: the disease was therefore formerly often called Asian cholera.

When did the first cholera epidemic take place? Ancient Sanskrit writings from 500 BC talk about cases of a disease resembling cholera. But did the disease occur in the form of epidemics so early? The Portuguese explorer Vasco da Gama landed on the southwest coast of India in 1498, after having sailed round the Cape of Good Hope. One of his officers, Gaspar Correa, relates that there must have been a local cholera epidemic in India in 1503, with 20,000 deaths. We estimate that similar epidemics unquestionably raged both before this and during the succeeding centuries, but were limited to the Indian subcontinent – until the fateful year of 1817.[121]

The seven pandemics

After the cholera bacterium had ravaged India for centuries, perhaps millennia, it set out in 1817 for other countries and parts of the world. This was to mark the beginning of a total of seven veritable pandemics.[122] After each of the first six, the bacterium appeared to retreat to its homeland, India – to be more precise, the considerable delta areas at the mouth of the Ganges in the Bay of Bengal, which for a long time was the 'headquarters' of the cholera bacterium. But the seventh pandemic is ongoing and does not give any impression of losing its hold in various parts of the world.

Without going into too much detail, we will look briefly at the seven pandemics and how widely they spread before considering their consequences. The global spread of cholera in these pandemics illustrates a number of the environmental factors involved in the interaction between man and microbe. There is some disagreement among historians about the precise dating of these pandemics, but that is of lesser importance in this context.

The *first pandemic* started in 1817 in the established core area for cholera in the Bay of Bengal. A major epidemic then broke out in the major city of Calcutta (now Kolkata), and cholera spread rapidly during the following months to most of the Indian subcontinent. Some of this was connected to the redeployment of military forces of the East India Company, which then controlled large parts of India. It is possible that this was the first time that the cholera bacterium had led to an extensive epidemic, perhaps because it had now fully adapted itself to the human race.

In the following years the epidemic spread both eastwards to Thailand, Burma, Malaya, Indonesia, China and Japan, and westwards to the Middle East, as far as the Syrian Mediterranean coast. It also penetrated the southernmost part of Russia. Europe was not attacked during the first pandemic, which burned out in 1824, except in its 'homeland', where it continued to remain active.

The *second pandemic* started once more in the Indian core area in 1827 and quickly spread westwards through Afghanistan and Persia to Russia along the trade routes. This time it did not stop at the Russian border areas but spread inexorably through Russia. From there it moved on westwards to Poland (partly via Russian troops), and then to Germany and the Baltic states. It then spread across to England, and in 1832 Western Europe, including France and particularly Paris, were badly affected. Over the next couple of years the pandemic spread to Southern Europe.

During this second pandemic, the rest of Asia west of India got off lightly. But, running parallel with the cholera attack on Europe, the pandemic had this time spread to the Middle East. There, in connection with the Muslim *hajj* (the pilgrimage to Mecca), the hosts of pilgrims contributed to a considerable extent to the spread of cholera from Mecca to the pilgrims' various home countries in the Middle East and Africa. In spring 1831 there were possibly almost 30,000 deaths in the holy cities of Mecca and Medina alone. Cairo may have lost 15 per cent of its population to the epidemic.

This time, however, *Vibrio cholerae* did not content itself with the Old World. In the summer of 1832 it arrived in Canada and the USA, and in the following year the West Indies and Latin America were affected.

It was, then, during the second cholera epidemic that Europe and North America for the first time made the acquaintance of this dramatic infectious disease. This had psychological, political and cultural consequences that had not been surpassed since the Black Death. The mortality rate was considerable in all the affected countries. In Paris alone, which at the time had around 800,000 inhabitants, there were 18,000 deaths from cholera in 1832, and in April of that year there were 700 deaths a week.

By 1837 this pandemic was on the point of dying out outside India, and many people thus consider this to be the year it ended.

The third pandemic broke out in 1839, with India once more the core area. Once again it was sections of the British army that were responsible for the first spread of the disease. British troops brought cholera to Afghanistan and to South West Asia and China during the First Opium War, when the British forced China to open up opium trading. Cholera then spread westwards from China to Central Asia. At the same time,

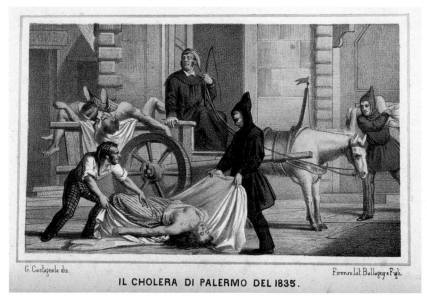

IL CHOLERA DI PALERMO DEL 1835.

The town of Palermo on Sicily was hard hit during the second cholera epidemic, which started in 1827 and lasted until 1837.

the cholera bacterium took the sea route westwards from India to Iraq and Arabia, where once again Muslim pilgrims were affected. Once more the disease spread westwards to most of Europe and then to the USA in 1848. Gradually the West Indies and several countries in South America were affected.

In 1854 French troops on their way to the Crimean War brought cholera to Greece and Turkey. It contributed to the many infection problems during the hostilities in 1853–6, during which Florence Nightingale, among others, made great efforts to improve the sanitary conditions in the military hospitals.[123]

The year 1854 was one of the worst for cholera in Europe. It was during this year that John Snow made his discoveries in London, but his conclusion that the infection was waterborne was not immediately accepted. From 1856 onwards this pandemic burned out nearly everywhere with the exception of Japan, which in 1858 was hit via the one port that was open to trade with the West, Nagasaki.

The *fourth pandemic* broke out in 1863, once more from India. Cholera spread by sea to Africa and northwards through the Red Sea to the centres of the *hajj*: Mecca, Medina and the port of Jedda. Of the 90,000 pilgrims in Mecca in the spring of 1865 some 15,000 died of cholera. From there the disease was taken back to the pilgrims' home countries in the Middle East and North Africa: 60,000 died in Egypt in the course of just two months. From there the bacterium crossed the Mediterranean and attacked most European countries before spreading to the USA and the West Indies.

Religion played a considerable role in the spread of cholera in India via the large pilgrimages in connection with Hindu festivals. Three million people gathered at a holy site beside the River Ganges in 1867: 250,000 pilgrims became infected and half of them died. In the course of 1874, however, the pandemic ebbed away.

The *fifth pandemic* started from its usual base in India in 1881 and lasted until 1896. It spread to a number of countries in East Asia as well as westwards, also via Muslim pilgrims on their way to Mecca, which once again was hard hit. From there cholera struck Egypt, with 58,000 deaths in 1883. It was during this pandemic in Cairo that Robert Koch and his colleagues carried out the fundamental investigations that led to the detection of the cholera bacterium. Once again, the disease

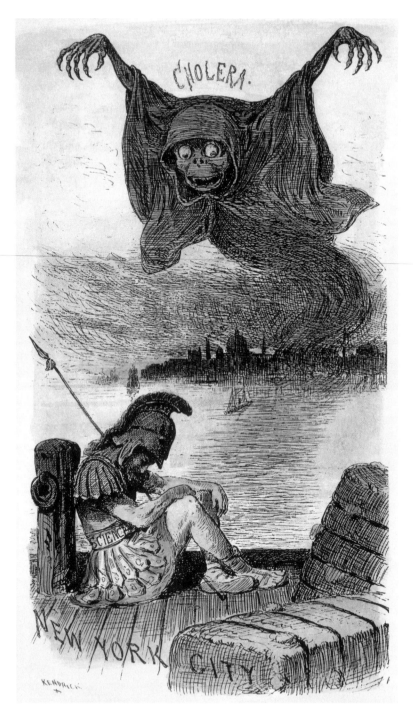

American drawing from 1883 that shows how the authorities (and science) sleep while the cholera ghost threatens them. The fear of cholera was considerable in the population.

crossed the Mediterranean, starting epidemics in a number of European countries, and crossed the Atlantic to several South American countries. North America got off lightly thanks to active countermeasures, including quarantine.

In Naples cholera struck in 1884 with a violence that almost paralysed the city. The young Swedish doctor and writer Axel Munthe sent gripping reports home to Swedish newspapers and also described the epidemic in Naples in the book that made him famous, *Boken om San Michele* (The Story of San Michele).[124]

The *sixth pandemic* broke out in India with great violence in 1899 (10 per cent of all deaths in India in 1900 were due to cholera) and lasted until 1923. The pandemic spread eastwards to South East Asia, Indonesia, the Philippines and China, and westwards, initially to the Middle East and Russia. After a pause of a couple of years, it moved into the Balkans and Italy. It gained new breeding grounds during the Russian Revolution and the First World War. This time the American continent was spared a pandemic.

The *seventh pandemic*, which began in 1961, differed in several ways from the previous ones.[125] First, the cause was a variant of the cholera bacterium that was given the name *El Tor* after the small Egyptian town where it was first detected among some Muslim pilgrims to Mecca.

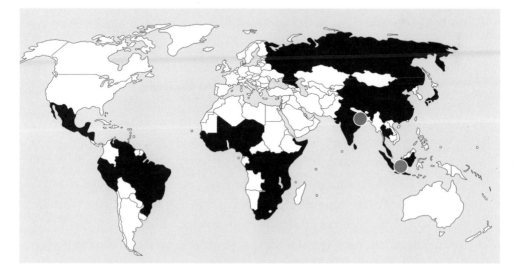

The first six pandemics all started in the Bay of Bengal (red circle), while the seventh originated in Indonesia (blue circle). Black areas indicate the spread of this ongoing pandemic.

Second, it did not start in India as had the previous six, but in Indonesia. Third, it was shown in a number of examples that this time the bacterium had spread via air travel, while the others had all followed traditional land and sea routes.

In the first phase of the pandemic a number of countries in East Asia were hit, but the disease also travelled westwards to India and the Middle East, and followed 'old' paths into the Soviet Union and from the Arabian Peninsula to East Africa. But now a number of countries in West Africa were also hard hit, via passengers arriving by air from Asia. Spain, Portugal and Italy were next in line.

In 1991, thirty years after the pandemic had begun, the cholera bacterium struck with violent force in Latin America, first in Peru, but then spreading to several other countries. By the end of the year there were 391,000 cases in Latin America, equivalent to two thirds of all the cholera cases in the world.

This latest pandemic also differed from earlier ones in that there was now far greater knowledge about cholera, particularly when it comes to prevention and treatment.[126] We now know that simply administering a large amount of fluid has a striking effect on recovery from this intestinal infection. For that reason, the case fatality rate from cholera is now far lower, perhaps 2 or 3 per cent as against 50 per cent in earlier times. Even so, cholera has a firm stronghold in many places around the world outside India: it has become what is called endemic. More or less widespread local epidemics break out at regular intervals at various places in the world whenever the now well-known ecological and environmental factors are favourable.[127] Examples are Haiti, where cholera broke out in 2010 after the destruction caused by the earthquake, and Yemen, which has an ongoing epidemic in the wake of the war there.

Miasmas or contagion from person to person?

When the cholera bacterium arrived in Europe and North America at the beginning of the nineteenth century, it came, so to speak, to a table ready laid. The sanitary conditions in the towns, which since the early Middle Ages had been extremely poor, became even worse during the Industrial Revolution.[128] The influx of industrial workers from the rural areas had created widespread slum areas where the poor population lived in very cramped conditions and had limited access to clean water and terrible sewage problems. Excrement was often thrown out onto the streets or into open ditches and holes, or was sometimes even stored in cellars. The potential for pollution of wells with human faeces was great. Drinking water was often fetched from rivers and other sources that were highly polluted with human refuse. Personal hygiene in these slum areas was also extremely bad. All the conditions were set for the cholera bacterium to spread in a highly effective manner, which is what happened from the second pandemic onwards, when the disease hit Western countries with full force.

Although no stratum of the population got off scot-free, it was quite obvious throughout the nineteenth century that it was in particular the lower social classes that were worst hit by cholera. This was partly due to the conditions in the slum areas, and partly to the fact that many groups of working people were in regular contact with infectious material of various types.

We have seen earlier that the struggle between the two most important explanatory models for infectious diseases and epidemics – miasmas and person-to-person infection – was fierce throughout much of the nineteenth century until the results of the bacteriological revolution were finally generally accepted, something which actually took some time even after the epoch-making discoveries of Koch and Pasteur in the 1870s and '80s.[129] It was not until the fifth pandemic that the cause of cholera and the method of infection were clarified.

More than any other infectious disease, cholera became central in the debate between supporters of the miasma theory in various guises and those who believed that it was a question of infectious materials that were transmitted from one person to another. The contrasting views naturally had consequences for the practical efforts made to combat cholera. Various forms of quarantine (measures that attempt to keep possibly infectious persons separate from the rest of society for a certain period of time) had been used as far back as the fourteenth century when combatting the plague, but quarantine had gradually become less frequently used.[130] Most countries now brushed the dust off their old quarantine regulations. Forced isolation or commitment to a cholera hospital was used in certain places, as was the setting up of so-called cordons sanitaires, employing militarily guarded borders to prevent the traffic of infectious persons. Such measures often led to violent reactions in the population, and people quickly started to doubt that they had any practical value against cholera. There was also considerable resistance to the quarantine regulations from industry, which regarded the measures as detrimental to trade. Many representatives of the medical profession also opposed the infection theory for most of the nineteenth century. All of this means that most countries slackened the implementation of the various compulsory measures somewhat from the second cholera pandemic onwards.

As early as antiquity, the stench from garbage, polluted water and rotting waste seemed to reinforce the belief in the role of miasmas in diseases. People believed that pathogenic miasmas could arise under such conditions. This way of thinking was unquestionably important for the so-called sanitary movement, which in the latter half of the nineteenth century was extremely active in improving urban slum areas with better sewage, waste disposal and personal hygiene and ensuring a clean water supply.[131] These efforts, which began in Britain but inspired many other countries, could show major advances by the end of the century. Even though the miasma theory underlay it, it is certain that the work influenced the combatting of cholera and other important infectious diseases such as tuberculosis. These measures could also to a great extent be defended after the infection theories made their impact in the bacteriological revolution.

But there was considerable opposition from many quarters against drawing the necessary conclusions from the breakthrough of infection theory. A good example of this is the cholera epidemic in Hamburg in 1892, during the fifth pandemic.[132] Hamburg was in effect a city state and its authorities had cited the need to take its economy and economic interests into account as the reason to decline introducing aggressive health measures to combat epidemics. When cholera struck, with several thousand deaths, the city was therefore badly prepared. The imperial government sent Robert Koch in person, who was authorized to combat the epidemic according to all the new principles of bacteriology. A number of his measures, however, were sabotaged by the city authorities.

When the German government tried to pass a national law on epidemics, based on Koch's recommendations, the proposal was initially rejected by the Reichstag. The highly respected physician Max von

Pettenkofer, who had many supporters for a long time, fought tenaciously against Koch's cholera discoveries until he realized that the fight was lost and committed suicide.

War, class struggle and revolution

From the earliest times, war and epidemics have been linked together. This also applies to cholera. Throughout large parts of the nineteenth century, cholera was often connected to war and troop movements.

The nineteenth century was also characterized by considerable social and political unrest, in particular by strong class conflict that had been exacerbated by the Industrial Revolution.[133] On the one hand, an influential and self-aware bourgeoisie had come into being, and on the other there was a large, poor lower class. The marked political tension between the classes manifested itself time and time again in political unrest and revolutions – and cholera tended to strike during such political crises. Cholera swept across Europe in the wake of the July revolution of 1830, and again during the February revolution of 1848, which was perhaps one of the worst years for cholera in Europe in the entire century. It was not cholera that triggered the revolutions, but the cholera bacterium spread effectively in connection with streams of refugees and with troops that were employed to put down the revolutions.

Cholera could also trigger political unrest and disturbances in a more direct way. This was clearly seen at the beginning of the second pandemic in Europe in the 1830s. Many governments then implemented the 'old' type of compulsory measures in combatting the epidemic, including strict quarantine regulations. This was highly unpopular in many places, because it interfered with many people's jobs and the transportation of goods, which could lead to price increases and food shortages. In Paris the so-called *chiffoniers*, a workforce that scratched a living by combing through refuse, set about building barricades and committing acts of arson after the authorities, for sanitary reasons, introduced a centralized form of refuse collection as a means to combat the disease. This caused older Parisians to recall the great Revolution of 1789.

In St Petersburg unrest arose when the authorities began roughly rounding up all people who might possibly be infected, as well as any other undesirables, and interning them in special cholera infirmaries. One such infirmary was stormed by the mob, killing a doctor and 'liberating' in triumph the living and the dead. The tsar was obliged to call in the army to put down the disturbances.

In many places doctors were particularly exposed to aggressive responses from the population because they were regarded as the authorities' henchmen in imposing the many unpopular measures against the epidemic.[134] More paranoid ideas also led to attacks on doctors. In France the view became widespread that the doctors had been instructed by the upper class to poison the drinking water in order to get rid of the poor. Such views derived from the fact that the poorer classes were hit by cholera much harder than the bourgeoisie and the upper class.

In Britain, many people believed that the doctors were simply trying to acquire corpses for dissection when teaching medical students. This came in the wake of a court case against two notorious mass murderers, William Burke and William Hare, who had taken the lives of some sixteen people in order to sell their corpses to the medical faculty of Edinburgh University.

The marked polarization between the social classes in connection with cholera was also seen in the attitude of the bourgeoisie to this disease. Modesty and the denial of bodily functions has seldom reached the heights prevalent among the middle class of the nineteenth century. Few diseases challenged these attitudes to the same extent as cholera, where patients, fully conscious, spent their last hours bathed in their own violent diarrhoea. People spoke of cholera involving a *mort de chien* ('a dog's death'), not the beautiful death that fascinated people of the time in literature and art. Since the epidemics affected the poor to such an extent, middle-class people felt that this highly unaesthetic disease must have its roots in filth and a directly immoral lifestyle; the poor clearly had only themselves to blame. The claim that the epidemics originated in India, where the indigenous population were particularly hard hit, also led to the British stigmatizing the native people in a similar way.

The nineteenth century was a time of growing imperialism among the major European powers. The threat that cholera represented to Europe led to the colonial powers combatting the epidemics with full force outside Europe, both in countries totally under their political control and in a number of independent states.[135] Large-scale Muslim and Hindu pilgrimages were particularly important in spreading the cholera bacterium in several of the epidemics. During the fifth and sixth epidemics the major powers struck with attempts to impose strict quarantine measures against pilgrims, for example in India, which was under British control, and in Persia (present-day Iran). The British also established a quarantine station at the southern tip of the Arabian Peninsula in order to monitor pilgrim traffic to Mecca. All these measures led to considerable discontent among those affected, since they regarded them as an arrogant infringement of their rights by Europeans.

The capricious behaviour of the cholera bacterium in nature

The cholera bacterium (*Vibrio cholerae*) was to prove to have far more secrets than Robert Koch and his successors were aware of. The highly complex life and behaviour of the bacterium in nature are still far from being fully understood.

The bacterium causes the life-threatening diarrhoea illness primarily because it has the ability to reproduce actively in the human intestines and produce a special toxin that affects the mucous membrane, making it unable to absorb water from the intestines as it normally does, which results in a highly fluid diarrhoea.[136]

The common conception of the way in which the cholera bacterium infected was that it behaved like so many other microbes that are transmitted from person to person via what is called faecal-oral infection, by ingesting food and drink that has in some way been polluted by faeces containing bacteria. This is still accepted, but in recent decades it has become clear that this is not the whole truth. It transpires that the cholera bacterium, which it was assumed only affects humans, is in fact a water bacterium that can happily live in both salt and fresh water if the right conditions are present.

In water, the cholera bacterium can swim freely, but this makes for a dangerous existence. It has therefore adapted itself to a more protected life by allying itself to living organisms in water, in particular to tiny crustaceans that are part of the plankton in the sea, and also to algae, insect eggs, large crustacea and fish.[137] In these protective environments the bacterium has considerably improved its chances of survival, and it can also get free transport over shorter and longer distances via plankton streams, insects and even birds.

Are all the cholera bacteria we find in water dangerous and pathogenic? No: there are more than two hundred variants of the bacterium, and only three of them cause cholera, because it is only these variants that have the necessary genetic equipment to produce the cholera toxin and the other virulence factors necessary for the bacterium to be able to cause infection in human intestines. The disturbing thing, however, is that the cholera bacterium, like many others, has a number of possibilities for changing its genetic make-up by, quite simply, picking up new genes from its surroundings.[138] Special DNA molecules (plasmids) can, for example, transport new genes into a bacterium as a supplement to those that are already there. This can also take place precisely with the genes that are needed for an innocent cholera bacterium to transform into a life-threatening cause of epidemics. If the conditions for this are right, such arming of previously harmless bacteria can without question take place in the aquatic existence of the cholera bacterium.

The important new knowledge about the existence of the cholera bacterium in water was first acquired by examining water from the Bay of Bengal, the original home of the bacterium and the area where the first six pandemics all started. Cholera epidemics have undoubtedly started there for centuries. What has triggered them? How have the bacteria from the Bay of Bengal, so to speak, gone ashore and initiated the person-to-person infection that has long been believed in? Recent research has shown that ecological conditions, linked to climatic variations, probably play a key role.

Somewhat simplified, one could say that the connection between climate and cholera epidemic seems to be that, when changes in the climate increase the temperature of the water and improve the nutritive conditions for plankton and other aquatic organisms, a marked growth increase takes place in the plankton and its 'stowaways', the cholera bacteria.[139] Not only that – the same climatic changes increase the tendency of the cholera bacteria to alter their genes, which can lead to the number of pathogenic cholera bacteria increasing in the water. This can trigger a cholera epidemic.

Humans have an important protective mechanism against cholera bacteria: the acid gastric juice that kills a great many of the cholera bacteria that are swallowed. It is estimated that at least 100 million bacteria must normally be swallowed to cause an infection. If climatic changes have led to a considerable increase in the pathogenic bacteria in water, this limit can be reached when sources of drinking water are contaminated. This can be the start of an epidemic, especially where poor sanitary conditions for dealing with human excrement and limited access to clean drinking water mean that person-to-person infection gets underway.

In the core area for cholera, present-day Bangladesh, conditions have always been optimal for these underlying cholera mechanisms. During the seventh pandemic, it turns out that the cholera bacterium is now also present in coastal water in many parts of the world, including North and South America, Africa and Asia. There is still a certain amount of disagreement as to the importance of the water in these areas as a reservoir for the cholera bacterium, since some still believe that epidemics are only triggered when new carriers of infection enter from other countries where cholera still occurs. It is nevertheless a fact that major epidemics are extremely often preceded by changes of climate, including the El Niño phenomenon, which lead to increased water temperatures and increased precipitation that prepare the way for the sudden surge in pathogenic cholera bacteria in water.[140]

Natural disasters such as earthquakes, volcanic eruptions, tsunamis and floods can also trigger cholera epidemics. In such cases, the most important factor is probably a major breakdown in sanitary conditions, with a considerably increased risk of cholera infection in the usual way by faecal-oral infection.[141]

There is still a great deal we do not know about the complex life of the cholera bacterium in nature and the factors that pave the way for epidemics caused by this unpredictable microbe. A few researchers believe that systematically checking the water condition of cholera-prone locations can provide a kind of cholera warning, perhaps through using such hi-tech methods as satellite surveillance of plankton and algae.[142]

We are by no means finished with cholera, even though our Western societies are no longer threatened by major epidemics, thanks to modern sanitary conditions. Nevertheless, 3–5 million people per year contract cholera, resulting in 100,000 deaths. This is completely unacceptable if we consider that a cholera patient can be saved using very simple means, supplying oral fluid in less severe cases or intravenously in more serious ones, supplemented by antibiotics.

The fear of global warming, which will bring about increased temperatures in seawater, also gives grounds for concern regarding the spread of the cholera bacterium via plankton streams to more northern waters, even to the coasts of Scandinavia.

Measles: Not Just a Harmless Children's Disease

Before vaccination against measles was introduced in the late 1960s, practically everyone contracted measles during childhood. This infection is therefore a typical example of so-called children's diseases. Infection with the measles virus also illustrates a number of other interesting facets of the interaction between man and microbe.

When did measles appear on the scene in the history of human infection? This virus is a typical example of a microbe that causes what are referred to as 'crowd infections'. These are microbes, often viruses, that cause acute infections that either lead to complete recovery with lifelong immunity or to death, and therefore they are completely dependent on constantly infecting new individuals if they are to remain 'floating' in the population. Such infections can only occur in populations of a considerable size.[143]

This means that the measles virus cannot have appeared as a cause of illness in *Homo sapiens* before large societies had emerged after humans had become settlers with agriculture and animal husbandry. Such conditions were first fulfilled around 5,000 years ago in Mesopotamia and some time later in other parts of the world.[144] In other words, the measles virus can hardly be more than 5,000 years old: ancestors from earlier times – hunters and gatherers – did not get measles.

Why did measles arise after the first epidemiological transition to societies that were populous enough? We have obtained the probable answer to this from what we call comparative virus research, investigations of related viruses in various animal species. The measles virus must have come from a species of large animal with which humans had regular contact. It belongs to a family with various representatives in many different animals, including dogs, cattle, pigs, goats and seals. Some of these viruses are so similar to the human virus that it is probable that they have a common progenitor and that they have subsequently developed in different directions. The virus in the animal world that is most similar to the measles virus is the so-called rinderpest virus, which causes an acute infection in cattle.[145] The common progenitor in all probability caused the infection in cattle and then, probably after many unsuccessful attempts, managed to hop over onto humans and adapt to its new host. Today's measles virus, under natural conditions, only causes infection in humans, not other animal species.

There are reasons for believing that the measles virus down through the ages may have changed its characteristics to a certain extent, and perhaps the virus in former times was a deal more dangerous than the present one.

Not just an innocuous disease

The term 'childhood disease' in present-day usage signals a fairly harmless illness that most children have to get through without there being any cause for alarm. In most cases in the developed world, the course of the disease corresponds to this description.

Measles is a highly infectious disease. The virus is found in considerable amounts in the patient, including the respiratory tract. Infection takes place if the virus is flung out into the surroundings when the patient coughs, sneezes or talks, either in the form of droplets or in extremely small air particles, aerosols, which are then breathed in by other people. The majority of those who are exposed will become ill. Airborne transmission can occur over quite large distances.[146]

Between ten and fourteen days after infection, the patient gets a fever and shows signs of air-passage infection, with coughing. After a few days a rash appears with red dots that gradually merge. The rash begins in the face, spreads down to the rest of the body and lasts around five days. The fever increases with the arrival of the rash. The entire illness lasts between seven and ten days.

The patient can be severely affected for a few days, even if the course of the disease is not serious. Quite often, however, complications set in. The most common are bacterial infections in the air passages, such as inflammation of the middle ear and pneumonia. A rare but serious complication is acute inflammation of the brain (encephalitis) when the patient is in the recovery phase. A considerable number of these patients suffer chronic damage to the nervous system. Also, although extremely seldom, a chronic inflammation of the brain may develop many years after the acute infection: it is always fatal.[147] In the Western world the most serious cases of measles in people who have previously been healthy are seen in children under five and adults over twenty years of age.

The patient can infect others from two to three days before the rash breaks out and until four days after. Measles usually results in lifelong immunity. If one contracts measles, the virus invades nearly all parts of the body and also the cells of the immune system.[148] This is probably why a measles patient during and just after the infection has a weakened immune system to other microbes, which can bring about other infectious complications, most often involving bacteria. It was well known to doctors in the late nineteenth century, when tuberculosis was extremely widespread, that it could worsen if the patient caught measles. Signs of syphilis could also increase during measles.

The course of the disease described above applies to patients who are healthy beforehand. If the patient has an illness or is receiving treatment that leads to a weakened immune system, measles can be far more serious. We see this in children and adults with cancers and in HIV patients. Here mortality can be between 40 and 70 per cent. Not infrequently, such patients do not have a rash. Pregnant women also have a tendency to get a more serious form of the disease, probably because the immune system during pregnancy is slightly weakened.

As a curiosity that illustrates the suppressive effect of measles on the immune system, one could mention that doctors observed that patients with the kidney disease nephrotic syndrome, which today we know is due to an attack on the kidneys by the immune system, showed a marked improvement if the patient contracted measles. Until the mid-twentieth century patients with this syndrome were actually deliberately infected with measles.[149] Today, however, drugs are used that reduce the immune response.

In the poor parts of the world, where measles is still very widespread, we often see more serious cases of measles in children.[150] A probable explanation is that undernourishment results in a weakened immune system. In these cases the rash is often intense, with skin bleeding; this is sometimes known as 'black measles'. Violent diarrhoea is usual and contributes to a fatal outcome.

All in all, it is clear that measles is not necessarily 'just' a harmless children's disease that there is scarcely any reason to vaccinate against, as certain opponents of vaccination claim. If we look back through history, we find that measles epidemics have often had tragic consequences.

Did the Romans have measles?

We believe that the measles virus is several thousand years old. However, we are not able to establish with any degree of certainty when the first measles epidemic took place.[151] Hippocrates, who describes so many conditions of illness, cannot help us here; in his writings we find no description of an illness that resembles measles. An important problem is that physicians down the centuries have not managed to distinguish clearly between other illnesses involving rashes, such as smallpox, and measles. The person given the honour of having shown that measles was a distinct disease is one we came across earlier, the Persian physician Rhazes, who thoroughly described this infection at the beginning of the tenth century AD.[152] In all honesty, however, he himself credits a Jewish physician, Al-Yahudi ('the Jew'), who lived three centuries before but whose written description of the illness has not survived.

Did measles enter Europe as early as the time of the Romans? The historian William McNeill believes so and suggests that the Antonine plague at the time of Galen in the second century AD may have been measles.[153] In my opinion his arguments are not convincing, but we can probably reckon on measles already having arrived in Europe in the sixth or seventh century, since El Yahudi seems likely to have described the illness at that time.

Throughout the Middle Ages and up to the seventeenth century, however, many physicians still did not manage to distinguish between measles and smallpox, since Rhazes' writings were unknown. During this period, measles without a doubt became a children's disease in Europe. It was perhaps more serious than in present-day Western societies on account of widespread undernourishment in poorer parts of the population.[154]

The measles virus as a cause of historical tragedies

The great tragedies resulting from the measles virus were enacted in connection with the Age of Discovery, particularly the incursion of the Europeans into the New World, where measles did not exist before the Spanish conquistadors brought it with them from Europe. Hard on the heels of the first violent smallpox epidemic, which almost paralysed the indigenous population in Central America and Peru, came measles, and it was no mere harmless children's disease. The native population had no immunity against the virus, and individuals of all ages were affected, with very high mortality to which, in all probability, under-nourishment contributed. Two-thirds of the native population of Cuba died of measles in 1531, a year that also saw measles as the cause of many deaths in Mexico. Two years later, unbelievably enough, half of the population of Honduras died of measles. So it is indisputable that the illness contributed greatly to the weakening of indigenous societies after the Europeans brought infectious diseases with them from the Old World.[155] There were several measles epidemics among both European colonists and indigenous people, with mortality most often worse among the latter group. There are examples of whole tribes being obliterated by the illness.[156]

The dramatic consequences of measles on the American continent were repeated on several occasions when the virus was introduced into societies that had previously been completely isolated from the rest of the world. A familiar example of this is the measles epidemic in 1875 on the islands of Fiji, which had recently been annexed by the British. In connection with the takeover, a meeting had been held in Sydney, Australia, in which the supreme Fiji chieftain participated. During the voyage home on a British warship several people in his retinue contracted measles. On arriving home, great festivities had been planned to which chieftains from many of the islands, along with their retinues, had been invited. Measles broke out with a vengeance: about 36,000 of Fiji's population of 135,000 died of it. For several months the islands were completely crippled. Many of the natives believed that this disaster must have been sent by vengeful gods.[157]

Perhaps the best-known and most-studied example of the course of a measles epidemic in an isolated population without immunity is that on the Faroe Islands in 1846. These islands, which had belonged to Norway in the Middle Ages, became part of the Union with Denmark, and remained Danish after the dissolution of the Union in 1814. The islands were quite isolated, with few ships putting in there. In 1846 a Danish carpenter sailed from Copenhagen to Torshavn on the Faroe Islands. He was already infected with measles before he set out, and this unleashed an epidemic in which 6,100 Faroese out of a population of 7,864 were infected, and 102 died.[158]

This epidemic contributed greatly to our knowledge of measles, thanks to the efforts of a 26-year-old Danish doctor, Peter Panum, who was sent by the Danish authorities to take control of the epidemic. His acute observations made it possible to establish a series of important facts about the disease: that the infection is transmitted person-to-person, that it takes place via the air passages, that it takes ten to fourteen days before the illness breaks out after infection, that the patient can already spread infection before the rash breaks out and for almost a week afterwards, and that the result is a lifelong immunity after infection. Panum was able to deduce this last fact because the epidemic did not affect anyone over the age of 65, and there had been a measles epidemic on the island 65 years previously. Panum's experiences, which he later published, laid down the central characteristics of the measles infection and formed the basis of further work on the virus.[159]

Although measles has not perhaps had the same role as typhus and the plague in history during wartime, this infection has also had consequences for important military operations. When recruits were mobilized, partly from remote areas where people had not been in contact with the virus, it was almost inevitable that they became infected in the army camps where they were posted. This was seen during the American Civil War. No less than two-thirds of the 660,000 who died during this war died of infectious diseases; of the 67,000 who contracted measles, 4,000 died. Experienced generals avoided sending newly enlisted soldiers into battle before they were 'matured' – that is, had survived measles.

The eradication of measles – an unrealistic dream?

For almost sixty years we have had effective measles vaccines that have practically eradicated measles in Western countries. Until now developing countries have not had the economic capabilities to carry out nationwide vaccination, so measles remains a considerable problem in these countries. Annually 120,000 people die of measles in the world, of which the great majority are children in developing countries. Given the existence of vaccines, this ought to be unnecessary today.

Since the effectiveness of comprehensive vaccination became evident, the hope was that the measles virus could be eradicated globally, just as the smallpox virus has been.[160] That would be a fitting end to an infection that for centuries has been confused with precisely the smallpox virus.

The hope of eradication, however, is much fainter today. We can now see that measles is not only still raging in developing countries, where this infection is only one of many that are not under control. In the Western world too it now looks as if measles is on the advance. Since 2016 there has been a disturbing increase in the infection in Europe, with a number of deaths. These deaths, which are seen among non-vaccinated people, are often a result of resistance to vaccination, for which there can be many causes. If this tendency cannot be reversed, measles may once more become a major problem in Western countries as well.

Yellow Fever: A Deadly Threat for Centuries

Yellow fever well deserves its place among the epidemics that have had a great influence on the history and health of the human race. The disease has never been a major problem in Europe, so it has never acquired the same place in people's consciousness as the plague and cholera. This is because of the particular way in which the disease infects humans. It is first necessary to understand this before tracing the path of yellow fever through history.

Jungle and town alike

Yellow fever is caused by a virus that is transmitted to humans via the bites of the various kinds of mosquito carrying it.[161] A few days after being bitten, the patient gets a high temperature and displays influenza-like symptoms, after which the patient appears to improve and the temperature falls again. Some patients then get better. Others, those who develop a serious illness, feel increasingly ill once more after a few days, with a high fever, headache, and muscular and stomach pains. Nausea and vomiting are common. The patient's skin and eyes then turn yellow, because of an accumulation in the blood of the bile pigment bilirubin, since the liver is being attacked. Then bleeding of both the skin and inner organs takes place, with the patient often vomiting blood. The kidneys and the heart are attacked in serious cases. The patient can often become confused and have cramping fits. Death normally occurs in the second week of the disease. If the patient survives, bacterial complications such as pneumonia may occur. In these serious cases of yellow fever, mortality can be up to 50 per cent.[162] Certain cases of infection by yellow fever do not lead any symptoms to develop. Young children are normally less seriously attacked than adults.

The virus is present in large quantities in the patient's blood during the first days of the illness. If a mosquito bites the patient, it sucks up the virus in the blood. The virus then reproduces in the mosquito, to which it is adapted through evolution. A couple of weeks later the mosquito becomes a transmitter of the disease. If it then bites a healthy human, the yellow fever virus can be transmitted to the person via the mosquito's saliva. The insect will be able to infect people for the rest of its life. In addition, the yellow fever virus can be passed on via its eggs to the next generation of mosquitoes.[163]

There are many species of mosquito that can transmit the yellow fever virus in this way. One particular species, however, *Aedes aegypti*, is particularly adapted to humans. This species has a form of life that means it likes to be in the proximity of humans, where it depends on water in pools, receptacles and tanks for its propagation.[164] It is also extremely home-loving, and seldom flies more than a few hundred metres from its base. If it is to transmit the disease effectively, this must be in densely populated, urban surroundings. One form of the disease, called urban yellow fever, is particularly responsible for epidemics in cities both large and small. The *Aedes aegypti* mosquito plays a decisive role here. For a long time it was thought that this was the only form of yellow fever and it was only this particular mosquito that transmitted it. Furthermore, it was believed that the infection only affected *Homo sapiens*.

It was not until the 1930s that it was discovered that various kinds of apes living in the wild are exposed to the yellow fever virus.[165] Here too the virus was transmitted by mosquitoes, but by other species than the insidious companion of human beings, even though they were related to it. These species of mosquito and the apes from which they suck blood are found in the jungle in both tropical Africa and South America, although they are not identical species in the two continents. In Africa the apes do not on the whole fall ill from the virus, while the apes in the New World often die. Frequent finding of dead apes in the jungle is therefore an indication that a yellow fever epidemic is ongoing among them.

The species of mosquito that have specialized in apes can also, if the opportunity arises, bite humans, even though this is not their first choice. For that reason, isolated cases of yellow fever occur among people in the jungle, particularly among forest workers. This form of yellow fever is known as jungle yellow fever, to distinguish it from urban fever. Both the species of mosquitoes involved and the apes that are their victims are normally found in the treetops. In the event of massive tree-felling in the jungle, there is increased risk of humans in the vicinity being infected by mosquitoes now on the ground. Deforestation of the jungle also increases the number of pools of water that provide breeding grounds for yellow-fever-infected eggs. Once again, we see an example of human activities triggering problems with infection because of altered ecological conditions.

The carrier of urban yellow fever, *Aedes aegypti*, is now found in all inhabited parts of the world and it has displayed an exceptional ability to expand its territory from Africa to the Americas, where it was not originally found.[166] The fact that this mosquito is present in an urban community does not necessarily mean that a yellow fever epidemic is inevitable, for the virus first has to be introduced into the population. But this situation is unstable and risky. If one or more patients with incipient yellow fever come to town, the conditions exist for a devastating epidemic. Here we have the connection between jungle yellow fever and the urban form: jungle yellow fever gives rise to patients who can start an epidemic in an urban community. The spread of jungle yellow fever from jungle to town has repeatedly taken place both in Africa and the Americas.

Slaves and mosquitoes

The history of yellow fever is fascinating. For much of our knowledge in this field we can thank modern molecular biology, whereas earlier we mainly had to work from historical sources, which can of course be misleading when it comes to the history of infection.

Until recently there was disagreement among historians about the geographical origins of yellow fever.[167] Some claimed that the virus comes from Africa; others that it arose on the American continent. Today, the supporters of Africa have won.

The first epidemic which the historical sources quite clearly identify as yellow fever hit Barbados in the West Indies and Yucatan in Mexico in 1647–8.[168] In a Mayan manuscript the disease is called *xecic* (heavy vomiting), which is typical of the most serious form of yellow fever, where the patient coughs up blood. It is possible that a yellow fever epidemic struck Haiti as early as 1495, only three years after the arrival of Columbus, but this is less certain.

The first reasonably well-documented epidemic in Africa afflicted British soldiers in Senegal in 1778. Yellow fever had ravaged Africa for centuries before this, but these cases have probably been drowned out by other diseases, including malaria. For that reason, yellow fever was not 'discovered' in Africa at an early date. The African population in regions exposed to the disease has probably also built up a considerable immunity against the virus, which only produces a mild illness during childhood. That African apes, unlike those in South America, do not fall ill from the virus also indicates a long period of adaptation to it. In Africa it was mainly white traders, seamen and explorers who were particularly hit by serious yellow fever, since they had not already become immunized via contact with the virus when children.[169]

The final proof that the virus originated in Africa comes from recent molecular-biological studies in which virus types from patients in both East and West Africa have been compared with those from the American continent.[170] The conclusion is that the virus probably originated in East Africa at some time during the past 1,500 years. The virus from the New World displays far greater similarities with that from West Africa than with that from East Africa. The finds indicate that the West African virus came to the Americas between three and four hundred years ago, at the time when large-scale slave-trading began, with the transportation of tens of thousands of slaves from West Africa to the Americas. In all probability, the virus came with the *Aedes aegypti* mosquito, which could survive for several months on board on the voyage across the Atlantic, together with its virus-infected eggs.[171] This mosquito adapted rapidly to the conditions in the New World, where it continued its existence close to human beings and caused epidemics. There the virus found a great many new victims, both the indigenous population and the Europeans, who had no immunity against the virus and were easy prey. This resulted in repeated epidemics with a frighteningly high mortality.

But the newly imported virus from Africa did not only attack humans on the American continent. It also spread to various American species of ape.[172] Several local species of mosquito showed themselves to be cooperative as regards the yellow fever virus and took over the spread of infection in apes, as was the case in African jungles. And just as in Africa, sporadic infections of humans occurred when they were bitten by the species of mosquito that attacked apes: America had gained its own jungle yellow fever. When such victims came into contact with urban communities where *Aedes aegypti* was already resident, the conditions were ideal for devastating epidemics.

Yellow fever initially gained a foothold in the West Indies, but it rapidly spread to the mainland. Epidemics ravaged cities in South and Central America and also spread to North America, where the virus actually got as far as Quebec in Canada. Europe did not escape either. In the eighteenth and nineteenth centuries, cities such as Lisbon, Porto and Barcelona were hit, and the virus even reached Madrid on one occasion. Lesser outbreaks also affected a few French and British towns. It was generally infection from the West Indies via trading ships that was the cause of these European outbreaks.[173]

Slave revolts and Napoleon's dreams of empire

For centuries the West Indies was an arena where British, French, Spanish and later North Americans in various alliances were constantly at war with each other. This meant that new soldiers without yellow fever immunity were always appearing on the scene. This led to repeated outbreaks of yellow fever with a high mortality rate among the soldiers, a fact that often influenced the military operations.

Major political consequences were felt on Haiti, where half of the island at the time was French and was called Saint Domingue. During the French Revolution, the black slaves on the sugar plantations rebelled against their French masters and chaos resulted on the island. The British then seized their chance to invade the island in 1793. This was the year before the Reign of Terror in Paris, but the mortality rate was higher among the British soldiers on Haiti than among the aristocrats in

France. Over half of these soldiers died of yellow fever, and the British forces were eventually withdrawn.[174]

In 1801, when there was a short period of peace during the Napoleonic Wars, Napoleon decided to recapture Haiti from the rebels, who had set up an independent republic.[175] Haiti was of great economic importance to France, since more than half of the world's production of sugar took place there. There is also reason to believe that Napoleon planned a major offensive in North America, where France already owned Louisiana. He sent an invasion force led by his brother-in-law General Charles Leclerc, who was married to the most beautiful of Napoleon's four sisters, the frivolous Pauline. The rebel forces were led by a liberated slave, the charismatic Toussaint L'Ouverture. Initially the

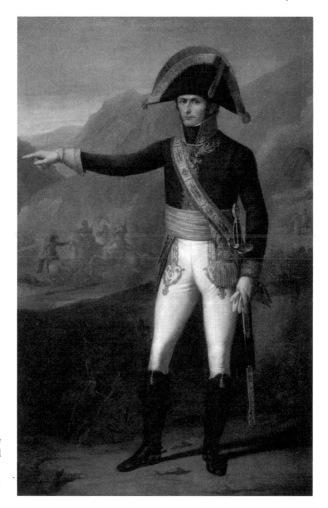

General Charles Leclerc, Napoleon's brother-in-law, seen here in a painting by François Kinson from 1804, was sent to Haiti in 1801 to put down the rebellion, led by the ex-slave Toussaint L'Ouverture. After a certain amount of initial success, the French army was badly hit by yellow fever, with a high rate of mortality. Leclerc himself also died of yellow fever in 1802. After a while the French army had to withdraw from Haiti, which became independent.

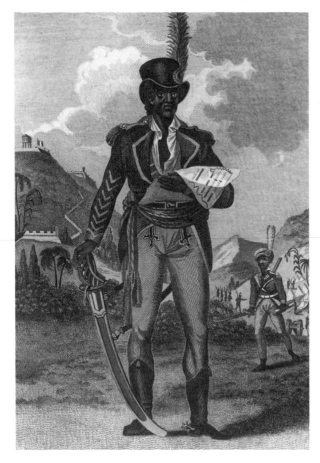

Toussaint L'Ouverture in an engraving by J. Barlow, 1805. A charismatic and able ex-slave, L'Ouverture led the slave rebellion on Haiti during the French Revolution and later the fight against the French invading army under General Charles Leclerc. He died in prison in France in 1803.

French enjoyed success, but then yellow fever struck. Within a relatively short time 25,000 of the 35,000 soldiers of the invasion force had died, mostly of yellow fever. General Leclerc also succumbed. L'Ouverture was taken prisoner and sent to France, where he died in prison of tuberculosis. Subsequently he has acquired a kind of hero status and been called 'the black Spartacus', a reference to the legendary leader of the great slave rebellion in the Roman empire in 73–71 BC. The devastated French force, however, had to withdraw. Haiti became the second republic in the Americas to have broken free from its European masters, and the only state based on the result of a successful slave rebellion.

Napoleon's defeat in Haiti caused him to abandon his dreams of expanding his empire across the Atlantic, and in 1803 he sold Louisiana to the USA. Indirectly, yellow fever undoubtedly played a role in his change of plans.[176]

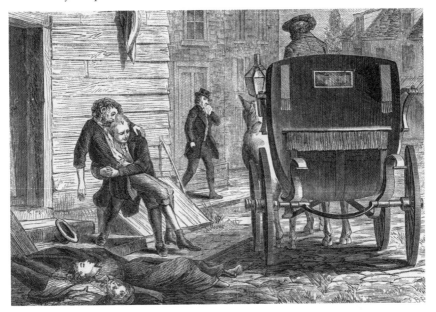

In 1793 a yellow fever epidemic broke out in Philadelphia, introduced by French refugees from the slave rebellion on Haiti. '[Stephen] Girard's Heroism', engraving in James D. McCabe Jr, *Great Fortunes, and How They Were Made* (1871).

Pauline did not grieve long over her dead husband, General Leclerc. A few months later she married the rich Italian prince Camillo Borghese. She can today be admired in the marble statue of her as *Venus Victorious* (1804–8) by Antonio Canova in the Galleria Borghese, Rome.

The dramatic events on Haiti also had repercussions for the young republic of the United States.[177] As a result of the rebellion and acts of war after the British invasion, many French colonists fled headlong from Haiti in 1793 to such cities as Philadelphia. The yellow fever virus accompanied them, and a violent epidemic broke out among the 51,000 inhabitants of the city, from which 20,000 people fled. Of those remaining, 5,000 died.

Yellow fever raged in the USA between 1668 and 1870. There were at least 25 epidemics in New York alone. In 1853 yellow fever struck New Orleans, with 9,000 deaths. In 1878 the virus hit the Mississippi valley, with 100,000 cases and 20,000 deaths. Hardest hit was the central commercial city of Memphis. The administrative apparatus of the city almost entirely broke down as the city council members fled, and a third of the police force deserted. But the city's doctors stood firm, an impressive example of a sense of duty and professional ethics.

The 111 doctors of Memphis did not flee the city and 60 per cent of them died from the disease.

The yellow fever code is cracked, but at a cost

On the American continent, yellow fever was the most important epidemic illness during the nineteenth century, but even in Europe people were concerned about this threat to both trade and military operations in America and Africa.

As with cholera, yellow fever became a central issue in the ongoing discussion about the causes of epidemics.[178] The miasma theory had strong support, which led to the authorities in a number of cities making efforts to improve sanitary conditions in the fight against yellow fever. But many others were convinced that there had to be some form of contagious disease, since there were clear examples of yellow fever often breaking out in a city after the arrival of people from areas ravaged by the disease. This was the case with the refugees from Haiti to Philadelphia in 1793. For that reason, quarantine measures of various kinds were still used, both as regards shipping and on land. The slang term for the disease 'Yellow Jack' comes precisely from the yellow flag that signalled quarantine, which often applied to yellow fever. It was North American and European ports in particular that imposed quarantine on ships from the West Indies, where such measures were much more lax.[179]

After several centuries of repeated yellow fever epidemics that came like bolts from the blue, acute observations by certain doctors led to a mosquito being identified as a transmitter of the disease. It was the Cuban doctor Carlos Finlay who first advanced this theory in 1881, only three years after the violent outbreak in the Tennessee valley. He concentrated on precisely the mosquito *Aedes aegypti*, carrying out a long series of experiments to prove the role of the mosquito in yellow fever, although his results were not convincing.[180]

In 1898 the USA was at war with Spain and the fighting took place on Cuba, which was Spanish at the time. Following a serious outbreak of yellow fever among the American soldiers stationed on Cuba, the U.S. government sent a group of researchers in 1900 to the capital, Havana, to crack the riddle of the disease. This so-called Yellow Fever Commission was led by the army doctor Walter Reed, with three highly dedicated colleagues under him. They were particularly inspired by

Carlos Finlay's mosquito theory and sought to prove him right via experiments. The theory had also become increasingly topical, because it had recently been demonstrated that another microbe, the malaria parasite, is transmitted via mosquitoes, and there were also certain other tropical infections where it was strongly suspected that insects were involved in infecting humans.

Since it was not then known that species of animals other than humans can contract the disease, the Yellow Fever Commission chose to carry out experiments on humans. Among the volunteers were Reed's three colleagues. These human guinea pigs allowed themselves to be bitten by mosquitoes that had first sucked blood from a yellow fever patient. One of them, Jesse Lazar, died of classic yellow fever, but James Carroll managed to survive, as did a number of the other volunteers after contracting yellow fever. These first experiments were not completely unequivocal, and were now followed up by well-controlled new experiments using volunteers. The total result demonstrated conclusively that yellow fever is due to a pathogen transmitted by a mosquito bite. It was also shown that this pathogen had to be smaller than bacteria, since it passed through filters that stopped bacteria from passing. There was still no possibility of directly proving the existence of the virus; this could not be achieved until the electron microscope was available around 1930.

Lazar's death on Cuba was not to be the last death among yellow fever researchers. In the latter half of the 1920s four researchers sent out to Africa by the Rockefeller Foundation died while seeking to prove the existence of the virus.

The Panama Canal and the fight against yellow fever

The success of the Yellow Fever Commission on Cuba quickly led to important consequences in the fight against the virus. Reed and his colleagues had already indicated a series of necessary measures against the mosquito *Aedes aegypti* in combatting infection.[181] Reed, however, died in 1902. He was succeeded by another army doctor, William Crawford Gorgas, who implemented intensive action against all the potential breeding grounds of the mosquito in Havana by draining swamp areas, filling ponds and spraying disinfectants. All yellow fever patients were isolated in their own barracks, protected against mosquitoes. These measures proved a success. In the course of three months, yellow fever had disappeared from Havana.

This was only the prelude, however, to Gorgas's fight against the disease. His next success was to have historic consequences for international shipping and trade. A sea voyage from the Atlantic to the Pacific then had to follow the highly hazardous route round Cape Horn at the southern tip of South America. The Frenchman Ferdinand de Lesseps had become famous as the engineer who built the Suez Canal, which was opened with great festivities in 1869. De Lesseps wished to follow up his success by building a canal through the Panama isthmus and thereby link the Atlantic and the Pacific.[182] A company was formed to raise capital for the venture, which was known as 'La grande entreprise'. The project started in 1881 and France invested not only money but its national prestige in the plans.

The obstacles, however, proved to be enormous. There were considerable financial problems, but even more serious were the formidable infection problems that faced Europeans working on the canal. Malaria

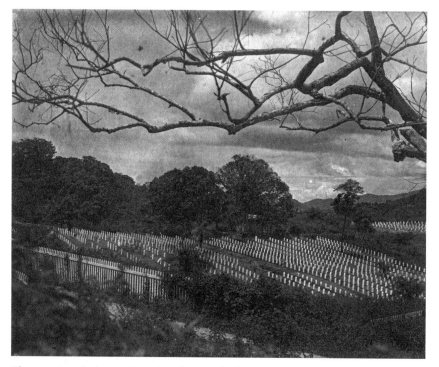

The cemetery in Ancon, Panama, close to the hospital where the yellow fever patients lay – and died. Photograph by W. R. Newbold Jr, 1908.

was a problem, but it was yellow fever in particular that was raging. The area for the construction of the canal was an eldorado for mosquitoes, with countless breeding grounds. The death toll of the victims of yellow fever rapidly rose. After a couple of years, two hundred workers were dying every month. All but one of seventeen newly arrived engineers died within a month in 1885. Attempts were made to conceal these figures so as not to hinder the recruitment of new engineers and labourers as well as the further financing of the costly project, but without success. In 1889 the project went bankrupt.

But the idea of the canal lived on. In 1904 the USA took over the construction of the canal. The man who led the medical side of the project was none other than William Gorgas, who had so effectively solved the yellow fever problem on Cuba.[183] He wished to employ a simi-lar strategy in Panama, beginning a full-scale war against the mosquito by draining the swamps, filling in ponds and spraying with disinfectants – and isolating yellow fever patients. Initially there was considerable resistance from the local authorities, but his will prevailed and he waged war against the mosquito in the Canal Zone with the same success he had achieved in Cuba. The last fatal case of yellow fever there was recorded in 1906. When the canal was opened in 1913, mortality from all diseases was lower in the Canal Zone than in all of the USA. This achievement is one of the most impressive examples of the successful application of research results in solving a serious medical problem. William Gorgas ended his brilliant career as Surgeon General of the U.S. Army in the First World War.

Racism and yellow fever

Early writers of accounts of yellow fever epidemics in the Americas and the majority of historians in our own time have agreed that Africans and people of African ancestry have an innate resistance to the disease. Ostensibly, the disease assumes a milder form in Africans and has a lower mortality rate. With our modern understanding of genetics this can be explained by the fact that hundreds, perhaps thousands, of years of contact with yellow fever in Africa have led to genetic changes that have increased resistance to the virus. This is a calculated evolution-ary adaptation to yellow fever similar to those we have identified with regard to malaria.[184] The hereditary condition of sickle cell disease (SCD) has arisen and remained present in certain regions of Africa precisely because it protects against malaria.

After his success with the Panama Canal, William Gorgas stated that tropical regions could now be made safe for the white man. There was probably nothing racist intended by this remark, but nonetheless Gorgas's statements and similar ones subsequently expressed by others have been attacked as racist. Even the concept of a hereditary, innate resistance to yellow fever in Africans has been rejected with scorn.[185] Various arguments have been used by these critics, including that Africans are more often infected during childhood, when the disease is most often mild and gives lasting immunity. This can naturally explain why Africans in yellow fever areas are to a much lesser extent hit by serious cases of yellow fever than white people travelling to the area. This argument is less convincing for the population in American yellow fever areas, where white children have also been exposed to mosquito bites and infection for centuries. In these areas too yellow fever has raged more among whites than among Blacks.

Critics of the theory of hereditary resistance to yellow fever in Africans have also claimed that down through the ages there has been so little interest in the state of health of the African slaves that serious cases of yellow fever have simply been overlooked. I do not feel that this argument carries much weight either, since the slaves had considerable economic value for their owners, even though one may prefer to deny the existence of any human empathy towards the slaves on their part.

Several yellow fever epidemics have also been referred to where Africans were greatly affected, particularly in Africa. But this may have to do with population groups outside the 'classic' yellow fever areas, where the disease has been 'imported' from outside. Lastly, certain critics have also based their arguments on the claim that yellow fever originated on the American continent, so that Africans have simply been unable to develop any hereditary resistance. This argument can now be rejected, since everything points to an African origin of the virus.

All things taken into consideration, I do not think that the hypothesis of a more or less pronounced resistance to yellow fever in certain African population groups can be discounted. It is possible that genetic research into the human immune defence against the yellow fever virus will be able to give a definitive answer to this question.

Yellow fever is still lurking in the wings

The striking results of the campaigns against yellow fever on Cuba and in Panama provided support for similar campaigns in the twentieth century against the *Aedes aegypti* mosquito in a number of big cities on the American continent where yellow fever had been rampant.[186] Here too there was great success: *Aedes aegypti* disappeared from these cities in the 1940s and '50s, thus marking the end of urban yellow fever. During the whole twentieth century there were generally only lesser outbreaks of yellow fever that could be traced back to the jungle variant through species of mosquito other than *Aedes aegypti*, which were now realized to be a problem. It is not possible to eradicate jungle yellow fever.

In recent years, however, *Aedes aegypti* has been advancing once more, particularly in a number of cities in Central America.[187] One cause of this is probably that people have gradually become more lax about combatting mosquitoes than when the heroic spirit of Gorgas prevailed. Either way, this is a worrying situation since it might form the basis of new epidemics of urban yellow fever.

Something else that gives cause for concern is that the Asian continent has until today been spared the disease, without anyone really knowing why. Asia has numerous species of ape that could be attacked by the virus, and the *Aedes aegypti* mosquito is strongly represented in many Asian countries. Why has yellow fever not attacked Asia with jungle outbreaks and urban epidemics as we have seen in Africa and America? A number of theories have been aired to explain this.[188] It seems possible that the Asian variants of the mosquito are slightly less effective at transmitting the virus than their American and African relatives. There are also many other pathogenic viruses in Asia that are related to the yellow fever virus. It is conceivable that immunity against these viruses after earlier contact also protects people against the yellow fever virus, which makes it difficult for the virus to gain a foothold in Asia. But it is still possible for yellow fever to strike in Asia, with similar consequences to those we have seen in Africa and America.

Syphilis: A Gift from the New World?

'Mother, give me the sun!' Osvald declares to his mother in the last act of Henrik Ibsen's gloomy drama *Ghosts* (1881). With this line Ibsen indicates that Osvald is infected with syphilis and has the dreaded encephalitis, which not infrequently is the fate of patients with syphilis in its final stage. Ibsen's mention of this disease caused quite a furore at the time. Syphilis was simply not talked about in polite society, despite the fact that it was widespread in nineteenth-century society and had many similarities with the AIDS pandemic of our time. The means of infection were the same, the course of the disease was chronic, with many long periods without symptoms, and the indications of the disease varied greatly. Both diseases were considered extremely shameful, and the fear of infection in the population was strong.

Syphilis has occupied a special place in the history of medicine for five hundred years. This is not only due to the factors already mentioned. A great many famous people were afflicted by syphilis: kings, heads of state and politicians, authors and musicians.[189] The origins of syphilis are also mysterious and have been the subject of lively debate for centuries.

The great imitator

The cause of syphilis is an infection by the *Treponema pallidum* bacterium.[190] The most usual means of infection is sexual contact (intercourse in one form or another). The second important means of infection, which is very rare in Western countries today, is an infection from mother to foetus during pregnancy. This was the basis of Osvald's tragedy in *Ghosts*. In a few exceptional cases infection can take place in other ways. In the event of sexual infection, we talk of three stages of the disease, unless the patient receives treatment.

The *first stage*, which on average starts three weeks after the time of infection, can be a small, painless sore, usually on the genital organs or around the rectum, more rarely in the mouth. Apart from this, the patient feels healthy.

The *second stage* normally comes six weeks after the time of infection, but can come as early as two weeks or up to ninety days afterwards. The signs of the disease vary a great deal. At this stage the syphilis bacterium reproduces rapidly and spreads to nearly all parts of the body. The commonest find is a widespread rash with various kinds of red spots, but most parts of the body can be attacked, including the nervous system, eyes, kidneys and joints. The patient often has a high fever and feels ill. This stage can last several weeks or a few months. The great variety of the disease picture means that syphilis has been called 'the great imitator', since it can resemble a great many other conditions. Doctors of earlier times also used to say that 'the person who knows syphilis knows the medical profession.'

The patient then moves into the lengthy *third stage*. During the first years the infection is latent, completely without symptoms, but the patient can still infect others. After a number of years two-thirds of patients manage to become free of the bacterium and have no further signs of the disease. The remaining patients can later develop a serious illness, up to thirty years after first having been infected.

The disease pictures of the late phase of this third stage can also vary greatly, but disease of the heart and blood vessels and in the brain and spinal cord is the most prevalent. The aorta is often affected, and this frequently affects the heart, damaging the valves. The patient can suffer strokes, because the syphilis bacterium causes inflammation of the blood vessels. It can also attack the brain tissue directly and cause personality disturbances, psychoses, dementia and paralysis. One form of brain disease is so-called *paralysis generalis*, with the patient having bizarre illusions of grandeur, imagining himself to be Napoleon or Caesar, for example. If the bacterium attacks the spinal cord, this can lead to what is known as *tabes dorsalis* and result in intolerable pain and disturbed gait, sometimes even to complete paralysis of the legs.

Our knowledge of the natural (untreated) course of syphilis comes to a great extent from meticulous studies of large groups of patients over many years. That was possible until the beginning of the twentieth century, before we had any really effective treatment for the disease. A very important study, one that is internationally famous, was the so-called Oslo study, carried out in Norway.[191] The Norwegian dermatologist Cæsar Boeck, justifiably, had little faith in contemporary treatment of syphilis with a mercury cure, which was both without effect and damaging, and chose instead to follow 1,400 untreated patients who had been reported as in the first and second stages of the disease in Kristiania (Oslo) from 1890 to 1910. These patients were subsequently followed

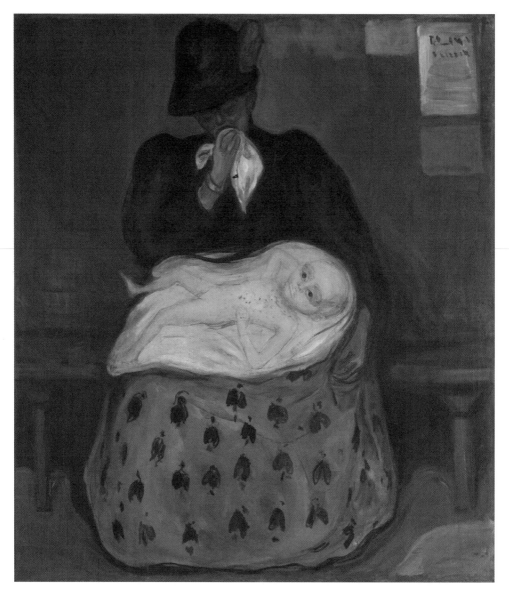

Edvard Munch, *Inheritance*, 1897–9, oil on canvas. A weeping mother sits with her extremely ill child, who has inherited syphilis and has a deformed body and a rash. Munch found inspiration for the picture in a visit he paid to a hospital in Paris.

Syphilitic Man, one of the first woodcuts by the German artist Albrecht Dürer (1471–1528). It shows a man with bad syphilitic skin wounds. His clothes indicate that he is a *Landsknecht* – one of the many mercenaries who in the 16th and 17th centuries contributed to the spread of syphilis in Europe. The representation of the sign of the zodiac above the man refers to the astrological theories of the time regarding the basis of the new disease.

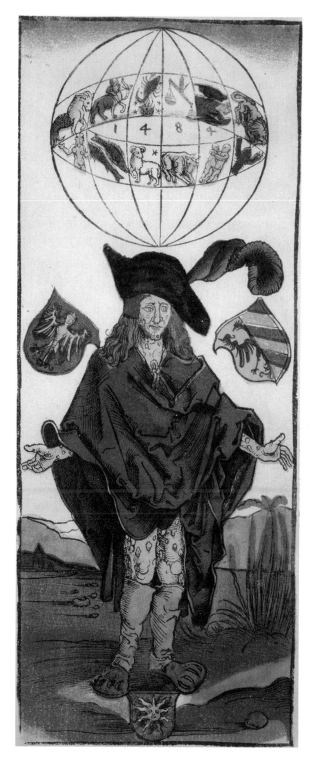

right up until 1948, providing material that secured invaluable knowledge about the course of syphilis.

Unfortunately, similar long-term studies were also carried out later, even though effective treatment was available by then. This is, of course, a breach of fundamental ethical guidelines for doctors. We shall later look at two such studies.

A grim disease appears on the scene

Today we are able to state with a high degree of certainty when syphilis first appeared on the European scene.[192] At the end of the fifteenth century Italy was still being ravaged by warfare, the main countries involved being Spain and France, who entered into changing alliances with Italian city states and princes. In 1495 the French, under Charles VIII, conquered Naples from the Spanish. The victors, who had with them an army of sex workers, began long-lasting celebrations that gradually degenerated into pure orgies, with sections of the Neapolitan population also taking part. After several months the French pulled out of the city. Not long afterwards, an increasing number of soldiers in the French army were stricken by a highly acute disease with quite frightening symptoms: sores that began on the genitals and quickly spread to the entire body, after which deeper wounds developed that began to devour tissues and destroyed fingers, toes, lips, eyes and genitals. The disease was extremely painful. Mortality was high: patients often died after a few months.

The French army did not consist only of Frenchmen, but was augmented by mercenaries (*Landsknechte*) from Germany, the Netherlands, Switzerland, Italy and Spain. After the dissolution of the army, these mercenaries, with their entourage of sex workers, returned to their respective home countries, taking with them the new, horrible disease. It spread very quickly: in the course of five or six years most European countries had been affected. Fairly soon syphilis had spread to other continents as well, taken to India in 1498 as a result of contact following the first voyage of the Portuguese explorer Vasco da Gama. The epidemic moved on to China, and a short while later to Japan.

Syphilis probably arrived in Denmark as early as 1495.[193] A contemporary chronicler writes that in the summer of 1495 'a very great epidemic' that 'no one had heard of before' arrived, 'which took the lives of thousands of people'. It was given various names, including 'mercenary disease'. It was often also referred to as 'the pox'. In all countries people refused to take any responsibility and gave other countries and nations the blame for syphilis. The French called it 'the Neapolitan disease', while the Italians, Dutch, British and Norwegians talked about 'the French disease'. The Poles called syphilis 'the German disease', while the Russians used the term 'the Polish disease'. In Japan and the East Indies its name was 'the Portuguese disease'. In Portugal, one consoled oneself by calling it 'the Castilian disease'. Religion was also brought into it: in Turkey it was referred to as 'the Christian disease'.

The course of the disease in the first period after syphilis appeared was far more violent than that which we know today, as is clearly illustrated by a number of accounts from the first year of the epidemic.[194] Some of the writers had themselves been attacked by the new disease and give dramatic descriptions of the pathogenic picture. One example is an account that appeared in 1503 by Joseph Grünpeck, the young, university-educated private secretary to the Habsburg emperor Maximilian I. Seven years earlier, in 1496, Grünpeck had written the first printed account of syphilis. Now he himself had been infected at an evidently lively banquet 'where not only Bacchus but Venus was present', according to Grünpeck. He describes in horrifying detail his painful afflictions, with deep sores on his sexual organ and the rest of his body. He further tells of his disappointing experiences with both doctors and charlatans who were appearing in great numbers to make a profit from the new disease. Grünpeck did not die, but lived to be more than eighty years old.

A number of doctors wrote learned treatises about syphilis. The best known is by the Spaniard Gaspar Torella, who was private doctor to both Pope Alexander VI and his son Cesare Borgia. The Borgias were one of the most notorious families of Renaissance Italy, responsible for ordering numerous assassinations and committing incest. Torella's first treatise on syphilis in 1497 was dedicated to Cesare Borgia, which was appropriate as Cesare was seriously ill with syphilis and often wore a mask to hide the syphilitic sores on his face. During his own wedding he had to wear heavy make-up.

Over the course of the first decades of the sixteenth century the infection became less stormy and gradually acquired the chronic form typical nowadays, with a much lower mortality rate. This was, among

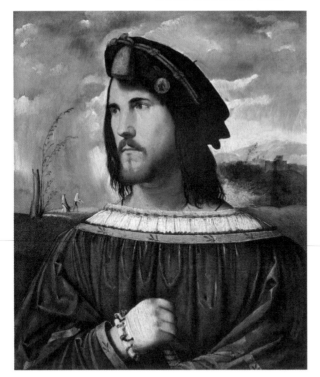

Cesare Borgia (1475–1507), seen here in a painting by Altobello Melone from 1515–20, was the son of Pope Alexander VI. He was a powerful and reckless military commander and politician who was infected with syphilis in early life, which at times gave him terrible skin afflictions and made it necessary for him to wear a mask.

other things, confirmed by Girolamo Fracastoro, who in 1546 published his famous work on contagious diseases, *De contagione et contagiosis morbis et eorum curatione*, in which he also mentions syphilis. As early as 1530 he had published his long poem *Syphilis sive morbus gallicus*. This poem, which in its very title blamed the French, not only has considerable poetic qualities (with some hyperbole, Fracastoro has been compared with Virgil), but gives a comprehensive and precise description of syphilis, even though it does not come up with anything essentially new in relation to the contemporary knowledge from other sources. The poem was highly successful and about a hundred editions were printed during the sixteenth century.

It was also Fracastoro who coined the term 'syphilis' in his poem. He writes about a shepherd by the name of Syphilus, who offended the sun god and was punished by the disease named after its victim.[195] In spite of Fracastoro's fame, however, the term did not catch on before the end of the eighteenth century.

Sex, planets or divine punishment?

Naturally enough, the frightening new epidemic led to many theories about possible causes.[196] As with earlier great epidemics of history, including the plague, there were many people who believed that the new disease was God's punishment for human failings and sinful life-style. We find a trace of this belief in Fracastoro's account of the shepherd Syphilus. Emperor Maximilian I issued a proclamation in 1495 in which he stated that the new disease was a punishment for the blasphemy of the age. Some people, including Joseph Grünpeck in his first work on syphilis, proposed that special alignments of the planets played a role. Such theories could also be combined with ideas that the disease was divine retribution.

There is no doubt, however, that a great many people, even from the earliest stages of the epidemic, were convinced that the disease was a form of contagion transmitted from person to person by sexual acts.[197] No one knew anything about what this contagion consisted of, but a great many people thought it had to do with the transmission of a kind of poison that caused sores and spread throughout the patient's body. We also recall Fracastoro's fascinating description of *seminaria*, invisible particles that can transmit disease, including syphilis.

The theories of contagion that gradually dominated the concept of syphilis also had practical consequences. Early on, sex workers were seen as dangerous carriers of disease that needed to be controlled in various ways. Brothels and bath houses, where prostitution often took place, were often closed down, or attempts were made to isolate syphilis patients, with special hospital-like institutions set up to treat the disease.

From Venus to Mercury

As Grünpeck noticed early on, syphilis gave rise to a flourishing market of suggested treatments, ranging from the activities of charlatans to more serious forms of treatment.[198] There was a widespread view that it was good for the patient to get rid of as much sweat and 'phlegm' (mucus) as possible, and various methods of treatment addressed this. Two forms of treatment that were often used were a decoction of bark from the guajac tree, which grows in the West Indies, and one using mercury preparations.[199]

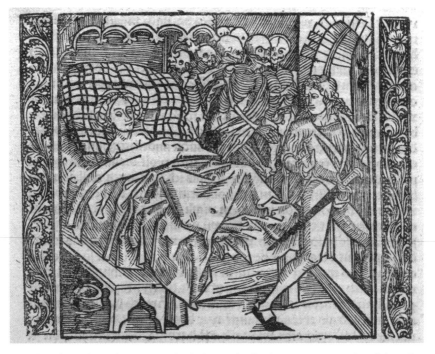

Woodcut from the 16th century which shows the fatal consequences of syphilis. The disease is represented by a young woman who is gazing at her young lover leaving the bed. Behind stand the skeletons of her dead lovers.

The guajac cures were combined with fasting for over a month and were considered pretty brutal. Just as brutal were the various forms of mercury treatment. This could be carried out in various ways. Often the patient was exposed to inhalation of mercury vapours in a kind of oven with a very high temperature. This treatment was given daily, often over a month. Ointments containing mercury were also used and mercury pills for internal use were gradually introduced. Many patients showed signs of mercury poisoning that could be serious and even lead to death. The brutal mercury cures were often repeated later. With a reference to the Roman gods Venus and Mercury, from whom quicksilver acquired the name mercury, people said: 'One night with Venus – a whole life with Mercury.'

The German aristocrat Ulrich von Hutten, who contracted syphilis, also wrote a book about the suffering caused by the disease, and particularly by the mercury treatment that he underwent on many occasions. He died at the age of 35, possibly of syphilis and the treatments he underwent.

Eventually people stopped using the guajac treatment, which in all probability had no effect whatever.[200] Treatment using mercury may possibly have had some effect in subduing the symptoms of the disease in the first and second stages of syphilis, and it was used right up until the end of the nineteenth century. The side-effects experienced by many patients, however, could be even worse than the disease itself: there are examples of syphilis patients who committed suicide rather than face a mercury cure.

Both physicians and charlatans became rich from treating syphilis, and it must be admitted that the boundary between these two groups was sometimes unclear. It is said that a prominent French doctor was

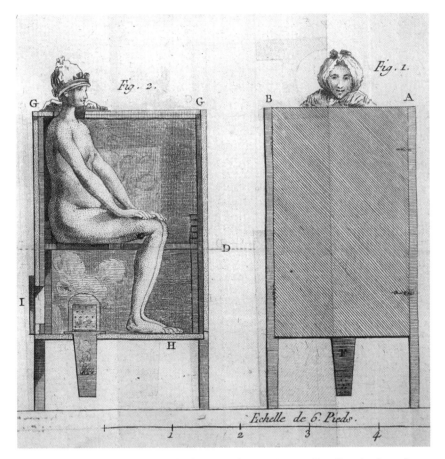

Mercury was used to treat syphilis for several centuries, until well on in the 19th century. Often the patient had to inhale mercury vapour in a kind of oven at a very high temperature. Engravings from Pierre Lalouette, *Nouvelle méthode de traiter les maladies vénériennes, par la fumigation* (1776).

surprised by a friend while kneeling in front of a statue of Charles VIII in a cathedral. 'But the king was no saint,' the friend objected. The doctor replied: 'Perhaps not, but I can never thank him enough for having introduced into France the disease from which I have earned my fortune.' It was probably syphilis that led to truly commercial marketing of medicines for illness. One of the richest business dynasties in Europe in the Renaissance, the Fugger family in Augsburg, Germany, earned enormous sums from importing guajac.

From a raging epidemic to a constant social evil

The sixteenth century, when the syphilis epidemic spread like wildfire, was characterized by a considerable dissolution of norms, particularly within the area of sexual life. This particularly applied to the upper social classes, where sexual promiscuity was extremely common. Included in this category were many of the clergy, for whom sexual debauchery was no rarity, even in the highest offices. It was not surprising that syphilis became widespread among the clergy early on. Cesare Borgia was already a cardinal when he became infected at the age of 22.[201] Cardinal Giuliano della Rovere, who later became Pope Julius II, is another example.[202] Cesare Borgia's father, Pope Alexander VI, whose life was typified by excessive debauchery, with numerous mistresses and illegitimate children, invited pilgrims from the whole world in 1500 to celebrate the Holy Year, an event that took place every 25 years. There they were received and serviced by thousands of Roman sex workers without any protest from the Church. The sexual wildness that followed shocked those who did not hold the prevailing view of sex, which even the Holy Father shared. One of those who arrived was a young German monk, Martin Luther, and it is highly probable that his experiences in Rome in 1500 contributed to his contempt for the Papal Church, which led to his break with it and the Reformation that followed.

In the prevailing atmosphere of the sixteenth century, it does not seem as if syphilis was a serious social burden for its victims. But this changed in the seventeenth century with the increasing religiosity that came to characterize the higher strata of society. Syphilis was now regarded as the shameful result of a sinful life. This naturally did not prevent the spread of the disease, but it was talked about a great deal less. It has been claimed that the loss of hair that is often observed with syphilis, and which patients therefore frequently tried to hide, contributed to the fashion for shoulder-length allonge wigs during the reign of Louis xiv.

Moralizing about syphilis became a bit more relaxed in the eighteenth century, and fear of the disease had also decreased since it had become less aggressive over the years. But syphilis was still widespread in all social strata of the population.[203] This can be seen, for example, from the autobiography of the Venetian adventurer Giacomo Casanova, whose countless stories about women made him a natural potential victim of venereal diseases. Without beating about the bush, he relates that he had the disease at least ten times, although some of these attacks must certainly have been gonorrhoea and not syphilis. Casanova did not distinguish between the two diseases – nor did anyone else, including the doctors, before the nineteenth century. And quacks and charlatans were still doing good business in the eighteenth century, when gullibility and superstition existed side by side with the rationality of the Enlightenment period.

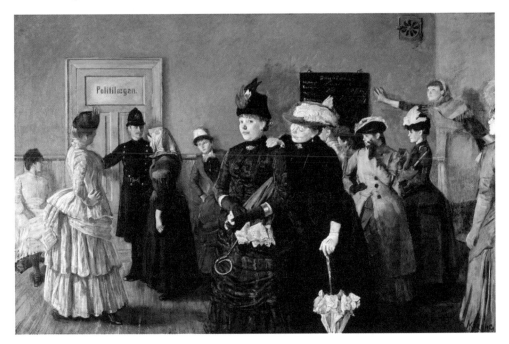

Christian Krohg, *Albertine to See the Police Surgeon*, 1887, oil on canvas. The picture shows the compulsory gynaecological examination of sex workers that was part of the fight against syphilis in many countries. Syphilis was regarded as a major social problem, with sex workers a key factor.

It was not until the nineteenth century that real progress was made in the medical view of syphilis.[204] Among the problems created by industrialization and urbanization was increased prostitution in the cities. In the middle of the century, one of the important figures in the history of syphilis, the French doctor Philippe Ricord, showed that syphilis and gonorrhoea were two different diseases by injecting pathogenic patient material into seventeen inmates of a Paris prison, an experiment that would hardly be approved today. He also described the three main stages of the disease. Ricord became famous, was appointed Napoleon III's personal physician and had a hospital named after him.

Of even greater importance in the fight against syphilis was Ricord's pupil Alfred Fournier, a researcher, doctor and strategist. He described the serious cerebral and spinal cord complications that affected patients in the third stage. He also realized that all the seriously proposed forms of treatment employed were virtually useless. He regarded syphilis as a social evil on a par with alcoholism that had to be combatted with far-reaching preventive measures, which included prostitution. He was also interested in the threat to marriage posed by husbands infecting their wives, who in turn infected their children. People began to talk about the 'innocent infected victims'. In Ibsen's *Ghosts* it is precisely Mrs Alving and her son Osvald who are examples of this. Ricord's efforts led to syphilis medicine, syphilology, becoming a recognized medical specialty – in fact the first – and he was awarded the first professorship in the field.

Among the many treatments tried out on syphilis in the early nineteenth century was a curiosity called syphilization.[205] This involved 'vaccinating' patients with material from 'soft chancre', a sore caused by a venereal disease that people then erroneously believed was a form of syphilis. The theory was that an overdose of the pathogenic material would have a favourable effect on the syphilis. The treatment had no effect and after a while was condemned in France as being directly dangerous. Despite this, it was used a great deal in Norway by Professor Carl Wilhelm Boeck. He was the uncle of Cæsar Boeck, who led the Oslo investigation of syphilis mentioned earlier. Carl Wilhelm became internationally famous for syphilization, which he wrote about in many languages in international journals and lectured on at conventions.[206] The treatment, fortunately, died with him in 1875. It was based on a

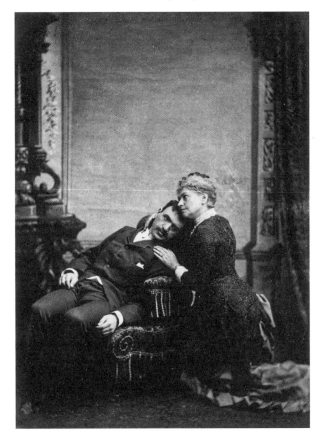

From the final act of Henrik Ibsen's play *Ghosts*. The young Osvald has congenital syphilis which is now affecting his brain and he cries out to his unhappy mother, widow Alving: 'Mother, give me the sun!' (The roles are played here by August Lindberg and Hedvig Winterhjelm, 1883.)

serious misunderstanding, since soft chancre has nothing to do with syphilis, but is connected to a completely different bacterium.

The bacteriological revolution also led to a hectic pursuit of the cause of syphilis, with many disappointments.[207] In 1905, however, Fritz Schaudinn and Erich Hoffmann in Berlin managed to detect the spiral-shaped bacteria, which they called *Treponema pallidum*. The following year another German bacteriologist, August Paul von Wassermann, invented a blood test, known as the Wassermann reaction, to detect syphilis in all its stages, including in cases where the patient was symptom-free. This blood test remained in use until recently, but has now been replaced by better ones.

World wars, medical breakthroughs – and medical molestation
At the beginning of the twentieth century syphilis was still an enormous problem. It has been claimed that 10 per cent of Europe's population

was infected. Probably a third of all the hospitalized syphilis patients on psychiatric wards had serious late complications from cerebral affection.

As in former ages, syphilis cases greatly increased under war conditions. The disease raged among the soldiers during the First World War, despite active attempts by the authorities to combat it. In the mid-1920s 60,000 men died each year from syphilis in England and Wales alone.[208] This was in spite of the fact that a new medicine to treat syphilis, Salvarsan, had been available since 1910. Unfortunately Salvarsan was not always effective, particularly in the later stages of syphilis, and it could have serious side-effects. Patients had also begun to be injected with vismuth, which admittedly had some results and at any rate caused fewer side-effects than Salvarsan.

During the Second World War syphilis erupted strongly again despite persistent attempts to combat it with eye-catching propaganda posters, in which warnings against sex workers were a constant theme. Such a poster showed a prostitute with a death's head walking arm in arm with Hitler and the Japanese emperor Hirohito, with a caption that said: 'She is the most dangerous of the three.'

In the early post-war years came the greatest breakthrough in the five-hundred-year history of syphilis, penicillin, which became generally available in 1947. Unlike Salvarsan, penicillin was extremely effective, with very few side-effects.

The extent of the syphilis problem in the first half of the twentieth century caused the American authorities to be very interested in clinical studies of the course of the disease. This led to one of the largest research scandals of recent times, the Tuskegee project.[209] In 1932 the U.S. Public Health Service started a study of 339 poor African Americans with untreated syphilis in the small town of Tuskegee, Alabama. The patients were not informed of their diagnosis, but were told that they had 'bad blood' and would therefore be followed medically. They received no treatment, not even when penicillin became available in 1947. The course of their illness, with eventual complications, was registered. This experiment continued for forty years until it was exposed by the press in 1972. A number of the patients had already died by that time, many of their wives had been infected and a number of their children had been born with syphilis. The study represents a clear breach of fundamental medical ethics, and it led to a tightening up of ethical rules for medical research. Naturally enough, it is linked to racist attitudes. In 1997 President Bill Clinton invited those still living from the Tuskegee experiment to the White House, where he apologized on behalf of the American authorities. For many of them, this apology came far too late.

This was not the only skeleton in the cupboard hidden by the u.s. Public Health Service. In 2010 it was revealed that between 1946 and 1948, in cooperation with the authorities in Guatemala, it had deliberately infected 1,500 soldiers, prostitutes, prisoners and patients at psychiatric hospitals with syphilis bacteria.[210] The intention was to observe the effect of antibiotics on the infection. The project was broken off when the supplies of penicillin ran out. Many of the 'guinea pigs' later died of their syphilis. The American government later apologized to Guatemala.

Geniuses and princes

Down through the ages, syphilis has had an aura of sex, sin and death about it. This is probably part of the explanation why, when dealing with the history of this infection, people have eagerly concentrated on famous people said to have been afflicted by it, more so than with any other epidemic. Here we can see a certain similarity with the aids epidemic of our own time, where the general public was also particularly interested in famous victims. But there are probably reasons beyond a desire for sensationalism that explain why accounts of syphilis throughout history have often focused on celebrities within various sections of society. When it comes to princes and heads of state, there are many examples, as with other serious infectious diseases such as smallpox, of how there can be considerable political and historical consequences when such people are affected. This also applies to the chronic infection of syphilis, which can, among other things, cause cerebral affection, particularly during the third stage. If heads of state are involved, this can of course have serious consequences. Artists and writers have also provoked the curiosity of historians interested in the field of syphilis, and imaginative theories have been advanced about possible connections between infection and artistic creativity.[211]

I have earlier discussed the problems often encountered when identifying the causes of past epidemics. The problem becomes even greater when one wishes to propose a diagnosis in individual historical figures where the available information is often somewhat uncertain. This is especially difficult in the case of syphilis – the great imitator – which can produce symptoms that resemble a whole series of other conditions. In my opinion, the considerable literature within this area has taken too little account of this. This applies not only to the many airy, sensationalist accounts of syphilis in historical figures but to the presentation of serious writers with a medical background.

From the sixteenth century, when the syphilis epidemic was particularly virulent, we have already seen well-founded examples of individuals with syphilis, some of whom, such as Joseph Grünpeck and Ulrich von Hutten, described the story of their own affliction in detail.[212] This particularly applies to the Renaissance.

The list of princes and heads of state who have been given the syphilis diagnosis is extremely long. Cesare Borgia's syphilis is well documented. Pope Julius II definitely had syphilis and probably died of it. The assertion that the popes Alexander VI (Cesare Borgia's father) and Leo X (son of Lorenzo de' Medici, *Il magnifico*, in Florence) were struck down by syphilis is more uncertain, although their way of life was a standing invitation to the bacterium *Treponema pallidum*.[213]

Three rulers from the sixteenth century are constantly mentioned as examples of crowned carriers of syphilis: Tsar Ivan the Terrible of Russia, King Francis I of France and King Henry VIII of England.[214] What is the basis for their diagnoses?

Ivan the Terrible was born in 1530, the son of the Grand Duke of Moscow.[215] He gained power at the early age of fourteen and was crowned Russia's first tsar in 1547. Shortly afterwards he married the pious Anastasia. Ivan had lived a wild youth and was certainly exposed to syphilis infection. The couple had three sons; the first died after a few months. In the first years of his reign Ivan was a good and, by the yardstick of his age, fairly humane leader of the state. Then Anastasia died in 1560. Beside himself with grief, Ivan threw himself into excessive debauchery and made violent attacks on innocent friends. From 1564 his behaviour had all the characteristics of a serious mental illness, resulting in a string of massacres and killing members of the civil population, Church and nobility until his death following a stroke in 1584. He also killed his own son, the heir to the throne, with his own hands.

Ivan was succeeded by his surviving son, Feodor, who was mentally less gifted and had a physical appearance resembling that caused by

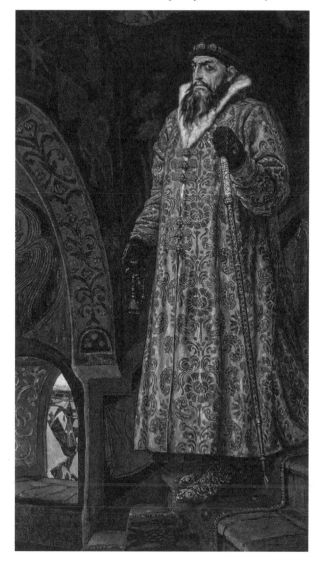

Ivan IV of Russia – Ivan the Terrible – was tsar from 1547 until 1584. There is some basis for believing that he suffered from syphilis, which might have changed his personality over the years and, among other things, have led to the many acts that brought about his nickname.

congenital syphilis. There have also been strong suspicions that Ivan's dramatic personality change in the early 1560s was the result of brain damage caused by syphilis contracted in his youth, but on its own that is not evidence that syphilis played a role in the Russian tragedy under Ivan.

In 1963 the remains of Ivan and his sons were exhumed and examined. It turned out that Ivan's body contained high concentrations of mercury. That could very well be an indication that indeed he had syphilis and that it had been treated with mercury, a common treatment at the time. The researcher who examined Ivan, on the other hand, interpreted this as the result of the use of ointments containing mercury, which had been used to treat the rheumatic pains in his legs that plagued Ivan during his final years. There were allegedly no discovered signs of syphilis. That remains the current position, with suspicions about this diagnosis but no certain evidence that Ivan had been a victim of the disease.

Francis I was born in 1494 and crowned king of France in 1515.[216] He was, in the best sense, the typical Renaissance ruler, highly interested in art, science and architecture. He founded a large library – and actually read many of the books. The famous Italian artists Leonardo da Vinci and Benvenuto Cellini were invited to his court. Cellini, incidentally, also had syphilis, which he described vividly in his autobiography. Francis explained the formula for his dazzling court: 'A court without women is like a spring without roses.' He also eagerly plucked the roses and came to feel the thorns: at the age of thirty he contracted syphilis. He died 23 years later, possibly from the disease.

Did the illness have consequences for his life and the way he governed? Despite his undoubted intelligence and considerable knowledge, Francis had little good fortune with his major political decisions. He was unstable and easily influenced. In his later years he displayed increased despotic tendencies, including his brutal treatment of the Protestant minority in France. Were these changes of personality a consequence of syphilis? Some historians have claimed this, but it is pure guesswork.[217]

Another Renaissance ruler who was a contemporary of Francis, Henry VIII of England, has inspired heated debate about his state of health.[218] Did he have syphilis, and does that explain important features of his personality and policies in government?

Henry, who was born in 1491, was highly educated and spoke several languages. He was extremely interested in literature, science and art, and was himself an accomplished writer, composer and musician. He was also much taken by women, and is especially remembered for his six marriages and many mistresses. As a young man he was charming and stately, and also proficient in many sports.

As the years passed, a dramatic change occurred both in his outward appearance and in his personality. From around the age of forty he became increasingly labile, with growing signs of paranoia. Possibly he was partly psychotic. At the same time he developed an increasingly despotic form of government, ordering the execution of supporters of religious minorities and others who had aroused his displeasure. Among these were two of his queens, Anne Boleyn and Catherine Howard. Was this a result of a brain disease caused by syphilis contracted during his early manhood? Let us look at the arguments advanced about his syphilis diagnosis.[219]

Henry's first two wives had a striking frequency of stillbirth and children who died in early infancy. His first queen, Catherine of Aragon, had seven pregnancies, but these produced only one child who survived longer than a few hours or days, the later Mary I. Since syphilis increases the risk of miscarriages and stillbirths, it has therefore been claimed that Henry had infected Catherine with syphilis. If this is correct, syphilis was to have major political consequences. Because he had not produced a male heir who lived beyond 52 days, Henry wanted the pope to annul the marriage so that he could marry a new wife, Anne Boleyn. When the pope refused, Henry broke with Rome and established the independent Anglican Church, with himself as its head. The pope's refusal was probably due to the influence of the Habsburg emperor Charles v, who was Catherine of Aragon's uncle. Charles v was a dominating force in Italy after having overcome a French army weakened by syphilis, as described earlier.

Supporters of the theory of Henry's syphilis further claim that the striking physical and mental changes of his later years were an expression of syphilis in the third stage, with cerebral affection. He also had a vilesmelling deep wound in one thigh that has been considered syphilitic. His daughter Mary I, who reigned before her younger sister took the throne as Elizabeth I, is said to have displayed illness characteristics that could well be an expression of congenital syphilis.[220]

The arguments in favour of Henry VIII having had syphilis are in my opinion rather weak and not based on tangible facts. We have quite detailed medical accounts from Henry's royal physicians, without it being mentioned anywhere that the king was given mercury treatment, which was well known in England at the time. The wound in his thigh could have been a chronic bacterial infection after an injury – an osteomyelitis. Henry had suffered quite a few such injuries, including one in 1537 when he fell off his horse during a tournament, injured his head and was unconscious for a couple of hours. After this injury he was no longer able to carry out any particularly physical activity. This, without a doubt, contributed to his constant increase in weight. During his last years he had to be moved around in a sedan chair. His marked mental changes may possibly have been a late consequence of an earlier head injury. Other illnesses have also been suggested, including diabetes and hormonal disturbances. Recently, it has been claimed that he might have had a rare blood group in the Kell blood group system, one linked to a particular illness, the McLeod syndrome. This causes cerebral affection, and the special Kell blood group could also explain Henry's problem in producing children capable of survival.[221]

Let us now move into the eighteenth century and take a look at another famous monarch who often features on the list of royal syphilis patients, Catherine the Great of Russia.[222] A minor German princess by birth, in 1745 she married the badly smallpox-scarred and not very gifted heir to the Russian throne, himself born in Germany. He became Tsar Peter III in January 1762 and was murdered six months later. From then until her death in 1796 Catherine ruled Russia as an absolute monarch, and governed well. She was intelligent, knowledgeable and well read, and a supporter of the ideals of the Enlightenment which, partially at any rate, she attempted to put into practice. Among her many interests was men. From her early twenties, she had a great many lovers, particularly officers.

What evidence is there that Catherine, one of the leading monarchs in Europe in the latter half of the eighteenth century, had syphilis? We have no evidence that she ever displayed symptoms that indicated it. On the other hand, people have focused a great deal on the pattern of her many pregnancies, where her husband can hardly be considered as having been the potential father. The first two pregnancies ended in miscarriages, the third produced a sickly boy, and the fourth a sickly girl who died after several months. She later had two normal pregnancies with apparently healthy children. Catherine's history of pregnancies is compatible with what is known as 'Kassowitz's law', which states that when a woman with syphilis has a series of pregnancies, the signs of congenital syphilis in the offspring become progressively weaker with each child. But Catherine's history of pregnancies is insufficient evidence for pronouncing a syphilis diagnosis.

Do we know anything about the health condition of Catherine's various lovers? Apart from the fact that most of them were officers, and some of them were given to debauchery, we have no information about any syphilis. Furthermore, Catherine herself was very much concerned about the risk of contracting a venereal disease and ordered her personal physician to examine all recruits to her bed to avoid this. In addition, one of her ladies-in-waiting had the task of 'interviewing' potential lovers. On one occasion, incidentally, this lady went a bit too far in testing the subject of her interview and was fired after having been caught in flagrante delicto.

Those who claim that Catherine had syphilis emphasize that she seemed to have a conspicuous interest in the subject.[223] This was clear from her preoccupation with the prevention and treatment of venereal diseases in Russia, where they flourished. She established the world's first specialized hospital for such diseases and insisted that the patients should be treated with respect and discretion. In this she was far ahead of her time. Is this a strong argument in favour of her having had syphilis herself? I remain unconvinced. As mentioned, she was very interested

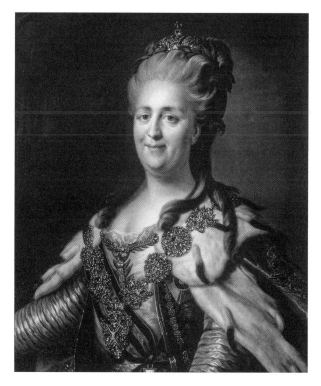

Catherine II, known as Catherine the Great, was tsarina of Russia from 1762 to 1796. There are some indications that she had syphilis.

in the ideas of the Enlightenment and attempted, with various degrees of success, to modernize what was, in many respects, a quite backwards country. Care for patients with venereal diseases was probably just one of many examples of this.

Several heads of state in modern times have probably had syphilis, even though the diagnosis must often be regarded as uncertain. When it comes, however, to the first leader of the Soviet Union, Vladimir Lenin, there is scarcely any doubt that he suffered from syphilis that eventually led to a serious brain disease.[224] Subsequent leaders tried for a number of years to conceal the fact.

Writers, philosophers and composers

Artists have always been the subject of public interest. This is not only because of admiration for their works but a certain fascination with their special way of life, which often runs counter to bourgeois norms. It is hardly surprising that people have also been absorbed by details of artists' sexual lives and their possible consequences – including syphilis. Another reason for this interest is that it has been claimed that the syphilitic cerebral affection may stimulate creativity and productivity in artists.[225]

History records a whole host of poets, writers and visual artists who have been said to have suffered from syphilis. But here we naturally ought to be critical about making diagnoses from a distance, since once again, on a closer observation of the facts, it often transpires that the diagnosis of syphilis is not always well founded. Despite this, there remain many instances where it probably holds water. Most of these cases are from the nineteenth century, which not coincidentally was the time when important new knowledge was gained about the disease and its various stages, even while there was still no effective treatment apart from the centuries-old and more or less inefficacious methods. As a result the infection often went through all the various stages, possibly down to the late complications.

One of the leading French poets of the Romantic period, Alfred de Musset, undoubtedly suffered from syphilis, and died from it at the early age of 46 in 1847. He had the typical cardiovascular complication with an enlargement of the aorta and damage to the heart valves. This gives rise to a very heavy pulse, so that the head nods in time with it. In medicine, this is referred to as 'Musset's sign', after the unfortunate poet.

The French poet Charles Baudelaire, best known for his collection *Les fleurs du mal* (The Flowers of Evil), contracted syphilis and died in his mother's arms with serious cerebral affection when also only 46 years old.

Another well-known French writer of the second half of the nineteenth century, Alphonse Daudet, contracted syphilis in his early youth and after some years developed the dreaded late complication *tabes dorsalis*.[226] The violent pains caused by this disease meant that he was strongly addicted to morphine in his final years. Daudet wrote an autobiographical account of his sufferings, *La Doulou*, known in English as *In the Land of Pain*, which was not printed until 1931, more than thirty years after his death. In this book, which many regard as his finest work, he writes that his afflictions resemble those suffered by another famous writer, the German poet Heinrich Heine.

From his mid-forties Heine developed increasing paralysis of the legs, which kept him bed-ridden for the last years of his life: he called it his 'mattress grave'. He was also in considerable pain and made use of morphine. Many people have concluded that Heine had syphilis with *tabes dorsalis*, although this diagnosis is uncertain.[227] Either way, one has to admire Heine, who despite his afflictions continued to write unforgettable works almost until the day he died. He also retained his sense of humour. Before he died in 1856, he jokingly asked his wife to promise him she would marry again, for, as he said: 'Then at least I will know for sure that there is one man who will regret my death.'

One of the best-known novelists of world literature, Gustave Flaubert, did not escape an encounter with *Treponema pallidum* either. Indeed he almost went in search of it. A journey to the Middle East, combined with unusually extrovert sexual behaviour, ended with a series of venereal diseases, including syphilis. Flaubert lost first his hair and then his teeth from mercury treatment. Even so, he was almost proud of his syphilis.[228] The same pride is found in another well-known French author, Guy de Maupassant, who enthusiastically exclaimed in a letter that he now had contracted the 'majestic' and 'elegant' syphilis that also 'Francis I died of'.

The elegant Oscar Wilde, the darling of London society until his tragic fall because of homosexual behaviour, then a punishable offence, probably contracted syphilis in his youth. It has been claimed that his treatment had damaged his teeth, which is why he refused to show them in any of the photographs taken of him. When he died in a shoddy hotel room in Paris in 1900, it was probably not because of syphilis. His wit did not desert him even on his deathbed, for when he looked at the hideous wallpaper, the old aesthete exclaimed: 'One of us must go.'

At the end of the nineteenth century a theory arose that the cerebral affection in the late stage of syphilis could have had an enhancing effect on creativity and productivity in artists and writers, with something called 'syphilitic toxin' stimulating the brain cells.[229] Maupassant was named as an example. Some have especially pointed to the German writer and philosopher Friedrich Nietzsche, whose highly productive career as a philosopher in the 1870s and '80s made him one of the most influential thinkers of modern times. This came to a dramatic end one day in January 1889, when he broke down in the street in Turin and, in tears, embraced a horse. From then on he was afflicted by increasing dementia and became in effect a long-stay geriatric patient until his death in 1900.[230] For many years it has been regarded as almost an incontrovertible fact that his cerebral disease was a dreaded late complication of syphilis, *paralysis generalis*. During the last couple of years prior to his breakdown, Nietzsche had displayed tremendous creativity, which has been taken as further proof of the idea that cerebral syphilis, for a while at least, can stimulate creativity. In recent years a number of people have questioned this syphilis diagnosis. Perhaps he had a congenital cerebral disease that causes dementia?[231]

The Danish writer Karen Blixen was infected with syphilis by her husband and, like Alphonse Daudet, developed the late complication *tabes dorsalis*, which had a drastic effect on her later years, just when she was gaining international fame.[232] It is interesting that she too believed that syphilis had a positive effect on her writing: 'Now that I have also lived through this, I approach greater things.'

Nor do we find any basis for a connection between syphilis and creativity in famous painters or composers.[233] This applies, for example, to the French painter Édouard Manet, who died with symptoms of a syphilitic neural disease. The Austrian composer Franz Schubert, who died when only 31 years old, probably had syphilis and underwent mercury treatment. There is disagreement as to whether he died of his syphilis or of a bacterial intestinal infection. Apart from the fact that the

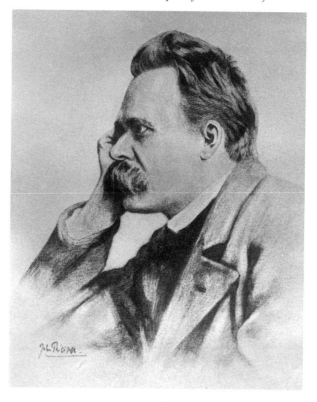

German philosopher Friedrich Nietzsche. For many years it was assumed that he suffered from the dreaded late complication of syphilis known as *paralysis generalis.*

compositions of his final years often have an air of melancholy about them, it is difficult to see any connection between syphilis and his art. Schubert's colleague Robert Schumann contracted syphilis at a young age and had both neurological functional disturbances and symptoms of a severe mental illness. Whether he died of syphilis in the third stage or of a mental affliction after two years in an institution is uncertain. Either way, his syphilis cannot be said to have had any positive effect on his artistic activity.

The fact of the matter is that there is no basis for asserting that the syphilis infection in itself can stimulate brain cells and increase artistic activity. The consequences of syphilis are generally speaking tragic both for geniuses and for ordinary people. Whether suffering and adversity can have certain positive effects on creative artists is, of course, a completely different question.

Was syphilis a gift from the New World?

After Columbus 'discovered' America, the continent was ravaged by a series of infectious diseases from the Old World. Did Europe, on the other hand, get syphilis in return? This has been claimed by many, almost from the start of the syphilis epidemic in the sixteenth century. Many others, however, have disagreed, and the discussion has been carried on with considerable vigour right up to the present day.

Those who are convinced that syphilis originally came from America – what we can refer to as the Columbus theory – point to the fact that this disease had not previously been seen in the Old World. One searches in vain in the writings of Hippocrates and Galen for any mention of such an illness. The fact that syphilis erupted so violently in the first decades of the sixteenth century in Europe has also been seen as proof that it hit a virgin population without any previous immunity, as we have seen with such epidemics as measles.

The Spanish physician Ruy Díaz de Isla stated that he had personally treated several members of Columbus's crew for the new disease. This claim appears in a book first published in 1539, although there is a manuscript copy dating from 1521. Nonetheless, that still places it nearly thirty years after the events and many doubt the statement's reliability.[234]

Until quite recently it was not possible to analyse DNA from *Treponema pallidum* in human archaeological finds, unlike with the plague, where DNA finds have been invaluable. On the other hand, a syphilis infection will, in many patients, produce typical changes in the skeleton after a number of years that experts claim to be able to distinguish from other diseases that affect bones. Such changes have been found in skeletal remains in the Americas long before the arrival of the Europeans, while the few corresponding finds asserted to have been made in Europe from the pre-Columbus era are highly controversial.[235]

This 'bone proof' has been given great weight in the discussion on the origins of syphilis as an important argument in favour of the Columbus theory. But the situation is unfortunately more complex than this. In the family of bacteria with the family name *Treponema* there are several members that are extremely closely related to the syphilis bacterium, but that cause less serious diseases.[236] In Africa, for example, there is the bacterium that causes the disease yaws, which often leads to deep, chronic wounds of the skin, and in the Middle East there is the disease bejel, which also causes a skin disease.

These other *Treponema* diseases, which are not sexually transmitted but come from close physical contact, existed in Europe before Columbus, possibly from ancient times. A few researchers who doubt the Columbus theory believe that the syphilis bacterium may have arisen from one of these close relations in the Old World. The pathogenic picture they have produced has perhaps not differed all that much from many other diseases in the Europe of the time, such as leprosy. That the mutation that allegedly led to the more dangerous syphilis bacterium happened around the time Columbus returned from America may be coincidental. The special conditions in the sixteenth century with the relaxing of norms and the increase of sexual promiscuity without a doubt enhanced the chances of a sexually transmitted bacterium of the *Treponema* family spreading. If this theory is correct, we have a fresh example of the considerable capacity of microbes to adapt to changed conditions in their surroundings.

New research results that focus on the origin of syphilis appear regularly and the last word has yet to be said. At the moment, the tendency among researchers is to believe that the syphilis bacterium comes from the American continent, where the *Treponema* family has existed for thousands of years, probably since the first humans came to the continent from Asia via the Bering Strait, bringing the microbes along with them.[237] Recently, however, it has proved possible to detect DNA from the various *Treponema* variants in human remains that are several hundred years old.[238] Gradually, perhaps, such methods will shed new light on the long-lasting debate regarding the origin of syphilis.

Syphilis has a five-hundred-year history, but it is by no means a closed chapter. The infection is on the increase in Europe, North America, China and Australia.[239] In 2009 almost 11 million new cases were reported in the world. It would seem that syphilis epidemics come in waves with intervals of between ten and fifteen years. This may be partly due to the relaxing of control measures. It may also be a consequence of new forms of sexually risky behaviour developing. It is further possible that the immunity of the population also moves in waves. But syphilis no longer has the same dreadful disease picture it had at the beginning of the sixteenth century, and today it can be treated effectively.

Tuberculosis: The White Death

Tuberculosis is no longer a disease that preoccupies significant numbers of people in the Western world. Until the first years after the Second World War, however, the situation was completely different. Tuberculosis was previously a very common cause of illness and death. Most people had relations who had been affected. In rural areas it was possible to point to farms where tuberculosis had struck one generation after the other. This disease has been the lot of humanity for thousands of years. The tuberculosis bacterium has probably been humanity's companion ever since *Homo sapiens* roamed the African savannahs. In all probability, this bacterium has taken the lives of more humans than any other microbe, with the possible exception of smallpox and malaria. The history of tuberculosis also excellently illustrates how ecological and environmental factors are involved in the never-ending duel between man and microbe. Before embarking on this history, let us look more closely at the disease itself.

From enchanted sleep to rampant disease

The cause of tuberculosis (TB) is *Mycobacterium tuberculosis* (MTB), the bacterium that Robert Koch discovered in 1882.[240] It belongs to a large family of mycobacteria, which are widespread in nature in earth and water. Some can cause disease in various species of animals and a few are so closely related to MTB that they can even cause tuberculosis in human beings, but such cases are very rare. The vast majority of cases of tuberculosis have been caused by MTB, which is normally only found in humans, although it can, in special instances, also infect animals such as apes.

MTB mainly causes infection in the lungs. Most people become infected when a patient with pulmonary disease ejects bacteria when coughing, sneezing or simply talking. The bacteria exist in tiny particles, aerosols, which are breathed in by others and cause infection of the lungs. Tuberculosis bacteria can survive for several months outside the lungs in dust particles. Fewer than ten single bacteria can be sufficient to start a new infection if inhaled. In most cases, the recipient's immune system will take care of the bacteria and either neutralize them or 'encapsulate' them in lung tissue with a wall of various immune cells and tissue. This is what happens in perhaps 95 per cent of cases. By being encapsulated in this way, they can lie in a kind of enchanted sleep for many decades, perhaps the patient's entire lifetime, without doing any damage.[241]

Occasionally, however, the bacteria can wake from their torpor because the immune system for some reason or other has relaxed its grip and can no longer keep them in check. The bacteria can then start to damage the lung tissue and spread through the lungs and possibly to the rest of the body. Untreated, the lungs will gradually be ruined, often resulting in death. An important characteristic of the pulmonary disease is that it forms larger and smaller cavities that contain large quantities of bacteria. These changes considerably increase infectiousness.

Disease of parts of the body other than the lungs can also result. The skeletal system is then often attacked. In former times one often saw tuberculous infection of the lymph nodes in the neck. This was called scrofula. Skin infection was also quite common and was known as *lupus vulgaris*.[242]

Why do the encapsulated tuberculosis bacteria occasionally become active and cause illness? Apart from weakness of the immune system, various other diseases or forms of treatment that weaken the immune system can also revive the bacteria. This is seen in connection with HIV infection and diabetes, and with patients who suffer from rheumatic diseases and are given cortisone or other medication in order to reduce harmful immune reactions.[243]

The immune system plays a complex double role in connection with tuberculosis. On the one hand, the immune defence system is important to stop infection initially, but when the bacteria revive and start to cause the illness, much of the damage to the tissue is caused by an over-reaction of the immune system, which hammers away in vain at the bacteria, thereby causing inflammation.[244]

Active tuberculosis of the lungs results in coughing, high temperature, a gradually increasing loss of weight and, in the later stages, coughing up blood. Although tuberculosis normally develops relatively slowly, one sometimes sees more dramatic instances where the lung disease gets rapidly worse, as in 'galloping pulmonary tuberculosis', or where the bacteria rapidly spread through the blood to most tissues and organs, as in so-called miliary tuberculosis (the term 'miliary' comes from the

Latin word for millet seed, since in this form of the disease there are numerous small nodes the size of such seeds in many tissues and organs).

Egyptians, Romans and sea lions

We know that tuberculosis is a very old disease. In mapping the fascinating history of this disease it is possible to use all the means at our disposal when studying historical epidemics: written accounts, archaeological finds from examining skeletons and modern molecular-biological methods. This is an active field of research where new finds are regularly being published, and where there is still disagreement among researchers concerning interpretation. We do not have all the answers yet regarding the origin and history of tuberculosis. Nevertheless, we can distinguish the major lines in its history to quite a large extent.

In written accounts from former ages it is mainly descriptions of diseases resembling pulmonary tuberculosis that we can build on. More or less long-lasting disease descriptions are found in writings from a number of civilizations.[245] The earliest of these come from the Indian Veda literature written in Sanskrit as early as 1500 BC, where there also appear the first descriptions of scrofula. The law code of the Babylonian king Hammurabi, recorded in cuneiform writing on a stele from the years up to 1750 BC, contains a quite clear reference to 'a wasting disease'. Chinese writings in the first millennium BC mention diseases that were probably pulmonary tuberculosis. In the Bible, on the other hand, there are extremely few references to anything that could possibly be tuberculosis.

Nor was tuberculosis unknown in ancient Greece, where the disease was called *phtisis* ('wasting' or 'consumption'; the Greek verb *phtiein* means 'to waste away').[246] The designation 'consumption' has followed the disease right up to recent times, both in medicine and in the vernacular. As far back as Homer's *Odyssey* there is mention of 'serious wasting that takes the soul from the body and causes the sufferer to lie sick for a long time and wither away'. But we have to turn to Hippocrates once more for the first comprehensive description of the disease, both of the pulmonary disease and mention of attacks on the spinal column. From his writings, we can conclude that tuberculosis was quite common at the time. His contemporary, Plato, also mentions

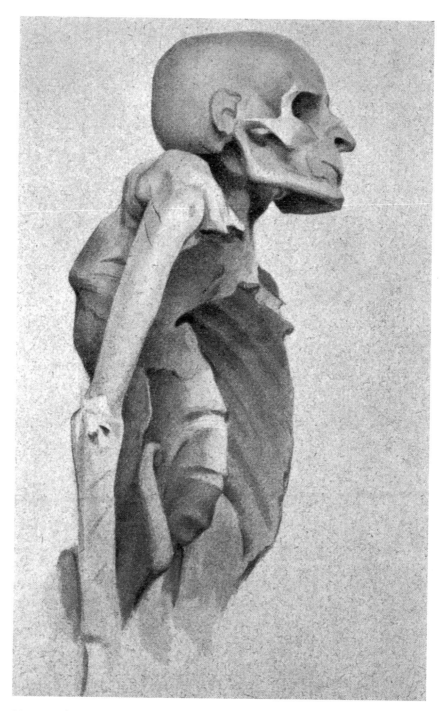

Mummy of a priest of the god Ammon, with tuberculosis of the spinal column and the formation of a hump known as Pott's disease. The mummy is from the 21st Dynasty, *c.* 1000 BC.

the disease, which he believed was one that no one could or should even attempt to treat.

The ancient descriptions are of course not always unambiguous. Certain other diseases can at times give rise to chronic cases of pulmonary illness. Are there any more reliable bases for our description of the history of tuberculosis?

Archaeological investigations of human remains have contributed to a considerable extent to our knowledge of the history of tuberculosis. Skeletal finds in particular have proved useful since bones are better preserved than other organs.[247] When tuberculosis attacks the spinal column, a deformity often occurs that produces the typical hump. This condition is known as Pott's disease. Such changes have been found in many Egyptian mummies. In a number of such cases, the tuberculosis diagnosis has been confirmed by the detection of DNA from MTB. Since only a lesser proportion of tuberculosis patients, perhaps between about 5 and 10 per cent, have such skeletal changes, we can assume that tuberculosis was a common disease in ancient Egypt from the fourth millennium BC onwards.[248] Egyptian art also depicts people with the characteristic hunchbacked deformity we connect with tuberculosis. There are reasons to assume that there were special sanatoriums for this disease in Egypt as far back as 3,000 years ago.

The most famous of the ancient Egyptians to have been given the tuberculosis diagnosis is one of the most powerful of all the pharaohs, Rameses II, who died about 1200 BC. His mummy was transported to France in 1976 for thorough examination, and evidence of tuberculosis was found. It created well-justified interest. Bruno Latour, the postmodern philosopher of science, claimed that Rameses could not have had tuberculosis, since MTB was not discovered by Robert Koch until 1882! Latour believed, absurdly enough, as did certain other extreme postmodern intellectuals, that scientific facts do not have any real validity, but are merely constructions.[249]

The very oldest well-documented finds of MTB in humans to date are from Syria and are 9,000 years old.[250] But tuberculosis is probably far older. Single finds suggest that precursors of the tuberculosis bacterium earlier produced the disease in the apemen ancestors of *Homo sapiens.* It is perhaps suggested in what is probably tuberculosis in a 500,000-year-old representative of *Homo erectus,* one of our forefathers, but the skeletal changes have not been confirmed by DNA analyses. Some researchers claim that MTB originally comes from East Africa.[251] The progenitor of the bacterium may have been a soil bacterium that learned how to infect humans and has since followed us and gradually adapted itself to human development and external, ecological changes.

The tuberculosis bacterium has characteristics that enable it to get by under a wide range of changing conditions. When humans were hunters and gatherers in small groups, it was to the bacterium's advantage that it led to a long-lasting, symptom-free illness, so that it did not die out in that small group. After the first epidemiological transition, when humans settled and engaged in agriculture and animal husbandry, the bacterium had new chances that it could exploit by changing its characteristics. By means of its capacity for airborne infection of a large number of people living close together, it is not improbable that the bacterium became more dangerous, more virulent, for now it had a far greater number of potential victims and no longer needed to be 'cautious' in its treatment of them. From then on, tuberculosis became a much more common disease than it had been in humanity's earlier existence as hunters and gatherers.[252]

One of the mycobacteria that very closely resemble MTB is *Mycobacterium bovis*, which can cause illness in both humans and cattle, as well as a whole range of other animals. Until recently people believed that MTB came from this cattle bacterium, which 'jumped' over to humans after animal husbandry became common, as we have seen with many other infections. Modern molecular biology has disproved that theory.[253] MTB is much older than *M. bovis*, but the latter bacterium has without a doubt contributed to tuberculosis in humans in former times, for example via infected milk. Today it is still a considerable problem for those who keep cattle in many countries, partly because wild animals that carry the bacterium may be a constant source of infection for the cattle. This applies, for example, to the badger in England.

New finds show that the emergence of the Roman empire, the most comprehensive empire to have arisen in Europe until then, might have played a major role in the increase of tuberculosis.[254] At the beginning of the second century AD, the empire under Trajan included the entire Mediterranean area, with parts of the Middle East, North Africa, and large sections of Central and Western Europe, including Britain and the

Balkans. Pax Romana – the Roman peace – guaranteed transport within the empire via both a superb road system and extensive shipping. But this also meant that tuberculosis could spread much more easily than before. The spread may also have taken place because Roman legions were constantly being shifted inside the empire to counter the threat of attacks from surrounding peoples.

It was probably just as important that a number of aspects of the Roman lifestyle were highly favourable for tuberculosis infection. More and more people lived close together in ever-growing cities. Rome had now become the largest city in the world, with more than a million inhabitants. The lower class lived in densely populated tenements, and Roman baths and markets were popular meeting places where microbes could also be exchanged. Numerous archaeological finds show that tuberculosis in Roman Europe became quite common.

Did tuberculosis exist in the New World when Columbus arrived in 1492? Yes: the disease had probably been in the Americas as long as *Homo sapiens*. When our forefathers emigrated from Africa 60,000–100,000 years ago, they were very likely accompanied by the tuberculosis bacterium, which then gradually spread to all continents.[255] It presumably came to America along with the first humans, via the Bering Strait. There are many early finds of what is probably tuberculosis in North and South America.

It caused quite a stir when researchers were able to show a few years ago that tuberculosis, detected in some skeletons from the west coast of Peru, was due to *Mycobacterium pinnipedii*, a bacterium that is closely related to the human bacterium, but found mainly in seals and sea lions.[256] These researchers suggested that the bacterium had perhaps spread with, for example, seals from Africa in the course of the last two thousand years. We know that this bacterium can cause tuberculosis in humans as well: infection from sea lions in zoos has sometimes taken place, for instance. But this form of the disease cannot be spread from human to human. Most researchers therefore believe that these Peruvian victims must have been special cases, and that tuberculosis in America, also prior to Columbus, was due to the 'classic' MTB, and came with the immigration of humans to the continent.

In the centuries before Columbus arrived, it would nevertheless seem as if tuberculosis was very much on the retreat in the indigenous

American population. With the Spanish conquistadors and later immigrants from Europe, the original American population received a highly unwelcome 'topping up' of tuberculosis, which was naturally added to the many other infectional tragedies that occurred in the wake of the European invasion.

'The king's evil' and the consequences of industrialization

After the Western Roman empire collapsed at the end of the fifth century AD, social and political relations changed radically, with Europe entering what have sometimes been called the Dark Ages. During this first part of the Middle Ages, the conditions for the spread of tuberculosis were no longer as favourable as during the Roman period, even though we know little about the extent of the disease in those centuries. From the High Middle Ages onwards, however, we estimate that tuberculosis was a fairly common disease. We know of at least one famous twelfth-century tuberculosis patient, Francis of Assisi, who exposed himself to infection through his indefatigable work on behalf of the poor and wretched in society.[257]

Tuberculosis increased during the seventeenth century. A key to this is the historical information we have about scrofula. This tuberculous infection of the lymph nodes in the neck once received considerable attention because there was a widespread belief in both France and England that a lawful king could cure the disease by placing his hands on the sick person's neck. Scrofula was therefore referred to as 'the king's evil.'[258] Clovis I, the Merovingian king of the Franks, was probably the first king to carry out this treatment at his coronation in AD 496, and he was followed by French kings for more than a thousand years. Louis XIV is said to have 'touched' 2,500 victims. His record, however, is surpassed by his contemporary, the British king Charles II, who during a twenty-year period touched no fewer than 9,500 victims. The Church of England even developed a special liturgy for this ceremony. William Shakespeare writes about this in *Macbeth*, anachronistically describing the ritual as if conducted by Macbeth's contemporary, Edward the Confessor of England:

'Tis call'd the evil:
A most miraculous work in this good king;
Which often, since my here-remain in England,

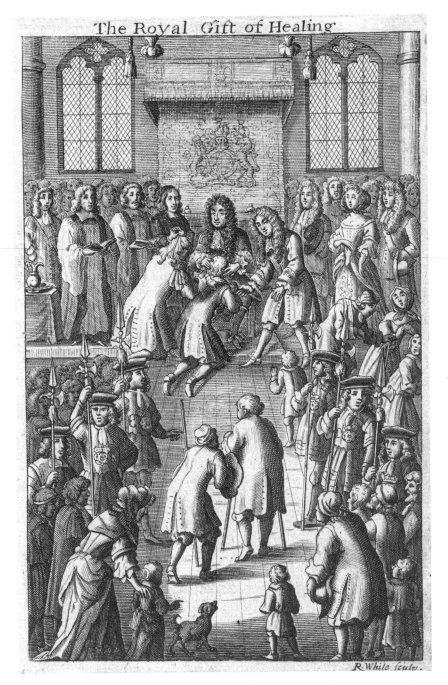

The Royal Gift of Healing

R.White sculp.

Charles II touches patients with scrofula in order to cure them in an engraving by R. White, *c.* 1684. Belief in the royal 'treatment' was more than 1,000 years old, and scrofula was therefore referred to as the 'king's evil'.

I have seen him do. How he solicits heaven,
Himself best knows; but strangely-visited people,
All swoll'n and ulcerous, pitiful to the eye,
The mere despair of surgery, he cures,
Hanging a golden stamp about their necks,
Put on with holy prayers, and 'tis spoken,
To the succeeding royalty he leaves
The healing benediction.[259]

There are reasons to believe that scrofula was common during the late medieval period and the Renaissance. Since this special form of tuberculosis only represents 5 per cent of all forms of the disease, we can multiply by twenty to calculate the approximate total of tuberculosis cases.[260]

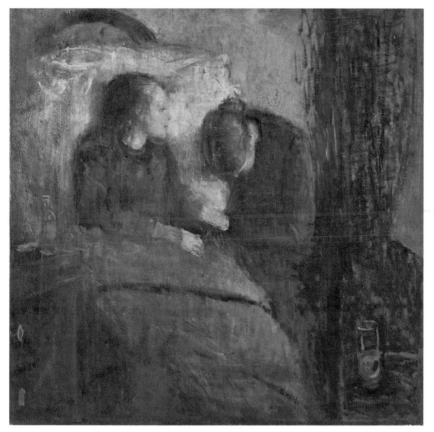

Edvard Munch, *The Sick Child*, 1885–6, oil on canvas. The usual view is that the pale child with the glazed look represents Munch's elder sister, who died of tuberculosis when he was fifteen years old. He never confirmed this himself.

In the course of the eighteenth century tuberculosis steadily increased throughout Europe, peaking in the first half of the nineteenth century. As mentioned, the process of industrialization, which began at the end of the eighteenth century, led to an increased influx into the emerging towns, where living conditions for the vast numbers of poor in the slums were wretched.[261] Undernourishment, crowded housing conditions and bad sanitation were all fertile ground for infectious diseases, particularly tuberculosis. Already by the end of the eighteenth century more than one per cent of the English population, irrespective of age, died annually from the disease. When Robert Koch gave his historic speech in 1882 about the discovery of the tuberculosis bacterium, he stated that one out of seven died from the disease, and among the working population no fewer than one out of three. In fact, the entire population of Europe was infected in the nineteenth century, though far from everyone developed symptoms.

Inheritance, miasma or infection?

Although pulmonary TB with its special symptoms has been known and mentioned in writing from the earliest times in many civilizations, it did not become clear until the nineteenth century that the various forms of the disease we know today, in their effect on the skeleton, skin and lymph nodes, for example, were all part of the same disease and derived from a single cause.[262]

As early as the age of Hippocrates, possible causes of TB were being discussed.[263] In ancient Greece there was a widespread view that it was a congenital disease, since entire families could be seen struck down by it generation after generation.

We have seen earlier how theories of contagion in certain diseases have existed down through the centuries alongside the classic explanations that were dominant among scholars, the concept of miasmas and the theories of the four humours known from the writings of Hippocrates and Galen. Ideas that tuberculosis was also transmitted from person to person existed as far back as antiquity and were held by certain scholars. Aristotle expressed this view, as did Galen. The same applies to certain prominent scholars in the Muslim world, such as Ibn Sina, known as Avicenna in Europe, who was active after about AD 1000. Girolamo Fracastoro, who developed theories of infection for syphilis and other infections in the sixteenth century, believed that TB was transmitted from person to person. In the seventeenth century a number of cities in Italy and Spain responded to this theory by introducing preventative measures for TB, which, however, gradually fell into disuse. In northern Europe the theory of heredity was predominant until Koch's experiments proved that TB was caused by the bacterium *Mycobacterium tuberculosis.*

Considerable advances in research into the disease had, however, already been made in the nineteenth century many years before Koch's epoch-making discovery. To a great extent, this is due to the fact that a number of French physicians based new theories on autopsies of patients who had died of TB. Such patients were easily accessible in Paris at the time. The physician who made much use of this material was René Laënnec, one of the great names in French medical history.[264] Laënnec carried out rigorous studies of patients, comparing what he had found from his autopsies with what could be gleaned from symptoms and signs of disease when examining living patients. He developed medical examination into a fine art, employing a new aid that was later to become part of a doctor's standard equipment, the stethoscope. Laënnec was able to prove that TB was a single disease, no matter whether it attacked the lungs or other parts of the body, and he described how pulmonary tuberculosis develops in the individual patient.

Laënnec also believed that TB was hereditary, not infectious. By a cruel twist of fate, he himself became infected when at the age of 25 he cut his hand while carrying out an autopsy on a victim of TB and acquired an infection that later spread to other parts of the body. Laënnec died of his TB in 1826, only 44 years old.

It had been known for a long time that small nodes, also known as 'tubercles' (from Latin *tuberculum*), were typically found at an early stage in the lungs of a patient. This was why the term 'tuberculosis' came to be used, first proposed by the Swiss doctor Johann Lukas Schönlein in 1834.[265] The medical term was formerly 'phtisis', which dates back to the time of Hippocrates, while most people used to speak of 'consumption', a term that has persisted right down to the present day.

The theory of contagion for TB was victorious following Koch's discovery and those of partially forgotten precursors, such as Jean-Antoine Villemin. Today, it goes without saying, no one doubts that

TB is an infectious disease, but this does not mean that the former strong convictions that it is hereditary are completely baseless. Koch and his colleagues were possibly over-enthusiastic about their bacteriological discoveries and somewhat one-sided in their emphasis on the microbe's importance in the development of the disease, tending to ignore individual factors in the patient. Louis Pasteur, probably Koch's greatest rival, touched on this when he stated: 'The microbe is nothing, the terrain is everything.' Today we know that the final outcome of a whole series of infectious diseases is determined *both* by the characteristics of the microbe and factors within the patient, with genes playing an important role. Tuberculosis does not seem to be an exception to this. Examinations of twins, in particular, have shown that there is a considerable *genetic* component in our innate defence against MTB. But the situation is a complex one, with many genes involved that have not yet been finally mapped.[266]

The Lady of the Camellias and the tuberculous genius

At the time of Laënnec, TB was widespread in all classes of society. This was the age of Romanticism, when feelings and aesthetic were very much in people's minds. The disease picture of TB was also seen from an aesthetic point of view.[267] Although the final stage can be harrowing, with violent bleeding from the air passages, the sick person shows no repellent signs of the developing disease for some considerable time. The pallor and emaciation that were typical of many patients were seen as fascinating, and strongly influenced contemporary ideals of beauty. At the same time, the inexorable development of the disease and the inevitable fatal conclusion, often at a young age, appealed to the fundamentally melancholic mood of Romanticism. It now became fashionable for young women to cultivate this ideal of beauty – one was to be deathly pale and thin, with an ethereal look. Women with such a physical appearance became a favourite motif in the art of the period. But we also have examples from earlier ages of painters preferring young, tuberculous women as a motif. One example is Sandro Botticelli's famous *Birth of Venus*, where the model for Venus emerging from the sea has been claimed by some to be Simonetta Vespucci, a renowned beauty in Florence who died of TB at the age of 22 (although it should be remembered that the painting dates from nearly a decade later).

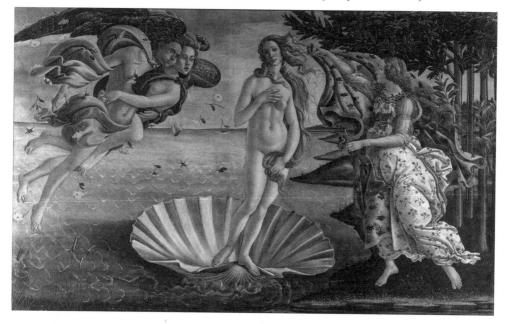

The commonly held view is that the model for Venus in Sandro Botticelli's painting from 1485, *The Birth of Venus*, was Simonetta de Vespucci. Vespucci, who was regarded as the most beautiful woman in Florence, died at the age of 22 from tuberculosis. She illustrates the ideal of beauty connected with this disease, one which was extremely popular during the Romantic period of the 19th century.

Young men in the nineteenth century also began to cultivate the tuberculosis-inspired ideal of beauty. Lord Byron, the poetic hero par excellence of the Romantic period, once stated to a friend: 'I think I wish to die of consumption, for then all women would say, "Just look at the unfortunate Byron – doesn't he look interesting as a man who is dying?"'[268]

The robust and larger-than-life Alexandre Dumas *père*, author of such classics as *The Three Musketeers* and *The Count of Monte Cristo*, remarked with mild disdain: 'Everyone had to have consumption – especially poets. It was fashionable to spit blood when experiencing strong emotions, and to die before one was thirty years old.' His own son, Alexandre Dumas *fils*, was, ironically enough, to contribute to a great extent to these attitudes with his novel *La Dame aux Camélias* (1848), which was based on the author's own passionate but brief love affair with the courtesan Marie Duplessis (whose real name was Alphonsine Plessis).[269] She was regarded as the most beautiful woman in Paris and lived a life of luxury financed by her rich lovers. But she also had TB,

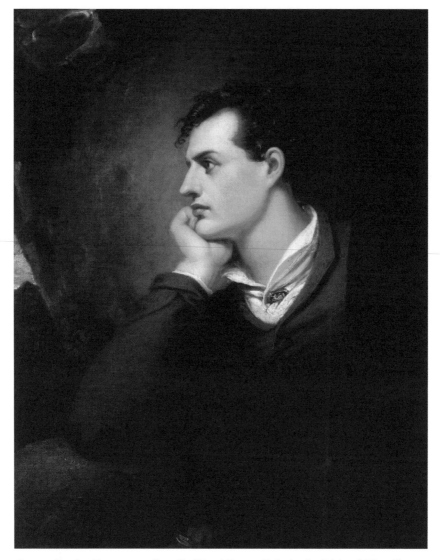

George Gordon Byron, usually called Lord Byron. Painting by Richard Westall, 1813.

with its classic physical appearance. She completely ignored her illness and died at the young age of 23. Dumas' book was a great success, and he adapted it for the stage in 1852. Many of the finest actresses of their day, from Sarah Bernhardt and Eleonora Duse to Greta Garbo and Isabelle Huppert, have played the role on stage or screen, often under the title *Camille*. The year after *La Dame aux Camélias* first appeared on stage, Giuseppe Verdi's opera *La traviata*, which was based on the book, premiered in Venice.[270] The heroine, here named Violetta Valéry, renounces her young lover when urged to protect his sister's reputation and dies in poverty, expending all her remaining strength when he returns.

Another of the most popular operas of the nineteenth century, *La bohème* by Giacomo Puccini, also has a tubercular heroine. This opera was based on a partly autobiographical novel, *Scènes de la vie de bohème* (1851) by Henri Murger, who himself died of TB at the early age of 38. The poor seamstress Mimi has a number of coughing fits in the course

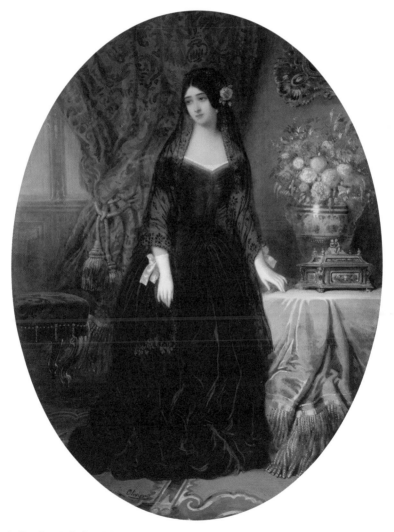

Marie Duplessis (née Alphonsine Plessis) was a courtesan regarded as the most beautiful woman in Paris. She also had tuberculosis and illustrates the tuberculous ideal of beauty at the time: extremely thin, with a pale, ethereal look.

of the opera, but here her life slips away while the audience's attention is on her friends. In my opinion, it is a travesty that certain modern opera directors have chosen to have Mimi die of cancer instead of TB. This is to ignore the Romantic cultivation of TB that characterized large parts of the nineteenth century.

The Romantic view of the disease, however, was not only linked to aesthetics. As far back as antiquity, there were some who claimed that the pulmonary disease phtisis (consumption) stimulated the intellect. In the nineteenth century many people believed that TB was connected to genius in artists and writers.[271] Supporters of the view could point to a large number of examples of excellent poets and musicians who suffered from TB and who often died young after a period of great creativity. An example of this is one of England's greatest poets, John Keats, who died in 1821 at the age of only 25. During the last year of his life he constantly coughed blood and knew what that meant: 'I know the colour of this blood: it is arterial blood . . . that drop of blood is my death-warrant. I must die.'[272] Within a year he was dead. The last year before the disease became obvious was characterized by tremendous artistic activity. The doctors had for a long time been using the Latin term *spes phtisica* (the hope of the consumptive) about the particularly optimistic state of mind they felt typified many with TB. Some even believed that this in itself could stimulate artistic activity.

Another famous example of a possible connection between TB and creativity is the English Brontë family, in the first half of the nineteenth century. Three sisters, Charlotte, Emily and Anne, became well-known novelists and poets (although their works were first published under the names Currer, Ellis and Acton Bell, respectively), but both Emily and Anne died young of TB.[273] Charlotte's death shortly before her 39th birthday has also been attributed to TB, although in recent years it has been suggested that she died after complications in what was her first pregnancy.

The Norwegian Niels Henrik Abel, one of the greatest geniuses in the history of mathematics, died of the disease in 1829 at the young age of 26 years.[274] He too displayed impressive creativity during the last two years of his life.

There were also well-known artists who lived with their illness for many years. One example is the prolific Scottish writer and poet

Robert Louis Stevenson, who is best known for his works *Treasure Island* and *The Strange Case of Dr Jekyll and Mr Hyde*.[275] The former book contains the unforgettable figure of the sinister one-legged pirate Long John Silver, based on a friend of Stevenson's who had had one leg amputated because of TB. Stevenson died at the age of 44 on Samoa in the Pacific of heart disease, not of his TB.

Nor did all playwrights escape the white plague. France's greatest writer of comedies, Molière, had pulmonary tuberculosis.[276] While acting in his final play, *The Imaginary Invalid*, in 1673, he suffered a violent haemorrhage. He insisted on carrying on acting, but coughed up blood once more and died a few hours later.

Less dramatic was the death from TB of the Russian playwright, short-story writer and doctor Anton Chekhov in 1904. On his deathbed he raised a glass of champagne, drank, and then lay down and died.[277] A beautiful death, many would say.

There are examples of famous musicians who succumbed to tuberculosis. The Polish composer Frédéric Chopin, who lived in France, is a well-known case.[278] He had the classic physical appearance – pale, handsome and thin – which made a deep impression on women,

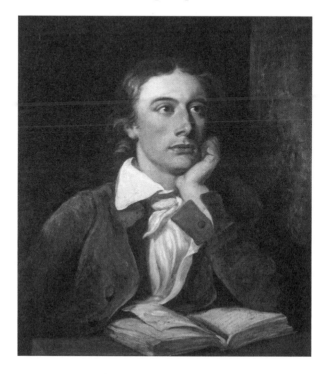

William Hilton after Joseph Severn, *John Keats*, c. 1822, oil on canvas. One of England's greatest poets, Keats died from tuberculosis at the age of 25 in 1821.

including the female writer George Sand, whose real name was Aurore Dudevant and who became his mistress. She called him her 'poor melancholy angel', and wrote that he 'coughed with endless elegance'. During a stay on Mallorca in 1838, the pair found themselves the victims of the theories of infection that were prevalent in southern Europe, for the locals were unfriendly and avoided them, fearing the risk of infection. In addition, it rained constantly. Chopin continued to cough and compose, including the famous 'Raindrop' prelude (Op. 28, no. 15). Although his tuberculosis diagnosis has been questioned by some, it can be regarded as fairly certain.

Another example from the early nineteenth century is the Italian Niccolò Paganini, the most famous violin virtuoso of all time.[279] He had contracted TB in his youth, which gave him a pale, demonic appearance that led to people whispering that his virtuosity came from having sold his soul to the Devil. He finally died of his TB – and incidentally also had syphilis.

Paganini is an example of a formerly widespread belief that tuberculosis could lead to increased sexual attractiveness. He had a long series of erotic relationships, including one with Napoleon's sister, the

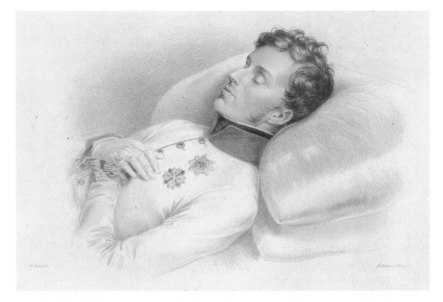

Napoleon's only legitimate son – the king of Rome – was born in 1811. After the fall of his father in 1815, he lived in Vienna under the title of Duke of Reichstadt. He died in Vienna of tuberculosis in 1832. The picture shows him on his *lit de parade* in an engraving by Franz Xaver Stöber.

lovely Pauline, whom we have already met as General Leclerc's widow after his death on Haiti. Pauline was yet another victim of pulmonary tuberculosis, dying at the age of 45.

Pauline was not the only one of Napoleon's family to be struck down by TB. Napoleon's only legitimate son was born in 1811 and was given the title King of Rome by his father. After the fall of Napoleon, his son, known to the Bonapartists as Napoleon II, lived almost as a prisoner of his maternal grandfather, Emperor Francis I, at Schönbrunn Palace in Vienna, where one can still see his rooms and effects, including his dear stuffed parrot. He died of TB as early as 1832.[280] His wretched fate inspired the French writer Edmond Rostand to write the tragedy *L'Aiglon* (The Eaglet, 1900).

Not all creativity is necessarily positive – it can also be destructive. If one believes in the connection between TB and creativity in a broad sense, one can find an important example in Sarajevo, Bosnia, on 28 June 1914.[281] There the heir to the Austro-Hungarian empire, Archduke Franz Ferdinand and his wife, Sophie von Hohenberg, were murdered by the young student Gavrilo Princip. A few minutes prior to the assassination, his fellow conspirator Nedeljko Čabrinović had unsuccessfully attempted to kill them with a bomb. Both of them had TB and knew they had only a short time to live – and they also died of it a few years later in prison. The assassination in Sarajevo triggered the First World War. Perhaps MTB ought to be included on the list of the many factors that led to that disaster, an issue about which historians still disagree.

The mysterious success

The problem of tuberculosis was not solved by Robert Koch's spectacular proof of the bacterium. About sixty years were to pass before the first effective medications to combat the disease – streptomycin and para-aminosalycic acid (PAS) – were discovered. Even so, it is a fact that MTB, which had kept an iron grip on the world for centuries, had gradually been forced to ease that hold in Europe and other parts of the Western world long before medications to combat the infection were found. Today, most Western countries have effective control over the disease. This, unfortunately, does not apply to the rest of the world.

The mysterious thing is that the tidal wave of TB across Europe was already beginning to recede in the 1860s, twenty years before Koch's star turn in 1882. It is still unclear what factors were of vital importance for the successful combatting of the disease. We have earlier mentioned the English epidemiologist Thomas McKeown's claim that the recession of infectious diseases, including TB, in Europe during the past 150 years is first and foremost due to better nutrition. He categorically rejects the idea that medical science can share the honour for this. It is a common view nowadays that McKeown's explanation is an oversimplification. One cannot ignore the fact that a number of factors other than nutrition contributed to the decline in TB. They include social-medical advances such as improvements in housing and the work environment. The so-called sanitary movement, with a strong emphasis on sanitary conditions and hygiene, probably contributed to the prevention of infection.

When it comes to diagnosing TB and preventing infection, the work of one man, now practically forgotten, must be emphasized: the Austrian baron Clemens von Pirquet.[282] He worked as a paediatrician in Vienna at the beginning of the twentieth century and made a series of immunological discoveries that laid the foundation for our knowledge about allergies and the ability of the immune system to bring about illness. Within the context of TB, he discovered that a tuberculous infection can be proved via a skin test where a small amount of tuberculin (an extract from dead tuberculosis bacteria) is placed on a small scratch. If the patient is infected, a small or slightly larger node of inflammation will develop on that spot, which is an immune reaction caused by T-lymphocytes. This so-called Pirquet test and later variants of it have been used extensively and have been extremely useful in work on TB. By means of this test, it was now possible to prove tuberculous infection in patients who were without any symptoms of the disease.

As a proficient researcher and one of the world's leading paediatricians, Pirquet briefly took up a tempting position at Johns Hopkins University and after the First World War was even put forward as a candidate for the Austrian presidency. Then, one February morning in 1929, he decided to end a brilliant career at the age of 55 by committing suicide with his wife, using prussic acid. This act had been just as meticulously planned as his scientific experiments.

Other medical measures employed from the mid-twentieth century onwards have played a role in combatting TB.[283] From around 1860 sanatoriums started to be built in Germany to provide long-term treatment for patients with tuberculosis, including rest, a nutritious diet and controlled physical exercise in the fresh air. Similar sanatoriums were later built in many countries, often located in areas regarded as being particularly healthy, for example in mountainous countryside. Here the patients might spend years of their lives in a highly distinctive environment characterized by rituals linked to the treatment of the disease, where the doctors were dominant figures of almost divine authority.[284]

The German writer and Nobel Prize-winner Thomas Mann portrayed such a sanatorium in his novel *Der Zauberberg* (The Magic Mountain, 1924), based on his experiences of visiting his tuberculous wife at a famous sanatorium in Davos, Switzerland.[285] In the novel the young engineer Hans Castorp comes to the Alpine sanatorium to visit his sick cousin, but subsequently proves to be infected himself. He stays at the sanatorium for several years, and through his eyes Mann describes in precise detail the medical features of TB of which he had acquired in-depth knowledge. At the same time, many have also viewed the book as an allegory of the 'sick' state of European politics, including the emergence of fascism. An equally realistic description of the special, psychological atmosphere of sanatoriums can be found in a much less well-known book, *The Rack* (1958), written by Derek Lindsay under the pseudonym A. E. Ellis.[286]

It is still unclear what effect a stay at a sanatorium actually had on tuberculosis. Gradually, treatment was supplemented by direct medical measures.[287] As early as the end of the seventeenth century an Italian physician made the surprising discovery that patients with pulmonary tuberculosis improved after having been given sword-stabs in the chest. The effect of the sword tip was the same as the so-called pneumothorax treatment that was introduced at the end of the nineteenth century. In this treatment, air was injected into the thoracic cavity where the lungs were infected, causing the lung to collapse. This closed the tuberculous cavities formed by the infection, which in turn could reduce infectiousness and improve healing, for the tuberculosis bacterium thrives best in lung tissue that is rich in oxygen. From the 1930s onwards a surgical procedure was introduced called thoracoplasty, in which several ribs were removed so as to cause the lung to collapse.

In 1895 Wilhelm Conrad Röntgen discovered the electro-magnetic waves now known as X-rays, which provided a basis for a completely new method of diagnosis.[288] This gradually also became extremely important for TB diagnosis and treatment, since one could now directly 'see' the changes brought about by the infection.

In the 1920s a vaccine against TB was introduced, the BCG vaccine, which has had a certain preventative effect in the Western world. Then came the first medications – PAS and streptomycin – at the beginning of the 1940s, which revolutionized the treatment of the disease.[289] But the gradual decrease of TB in Western countries, which started as early as the mid-nineteenth century, must have other explanations. Are there things we are not yet aware of regarding the long-term epidemic patterns of MTB? It is thought-provoking that the extent of TB in Japan, which adopted the same measures as Europe in combatting the disease at an early stage, did not begin to show a decline until after the Second World War.

New threats from the white plague

As we have seen, during the first decades after the Second World War there was a widely held view that the great importance of infectious diseases was over. This also applied to TB to a high degree, since a number of new, effective medicines had been found. Some thought that it was now possible to eradicate the disease completely. Mortality from the disease was also strongly on the decline in Western countries. This led to a down-grading of the importance of tuberculosis, one of the consequences of which was that new medicines were not developed. The intensiveness of measures against the disease that had existed throughout the first half of the twentieth century weakened in Western countries, where it was no longer feared.

This attitude has proved itself to be extremely dangerous. Since the 1980s TB has once more been on the increase in the world. This is due to various factors.[290] The poorer parts of the world, which have been hit hardest by TB, simply cannot afford the investments needed to effectively combat this infection with the methods that are now available. Since the 1980s the situation has worsened further as a result of the impressive capacity of the bacterium to adapt to the outside world.

First, the bacterium has to a great extent become resistant to available drugs. In certain cases, the bacteria have become completely resistant not only to the usual medicines but to the few back-up medications that exist. Patients infected by such a bacterium are actually in the same situation as those before the breakthrough in treatment in the 1940s, and we have little to offer against the infection, which can prove fatal. Certain African countries are particularly hard hit by this problem. With the present scope for travel, patients from these regions can transport deadly bacteria to all parts of the globe. The extensive migration that is typical of today's world also contributes to the spread of TB, since many migrants come precisely from countries with considerable TB problems.

The other great problem that has arisen since the 1980s, when the AIDS pandemic exploded, is the deadly alliance between MTB and the HIV virus.[291] HIV patients who do not receive treatment develop a serious immune deficiency that weakens their resistance to the tuberculosis bacterium. Such an HIV patient is between twenty and thirty times more likely to develop active tuberculosis than one with a normal immune system.

After two hundred years of research, there is still a great deal we do not know about MTB and the mechanisms of the disease.[292] We need new medicines and a more effective vaccine than those we have been using for almost a hundred years. Even so, we must face the fact that TB is not simply a medical problem in the worst-hit areas of the world. Like many other infectious diseases, TB is also linked to poverty, wretched housing conditions, a poor diet and a lack of medical help. The slum areas of many large cities in such areas as Africa, which have experienced explosive growth, greatly resemble poor urban areas in Europe during the Industrial Revolution, where TB was rampant. If we are to combat the global epidemic of TB effectively in the years ahead, this will mainly depend on economic conditions. The basic medical know-how we already have.[293]

Leprosy: The Disease of Outcasts

Leprosy is no longer a medical reality in Western countries. But the word 'leper' lives on in the expression 'to be treated like a leper': that is, to be detested and avoided in every possible way. This expression is a faint echo of what for thousands of years has been part of everyday life for people who suffered – or suffer – from leprosy. Many infectious diseases have taken a far greater number of lives than leprosy and had far more dramatic and stormy courses of illness as epidemics and pandemics. Yet there is probably no infectious disease that has given rise to more stigmatization, discrimination and ostracism, and thereby to mental suffering.

If non-doctors today ever consider leprosy at all, it is probably in connection with the Middle Ages and the diseases that then threatened people. Some may be aware that leprosy still exists in tropical climes, but not many know that Norway actually had a leprosy epidemic as late as the nineteenth century and that this was where the disease held its last stand in Europe. Very few people know that Norway's last leprosy patient died in 2002, having lived with his secret since youth.[294]

From loss of feeling to leonine facies

The 'classic' microbe that causes leprosy is *Mycobacterium leprae* (often abbreviated to *M. leprae*), which was discovered by the Norwegian doctor Armauer Hansen in 1873. This bacterium is related to *M. tuberculosis*, with which it shares a number of similarities.[295]

In 2008 researchers made public that they had discovered a new bacterium that also can cause leprosy.[296] This bacterium was given the name *Mycobacterium lepromatosum* and is extremely closely related to *M. leprae*. The new bacterium is mainly found in Mexico and other countries in Latin America. From now on, the discussion will centre mainly on the 'classic' leprosy bacterium.

When the leprosy bacterium causes illness, it is always a chronic infection. If the infection proves fatal, it is normally not the bacterium itself that is the cause but complications of various kinds. The progression of leprosy is the result of an interaction between the microbe and the immune system, with the patient's immunological reactions to the bacterium playing a crucial role in the disease picture – for good or bad.[297] This interaction is highly complex, and we will only glance at the main characteristics so as to be able to understand the various disease pictures. It is first and foremost the T-lymphocytes of the immune system that are important for the disease progression.

Let us begin by stating that the majority of people will not develop symptoms even if they become infected with the leprosy bacterium. This is due to genetic factors that normally result in resistance to the bacterium. In a relatively small number of cases, where the unfortunate victims do not have this resistance, there is a whole spectrum of possible pathological pictures of various degrees of seriousness resulting from infection. Some patients have only very light symptoms after being infected (a few spots on the skin, which often disappear), and remain healthy. Others develop a chronic form of the infection, with various symptoms.

The two extremes of the chronic illness spectrum are known as *tuberculoid lepra* and *lepromatous lepra*. Recent research indicates that genes to a great extent determine which form of the illness a patient gets.[298]

With *tuberculoid lepra* the patient's immune system is relatively effective against the leprosy bacterium and manages to restrain and combat it to quite a high degree, so that the amount of bacteria in the patient's infected tissue is small.[299] But it does not totally prevent the disease. With this form of leprosy, it is mainly the skin and nerves that are attacked. On the skin the patient gets one to three large or small spots that are either pale or pink. These areas of skin are insensitive because the skin nerves in the area have been attacked, so that it is often possible to stick a needle into them without the patient feeling pain. In later stages of the disease more nerves can be attacked. The cause of this is that the bacteria have a preference for infecting a cell type that is intimately connected to the nerve fibres. The immune system of the patient then attacks these cells containing the bacterium, causing inflammation and nerve damage.

It is *lepromatous lepra* that causes the more serious pathological picture. In these patients the immune system is highly ineffective at combatting the bacterium, and the organs and tissues that are attacked contain large quantities of bacteria, which then spread throughout the body. Here the skin changes are far more extensive than in tuberculoid leprosy and can have various appearances. Quite often wounds develop in these skin changes and the areas attacked become badly coarsened. When this takes place in the face, it can produce a very unsightly appearance, a condition known as 'leonine facies' (*facies leontina* in Latin). All facial hair disappears.

Quite often even more disfiguring changes take place in the face because of the bacterium's ability to destroy osseous tissue. In the face it is particularly cartilage and bone in the nose and the upper jaw that are destroyed, causing the middle section of the face to collapse where the nose was and leaving only a gaping hole. This produces a grotesque

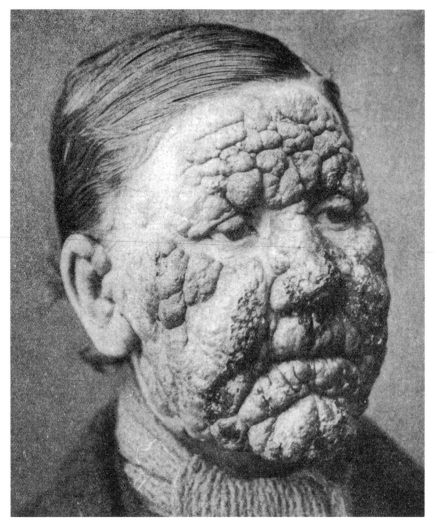

Patient with *lepromatous lepra*, from Norman Walker, *An Introduction to Dermatology*, 7th edn (1922).

appearance called *facies leprosa* (leprosy face). Other bones may also be attacked. Widespread nerve damage with loss of sensitivity can result in infected wounds that can lead to severe deformities such as 'claw hand' and similar changes to the feet that make walking difficult. Often the outermost joints of the fingers are gradually eaten away, and parts of the fingers can quite simply fall off.

The cartilage of the larynx can be attacked, which gives the patient a characteristically hoarse voice and speech difficulties. The eyes can be subject to infection, which can lead to blindness. Other organs can also be involved in this form of leprosy, including kidneys and testicles, so male patients can become sterile.

In its most advanced forms, the lepromatous type of disease can give the patient a quite repellent and sinister appearance, which without a doubt has strongly contributed to the stigma victims have experienced through the ages.

Until now I have described the two extremes of the disease spectrum. Most common, however, is a mixed picture somewhere in between, with features from both extremes. These intermediate forms can gradually move more distinctly towards one or the other extreme. The situation for leprosy patients is made even more complicated by a worsening of the symptoms as a result of more or less sudden processes of immunological inflammation. This is most often seen when one attempts to treat the disease by medication.

We still do not have a final answer as to how leprosy spreads. The common view is that infection is via nasal discharge, in which we find large quantities of bacteria in leprosy patients. These bacteria are inhaled by the recipient and then move to the skin and nerves near the surface of the skin, since they prefer somewhat lower temperatures than our usual body temperature. Infection via skin wounds can also occur. Infection requires close and long-lasting contact, for leprosy is not at all highly infectious.[300]

The origin of leprosy: Alexander the Great or Africa?

Leprosy is without question an extremely old disease. Where did it originate, and how has it spread to all inhabited parts of the globe? These are questions that have preoccupied people for two thousand years. We still do not have the final answers, but know a good deal.

As with research into the history of other epidemics, we have various methods to fall back on: historical accounts, archaeological finds of human remains, special parts of the skeleton and new molecular-biological methods. All of these have been made use of in investigating the history of leprosy, but their results do not always coincide.

One has to be critical when deciding what historical accounts can teach us about leprosy, for the disease descriptions are often vague and uncertain, as we have already found for other diseases. This is a particular problem in the case of leprosy, since changes to the skin are an important part of the pathological picture, but these symptoms can often be confused with many other skin diseases that have plagued humanity through the ages. It is the most dramatic symptoms, such as those of the lepromatous form, especially the changes to the face, that are the easiest to judge in old accounts.

Until the 1970s it was regarded as an established fact that the Old Testament described this infection (Leviticus 13). Many scholars, however, believe that the skin described here can hardly be leprosy. The mention here of what was thought to be leprosy has nevertheless had tragic consequences for later victims, because Leviticus states that those who have this disease are 'impure' and must be isolated until they regain their health. Since real leprosy cannot be cured without modern drugs, this would also seem to suggest that many cases mentioned in the Bible were not caused by the leprosy bacterium.

In Egyptian medical writings, of which there are many, we do not find any mention of leprosy. Among the many, detailed accounts of diseases in Hippocrates we also find absolutely nothing that is reminiscent of leprosy.

The oldest, quite certain description of this infection is found in an Indian source, *Sushruta Samhita* from 600 BC.[301] Here one gets the impression that it was a quite common disease in India. Descriptions in slightly later Chinese writings also seem to deal with leprosy.

When it comes to Europe, we have to consult Roman writers in the first two centuries AD to find any mention of leprosy, including the Roman natural scientist Pliny the Elder.[302] Pliny, who lost his life in the eruption of Vesuvius in AD 79 because his ungovernable interest in natural phenomena led him to get too close to the volcano, suggests in his writings that the disease had come to Rome when Pompey returned with his troops from a campaign in the Middle East in 62 BC. He believed that leprosy came from Egypt. Aretaeus of Cappadocia, an important physician who was forgotten for 1,500 years, provided a very detailed account of the disease picture of leprosy, including the leonine facies and the skin changes. The general view at the time was apparently that the disease was quite new in the Roman empire: the historian Plutarch writes that the disease came to Greece at a time that we calculate as being roughly 100 BC.

What do archaeological finds tell us about the history of the infection? The fact that leprosy affects the skeleton of many of its victims, particularly those who have the lepromatous form, is extremely useful when examining bones from archaeological excavations. A great many finds exist from Europe and the Middle East.[303] Recently an interesting find was made in India in a grave dating from 2000 BC where the skeletal changes strongly indicate leprosy, but this is still uncertain. In the Americas no skeletal finds have been made that suggest leprosy before the arrival of the Europeans with Columbus. This infection was probably part of the Columbian exchange, one that generally speaking did not favour the indigenous population.

Alexander the Great, the military genius from Macedonia who conquered the Persian empire and whose invincible army made it all the way to India, had a glorious career and shaped history for the succeeding centuries. In the last fifty years, however, he has been credited with something less glorious: bringing leprosy from India to Europe.[304]

This was first claimed by the Dane Johannes Andersen in 1969 and has since been accepted by many archaeologists, historians and leprosy researchers. Even so, there is scant evidence for this theory, except that the first leprosy finds in Europe date from a time after Alexander's return from the East in 326 BC. Some historians are therefore highly critical of the idea of Alexander's contribution to the introduction of leprosy to Europe, yet they still believe that the disease came from Asia, probably India, most likely taken by ship to Egypt, Arabia and East Africa. Both before and after the time of Alexander there was extensive trade by sea between Egypt and India. A popular commodity to Egypt from India was slaves, who might have carried the leprosy bacterium.

Most of the first skeletal finds of leprosy in the Mediterranean world are archaeological finds in Egypt and date to about AD 200. An increasing number of finds from succeeding centuries suggest that leprosy, probably still quite uncommon in the Roman empire during the first centuries AD, steadily increased in frequency. We must assume that it spread through the Roman empire in the same way as tuberculosis, with the communication possibilities that the Pax Romana had opened up for microbes.

In recent years molecular biologists have eagerly addressed the problem of leprosy and studied skeletal remains from a number of graves, especially in Europe and the neighbouring areas. The leprosy bacterium is well suited to such investigations, for its DNA is protected by the thick capsule that surrounds it. In some cases the diagnosis of leprosy based on skeletal changes has been confirmed using the new methods. All the finds are from the past 1,900 years: the oldest to be confirmed via DNA evidence is from a man laid to rest near Jerusalem in the first century AD.

Until now the modern molecular-biological methods have not provided any final answer when it comes to the origins of leprosy.[305] Some researchers believe that it is an extremely old infection in *Homo sapiens*, perhaps inherited from our ape-like forefathers. New examinations of the genetic make-up of the bacterium suggest that it adapted itself to humans over a very long period of time. It has apparently dropped a great many genes that were once important to it, since human genes can replace them during infection. A few researchers believe that the leprosy bacterium travelled with *Homo sapiens* when the species journeyed outside Africa 60,000–120,000 years ago and then spread out worldwide, along with the human race.[306] If that were so, however, we would have encountered it in the New World prior to Columbus, which is not the case.

Other researchers doubt that leprosy is that old and believe that it did not acquire good conditions for dissemination until after the first epidemiological transition, when greater population density came into being. Infection by the leprosy bacterium requires quite close contact. Perhaps the bacterium then became more virulent? It is to be hoped that new archaeological finds in various parts of the world will be able to provide better answers to the question of the age and origins of leprosy.

New molecular-biological research has also confirmed that leprosy on the American continent comes originally from Europe and Africa in the time after Columbus. Both slaves from West Africa and immigrants from Europe could have contributed to this. Researchers have actually claimed that the extensive immigration to the Midwest from Norway could have contributed to the occurrence of leprosy in the USA, since Norway had a serious leprosy epidemic in the mid-nineteenth century.[307]

Armadillo and squirrel

Until recently leprosy was regarded as an infectious disease that exclusively affects human beings, meaning that it is not a zoonosis with a reservoir in the animal world, of which we have so many other examples. We may have to reconsider this, because the leprosy bacterium has been

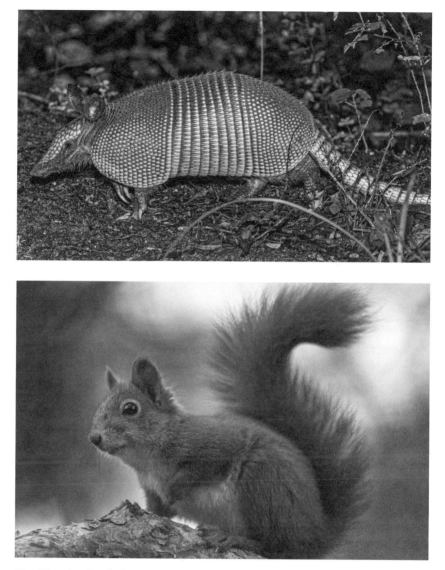

Top: The nine-banded armadillo found in large numbers in South and Central America and the southern parts of the USA is quite often infected with the leprosy bacterium. Probably, the armadillo was originally infected by humans, but now it can repay the compliment. This animal is important in leprosy research, since unlike most other animals it gets an infection with the leprosy bacterium that resembles leprosy in human beings. *Bottom*: The common squirrel, *Sciurus vulgaris*. In the British Isles it has recently been discovered that this species of squirrel bears both the common leprosy bacterium *Mycobacterium leprae* and the newly discovered *M. lepromatosum*.

found in a very special species of animal, the so-called nine-banded armadillo (*Dasypus novemcinctus*), which is found throughout Latin America and in the southern states of the USA. This strange little animal has developed a form of armour made up of keratinized scales, which gives it an appearance similar to the Ankylosaurus, which many dinosaur-loving children know about. The armadillo was originally infected with leprosy by humans, but recently it has become clear that the armadillo can do the reverse: infect humans.[308] Its susceptibility to the leprosy bacterium has made the armadillo very popular with researchers.

It has also become clear that not only the armadillo can be infected by humans, since the 'classic' leprosy bacterium has been found in species of ape in Africa and the Philippines. It is thought that they have been infected by humans, but, as with the armadillo, perhaps infected apes can 'return' the bacterium to humans in the event of close contact.

Perhaps the most surprising find has been that the native species of squirrel in the British Isles, the red squirrel (*Sciurus vulgaris*), is a bearer of both leprosy bacteria we know today: *M leprae* and *M. lepromatosum*.[309] The molecular type *M. leprae* found in squirrels is the same as that detected in English leprosy patients from the Viking period and the Middle Ages. Some researchers believe that the squirrel population in the British Isles has possibly been infected in the past via the considerable trade in skins carried out by the Vikings, including squirrel skins from Scandinavia. Has the squirrel then perhaps infected humans as the armadillo has done? Infection from squirrel to human has not yet been detected, but it has been claimed that the medieval English not only liked squirrel skins but kept the animals as pets.

The Leper King and the Living Dead

In the first centuries AD leprosy gradually spread across Europe, becoming a dreaded disease. The epidemic peaked in the period 1100–350, coinciding with the crusades.[310] Some people think that this is an important factor in its dissemination. There is no doubt that leprosy was very widespread in Palestine and the Middle East in general. We also know that crusaders became infected with leprosy, so it is highly probable that they returned home as bearers of the disease. Leprosy, however, had a solid grip on Europe prior to the crusades, which thus can hardly have played any major role in spreading the infection.

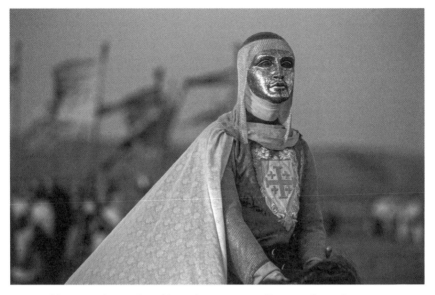

King Baldwin IV of Jerusalem (from the American film *Kingdom of Heaven*, 2005, directed by Ridley Scott) wearing a mask because of the pathological changes to his face. There is no historical evidence that the real Baldwin ever wore a mask.

Among the various orders of knights founded during the struggle for the Holy Land (Palestine) was the Order of St Lazarus, named after the patron saint of lepers. In addition to its role in fighting against the infidels, the order had the task of caring for leprosy patients. The hospitals they established in Palestine and various European countries were known as lazar houses, which is why some languages use variants of the word 'lasaret' for a hospital. Some of the knights of this order were themselves lepers, and it also received knights from other orders who had been infected with leprosy.

It was not only knights who were infected by leprosy in the crusader realm of Jerusalem, which existed for almost two hundred years. Baldwin IV was crowned king of Jerusalem in 1174 at the age of thirteen.[311] A year earlier the young king had been diagnosed with leprosy when his teacher discovered that he had insensitive patches of skin. The disease developed into *lepromatous lepra* over the succeeding year, with the horrible physical changes already mentioned.[312] The unfortunate king became increasingly disabled and blind, and gradually his face became so disfigured that, according to certain accounts, he wore a mask. Despite his afflictions, he was an impressive monarch, both politically, despite intrigues at court over his succession, since he was not expected to live long, and as a military leader. He was victorious over the Ayyubid sultan Saladin at the Battle of Montgisard in 1177 and took part in the battle itself, in spite of a lame right arm. In later years he had to be transported in a litter. He died in 1185 at the age of just 23 years.

The attitude towards leprosy patients in Christian countries during the Middle Ages and later was in many ways a continuation of the view found in the Old Testament. Fear of infection was undoubtedly widespread in the population of Europe and this was probably crucial for the strong wish to exclude leprosy patients from society. At the same time, there was felt to be something morally despicable about leprosy patients, for many people saw leprosy as God's punishment for an immoral life. Their tragic lot is depicted, for example, in Lew Wallace's novel *Ben-Hur: A Tale of the Christ* (1880), which was one of the best-selling books in the USA in the nineteenth century; the early stage adaptation and two classic film versions (1925 and 1959) have been a byword for spectacle, keeping the story alive.

It was often priests, sometimes with the assistance of physicians, who declared someone a leper, with the serious consequences that had for the individual. In 1179 the Third Lateran Council, the highest assembly of the Catholic Church, laid down a special ritual for when someone was declared a leper. He or she was declared dead to society, with a kind of burial ritual that could involve grave earth being thrown over the patient, or the person standing in a grave during the ceremony. The patient was also forbidden to touch children or young people, or to give them any of his or her personal belongings. Following the ritual the sick person's spouse was free to remarry.[313]

Now excluded from society, the leper was now in effect a living dead person, and was taken to a special institution called a leprosarium or lazar house. The first such institutions are found as early as the third century AD.[314] They were often run by the Church, and later also by local authorities, and were highly dependent on support from the local community. In the great majority of cases, the leper had to spend the rest of his or her life in such an institution. At the end of the Middle Ages there were at least 19,000 leprosaria in Europe.

Not all leprosy patients lived in a leprosarium. Where no such institutions existed, those with leprosy lived alone and eked out a living as beggars. Because of the fear of infection, they were nevertheless subject to a number of restrictions. They had to wear a yellow cross on their clothes. If they were out on the roads, they had to warn others with a bell or a kind of rattle and stand out of the way if they met anyone. They were not allowed to visit marketplaces, inns or other places where people gathered. Many towns also refused to admit anyone suffering from leprosy.

It does not take much imagination to picture the human suffering it must have involved to be declared the living dead and to have to leave one's home, spouse and children, and always to face the prospect of a frightful, disfiguring development of the disease. It is also a tragic fact that people with leprosy were occasionally subject to brutal persecution in crisis situations, since they were regarded as morally inferior. This was the case, for example, during the Black Death.

Although the attitude of Christian Europe to leprosy was characterized by Old Testament teachings, it is interesting that most other civilizations had similar attitudes, for example in India and China. There is, however, an important and interesting exception: in Islamic societies victims of leprosy were neither social outcasts nor regarded as morally inferior.[315]

The mysterious decline

The climax of the leprosy epidemic was between 1100 and 1350, after which leprosy gradually decreased in most of Europe. The decline started at roughly the same time as the second great plague epidemic, the Black Death, struck in the mid-fourteenth century. In the course of the next one to two hundred years leprosy almost disappeared from the continent and the British Isles, except for a few pockets in the Balkans and Scotland.[316] It survived, however, to a considerably greater extent in Scandinavia, especially in Norway. The reasons for this are unclear.

No one knows what caused this decline in leprosy, but many theories have been discussed.[317] That it coincided with the Black Death could, of course, have meant that the plague in particular struck patients in the leprosaria that had already been weakened by illness, but this cannot be the whole explanation. It is interesting that at the same time that leprosy started to decline, tuberculosis began inexorably to increase in Europe. Since *M. tuberculosis* and *M. leprae* are fairly closely related bacteria, one theory is that the 'weaker' leprosy bacterium could not gain a foothold in patients already infected with the tuberculosis bacterium because of so-called cross-immunity. Another possibility is that the reduced fertility in men infected with leprosy where the testicles are affected led to fewer people with the genes that determine susceptibility to this infectious disease. It has also been suggested that the leprosy bacterium could have become less virulent (that is, more 'benign'), but so far no evidence of this has been found.

Norway: the last bastion of the leprosy bacteria

In the Middle Ages leprosy was quite widespread. That includes Norway, where leprosaria were established in the major towns. In Scandinavia such an institution was often called a 'Skt Jørgensgård' (St George Leper Hospital), since the patron saint there, as also in England, was St George the dragon-slayer. A decline in the infection can be identified during the sixteenth century, but this was reversed in the seventeenth and the rate of increase was maintained until by the nineteenth century it had become a serious health problem in Norway.[318] By this time leprosy had become rare in most other European countries, including the rest of Scandinavia.

The interest in leprosy was great among politicians and doctors. In the mid-nineteenth century the need for leper hospitals in Norway had become so great that new ones were established. Research conducted at the two most important of these, in Bergen, gradually gained international recognition. Daniel Cornelius Danielssen and Carl Wilhelm Boeck, who was later a professor in Christiania (Oslo) and has already been mentioned as an eager champion of syphilization, wrote an extensive work, *On Leprosy*, which commanded international interest and won a prestigious prize from the French Academy of Sciences.

Danielssen and Boeck, like most doctors at the time, believed that leprosy was a hereditary disease. The belief in a form of contagious disease that had affected the view of leprosy since time immemorial, and that was still prevalent in the population, was now regarded as outdated in scientific circles. This, however, was not the opinion of Armauer Hansen, who also worked at the leper hospitals in Bergen. He ended the centuries-old debate by finally publishing proof of the existence of the leprosy bacterium in 1874.

No matter whether one believed in inheritance or infection, nineteenth-century Norway was keen to isolate leprosy patients in separate institutions, both in order to ensure they had good care and to combat the disease. Many supporters of the theory of heredity wanted to prevent leprosy patients from being allowed to marry, so as not to pass on their unfortunate legacy, and some even considered sterilizing young men with leprosy. The supporters of infection, who naturally gained a fresh impetus from Hansen's discovery, wanted patients to be isolated in special hospitals to prevent infection. The leper hospitals were also full.[319] Irrespective of the cause, it was possible to note a steady decline in leprosy in Norway during the second half of the nineteenth century. It then became possible to close a number of leper hospitals.

Leper colonies, medicines and modern saints

Over the past century leprosy has disappeared from Western countries in all but name. The rare cases that are discovered are always people who originate in other parts of the world where leprosy remains a serious problem. Every year more than 200,000 new cases are reported: most of the patients are found in India, Brazil and Indonesia.

Leprosy is still a disease that brands its victims and leads to exclusion from society.[320] This means that many victims avoid seeking medical help, even though since the mid-twentieth century we have had medication that can lead to a cure for a disease that was untreatable in former times.

Attempts have also been made in recent times to collect leprosy patients together in special areas as a continuation of the leprosaria of former ages. The best-known leper colony in Europe is on the small island of Spinalonga, just off the northeast coast of Crete.[321] Several thousand patients were isolated there between 1904 and 1957. Conditions during the first few years were wretched. Originally no one was allowed to approach Spinalonga, where a yellow flag waved as a sign of infection. During the Second World War, none of the powers involved in the war dared go ashore for fear of infection, and the leprosy patients became part of the resistance movement against the Nazi occupiers of Crete. Today, Spinalonga, with its small leper village, has become a popular tourist attraction.

Another famous leper colony lies on the other side of the globe, on the picturesque Hawaiian island of Molokai. From 1865 to 1969 thousands of leprosy patients were forcibly isolated there. In 2009 President

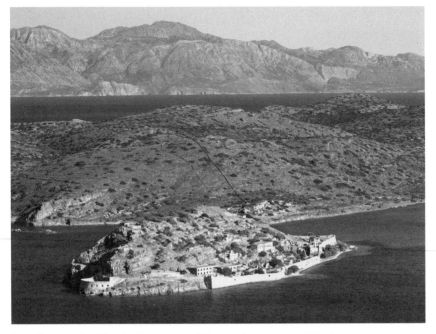

Spinalonga – the Island of Lepers – off the northeast coast of Crete.

Barack Obama, who was born in Hawaii, announced that a monument was to be raised bearing the names of all the unfortunate people who had spent their lives on Molokai. The Catholic Church recently recognized the dedicated work for the lepers of Molokai performed by Father Damian de Veuster, who himself contracted leprosy,[322] and the nun Marianne Cope. They were canonized by Pope Benedict XVI in 2009 and 2012, respectively.

It is an unfortunate fact that the care of leprosy patients has rarely been carried out by saints. The lives of lepers in those parts of the world where the disease is still common have been characterized by more than just prejudice and mechanisms to exclude them from society. The treatment of lepers in Japan has until recently been an example of how official attitudes to the leprosy problem have at times also been based on ignorance and a lack of humanity. Restrictive legislation with a strong emphasis on more or less enforced isolation for many years led to the Japanese government being ordered in 2001 to pay compensation to its leper patients.

Malaria: Fever and Death

Nowadays, malaria tends to evoke tropical climes to the great majority of people in Western countries. Few are aware, for example, that malaria existed in Scandinavia just a few generations ago. With the extent of present-day international travel, Scandinavians have also begun to encounter the malaria issue, since it is necessary to take malaria-preventative medicine before setting out for tropical regions. However, this infectious disease is not part of everyday health problems in much of the world.

For almost half of the world's population, however, malaria is still a threat, as it has been for thousands of years in the history of humanity. Malaria is perhaps the infectious disease that has claimed most lives down through the ages, in keen competition with tuberculosis and smallpox. At the same time, it displays convincingly just how impressive the adaptability of microbes is, as well as the crucial importance of ecological factors in humanity's never-ending duel with the world of the microbes. For these reasons, the history of malaria is well worth a more detailed look.

What is the real nature of malaria?

To comprehend the history of malaria and the many crucial factors involved, it is necessary to understand the main stages of the quite complex existence of the malaria parasites.[323] Malaria is an infection caused by members of the large group of microbes called protozoa, single-cell organisms that I referred to earlier as 'the first animals'. They much more closely resemble cells in animals and humans than the much simpler bacteria. The protozoa that cause malaria belong to a large family of parasites known as plasmodia. Four members of this family have been known for many years as causes of malaria: *Plasmodium vivax*, *P. falciparum*, *P. malariae* and *P. ovale*. Quite recently, *P. knowlesi*, a fifth member, was discovered to be a cause of malaria in Southeast Asia. The last of these also causes malaria in apes, while the other four have specialized in human beings. It is *P. vivax* and *P. falciparum* that dominate the world as a cause of malaria today. The various species of malaria differ from each other in various ways that are important for disease pictures and treatment. Let us first consider the similarities between them that result in the pathological pictures we sum up as malaria.

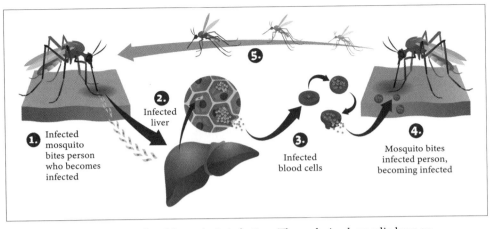

1. Infected mosquito bites person who becomes infected
2. Infected liver
3. Infected blood cells
4. Mosquito bites infected person, becoming infected
5.

The transmission cycle of the malaria infection. The malaria plasmodia have an alternating existence between the female *Anopheles* mosquito and a human being.

The malaria plasmodia live a quite complicated double life. They spend their lives in different hosts, one of which, unfortunately, is *Homo sapiens*. The other host is the female mosquito of the large family called *Anopheles*. This family has several hundred members, but only thirty or forty of them are important in a malaria context. Most of these species of mosquito suck blood from both animals and humans, but a couple of species have specialized in humans, and these are the most effective transmitters of infection.

Throughout their existence shared between mosquito and human being, the malaria plasmodia appear in a variety of forms, with different characteristics and names. We need not deal with the various terms here: even medical students find it hard to cram these names and normally forget most of them after the examination.

It is the female *Anopheles* mosquito that is responsible for the transmission of malaria from human to human. The forms of plasmodium that have developed in the stomach of the female mosquito move to the salivary glands of the insect. When the mosquito bites a human in order to suck blood, the malaria parasite sees its chance to move into the victim's bloodstream. The parasites make purposefully for the liver cells, where they mature in the course of a couple of weeks into new forms that in turn start to swim in the bloodstream. They have but one aim: to gain entrance to the erythrocytes – the red blood cells – to feed on the nutrients found there. During this feast inside the red blood cells the malaria plasmodia once more undergo change and increase in number, until after one to three days they cause the red blood cell to burst and once more enter the bloodstream to hunt down new red blood cells.

In typical cases of malaria, all the plasmodia synchronize their attack on the red blood cells, so that the bursting of the cells – the destruction – takes place at the same time. This produces an attack of fever. In malaria caused by *P. vivax* and *P. ovale* these attacks normally occur with a two-day interval in between, which is why this type of malaria is known as *tertiana*. In the case of *P. malariae*, known as *quartana*, the interval is one day longer. During an attack the patient suffers shaking chills, shivering and a fever that can be as high as 41°C. This lasts for five to six hours and is due to the release of many inflammatory substances. After a series of feverish attacks with the same rhythm, though of gradually lessening strength, the patient recovers, but without treatment further attacks can occur at any moment later. Malaria with *P. falciparum*, the most dangerous type, differs from the others in that the attack on the red blood cells is often not synchronized during the first few days, resulting in shaking chills and a fever that lasts longer and can occur quite irregularly.

P. falciparum also differs from the other forms when it comes to the degree of seriousness and level of fatalities. Malaria caused by this microbe is often called 'malign malaria', as opposed to the other forms, which are called 'benign'. In malign malaria, far more red blood cells are normally attacked in the patient, who often develops severe anaemia. In addition, the infected blood cells have a tendency to 'clog' the small blood vessels in many of the body's tissues and organs, which can cause extremely serious functional disturbances. When this occurs in the brain, we get cerebral malaria, which is a dreaded, life-threatening complication of malign malaria. All in all, more than 99 per cent of the deaths from malaria in the world come from this malaria species. Only rarely does infection with *P. vivax* cause serious illness and death.

Like other microbes, the malaria plasmodia constantly seek new victims so as to ensure the survival of the species. Once again, it is the biting female *Anopheles* mosquito that comes to the rescue. When such a mosquito bites a malaria patient with plasmodia in the blood, the mosquito ingests special variants of the parasites from the blood, which now further develop in the insect, where they are actually present in two sexes that mate. After a couple of weeks of highly active sexual life in the mosquito's stomach, the mature parasites are ready to attack a new human victim, and the round dance begins all over again when the mosquito once more sucks blood.

As we have seen, there are certain differences between the various types of malaria. Another important difference, in addition to those named, is that *P. vivax* and *P. ovale*, unlike *P. falciparum*, can descend into a kind of torpor in the patient's liver cells, where they can stay inactive for years during which the patient is completely without symptoms. The plasmodia can then wake up and once again produce classic malaria attacks. *P. malariae* also has a so-far-unexplained mechanism for surviving in symptom-free patients for up to thirty years, before once more becoming active and causing new attacks of malaria. It is well known that sailors in old age can get malaria attacks after voyages in tropical climes in their youth. *P. falciparum* is unable to remain in patients for long periods. If the patient survives the acute phase with this species, the malaria will burn out after a few months and the patient recovers. New infection can, however, occur in the same patient at a later date.

Does the patient's immune system not react to the malaria parasites? Yes, fortunately there is a response against plasmodia in patients.[324] This response can considerably reduce the seriousness of the symptoms and especially the mortality. In children from six months to five years old and in pregnant women, however, the immune response is weaker than in others. In these groups we therefore get the most serious course of the disease and the highest mortality rate.

To develop a really effective immune response that can protect one against malaria is not, though, done at the drop of a hat and it does not occur during the first round of infection. It needs repeated infections with plasmodia over a certain length of time, so that the immune system is constantly stimulated. In practice, therefore, this only occurs in regions where malaria is always present – that is, where it is endemic – and the immunity that develops is only short-lived unless it is kept going via new infections. After leaving the malaria area, the immunity will disappear after about a year, and the individual becomes unprotected against new infection if they subsequently return to that area.

It is the immune system that explains why the most serious cases of malaria are most frequently seen in individuals who have not stayed for a certain length of time in malarial areas.[325] Europeans newly arrived in Africa therefore have always been easy prey for the malaria plasmodia. It used to be reckoned that Europeans who came to work in certain parts of Africa suffered a case fatality rate (the proportion of people with confirmed infections who die) from malaria of almost 50 per cent. Indigenous Africans from areas with extremely low rates of malaria are in the same situation if they travel to malarial areas, for example as refugees or seasonal workers.

Even though the immune system responds to malaria plasmodia once it has had time to react, and protects against the most serious forms of the disease and dying from it, chronic malaria and repeated new infections nevertheless cause health problems, including growth and developmental disturbances in children, loss of weight, reduced capacity for work and sick leave from work and school. Chronic malaria also weakens the immune system and increases the risk of catching a number of other infectious diseases, such as pneumonia with bacteria. In the hardest-hit areas, malaria therefore leads to major social and economic problems.

The complex interaction between malaria plasmodia, mosquitoes and humans means that many ecological factors play a crucial role for the existence of malaria in various geographical areas. Climatic conditions, for example, are essential for the *Anopheles* mosquito to become an effective transmitter of the disease. A certain temperature and humidity are needed for the mosquito to be able to survive and reproduce and for the maturation of the plasmodia in the mosquito. In regions with malaria the number of cases increases after periods of rain, when the mosquito has plenty of opportunity to breed.

Malaria through history

How old is malaria as a human disease? And where did the malaria plasmodia arise that attack humans? These questions have been answered in different ways by researchers in recent years. Modern molecular-biological methods have also been increasingly used in malaria research in recent years – with somewhat varying results.

Let us first see what historical accounts can tell us about malaria, even though this infection definitely started before written sources became available. As always, we must look critically at the old accounts of diseases, which are often too imprecise for us to be able to identify the underlying illness with certainty. With malaria, we often find a description of fevers that recur seasonally with a characteristic rhythm, and other typical symptoms such as an enlarged spleen. In these cases we can say with a fairly high degree of certainty that we are dealing with malaria.

The earliest mention of malaria is to be found in the Chinese medical account *Nei Ching* (The Basis of Medicine), which is 4,700 years old.[326] In Chinese writings from the pre-Christian era, the plant quinghao, which contains the substance artemisinin, is mentioned as being effective against fever. This plant is today an important malaria medicine.

In ancient Egypt malaria was already common around 2000 BC. The disease is described in the so-called Ebers papyrus from 1570 BC. In 2008 researchers managed to detect DNA from *P. falciparum* in a number of mummies that were 4,000 years old.[327] And in 3,000-year-old Vedic writings from India we find quite precise descriptions of malaria, including an account of what was probably the *P. falciparum* malaria, described as 'The King of Diseases'.[328]

The Hippocratic writings indicate that malaria was common in ancient Greece. Hippocrates is clearly describing some of the common

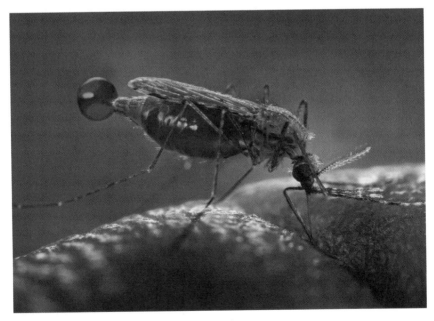

Female *Anopheles* mosquito biting a human being.

forms of malaria, although not the most malignant of them, *P. falci-parum* malaria. This type of malaria probably did not gain a foothold in ancient Greece until the centuries after Hippocrates, but then it had considerable consequences, causing depopulation of entire districts and a decline in agriculture and commerce. It is, however, doubtful if malaria contributed to any great extent to the decline and fall of classical Greek civilization, as some historians have formerly claimed.[329]

Nor did Rome escape malaria. Recent research indicates that malaria plasmodia came to the Roman empire during the last couple of centuries BC, most probably imported from Africa via sea trade, perhaps involving slaves. Malaria may also have come from Greece, but as in that region the 'more benign' forms probably came before the malign form. Molecular-biological methods have detected DNA from *P. falciparum* in human remains from the time of the early emperors (first century AD). Malaria then gradually increased and by the time of Galen in the second century AD it was a serious health problem for Romans.

Galen describes the various forms of malaria in detail.[330] He was clearly aware that malaria was most prevalent close to low-lying swampy areas and ascribed it to the miasmas that came from them. Today we know that the malaria mosquito had its breeding grounds there. By then the Roman upper class had known for a long time that it was wise to build their villas in more elevated areas. Galen emphasized that Rome and the areas around the city suffered greatly from this 'malignant fever', which came especially in the autumn. This is hardly surprising, for the notorious Pontine marshes outside Rome had become an ideal breeding ground for mosquitoes and malaria. This also applied to Rome itself, where stagnant water between the seven hills and the many gardens were an open invitation to the *Anopheles* mosquito.[331]

The comprehensive Roman building projects around Italy also provided ideal conditions for malaria: newly built roads ruined drainage conditions, and comprehensive deforestation created new, water-filled breeding grounds for various types of mosquito. In all probability, malaria was carried round the widespread empire by Roman legionaries and by trade and shipping during the years of peace known as the Pax Romana.

When the Western Roman empire collapsed at the end of the fifth century, malaria had become a major problem in Italy. The ruinous consequences of the constant invasions of Italy during the great migrations that followed the fall improved conditions for malaria even further. The Roman Campagna, which surrounded the city and included the Pontine marshes, was ravaged by malaria right up until modern times.

We do not know all that much about malaria in the Middle Ages. Written accounts from this period are frustratingly imprecise about the disease. The writer Dante Alighieri, however, had a good knowledge of malaria: in his *Divine Comedy* we find no fewer than three descriptions of the disease, suitably enough in his account of the Inferno. Dante himself died of malaria in 1321.[332]

From the Renaissance we have good sources showing that the city of Rome was still haunted by malaria, known as the Roman fever, particularly during the autumn, when the mortality rate was considerable. Without a doubt it was *P. falciparum* that took the lives of pilgrims, cardinals and several popes, including Cesare Borgia's father, Pope Alexander VI, who died of malaria in August 1503. Fate also had it that Cesare, whom we earlier met as a victim of syphilis, was seriously ill with malaria when his father died.[333] For that reason, he was unable to ensure his position of power at this critical moment. He not only lost the support of his father, but the successor to the papacy, Giuliano della Rovere, who took the papal name Julius II, was his bitter enemy. This may well have had historical consequences, since Cesare Borgia had great plans to bring together the states of Central and Northern Italy. Who knows what he could have brought about if malaria had not struck him down during these fateful days: he was, after all, the model for Machiavelli's study of power, *The Prince*.

The seventeenth and eighteenth centuries would seem to suggest that the malaria problem gradually grew worse in Europe, not only in the south but in northern Europe, including the southern parts of Scandinavia.[334] It was probably *P. vivax* that spread, since this form is particularly well adapted to temperate climes. Malaria was especially prominent in Scandinavia in the nineteenth century, when Denmark and Sweden had major epidemics that involved high mortality. In Norway there was a certain amount of malaria during most of the nineteenth century in southern coastal areas, particularly along the Oslo fjord, especially the Hvaler islands and the area around Fredrikstad. Such 'swamp fever', as it was called, was mainly in evidence during the summer months.

In the twentieth century Scandinavia has been free of malaria, except during the Second World War, when malaria shifted northwards and affected both warring sides in the battles between Russian and German forces in Karelia. Malaria was imported to the battle zone by Russian soldiers who had been transferred from Central Asia.

A number of countries in the rest of Europe had considerable problems during the first half of the twentieth century, when malaria affected not only southern Europe but Poland, the Netherlands, Germany and the former Soviet Union. From 1975 onwards malaria has been considered to have been eradicated from Europe after active campaigns. The new cases that are occasionally seen have been imported from other parts of the world where malaria is still a major problem.

War and malaria

For thousands of years, the malaria plasmodia have greatly interfered with the plans of army leaders and often had a decisive effect on the outcome of military campaigns. In 323 BC, after withdrawing his army from India, Alexander the Great died following a short illness in the capital of the Persian empire, Persepolis. His death had major historical consequences for the development of the Mediterranean area during the following centuries. Some eminent historians have claimed that malaria caused his death, though a number of other theories have also been advanced.[335]

When malaria had firmly tightened its grip on the Roman empire, it transpired, paradoxically enough, that this had a certain protective effect against the barbarian invasions of Italy. The Visigoth king Alaric I died shortly after he captured Rome in AD 410, probably of malaria, and his army then withdrew from Italy. Many examples during the following centuries also showed that malaria was a serious opponent for armies invading Italy. Holy Roman emperors were among those who had to stop their campaigns because malaria broke out in their army.[336]

In modern times we also have numerous examples of the importance of malaria for waging war. During the American War of Independence against Britain in the late 1770s, the British forces were severely hampered by malaria, against which the soldiers had less immunity than their American opponents. At the time of the American Civil War, American soldiers were also hard hit: between 1861 and 1865 it was recorded that more than 1.3 million soldiers from both sides succumbed to the disease, with 10,000 deaths.[337]

During the First World War both sides on the Macedonian front in the Balkans were almost paralysed by malaria. A French general replied, when given the order from headquarters to attack: 'I regret to say that my army is in hospital with malaria.'

Malaria was also an enormous problem during the Second World War for those posted outside Europe, especially in the Pacific area. General Douglas MacArthur, who led the American fight against the Japanese, stated: 'It's going to be a very long war if for every division I have facing the enemy, I have one sick in hospital and another recovering from this dreadful disease.'

The problems with malaria during the Second World War were of crucial significance for the development of new medicines to replace quinine. The main source of quinine prior to the war had been the large Dutch plantations of Cinchona trees on Java. When the Japanese took Java, the supplies of quinine were cut off. The warring powers then made great efforts to develop new, synthetic medicines against malaria, which were gradually introduced.

How did the malaria plasmodia come into being?

At some point in the distant past the 'progenitor' of the malaria plasmodia was probably a free-living microbe, a protozoon. It then started a new life as a parasite in the intestines of certain insect larvae that lived in water. Some of these insects gained nutrition from sucking the blood of various species of animals. Gradually the 'malaria progenitor' managed to infect these animals too with the aid of the host insect's sucking. Through evolution, this parasite established a dual existence like the one we know today in malaria in human beings: it spends part of its life in blood-sucking insects, and the other part in the animals from which the insects suck blood. Today most vertebrates have their own form of malaria.[338]

When and how did the malaria plasmodia evolve that have specialized in *Homo sapiens*? Down through history, we know that all inhabited continents have been ravaged by malaria, but which one is the cradle of the disease? And when did malaria start to become a threat to humanity?

It is highly likely that our ape-like forefathers also had their own malaria problems. Perhaps the types of malaria we have today are a further development of the plasmodia of our forefathers, a kind of legacy. In that case, 'our' plasmodia might be several million years old, as certain researchers have claimed. Today, the majority of them believe that *P. vivax*, *P. falciparum*, *P. malariae* and *P. ovale* as a cause of malaria in human beings are quite a bit more recent. There are various factors that seem to suggest this.

Before the first transition in our history of infection, when our ancestors began to settle and take up agriculture and animal husbandry, they lived in small groups as hunters and gatherers. This did not provide all that favourable conditions for the malaria parasites.[339] *P. malariae*, which can live in the patient's body for a number of years, was perhaps able to survive under such conditions, but it can hardly have played a major role. *P. vivax* and *P. ovale* would have had even worse chances of staying alive in these small groups. *P. falciparum* would be severely handicapped in the hunter and gatherer groups, because the transmittance of this variant of malaria is actually fairly ineffective. Many researchers therefore believe that *P. falciparum* can hardly have existed for any length of time before the first transition in the history of human infection – and at any rate cannot have played any major role as a cause of malaria in humans. Why then has this 'malignant malaria' become as deadly as it now is, particularly in Africa, south of the Sahara?

The key to this is without doubt the radically altered conditions arising from the first transition, which not only changed human beings' life situation but the ecological conditions around the new permanent settlements. First, the much larger population groups led to far more human *Anopheles* victims and thus made infection easier. Second, many breeding grounds for mosquitoes were established close to human dwellings because of deforestation. Third, the *Anopheles* species that preferred humans to other animals gained a survival advantage when competing with other species and further adapted itself to this role. With such mosquito species, *P. falciparum* at last gained an opportunity that it eagerly grasped and ushered in an era as one of the major killing machines in the history of human infection. In all probability, this process took place in Africa, partly because the climatic conditions were particularly favourable there, but mainly because it was there that the *Anopheles* species that had specialized in humans developed. The new permanently resident farming communities that arose in Africa had far fewer domestic animals that could compete with humans as 'prey' for the *Anopheles* mosquito than similar agricultural communities outside Africa.

New molecular-biological finds also strongly suggest that *P. falciparum* arose in Africa.[340] It transpires that a host of malaria plasmodia are to be found in African apes. A type of plasmodium recently found in gorillas in West Africa is very similar to *P. falciparum* in humans. It is highly likely that our type of *falciparum* is due to infection from the gorilla. Perhaps this happened only once with a somewhat special gorilla variant that managed to get a foothold with humans. Some researchers believe that this infection from gorilla to human may have taken place relatively late, perhaps during the last 10,000 years.

What about the other species of malaria that is so widespread in the world today, *P. vivax*? Until recently it was thought to have originated in Southeast Asia, since there is a quite similar type of plasmodium there in a macaque ape that could be the source. This theory has now been abandoned. The place of origin for this type of malaria is probably also Africa. A group of researchers recently discovered a number of African types of ape, both chimpanzees and gorillas, that are infected with malaria plasmodia extremely like *P. vivax*. So it seems reasonable to assume that we too have received this type of malaria as a gift from our ape relatives. It is, however, difficult to ascertain when precisely this took place.

We can also deduce that *P. vivax* originated in Africa from completely different research finds. The occurrence of special genes in humans can in fact tell us a great deal about the history of malaria.[341] The *P. vivax* variant is found worldwide, but it is quite rare in large areas of West and Central Africa, where other forms of malaria are common. Nevertheless, the variant is thought to have originated in Africa. The explanation for this, which we touched on earlier, is that the population in these regions has, over several thousands of years, gradually increased its hereditary resistance to the *P. vivax* that originally existed there. This is due to an increased occurrence of a special blood type in the so-called Duffy system, which prevents the *vivax* plasmodia from entering the red blood cells, which parasites are completely dependent on to cause infection. Human beings with the gene for this special blood type have therefore had a survival advantage because of their resistance to *P. vivax* compared to individuals who lack this specific gene. As this resistant group in the population has gradually increased, this type of malaria has therefore lost a great many of its potential victims and become rare in the areas concerned. Once again, we see an example of the influence of evolution on the duel between man and the microbe. This process has probably taken several thousands of years. Since we usually do not find this special blood type that protects against *P. vivax* outside Africa, it fits the theory extremely well that this type of malaria originated in Africa and had the longest time to influence the genes of *Homo sapiens* there.

We have similar examples of the interaction between genes and malaria when it comes to *P. falciparum*. In our red blood cells (erythrocytes) there is an important protein, haemoglobin, which binds oxygen in order that the blood cells can transport this vital molecule to tissues and organs in the body through the blood vessels. There are various hereditary variants of the haemoglobin molecule. Some of these variants provide a certain resistance to *P. falciparum* itself, although it is not 100 per cent. An example of this is the congenital disease 'thalassemi' (*Thalassa* is the modern Greek word for sea), also known as 'Mediterranean anaemia'. As the name indicates, this disease causes various degrees of anaemia, but offers a certain protection against *P. falciparum* malaria. The disease is quite common in the Mediterranean area, but is also found in certain regions of Africa and Asia.[342]

Another important example is the hereditary haemoglobin variant haemoglobin S, which causes 'sickle cell disease', where the red blood cells resemble sickles. In a double dose – that is, when the gene has been inherited from both father and mother – this gene causes a severe disease with a reduced lifespan, but a single dose provides considerable protection against 'malignant' malaria. This has led to a great increase in individuals with the sickle cell gene in the malaria areas in Africa; it is now also frequently found in African American descendants of African slaves.

Malaria provides a number of examples of the duel between man and the microbe over many thousands of years that has also influenced human genes. Scientific finds are never ultimate conclusions, for new discoveries can always change our conceptions. Today, though, it is regarded as fairly certain that the malaria plasmodia that attack *Homo sapiens* originated in Africa, including *P. ovale* and *P. malariae*, which probably originally came from apes.

Out of Africa with Homo sapiens

When *Homo sapiens* moved out of Africa between 60,000 and 120,000 years ago, malaria was part of its luggage.[343] These parasites often found new, local species of *Anopheles* that could take care of transmitting infection. But species of mosquito also roam and can adapt to new geographical and climatic conditions. As humans spread out to the various continents, malaria did too. As we have seen from written accounts, malaria is many thousands of years old in both Asia and Europe – with the New World as an exception.

As in other areas of malaria research, there has also been disagreement about the arrival of malaria on the American continents. Some researchers have claimed that malaria was well established long before Columbus arrived in 1492. One of their arguments has been that in the apes of South America there are malaria plasmodia that closely resemble *P. vivax* and *P. malariae*. It has therefore been claimed that these plasmodia variants are due to infection from humans to apes with *P. vivax* from South East Asia and *P. malariae* from West Africa, and that this infection took place long before Columbus. This theory presupposes risky sea voyages over large expanses of ocean with somewhat primitive vessels, and there is no evidence of this whatsoever. We know that the Vikings arrived on the east coast of North America over a thousand years ago, but it is highly improbable that they had malaria with them since this infection did not exist in their home country. Nor is it likely that malaria arrived with the first humans who crossed from Siberia via the Bering Strait between 20,000 and 30,000 years ago. The climatic conditions hardly made malaria possible in that part of the world.[344]

Another argument that would seem to refute the idea that malaria was already present is that we do not see any signs of the malaria plasmodia having influenced the genes of the indigenous human population, of which there are several examples in Africa, as we have seen.

Most researchers today are convinced that malaria – *P. vivax*, *P. falciparum* and *P. malariae* – came to the American continents *after* Columbus, with Europeans and slaves from West Africa who were regularly imported over the succeeding period of almost three hundred years. There were several local species of *Anopheles* in America that could start the transmission of infection, which led to the malaria plasmodia spreading both to local apes and to the indigenous population.[345] Malaria first gained a foothold in the West Indies and in Central and South America. From the mid-eighteenth century, with the slave-based economic growth of the southern states of the USA, the disease spread extremely fast in large sections of North America, where the vast increase in agricultural areas with breeding grounds abounding in water for mosquitoes were ideal for the plasmodia.

Malaria joined the long list of disease-causing microbes that were a gift from the Old World to the New after Columbus. By a quirk of fate, the return gift of the New World was the first effective medicine to combat malaria – the bark from the cinchona tree.[346] The powder or extract from this bark, which we know to contain the active substance quinine, was brought from Peru to Europe in the seventeenth century by the Jesuits, and until the twentieth century it was the only efficacious medicine against malaria that one had. Quinine, however, only suppresses the symptoms and neither prevents nor cures. In addition, there was considerable variation in the quality of the bark that was marketed, quite often because of falsification. So it was a great step forward when French researchers found in 1820 how to produce a pure form of quinine from the bark of this tree.

In the mid-nineteenth century, the world malaria pandemic reached its peak: never before or since have the plasmodia caused so much disease and death. More than half the world's population lived with a considerable risk of being infected, and at least a tenth of those who became infected died.

Military doctors crack the malaria code

The everyday life of a military doctor in peacetime is hardly ever interesting, but the history of infection medicine also provides examples of military doctors facing major and fascinating challenges and coming up with results that have had wide-ranging consequences. The discovery of the cause of malaria is a good example of this.

Ever since the time of Hippocrates, people had believed that malaria was linked to miasmas from unhealthy swamp areas that influenced the balance of the four humours. The miasma theory survived right up to the time of Koch and Pasteur. With the bacteriological revolution the hunt began for microbes as a cause of malaria. In 1884 two researchers believed they had detected a bacterium in water in the Pontine marshes outside Rome, where malaria was extremely common. The bacterium, which they called *Bacillus malariae*, caused fever when they injected rabbits with it. Robert Koch, however, was sceptical and set off to Italy to study malaria, in direct competition with the Italian researchers within the field. On that occasion he had no success and what the Italians regarded as his arrogant behaviour caused great offence.[347]

As early as 1880 a military doctor stationed with the French foreign legion in Algeria, Charles Louis Alphonse Laveran, had found some strange organisms in the red blood cells of soldiers suffering from malaria.[348] He discovered that these organisms disappeared after treatment with quinine and thought he had found a protozoon that caused malaria. For several years he tried without success to convince Koch and other prominent bacteriologists, but in 1884 an active Italian group of researchers accepted his discovery and then developed his findings. By 1890 it had become clear that malaria attacks were due to protozoon-infected red blood cells bursting and releasing parasites. The Italian researchers, with Giovanni Battista Grassi as a key figure, had by then already discovered three of the most important malaria plasmodia: *P. vivax*, *P. falciparum* and *P. malariae*.

As yet, however, no malaria researcher understood how the infection took place via the malaria plasmodia. This is where the Englishmen appear on the scene. The English mission doctor Patrick Manson, who is regarded as the father of the discipline of tropical medicine, had, during his many years in the East, made the important discovery that a troublesome infection with the intestinal worm *Filaria*, which produces so-called elephantiasis, causing tremendously swollen legs and genitals, is transmitted by mosquitoes. Manson thought it was possible that malaria could be transmitted in a similar way. He then convinced Ronald Ross, a military doctor who worked in India, to test this mosquito theory about malaria.[349]

Ross was not an obvious candidate to solve the malaria enigma. He had not done well in his medical examinations and had no special scientific background. He was actually most interested in writing poetry and novels, which were nearly always turned down by publishers. Nor did he know anything about species of mosquito: it is said that his only work that dealt with insects was a book on fly-fishing. He did not initially attach much credence to Laveran's findings, but he took up Manson's challenge as far as his duties as a military doctor allowed. He started to dissect mosquitoes to see if he could find Laveran's protozoa, but even after thousands of experiments he found none. We now know that he had begun by examining the wrong kinds of mosquito, ones that cannot transmit malaria. One day in August 1897, however, when in a semi-torpid state in oppressive Indian heat, he was looking at yet another mosquito under the microscope and was startled to see organisms similar to Laveran's in its alimentary canal. By chance he was then looking at an *Anopheles* mosquito that had bitten a malaria patient. He immediately wrote a poem in several verses about the discovery, in which he enthused about the new possibilities it had opened up.[350]

But the crucial question remained: how did the transmission of infection take place from mosquito to human being? Ross doubtless knew that Italian malaria researchers had also detected malaria in birds, and he now decided to make use of various species of bird in his experiments in order to map the infection mechanism of malaria. He then discovered that the plasmodia, during their maturation in the mosquito, gradually shift to the salivary glands and are transmitted to the next victims with the saliva when the mosquito sucks blood. He expected this was also what took place with humans.

Meanwhile, the Italian researchers under Grassi's leadership had not been idle.[351] They probably knew about Ross's new finds. By systematic examination they quickly found that it had to be the *Anopheles* mosquito that was involved as the transmitter of infection to humans, and demonstrated that malaria is transmitted by this mosquito. They immediately published their results, unfortunately without mentioning Ronald Ross, who despite everything had been responsible for the breakthrough regarding the role of the mosquito in infecting humans. Ross never forgave them for this, and referred to his competitors as 'Italian pirates'. There was a long, bitter feud, as one unfortunately often sees with scientific breakthroughs where there is disagreement about priorities. The bitterness of the Italians did not lessen when Ross was the sole winner of the Nobel Prize in medicine in 1902. The reason why the prize was not shared between Ross and Grassi was probably because of statements made by Robert Koch, who had been appointed the neutral arbitrator. In 1907 Laveran was awarded the Nobel Prize. The Italian researchers, who had carried out systematic studies of malaria in humans for many years, were never awarded the prize. The lack of justice in this matter has been discussed ever since.

The battle against malaria: early victories and later defeats

When Ross, Grassi and the latter's colleagues made their epoch-making discoveries at the end of the nineteenth century, malaria had been on the retreat from Northern and Western Europe since the middle of the century. There are several reasons for this. One could perhaps have thought that lower temperatures made the situation less favourable for the *Anopheles* mosquito, but that is not the explanation. On the contrary, there was a tendency for the temperature to rise in Europe during the latter half of the nineteenth century.[352]

An important cause of the decline was in fact the increasing modernization of agriculture in Northern Europe, including better drainage that led to the mosquito having fewer breeding grounds.[353] Another important cause was a change in housing practice in rural areas, which led to a greater physical separation between livestock and humans, so that the *Anopheles* mosquito began to concentrate more on livestock, which it actually preferred. A general increase in the standard of living, including nutrition and housing conditions, may also have contributed to the decrease in malaria.

In Southern and Eastern Europe, however, malaria continued to flourish until the mid-twentieth century. The scientific discoveries that revealed the complex infection mechanisms had originally led to a strong hope that at last it would be possible to overcome this disease, which had ravaged humanity since time immemorial.

Initially, efforts concentrated on combatting the *Anopheles* mosquito with all possible means, so as to break the chain of infection.[354] First and foremost, the mosquito larvae were attacked in their breeding grounds, partly via the use of various chemical products and partly via comprehensive draining projects. Where this work was carried out intensively and with sufficient resources, it led to success. We have previously mentioned the American military doctor William C. Gorgas and his success in combatting yellow fever, first on Cuba and then in Panama during the construction of the canal. It was mainly the assault on the mosquito that was key to his success. Not only did this work for yellow fever, but it brought about a tremendous reduction in the malaria problem in the same areas. The Italian authorities in the interwar period used similar methods to eradicate malaria from the notorious Pontine marshes, where the spectre of the disease had threatened people since Roman times. This was regarded as a triumph for Mussolini's fascist state. There are also many examples of malaria being successfully combatted in other parts of the world in the years leading up to the Second World War, but the strategy employed needed lots of resources and was expensive, and a failure to maintain the measures often led to the return of malaria.

This was, for example, the case in the Soviet Union. The displacement of peoples, undernourishment and climatic conditions in the wake of the First World War and the Russian Revolution led to the largest malaria epidemic in modern times with both *P. vivax* and *P. falciparum*. It is thought that at least 10 million people were infected and 600,000 died. Malaria was common as far north as Arkhangelsk on the White Sea. After the authorities had gained a certain amount of control over the malaria situation in the following years, the destruction wreaked by the Second World War led to new, serious malaria problems, with at least 4 million people being infected.[355]

During this war, the initially highly promising insecticide DDT started to be used. The use of DDT in the fight against the mosquito larvae in their breeding grounds was so effective in the early years that people started to eye the possibility of completely eradicating malaria. A number of new and effective medicines had also been discovered for treating malaria. These advances led to the launch of the ambitious eradication strategy known as the Malaria Eradication Program (MEP) by the recently established World Health Organization (WHO) in 1955.[356]

The hope of eradicating malaria fitted in well with the optimistic belief of the post-war period that the era of infectious diseases was over. At last, *Homo sapiens* had secured the upper hand in the duel with the world of microbes. This, unfortunately, proved itself to be a case of hubris, which the Greeks believed always led to the gods taking revenge. In the field of malaria, this began to become clear during the first decade of the MEP. It was admittedly possible to point to certain successes, but generally speaking it was apparent that the WHO's programme had failed. At the same time, it became obvious that many species of mosquito had become resistant to the wonder cure DDT, and that this chemical also had many unintended harmful ecological effects. Resistance to the new anti-malaria medicines also developed at an alarming rate.[357]

Even though new strategies for combatting malaria gradually materialized, malaria is still one of the world's major health problems. About half the world's population is still exposed to malaria: in 2017 there were 219 million new cases in ninety countries, and 415,000 deaths. More than 90 per cent of both new cases and deaths were in Africa. The challenge from the malaria plasmodia, in other words, is enormous in the years ahead. Malaria is not going to loosen its grip on *Homo sapiens* for a long time to come.

Influenza: A Ticking Time Bomb from the East

Influenza is still part of our everyday lives, unlike such infections as smallpox, plague and malaria, which are most often perceived in Western societies as being historical phenomena. Influenza is nevertheless not seen by most people as being a serious threat to the individual. This is mainly due to the fact that the term 'influenza' is used quite uncritically about many forms of trivial, acute respiratory tract infections. For the small group of epidemiologists who are responsible for our response capacity to epidemics, on the other hand, influenza is a source of considerable unease. The influenza virus has caused some of the most serious pandemics of recent times, and there is much to suggest that this can happen again. That is one of the reasons why earlier pandemics involving the influenza virus have been subjected to a whole series of studies, and this is still a highly topical field of research. There can be no doubt that we both can and must learn from history if we are to prepare ourselves effectively for new pandemics involving this virus.

A virus with countless hosts and many victims

There are three main groups of the influenza virus, known as A, B and C.[358] Influenza virus A is of particular interest, since it can cause major epidemics and pandemics, so it is this group on which we intend to concentrate. The B group causes influenza but not pandemics, and the C group causes only a quite light form of infection of the upper respiratory tract. The B and C viruses exclusively affect humans, unlike the A virus. This virus is widespread not only in humans but in a large number of other warm-blooded animals, including numerous bird species, pigs, horses and dogs. Here, 'influenza virus' refers to the A virus, often called the IVA virus.

Among all the species of animal susceptible to the IVA virus, its true home is wild seabirds and wading birds. These are the species that are the reservoir of the virus in nature. In these birds, the virus causes a quite light infection in the intestines and is then excreted and can infect new birds. Normally, the host birds do not fall ill. From this natural reservoir, the virus can transmit infection from wild birds to other species of animal with varying results, depending on whether the virus is able to adapt itself to the new species and cause infection, and subsequently pass this on to others of the same species. If this happens, major epidemics can arise in the new host, normally resulting in illness. This can occur, for example, in domesticated birds such as chickens and ducks.

Influenza in humans

The disease picture of influenza in typical cases is an acute infection of the respiratory tract with sudden high fever, headache, aching muscles and limbs, a runny nose and coughing. The patient often feels extremely tired, with a strong sensation of being ill. The high temperature lasts between seven and ten days, but the lassitude can last for quite a while. All age groups can be affected. The most serious cases tend to be very young children, the elderly and people with other illnesses such as chronic cardiac and broncho-pulmonary complaints, diabetes, obesity and conditions with a weakened immune system. Pregnant women are also regarded as a high-risk group.[359]

Among the commonest complications is pneumonia, which may be due to the influenza virus itself, but is most often a consequence of a bacterial infection. In particularly serious cases of influenza, failure of the lungs can result in death in the course of a couple of days.[360]

Person-to-person infection can take place in various ways: droplet infection, in which droplets of nasal secretion containing the virus are spread to the surroundings via coughing, sneezing or speaking, or via human contact, in which the virus is transmitted either directly or indirectly via objects. Aerial infection from aerosols is also possible.

The IVA virus that has caused illness in humans for at least five hundred years comes, then, from wild birds and over the centuries has repeatedly adapted itself to *Homo sapiens*. The big question is *how* this adaptation has formerly taken place and will be able to do so again. What are the mechanisms behind this transition from wild birds to humans that constantly causes epidemics and repeatedly has also led to catastrophic pandemics?

We do not intend to examine the complex construction and characteristics of the influenza virus in detail here, but it is necessary to look at certain characteristics of the building blocks of the virus in order to understand why epidemics occur. Like other microbes, the virus has genes that control the production of certain types of molecule, antigens, which the immune system of the infected person regards as being alien. This can trigger an effective response that aborts the infection. The influenza virus has two particularly important antigens known by the letters H (sometimes HA) and N (sometimes NA). These antigen molecules sit like spikes on the surface of the virus and are essential for the capacity of the virus to invade cells. We reckon on there being eighteen variants of the H antigen, called H_1, H_2 and so on, and eleven N antigens, called N_1, N_2 and so on. All possible combinations of H and N antigens are found in nature, and the individual variant of the virus is typically named H_1N_1 or H_3N_5, for example.[361] When a new influenza epidemic is announced, the composition of the virus is normally named.

In addition to the two genes that control the production of the H and N antigens, the virus has genes that are important for other characteristics, including the capacity to pass infection on from one individual to another. This capacity is often adapted to the individual species of animal, so that a virus cannot necessarily pass on infection, even though it has been able to infect a new species. But adaptation to transmission in its new host can occur after infection, and this produces epidemics. There is still a great deal we do not know about the mechanisms underlying this adaptation, particularly how the influenza virus from birds can adapt itself to human beings. This is an active field of research that is of very great theoretical and practical importance, and also for the production of effective influenza vaccines.

The pig: the missing link?

In the natural reservoir of the influenza virus, wild birds, there are the greatest number of H and N combinations of the virus. The virus is extremely 'nervous' and unstable. This is shown by the fact that the individual virus variants have a distinct tendency to swap genes with each other so that new combinations arise, not only with regard to the genes coding for H and N antigens. This can occur if several virus variants infect the same cell in the host animal. This crossover of genes is known as 'gene reassortment'. Virus variants with completely new characteristics can arise in this way.[362]

So far, experience shows that the influenza virus from birds can occasionally cause infection in humans, but generally speaking it is not able to pass infection on further and cause major epidemics. The bird viruses are not initially adapted to human beings, and for that reason the infection of humans is a dead end for the virus. But we know that several variants of IVA must at some point have become adapted to humans, since infectious influenza virus can still cause epidemics among us, and sometimes pandemics.

Before discussing further how a bird virus can adapt itself to humans, we will take a look at how the already adapted human variants of IVA behave and create our everyday influenza problems. The virus is what we call endemic – that is, it never disappears, but roughly every year causes new epidemics, so-called seasonal influenza, mostly during the winter months. Under pressure from our immune response to the present virus in circulation, it changes to some extent through time as the result of mutations that cause a certain alteration of the virus antigens, the H antigen in particular. This leads to our immune system becoming less effective in the population against the 'new' mutated virus during the year, and to more people becoming susceptible to this virus in the following season. This is why an influenza vaccine has to be tailor-made for every fresh influenza season and is once more an example of the flexible adaptation of the microbes in the duel with humanity.[363]

These mutations that change the virus in circulation are normally quite small and do not lead to pandemics. Nevertheless, we had a number of pandemics in the twentieth century alone, and in all probability will have new ones in the twenty-first. The precondition for a pandemic is that a new IVA virus has come into being that has H and/or N antigens that are different enough for the world's population not to have an effective immunity against it. How can such a situation arise?

Normally a wild bird virus will not be adapted to humans. This means that further infection does not take place, even though such a virus would initially be able to infect a human individual. A bird virus that is adapted to humans, on the other hand, can come into being via gene reassortment, as mentioned. If a human virus infects the same cell as a bird virus in an animal, this crossover with genes can take place. There are, however, few species of animal where the cells are susceptible to both human and bird viruses. The pig is an exception, which is why it has come very much into the spotlight of influenza research.

Many influenza researchers believe that the pig can function as a kind of mixing bowl for human and bird variants of the virus, resulting in a new virus that has antigens against which humans lack any effective immunity, while the virus has retained the ability to spread via effective person-to-person infection. This was probably the recipe for some of the great influenza pandemics of history. It can also explain why so many influenza pandemics have started in China, where the special conditions in agriculture make extremely close contact possible between a large number of domesticated and wild birds, pigs and human beings. The conditions for the exchange of genes between various IVA viruses via gene-reassortment are particularly favourable there.

Even so, there is much to suggest that the adaptation of the virus to humans in special cases can take place via direct infection from bird to human – without the pig as an intermediary – although we do not have any cast-iron evidence of this as yet. Possibly, some of the pandemics have come about in this way.[364] We must in such cases assume that the bird virus, after having infected a human being, manages to adapt itself to humans via so many rapid mutations that further infection also becomes possible. Perhaps gene-reassortment between human virus and dangerous bird virus can occasionally take place in human cells? Certain research findings would seem to indicate this.[365]

A recent infection in human history

It is hardly likely that the influenza virus troubled our ancestors when they were nomadic hunters and gatherers. It would have been unable to maintain itself in such small groups where individuals would either die or become immune. So influenza probably did not appear on the scene until after the first epidemiological transition in the history of human infection, after the size of the population had become large enough a few millennia ago.[366]

We have very little information about possible early epidemics and pandemics, since written accounts are often imprecise and make it difficult to distinguish influenza from many other epidemic fevers. It is not clear whether Hippocrates mentions influenza in his writings. Historians disagree about what can be considered the first absolutely certain major influenza epidemic. An epidemic that quite possibly may have been influenza was written about in 1173, but it hardly spread outside Europe, so it was not a pandemic. The first quite certain influenza pandemic occurred in 1510.

The term 'influenza' probably originally comes from Renaissance Italy, where the infection was known as *ex influenza di freddo* ('from the influence of cold'). The term *influenza di stelle* was also used, since people believed the illness was due to a kind of influence from the stars. Later, the simplified form *influenza* came to be used.

A number of large influenza epidemics broke out in Europe in the sixteenth century. The last one, in 1580, was without doubt a pandemic as it affected Asia and Africa as well as Europe. In both the eighteenth and nineteenth centuries there were at least three pandemics, in addition to a number of major epidemics. Several of these pandemics were thought to have arisen in China. The last pandemic of the nineteenth century, in 1889–90, was also thought to have come from the East and was given the name 'Russian disease'. During this pandemic, 250,000 people died in Europe alone, and at least three times as many in the rest of the world.[367]

All in all, the influenza virus took far more lives in Europe in the nineteenth century than the much more feared disease of cholera. But since most of the victims were elderly, influenza did not have the same aura of dread and death as cholera did.

The influenza virus was yet another gift from the Old World to the New, for we have no information about influenza in the Americas before Columbus. It is likely that influenza epidemics contributed to the infection problems of the Native American people after their meeting with the Europeans.[368]

Spanish Flu, 1918: the mother of all pandemics

Nearly thirty years after the influenza pandemic of 1889–90, an influenza virus struck again, giving rise to a pandemic that has probably never been surpassed when it comes to the number of deaths in the space of just a few months.[369] Probably at least 500 million people were infected, a third of the world's population. This influenza was also uncommonly serious. Certain researchers have claimed that up to 100 million people died during this pandemic, although some new research reports have raised doubts about these extremely high figures.[370]

In 1918 the First World War was entering its final phase. Millions of young men had fallen on the battlefield, some in huge individual battles and some in the endless trench war on the European continent. And then the warring nations and their civilian populations were hit by a new disaster: an influenza pandemic that, in the course of a year, was to leave an indelible mark on most of the inhabited world. This pandemic was given the name 'Spanish Flu', and it had a number of characteristics that clearly distinguished it from normal influenza epidemics, of which people had a certain amount of experience. Why was it called the Spanish Flu? Quite simply because the warring powers, for tactical reasons, had censored information about the explosive new disease, while Spain, which stood outside the hostilities, had no restrictions placed on featuring the sensational news of the pandemic in the newspapers, with the Spanish king, Alfonso xiii, and several of his ministers going down with the illness.[371]

The pandemic developed in Europe in three partially separate waves with fairly short interludes – in itself something of a surprise.[372] The first wave started in March 1918. There is still considerable disagreement as to where the virus first appeared on the scene. A common view is that it did so at Camp Funston, a u.s. Army camp in Kansas, and that the virus was then spread by American troops transported to ports in France.[373] Others believe that the virus might have started in Europe, perhaps in a large British military camp in northern France.[374] This camp lay on an important route for migrating birds from East Asia, so the virus could have been brought by birds that infected local hens and geese. China has also been suspected as the country of origin, partly because a large number of Chinese migrant workers came to North America at that time, but there is little evidence to support this theory. Perhaps the geographical origins of the Spanish Flu will never be known.

The *first wave* of influenza spread rapidly during the following months to both warring parties and the civilian population, and then swiftly moved on to Asia. Many people became infected, but initially the symptoms were no more serious than with ordinary seasonal influenza. However, it was soon obvious that a strikingly large percentage of the most serious cases were people between twenty and forty years of age, who normally get off lightly with influenza.

Then the *second wave* struck in August 1918, at roughly the same time in Europe, North America and Africa. The virus now showed itself to be far more dangerous than during the first wave, with a much higher case fatality rate. Once again it was those between twenty and forty who were hardest hit. Mortality is normally highest among the youngest and oldest; now the highest mortality was *between* these extremes – in young adults. In all age groups, mortality was higher than for common flu, but strangely enough it was not so high among the elderly as among young people.[375]

The epidemic then decreased for a while, but this lull was replaced by a *third wave* from February 1919. This wave was clearly milder and smaller than the previous one. When the Spanish Flu subsequently burned out in 1919, in the course of one year it had left in its wake more deaths than any other known pandemic in human history.

The fear of such a catastrophe repeating itself with a new influenza virus probably partially explains why for the last few decades considerable research has been done on the Spanish Flu: its characteristics, the ways in which it spread and the social, economic and political consequences of the pandemic. A lot of interesting finds have been made, but many of the key questions have yet to be answered.

What do we now know about the influenza virus that was the cause of this catastrophe? Since the pandemic dates back a century, it might be thought that the virus no longer exists and could not be analysed. This is fortunately not the case, particularly due to the efforts of the American virologist Jeffrey K. Taubenberger and his colleagues, to old military medical archives of tissue from patients who died during the pandemic, and to the remains of patients buried in Alaska, which was very badly hit. In order to bury corpses in frozen ground, it had been necessary to call on miners who were experts in excavating in the permafrost. These conditions have preserved the virus in the buried bodies, so that it is still possible to analyse it in detail.[376]

Investigations have shown that the influenza virus that caused the pandemic was an H1N1 virus. It has also proved possible to reconstruct it in the laboratory and it has been used in animal experiments in order to study its effects. It turns out that this virus is closely related to bird virus, yet differs from both present-day bird virus and bird virus from the time of the pandemic. It is still a mystery how the virus that caused it arose.[377]

Nor have investigations of the genes of the virus and eventual mutations provided any clear answer to why this virus was so virulent and led to more serious infection than other types. The cause of death was very frequently pneumonia from bacteria that struck in the wake of the influenza.[378] Taubenberger and his colleagues have shown in the old tissue samples from patients at the time of the pandemic that the virus caused considerable changes to the air passages, which paved the way for bacteria such as pneumococci and streptococci, along with the common bacterium we now call *Haemophilus influenzae.* The last-named is of particular historical interest because the leading German bacteriologist at the time of the pandemic, Richard Pfeiffer, who was a pupil of Robert Koch, believed that precisely this microbe was the actual cause of influenza. Many shared this view at the time, but it was gradually abandoned because the bacterium was not usually found in influenza patients with pneumonia.[379]

The striking mortality rate of the Spanish Flu victims, however, was hardly solely due to bacterial infections as complications of influenza. Many of the particularly susceptible young patients died within a couple of days, with a highly dramatic pathological picture including a fatal failure of the lungs, with the patients' skin taking on a bluish tinge reminiscent of the heliotrope flower. People spoke of 'heliotropic cyanosis', since cyanosis is the ordinary medical term for a sickly, bluish-coloured skin.[380] There is much that could possibly indicate that

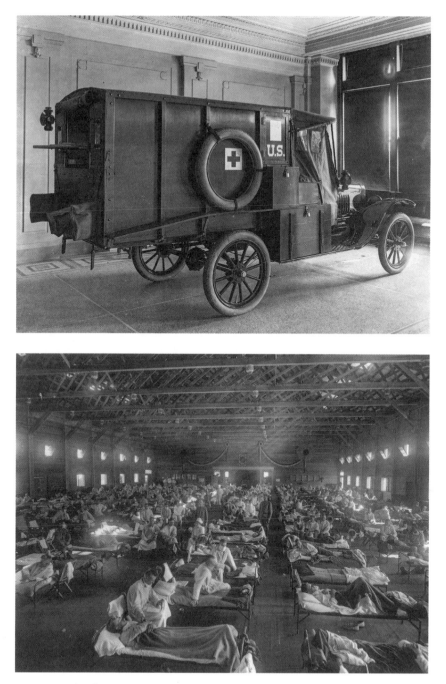

Top: Example of a 1917 Ford Model T U.S. Army ambulance used during the First World War. The transportation of wounded and influenza-sick patients with these ambulances provided good conditions for the spread of infection. *Bottom*: Improvised American military hospital with influenza patients during the Spanish Flu pandemic, Kansas, *c.* 1918.

this violent pathological picture was due to what is known as a cytokine storm, an explosive over-reaction of the immune system, which, among other things, involves a massive release of cytokines from the immune system that can cause life-threatening inflammatory reactions. Animal experiments with the reconstructed Spanish Flu virus have shown that it can cause precisely such reactions. This could partially explain, at any rate, the fatal effect of the virus on young adults, who normally have a particularly robust immune system. The fact that elderly people escaped more lightly could be due to the weakening of the immune system that takes place over time, so that a cytokine storm is less likely. But it is also believed that people over sixty years of age during the pandemic may have acquired a certain degree of immunity from contact with the earlier flu pandemic of 1889–90.[381]

The second wave of the flu, which struck from August 1918 onwards, was clearly more virulent than the first, so something must have happened to the virus, probably mutations that in the course of a few months had resulted in a more dangerous virus. The evolutionary biologist Paul Ewald has placed considerable emphasis on the conditions at the front in 1918 to explain the increased virulence of the virus.[382] In the trenches, where the soldiers fought shoulder to shoulder, the conditions were ideal for the spread of virus. The same applied to the conditions in which soldiers, both those wounded and those with influenza, were transported by ambulance back to overcrowded field hospitals. At the same time, the evacuated soldiers at the front were constantly being replaced by fresh soldiers who had no immunity, who in turn became infected. Under such conditions, the laws of evolution, according to Ewald, state that the influenza virus – which, like other microbes, exclusively prioritizes its own survival and dissemination – does not have any interest in causing a mild illness. On the contrary, it will prioritize mutations that ensure more rapid propagation and dissemination, and a more virulent virus. Similar conditions in army camps and troop ships will have contributed to this.

Even though the special conditions for military personnel may have led to the development of the virulent virus, the civilian population was also hard hit. In fact, the mortality was just as high among women as men. Pregnant women were especially vulnerable, with a very high mortality rate.

In the USA alone, 675,000 people died, more than the total of all military deaths in the country's wars anywhere in the world during the twentieth century, including the two World Wars.[383] Japan had 400,000 deaths from influenza.

Although the influenza virus affected all groups and social classes, it is a fact that economically under-privileged groups in all countries were hardest hit, because of their cramped living conditions, malnutrition and lack of care. This tendency was particularly in evidence in what we now refer to as the developing countries, where mortality was considerably higher than in the Western world. In India alone, almost 20 million people died, with a clearly higher mortality in the lower Hindu castes than in the higher strata of society. Normally Hindus are cremated on a funeral pyre on the banks of a river and the ashes then scattered on the water. Now there was no longer sufficient firewood for the cremations, and the rivers were full of corpses.[384] On Western Samoa in the Pacific, it is estimated that 25 per cent of the indigenous population died.

Despite the shocking figures for mortality from the Spanish Influenza in developing countries, they are probably still too low.

An age full of death

The Spanish Flu left a serious imprint on all societies affected by it.[385] All over the world, people were confronted with the deaths of many relations and friends because of what had initially been thought to be merely common influenza. An example of the hopelessness and fear this instilled is obvious in Sigmund Freud's words when writing to a friend: 'Do you recall any other age so full of death as this one?' He had just lost his pregnant daughter Sophie to the Spanish Flu. Since the pandemic was particularly brutal towards those between the ages of twenty and forty, there was a great increase in the numbers of orphaned children.

The infrastructure of society was also strongly affected in many areas. Doctors and nurses were often far too few and overburdened. Funeral parlours and burial services could not cope and mass graves for victims of the disease had to be introduced. A lack of staff could lead to the breakdown of ordinary public services, such as telephone exchanges and rubbish collection in urban areas.[386]

In many ways the Spanish Flu represented an enormous humiliation for the medical profession. The bacterial revolution had led to considerable optimism when it came to the prospects of gaining control over infectious diseases. Bacterial causes for a whole series of infections had already been clarified. Now medicine faced a pandemic with no known cause, even though for a time many clung to a belief in Richard Pfeiffer's bacterium as the cause. The reality was that doctors were helpless in treating the victims of the disease. Very little about viruses was known at the time: the influenza virus was first detected by American and British researchers in 1933. The historian Alfred Crosby, who has carried out thorough studies of this pandemic, has stated: 'The physicians of 1918 were participants in the greatest failure of medical science in the twentieth century or, if absolute numbers of dead are the measure, of all time.'[387] This damning judgement, in my opinion, is somewhat unjust. The fact is that the scientifically most advanced states at the time were engaged in a war. Medical staff were particularly involved in the treatment of the enormous number of wounded young men, and scientific activity in general was geared to the arms industry and other war-related objectives. Nor should we forget that certain medical researchers, in the midst of the chaos that prevailed, attempted to develop a vaccine against the unknown microbe facing the world. But in fact doctors probably played a more modest role in the treatment of influenza patients than nurses, who were also in short supply. Good, ordinary care was the most important thing that victims could be offered.[388]

Apart from this, the authorities in most countries introduced many kinds of preventative measures, with varying degrees of success. Schools, churches and theatres were closed in many areas. In San Francisco, for example, wearing masks in public spaces was made compulsory. Earlier quarantine measures were once more activated, but not always successfully, for the influenza virus was not easy to limit. Using effective quarantine measures, Australia managed to keep the virulent second wave of influenza at bay throughout the autumn of 1918. In most Asian and African countries, some of which were colonies, the measures taken to combat the pandemic by the authorities were far less energetic than in Western countries, mainly because of a lack of resources. In a number of countries in and outside Europe, the response of the authorities to the pandemic led to public disturbances because of a lack of, or unpopular, measures. This applied, for example, to India, where discontent with the British colonial authorities' quarantine measures led to riots.

Spanish Flu and the outcome of the First World War

There can be no doubt that the development of the influenza pandemic in 1918–19 and important events linked to the First World War were intertwined in many ways. This does not of course mean that the pandemic could not have come about in peacetime, but would it then have taken a different course? This we will of course never know, although it is certain that conditions in 1918 were almost ideal for the influenza virus. Already prior to the war, the national and international transport network was well established in large parts of the world through shipping and railways. To a high degree, this facilitated the spread of the virus over large parts of the globe.

The First World War itself was a fine breeding ground for the pandemic.[389] We have seen how conditions at the front were particularly favourable for the spread of the virus and probably also contributed to the increase of virulence in the second wave of the pandemic. The constant transportation of troops between the continents undoubtedly played a major role in the spread of the virus. And, as mentioned, a great many resources within medicine and research were focused on the war effort. It is also likely that the war led to a worsening of the civilian population's health and nutrition, which in turn increased the susceptibility to influenzas. Data from Germany would seem to suggest this.

Another interesting but more complex question is whether or not the Spanish Flu had a significant effect on the course of the war, especially on its outcome. Here the opinions of historians differ.[390] My impression is that the majority do not consider this to be relevant and therefore avoid adopting a stance on the matter: there are many historical presentations of the war in which the influenza pandemic is scarcely mentioned.

Among the historians who have been interested in the Spanish Flu, there are differing views on the pandemic's influence on the war's outcome. No one doubts that the illness raged among military personnel on both sides, for here there are clear statistics. According to the head doctor of the American army, about 1 million soldiers of the American Expeditionary Force (AEF), which was engaged in the fighting in Europe in 1918, were hospitalized. Of these, 775,000 had influenza, while 225,000 had war injuries. This had marked consequences on the fighting efficiency and strength of the divisions, and on the morale and combat

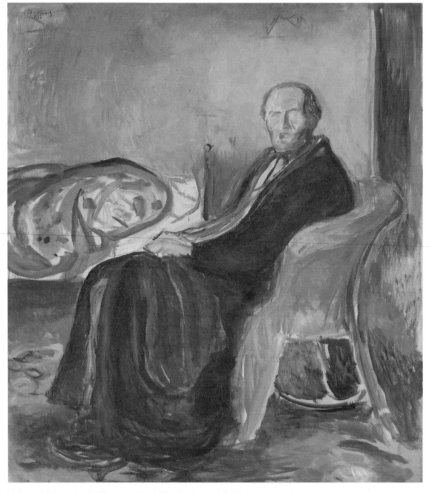

Edvard Munch, *Self-portrait with the Spanish Flu*, 1919, oil on canvas. At the very beginning of 1919, Munch went down with Spanish Flu and painted a number of pictures with this motif. In this picture he is sitting limply in a chair with a pale face that shows clear signs of the disease as well as of exhaustion.

willingness of the soldiers. The British army had more than 300,000 cases of influenza in 1918 with similar mortality to the civilian population, while France lost 30,000 soldiers during the pandemic.

The virus also raged among the Central Powers: Germany, Austria-Hungary, Bulgaria and Turkey. The German army was hard hit during the spring and summer of 1918, with more than 1.5 million cases of influenza. Certain divisions had up to 80 per cent of personnel affected by the disease. Without a doubt, this must have weakened the German war effort, with military transport and the supply lines also being partially undermined by the large number of cases. The German chief of general staff, Erich von Ludendorff, who was one of Germany's most powerful men, hoped to gain a final victory in the spring of 1918, since Russia was now out of the war. He initiated an enormous offensive in northern France in March and at first the German forces enjoyed great success, but then the offensive gradually ground to a halt, and at the same time the influenza virus struck. Another large-scale offensive in July, during the first wave of the virus, also proved unsuccessful. Ludendorff, who was himself plagued by illness, now lost faith in the possibility of a military victory and placed much of the blame on the influenza pandemic. Although some historians have dismissed this as wild exaggeration and attribute the lack of military success to Ludendorff's attempt to deny any responsibility, others are inclined to support his assessment.

Austria-Hungary was also hard hit by the pandemic, particularly by the second wave of autumn 1918. A couple of weeks after that struck, the old Habsburg empire started to disintegrate.

Historians who believe that the influenza pandemic exerted a decisive influence on the outcome of the First World War emphasize that the Central Powers, Germany in particular, were hit first, so that the major offensives during 1918, which possibly could have resulted in German victory, were unsuccessful.[391] It is also conceivable that the Central Powers might have gone on fighting longer if their armies had not been weakened by the influenza. The causes of their defeat are, of course, many and complex. Even so, it seems to me that the knowledge we now have of the Spanish Flu in 1918–19 suggests that it must be included in any assessment to a greater extent than most historians have done until now.

Even after the conclusion of peace on 11 November 1918, the influenza virus may have played a final historical role. The Treaty of Versailles of summer 1919 is generally acknowledged as having been excessively hard on Germany. This created a great deal of bitterness in Germany and a lust for revenge that, in the opinion of many historians, may well have contributed to the Second World War. President Woodrow Wilson of the USA was initially interested in getting as just a settlement as possible, while others, particularly Georges Clemenceau, the French prime minister (known as 'The Tiger' by his fellow countrymen), was first and foremost motivated by revenge and the imposition of merciless conditions on Germany. In the middle of negotiations, President Wilson went down with Spanish Flu, a condition worsened by a stroke. The sick president changed his attitude towards the peace process, allowing 'The Tiger' and those of like opinion to more or less have their way. Did the Spanish Flu, in this sense, perhaps sow the seeds for the Second World War?[392]

Spanish Flu was not the last pandemic

Gradually this H1N1 virus lost its terrifying characteristics and became a more common influenza virus that caused ordinary seasonal influenza. In 1957, however, a new pandemic occurred. This time it was caused by an H2N2 virus. The H1N1 virus apparently disappeared at this point, for it would appear that a new pandemic virus normally ousts already existing influenza viruses.[393] In 1977, however, the former H1N1 from the Spanish Flu pandemic reappeared, this time not only as the cause of ordinary seasonal influenza, without anyone being completely able to understand why. Some have suggested that it may be the result of a laboratory mishap that caused the virus to leak out into the population.

The new pandemic of 1957 is often referred to as Asian Flu, because it is thought that it originated in the Yunnan province of China. The H2N2 virus that was the cause was apparently the result of a reassortment of genes, probably among pigs. The virus that arose via this 'exchange deal' of genes between a bird virus and a human virus had H and N antigens from birds and other antigens from humans that made it highly infectious.

In the course of six months, Asian Flu had spread to most of the world. This was mainly via shipping traffic, so that ports were hit before the disease spread further inland. The virus came overland to Scandinavia via Russia, however. A special form of spreading took place when participants from various countries hit by the disease attended an international convention in Iowa in the USA. Two hundred participants were infected and took the virus home with them after the convention, resulting in further dissemination.

The Asian Flu virus was not as virulent as that of Spanish Flu, but still resulted in about a million deaths, particularly among the very young and very old, as well as pregnant women. A second wave came in 1958. Then the pandemic died out. Subsequently the H2N2 virus has only caused ordinary seasonal influenza.[394]

A new influenza pandemic came in 1968. This one was given the name Hong Kong Flu because it also started in China and quickly hit Hong Kong, which in the month of July alone had 500,000 cases. This new virus was an H3N2 virus. Here too it is thought it was the result of reassortment, possibly in pigs. The pandemic quickly spread to the rest of the world. It also came in two waves: the first wave in 1968 caused only moderate mortality in Europe, which was hit somewhat harder by the second wave in 1969. It is estimated that the global death figure was between 1 and 3 million. The 'old' H2N2 virus that had ruled the roost after Asian Flu was now replaced by the H3N2 virus, which also gradually ended up causing seasonal influenza.[395]

Both these two recent pandemics, then, were considerably milder than Spanish Flu and did not have the same 'abnormal' characteristics with young adults being the most vulnerable victims or dramatic pathological pictures with cytokine storms. The virus variants in both these pandemics had elements of the genes of Spanish Flu. That may explain why the number of influenza cases among elderly people was somewhat lower than expected, since this group probably had a certain immunity from contact with Spanish Flu in their youth.

The most recent pandemic, normally called Swine Flu, came in 2009. It was due to an H1N1 virus from pigs, where the virus was a result of several rounds of reassortment, with an exchange of genes between several virus variants, including a human virus. It proved capable of infecting from person to person. It first appeared in Mexico, where it resulted in serious illness. As the disease spread over most of the globe, the infection began to behave roughly as ordinary seasonal influenza.[396]

A ticking time bomb

It is said about heavyweight boxing world champions who have lost their title that they never come back. This, unfortunately, does not apply to the pandemic influenza viruses. Over the years *Homo sapiens* has seen repeated comebacks from the influenza virus, often with disastrous consequences. Formerly it was thought that there was a certain regularity about this, but that does not seem to prove true. It is fairly certain, though, that the world will face a new pandemic caused by the virus. It is difficult for us to forecast when this will take place. This is mainly due to the fact that our knowledge of the underlying mechanisms is still deficient.

Constant readiness to discover the first signs of an incipient pandemic with the influenza virus is necessary, so that vital measures can be implemented in time to combat new pandemics. Alfred Crosby called his book about Spanish Flu *America's Forgotten Pandemic*, because he felt that to a great extent we had forgotten this catastrophe.[397] The world cannot allow itself such a lapse of memory, for the consequences of new influenza pandemics in the future may be just as serious as they were in the past.

Poliomyelitis: A Feared Cause of Paralysis

Poliomyelitis, or polio as the disease is often abbreviated, is due to a virus that, in its most malignant form, attacks the nerve cells in the spinal cord that control our muscles. The destruction of these cells leads to paralysis. As a cause of major epidemics, the polio virus is a newcomer on the scene among the many microbes that have afflicted *Homo sapiens* down through the ages. We have only seen polio epidemics for just over a century. This closely corresponds to the way in which the spread of infection occurs.

From intestines to nerve cells

The polio virus normally invades the body via the mouth and initially infects cells in the plentiful lymph tissue in the mucous membrane of the intestines. The virus then spreads through the blood to lymph tissue in other parts of the body. In the vast majority of cases, the immune system deals with the infection without the patient having had any signs of the disease. But in some patients (less than 10 per cent) the virus spreads via the blood and the patient experiences a state of mild illness with a couple of days of high temperatures, perhaps also headaches, nausea and stomach pains – and then it is all over. In 1 or 2 per cent of patients, however, there are signs of cerebrospinal meningitis, with high fever, headaches, stiffness of the neck and back pains. This normally passes of its own accord and in the great majority of cases of infection with the polio virus there are no serious problems.[398]

In a small fraction of patients infected by the polio virus (perhaps 0.1 to 1 per cent), who have had a fever and displayed symptoms of the disease, paralysis takes place in various groups of muscles. There is often a short break after the first signs of the disease, during which the fever

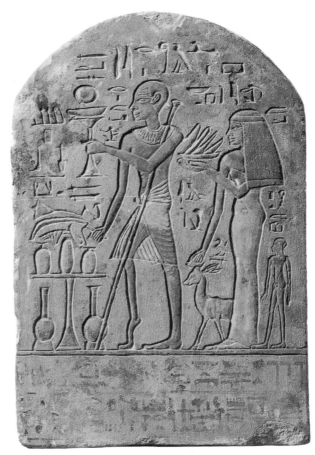

The Egyptian priest Ruma from *c.* 1500 BC (seen here on a stone tablet in the Ny Carlsberg Glyptotek in Copenhagen) has a crippled foot and uses a stick. This has been viewed as a sign of poliomyelitis.

falls, before rising once again with the beginning of paralysis, so that the temperature curve is biphasic, with two humps: a 'camel curve'. This is because the polio virus has now penetrated the central nervous system, normally the spinal cord, and has infected nerve cells that control the muscles, resulting in paralysis. The nerve cells sit in the grey matter in the spinal cord, and this is why the disease is called poliomyelitis, which is derived from the Greek word *polios*, which means grey, and *myelos*, which means marrow.

All combinations of affected muscles and all degrees of paralysis can be observed. Paralysis is often more serious if the patient has engaged in strenuous physical activity during the first days of the disease. The infection becomes life-threatening if the respiratory muscles are affected. With the early epidemics, when the only intensive-care medicine available was less advanced than today, the mortality rate in such cases was at least 10 per cent. Most of the patients who survived had permanent weakness in the affected muscles. Even in cases where the paralysis had completely retreated, patients could later develop a new weakness in the muscles that had originally been affected, and sometimes even in muscles that had apparently never been attacked. This is known as post-polio syndrome.[399]

As mentioned, the polio virus infects the mucous membranes of the intestines and is then excreted. It is virus from excrement that is the source of new infection, either via direct personal contact or indirectly via objects. This is an example of faecal-oral infection. Sanitary conditions and hygiene in the environment naturally play an important role here, and changes within this area probably explain the dramatic appearance of the polio virus as a cause of epidemics over the past hundred years.[400]

Was the pharaoh a sufferer?

Let us return to the early history of *Homo sapiens* as hunters and gatherers. Since it is hardly likely that acute infectious diseases of this kind affected such small groups of people where the virus would be unable to sustain itself, polio, at the earliest, must have come after the first epidemiological transition, when the size of the population had become large enough.[401]

We do not have descriptions of polio in ancient chronicles. Even so, it is often claimed that the ancient Egyptians were affected by the disease. The basis for such claims is representations of alleged polio sufferers on Egyptian wall paintings, as well as certain mummy finds. Reference has in particular been made to a stone slab or stele from about 1500 BC in the Ny Carlsberg Glyptotek in Copenhagen, which portrays the priest Ruma with one leg shorter than the other and walking with the aid of a stick. The mummy of the pharaoh Siptah from about 1200 BC shows a clearly deformed foot, which has been interpreted as a result of polio; this mummy was among those processed through the streets of Cairo in April 2021 in the 'Pharaoh's Golden Parade' before being rehoused in the National Museum of Egyptian Civilization. Viewed objectively, neither of these examples can be taken as final proof that polio existed in ancient Egypt. There are many possible causes for such deformities, ones that have been common throughout history.[402]

In 1789 the English doctor Michael Underwood gave an extremely precise description of the first individual cases of what was probably polio. It is the German doctor Jacob Heine, however, who has been given the honour of having painstakingly described a large number of patients with polio and publishing his results in 1840. The Scottish doctor Charles Bell described the first real polio epidemic, which struck Napoleon's final place of exile, St Helena. Bell was so well known for his keen powers of observation that he was allegedly the model for Arthur Conan Doyle's famous fictional detective Sherlock Holmes.[403]

Internationally speaking, however, it is particularly the Swedish doctors Oskar Medin and his pupil Ivar Wickman who have become known for having described polio as an acute infectious disease that occurs in epidemics. They also described the clear seasonal variation with polio epidemics in early autumn. Wickman in particular realized that milder cases of the disease without paralysis were also part of the epidemics, which he believed were due to a microbe that could be transmitted via direct contact. Polio is sometimes described as Heine-Medin's disease in order to pay tribute to two of the pioneers within the field. Wickman made a considerable contribution by identifying important characteristics of polio infection, but this has perhaps been slightly overshadowed by laboratory researchers within this field.[404]

In 1908 the Austrian doctors Karl Landsteiner and Erwin Popper published their discovery of the polio virus after they caused polio in apes by injecting them with spinal cord tissue from a polio patient.[405] Landsteiner was a versatile researcher and was granted the Nobel Prize in 1930 for his work on systems of blood groups.

The discovery of the virus was an important breakthrough that was rapidly picked up by other researchers, including a dynamic Swedish group under the leadership of Carl Kling. This group demonstrated the importance of intestinal infection by the polio virus, which makes further infection possible after it has been excreted.[406]

With all these epoch-making discoveries shedding new light on polio, everything ought to have been favourable for the development of a vaccine, inspired by the results of smallpox and rabies vaccines. Nevertheless, several decades were to pass before the first effective polio vaccine was introduced, in 1955, and in the intervening years major polio epidemics raged in Western countries. What were the reasons for this delay, which led to death or invalidity for tens of thousands of patients? An important reason was probably that there was little contact between the researchers in laboratories who carried out experiments with animals and clinical researchers who were working with patients. American researchers in particular, led by the powerful head of the Rockefeller Institute, Simon Flexner, mainly worked on apes, where the polio virus principally attacks the mucous membranes of the air passages and not those of the intestines, which in human patients is a central characteristic of the infection. Flexner believed that the virus from the mucous membrane of the nose directly infected the nervous system.[407]

Flexner and his colleagues ignored the findings of the Swedish researchers, who had clearly demonstrated the importance of the intestinal infection through studies of patients. Was this perhaps due to a certain element of major-power arrogance regarding the research contribution of a small country? Or maybe the well-known phenomenon in science that leading researchers are not always open to other people's theories? This unfortunate chapter in polio research also shows what can happen if powerful members of the research community focus attention exclusively on their own particular fields of research for a long time.

These experiences with the delayed development of the polio vaccine illustrate how important so-called translation research, based on close contact between clinic and laboratory, is in medicine. It is vital to build bridges over the gap that so easily opens up between laboratory research and clinical, patient-orientated research.

The polio epidemics: a result of improved hygiene?

Unlike the many other microbes we have discussed as causes of pandemics and major epidemics, the polio virus does not appear as a cause of an epidemic until the end of the nineteenth century, and it caused increasing problems up until the mid-twentieth century. What is the reason for this striking pattern of development? The polio virus as a source of infection in humans was hardly new and has quite possibly existed for thousands of years, so why did the first major epidemics occur in the nineteenth century in Scandinavia (in both Norway and Sweden) and a short time afterwards in the USA?

The key to understanding the onward march of polio epidemics probably lies in how the virus infected and the reaction to the virus of our immune system.[408] The virus is transmitted via faecal-oral infection. It is excreted from the bodies of infected people and spreads either by direct or indirect personal contact, infecting the mucous membrane of the intestines and possibly spreading further through the nervous system via the blood. In societies with bad hygiene and sanitary conditions, practically everyone is exposed to infection at a very early age. Once infection by the polio virus has been overcome an individual is granted lifelong immunity, which is mainly mediated by immune globulin molecules acting as antibodies. In the last stages of a pregnancy these antibodies are transmitted from mother to child, who therefore, after birth, has a 'stock' of protective antibodies that last the first six months of its life. When the baby is exposed to the polio virus, this normally does not lead to illness and grants the child lifelong immunity. The first person to realize this was probably Ivar Wickman in Sweden.[409]

The considerable improvement in hygienic and sanitary conditions that took place in Western countries from the late nineteenth century onwards was of great importance when it came to combatting many infectious diseases. It also, however, led to children's first contact with the polio virus being delayed until after they had lost the protective antibodies from their mother. This resulted in an increase in poliomyelitis, which came to be called 'child paralysis'. As hygienic conditions continued to improve during the twentieth century, cases of polio were delayed to higher age groups, even though children and young adults still dominated. This created the basis for polio epidemics, since a considerable proportion of the population had not become immune via contact with the virus during their childhood, thus making epidemic dissemination of the polio virus possible.[410]

The crucial importance of sanitary conditions for the development of polio epidemics has been obvious in a number of developing countries, where until recently polio infection has followed the same non-epidemic pattern we once had in Western countries. In an investigation of the occurrence of polio in Casablanca in Morocco around 1950, the indigenous population was compared with that of immigrant Europeans. One then found, as expected, that the number of cases with polio paralysis was far higher among the Europeans and took place at a higher age, since the Europeans had not been infected during childhood. Epidemics, however, have also occurred in the developing countries, particularly in more remote areas, where contact with the polio virus has not been as pervasive as elsewhere.

In the northern hemisphere, polio epidemics were extremely seasonal, with activity mainly during the months of August and September and almost no cases during the winter. The climatic factor that is crucial for this is not the temperature but air humidity. The polio virus stops being active after only a few minutes of relative humidity less than 40 per cent.

The regularly recurring polio epidemics, naturally enough, gave rise to considerable fear in the populations of Western countries. Every autumn there were many children who could not start school in the autumn because of polio infection. Even though the virus had been detected, the manner of infection was still disputed and this naturally contributed to unrest in the population. In medical circles, the possibility of transmission via insects was a great preoccupation, inspired by experiences gleaned from malaria and yellow fever. When Carl Kling and his colleagues presented their important findings about intestinal infection with the polio virus at a convention in the USA in 1911, it gave rise to little interest, while the claim by two Harvard professors that infection was spread by insects gained loud applause. In a few places, including the USA, people suspected that special low-status groups, such as immigrants, were particularly responsible for the epidemics because of their bad hygiene.[411]

Then came a breakthrough in 1955 with the presentation of Jonas E. Salk's vaccine, which led to a dramatic fall in the number of polio cases in all countries that began to use it. Church bells were rung throughout the USA to celebrate the publication of the vaccine results on 12 April. History's most famous polio victim, the American president Franklin D. Roosevelt, who was struck down in 1921 and had led the USA into the Second World War from his wheelchair, had strongly supported the massive efforts underlying the development of the vaccine.

Today it is a realistic hope that targeted work based on vaccination will enable the eradication of the polio virus from the world, so that it will follow the smallpox virus into the ranks of the microbial dinosaurs.[412] Perhaps one day we will be able to ring the church bells again to celebrate that the polio virus is no more.

FIVE

Mysterious Epidemics in History

Aconsiderable challenge when studying the epidemics of the past is that we often have highly incomplete information about them. The definitions of an illness can be inadequate and imprecise, and the course of the epidemic and its behaviour are not always well described. This naturally makes it difficult, if not impossible, to identify the microbe involved.[1]

There are also other reasons why we are not always able to interpret earlier epidemics. We cannot exclude the possibility that they were caused by unknown microbes that have since disappeared. Another possibility is that they may have involved microbes that still exist, but which through mutations have altered their characteristics when it comes to being pathogenic or infectious. Earlier epidemics with such microbes can therefore have a different appearance from those we see today.

In this historical detective work, modern molecular biology has proved extremely useful. New methods have enabled us to detect microbes in human remains from earlier epidemics of such diseases as tuberculosis and plague.

Nevertheless, it is frustrating that we now know of many former epidemics that both created major problems at the time and had considerable historical consequences without being able unequivocally to determine what kind of microbe caused them. Let us take a look at some of them.

The Athenian Plague

Classical Athens has occupied a key position in the cultural history of Europe. That has undoubtedly contributed to the fact that the so-called Athenian plague is the most famous of the mysterious epidemics of the past. A great many historians have written about the epidemic and have rarely agreed about the cause, which has still to be clarified.

In 431 BC Athens was at the height of its power. With the prestige gained after the victories over the invading Persian forces at Marathon in 490 BC and Salamis in 480 BC, Athens had become the leader of the so-called Delian or Attic League, of which a number of Greek city states were members. Sparta, the other major power in Greece, regarded Athens as a threat that had to be faced. This led to the outbreak of the Peloponnesian War in 431 BC. The war between the Delian League, under the leadership of Athens, and Sparta, which had a number of allies, lasted right up until 404 BC.

Athens and the city's port at Piraeus were both surrounded by walls and joined by a pair of 'long walls' that stretched 9 kilometres between them. The decision of the Athenian leader, Pericles, to bring his forces within the walls, along with much of the rural population of Attica, led to serious overpopulation and bad housing conditions in Athens, which was under repeated sieges during the hostilities. Pericles was unwilling to fight the war on land and allowed the Spartans to ravage the rural areas around Athens. He had decided on waging a war of attrition against Sparta because the Athenians had a strong fleet that constantly attacked the Spartan rural areas and ensured supplies to Athens via Piraeus.[2]

Then, however, something unexpected happened. In 430 BC Athens was hit by an epidemic, with terrible consequences for the population. We have a meticulously written account of this epidemic from the historian and retired general Thucydides, whose work about the Peloponnesian War also deals with the epidemic in great detail. He had first-hand knowledge of it, since he himself went down with the plague, but survived. Thucydides was not a physician, but was clearly well orientated in contemporary medicine. It is almost exclusively his description on which the continuing discussion of the epidemic has been based for the last 2,500 years.[3]

Thucydides writes that the epidemic originated in Ethiopia and spread to Egypt, Libya and the Middle East before arriving in the port of Piraeus and quickly moving on to Athens. It broke out in May 430 BC and lasted for four years, but came in several waves.

Infection started suddenly with a violent headache and red and inflamed eyes, tongue and throat. The patient became hoarse and started sneezing, followed by a hacking cough. Then came violent attacks of vomiting and cramps. Patients were plagued by an enormous thirst and an inner heat that led many to throw off their clothes and fling themselves into cold water. Many victims developed a rash that consisted of what some later historians have interpreted as being blisters and sores. The actual appearance of this rash is, however, uncertain, since it is unclear what Thucydides actually meant by the term he used for these special blisters, *phlyctainai*. This uncertainty is an important point in discussing the cause of the epidemic, since several microbes can cause characteristic skin changes.[4]

Many patients died after seven to nine days. Those who survived that far were often afflicted by violent diarrhoea, from which many more died. Those still alive often contracted gangrene in their fingers, toes and genital organs, while some went blind and lost their memory.

The disease picture was certainly dramatic and the spread of the epidemic extremely rapid. All sectors of the population were hit, but in particular those living in the overpopulated areas of the city, where housing conditions were worst. Both Thucydides and people in general were clearly convinced that it was a contagious disease. Physicians and those nursing the sick were especially badly hit. Entire families were wiped out. It was not possible to bury the numerous corpses as usual, and they often lay where they had died or were thrown onto other people's funeral pyres.

It is estimated that about 25 per cent of the 300,000–400,000 people behind the walls of Athens died during the epidemic.[5] Pericles lost his two sons and died himself in autumn 429 BC, possibly of the disease, although the course of his illness took longer than was usual.

In addition to his thorough description of the disease, Thucydides also made an important observation that those who survived an attack during the epidemic gained lasting immunity, at any rate for the four years that the epidemic lasted.[6]

Everyone believed that this disease was new in the Greek world. The physicians had no experience of it and were unable to do anything for the patients. It is said that Athens asked Hippocrates himself for help, but that he gave up and fled the city.

What was the cause of this epidemic, the deadliest we know of from ancient Greece? Over the past century, at least thirty different microbes have been mentioned as an explanation for the Athenian plague.[7] The individual candidates have been thoroughly discussed in the light of practically every word in Thucydides' description. My impression is that people tend to emphasize what suits their theory best, while suppressing and explaining away anything that does not suit their own explanation. Writers use the same method as Procrustes, the murderous innkeeper in Greek mythology who had only one bed to offer his guests: he either chopped off part of their legs if they were too tall or stretched them by force if they were too short. Let us take a look at some of the proposed causes of the epidemic.

Classic plague caused by *Yersinia pestis* has had its supporters, but is not particularly likely. The first known plague epidemic was the Plague of Justinian in the mid-sixth century AD. The plague bacterium was definitely older than this, but the pathological picture described by Thucydides does not really fit the plague. It is, for example, unlikely that he would have failed to describe the characteristic swellings (buboes) if the epidemic had been the real plague. When the argument is raised that the black rat hardly existed in Athens at that time, this is questionable, since recent research suggests that mechanisms of infection were possible beyond the 'classic' ones with rats and fleas. But it is highly doubtful that the plague caused the epidemic that afflicted Athens.

Smallpox has had, and still has, some supporters. When the virus attacks a virgin population without immunity, mortality is extremely high. The virus spreads rapidly via droplets, contact and airborne transmission, which is something that tallies with the Athenian Plague, as do the initial symptoms of a violent headache and inflamed eyes and throat. Many believe that the blisters in the skin (*phlyctainai*) and other parts of Thucydides' description of the rash can also apply to smallpox, but others disagree entirely. Another argument is that there are no grounds for the claim that this virus existed in ancient Greece, even though it was probably the cause of illness in other parts of the world. It is also striking that Thucydides does not mention the formation of scars, which are extremely common in smallpox.

Typhus caused by the *Rickettsia prowazekii* bacterium has also convinced supporters. This infection commonly arises during times of war, when large numbers of people are often crowded together under awful sanitary conditions. This was very much the case within the walls of Athens, and lice were common in Greece.

Many of the symptoms were compatible with typhus, including the initial fever, inflamed eyes and respiratory difficulties. A fuddled mental state is common. Vomiting and diarrhoea also occur. The gangrene complications also fit with the loss of fingers and toes. The problem, however, is that typhus hardly existed in ancient Greece, only appearing in Europe in the sixteenth century. Nor does transmission take place as rapidly as was seen in Athens, since it is dependent on transmission by bacteria-infected lice.

Measles is also one of the most discussed suggestions. Many examples in history have shown that mortality is extremely high if the virus affects a virgin population without any immunity. Airborne infection

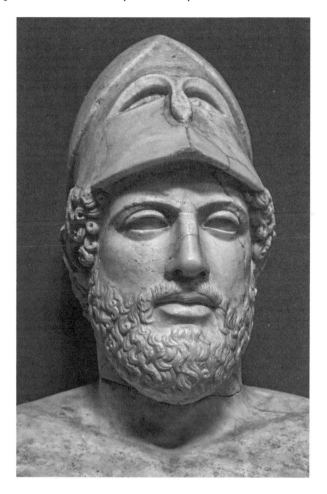

Pericles was the leading statesman in Athens during its heyday in the 5th century BC. He died in 429 BC, possibly of the Athenian Plague during the Peloponnesian War.

agrees well with the rapid spread of the epidemic, but many of the symptoms in Athens are hardly compatible with measles.

A considerable number of other suggestions have been made over the years to try and explain what caused the tragedy in Athens, including bacteria such as staphylococci, streptococci and the bacterium that causes anthrax. Some viruses that, as far as we know, only emerged in our own time have been advanced, using what I consider to be quite weak arguments. One historian has even suggested that the epidemic had nothing to do with infection at all, but rather was the consequence of ergotism due to poisoning with a substance from a fungus that can grow on corn.

One of the bacteria that has been put forward, *Salmonella typhi*, which causes the serious intestinal infection typhoid fever, recently gained impetus in the discussion of the epidemic in Athens after Greek researchers made use of new molecular-biological methods in examining remains of corpses from a mass grave outside Athens from the time of the epidemic.[8] In three of the corpses they found DNA from *Salmonella typhi*, and on the basis of this announced that they now had the correct answer. This has not been generally accepted, partly because of technical objections to the methods used, and partly because the number of corpses examined is so low.[9] This naturally does not mean that the Athenians under siege could not have been infected with typhoid bacteria, but it has scarcely been proven the main cause of the epidemic.

Even though new investigations using molecular-biological methods will probably be carried out, it is not certain that we will ever arrive at a definitive diagnosis of the Athenian Plague. We cannot exclude the possibility that it was due to several dissimilar microbes that flourished under the terrible conditions existing in Athens while under siege. It is also possible that the microbe responsible has disappeared, or that it has completely changed its characteristics during the thousands of years that have passed since the Peloponnesian War.

The Antonine Plague: Apollo's Revenge

A few historical accounts suggest that Rome was hit by an epidemic at the same time as Athens. We do not know if the same microbe was involved. Whether this was the case or not, the Roman empire was savaged by large epidemics over the centuries, two of which deserve a place on the list of mysterious epidemics with unclear causes.

The first of these is the so-called Antonine Plague, which raged for several years from AD 165 at a time when the Roman empire had reached the apex of its power. The empire stretched from the Euphrates and Tigris rivers in present-day Iraq to Scotland and from the Sahara to the North Sea. The empire was governed jointly by Marcus Aurelius, a philosopher as well as emperor, and Lucius Verus, the adopted son of their predecessor, Antoninus Pius. Verus' death in 169 left Marcus Aurelius as sole ruler.

The English historian Edward Gibbon called this period the happiest age of mankind. Internally, the empire was peaceful and prosperous, but its borders had to be constantly defended against attack, including from the Parthian empire in present-day Iran.[10]

In AD 165 the Roman army had just completed a successful campaign against the Parthians and returned home with considerable booty. The Roman legions also had with them a microbe that was to cause one of the most extensive epidemics of antiquity.[11] It was named the Antonine Plague after the emperor's full name, Marcus Aurelius Antoninus. As we shall see, it was not a plague in the precise sense of one caused by *Yersinia pestis*. The Antonine Plague is often overlooked when discussing Roman history, despite the fact that for a number of years it profoundly influenced the Roman empire and probably had lasting consequences.

The prevailing view among the Romans was that the epidemic started in AD 165 when the city of Seleucia, close to present-day Baghdad, was conquered and plundered by the Romans. It was said that the soldiers also looted the temple of the god Apollo. When they opened an old grave, however, allegedly plague-causing vapours emanated from it. In another version, this occurred when opening a gold casket in the temple. Since Apollo was linked to plague, in addition to his other characteristics, the religious Romans believed that the ghastly plague that broke out was the god's revenge for the Roman army having defiled his temple. Although Seleucia was originally regarded as the place of origin for the epidemic, this is not necessarily correct: some have suggested that it came from the area around the Red Sea, possibly Arabia.[12]

Irrespective of its origin, the epidemic quickly spread to large parts of the Roman empire, including the Middle East, North Africa and the

Roman part of Europe, including Britain. The lines of communication in the well-organized empire were ideal for the spread of infection via excellent roads and trade by sea. It is possible that we are looking at the first known pandemic here, for even distant China was hit by an epidemic at the same time, which could well have had the same cause. The Silk Road, which had long since been established as an important trading route between Asia and Europe, might have played a role in the spread of the disease.

How did the Antonine Plague develop? Unfortunately we know a lot less about this than the Athenian Plague because we do not have a source with the same degree of precision and quality as Thucydides' classic account. There are, however, some scattered notes made by the most famous physician of the Roman empire, Galen, who was right in the middle of the epidemic and treated a great many patients. For that reason, the epidemic is occasionally referred to as Galen's Plague.[13]

According to Galen, the illness started with acute fever, gradually followed by coughing and hoarseness. The most characteristic feature he describes is a widespread rash with pus-filled blisters, often also full of blood, which after a few days started to dry out and become scaly. The patient often excreted a black stool, probably a sign of bleeding in the intestines. Sometimes the patients coughed blood. Death normally came after nine or ten days, but some patients regained their health.

Historians have eagerly pored over Galen's somewhat ambiguous description of the disease. The majority have concluded that it must have been smallpox, and more precisely the form characterized by widespread bleeding, which also affected the skin. Mortality is extremely high in this form of the disease. Galen himself believed that it must have been the same disease as the Athenian Plague.[14]

Although many people have interpreted the Antonine Plague as a smallpox epidemic, I find this theory problematic for several reasons. As mentioned earlier, it is uncertain when the smallpox virus established itself in Europe. It may have taken place in the early Middle Ages, but does not seem to have caused any major problems before the Islamic armies brought the virus to Europe in the seventh and eighth centuries. If the Antonine Plague really was smallpox, one would expect the virus to have gained a foothold in Europe and caused regular epidemics long before the seventh century.

The Antonine Plague is usually said to have lasted from AD 165 to 180. Some believe that a new epidemic in 189 was a continuation of the main epidemic, but this is uncertain.[15]

Historians have arrived at widely differing figures with regard to the mortality of this epidemic: it has been estimated that between 2 and 50 per cent of the population died.[16] Figures varied considerably between the various parts of the Roman empire. The major cities, Rome in particular, were hard hit, and the same applied to the Roman army. Taken as a whole, the overall death rate was probably around 10 per cent, indicating that 7–8 million people died out of a total population in the empire of 75 million. This must have made a considerable impact on society.

Since it was commonly held that the epidemic was an act of revenge on the part of Apollo, attempts were made throughout the empire to appease the god through sacrifices and other religious rituals. In particular, his oracles were consulted, but the answers received about measures to be taken against the epidemic were clearly of no particular help except to sculptors, since they often included a suggestion to raise a statue of the god.[17]

The disease was not necessarily thought of as being contagious: even Galen took no precautions when examining patients. There are signs, nonetheless, that people felt there was a risk of person-to-person infection. An amulet against the plague found in London bears an inscription warning against kissing, which was a usual form of greeting at the time.[18] Particularly interesting is the account of Marcus Aurelius' deathbed in AD 180. He died of the plague in Vindobona (now Vienna), where he had spent his final years helping to defend the empire against invading Germanic tribes.[19] The emperor forbade his son and successor, Commodus, from entering the sickroom, fearing that he might contract the disease. With this well-meant act, paradoxically, the noble philosopher-emperor did a disservice to his subjects: the eleven years of Commodus' rule were a reign of terror, marked by a series of executions linked to real or imagined conspiracies against the emperor, who showed increasing signs of paranoia and megalomania. He insisted that the city of Rome be renamed Commodiana, fought as a gladiator in the arena and referred to himself as the demi-god Hercules. He was murdered at the age of 31 in AD 191.

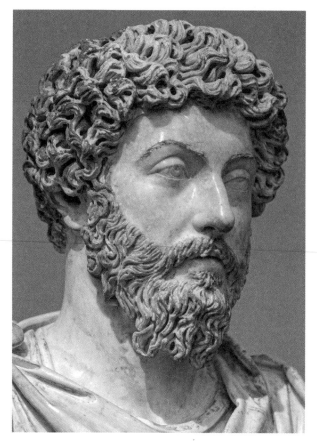

Marcus Aurelius Antoninus – the philosopher on the imperial throne – was Roman emperor from AD 161 until 180. He died during the epidemic which was named after him: the Antonine Plague.

All in all, there can be no doubt that the Antonine Plague put a great strain on the Roman empire, but there is still much uncertainty about its extent. This also applies to the possible after-effects it had on Roman society, about which historians still disagree.[20]

The Plague of Cyprian: The Forgotten Epidemic

For some reason or other, historians, maybe unconsciously, seem unwilling to include the major epidemics in their analyses of historical events. The American historian William McNeill brought about a change in this in the 1970s with his book *Plagues and Peoples*, but the barrier has undoubtedly continued to exist. A convincing example is the epidemic that ravaged the Roman empire in AD 249–70, which has been given the name 'The Plague of Cyprian'. For some reason this plague is practically never mentioned in accounts of the history of the Roman empire.

The Plague of Cyprian descended on the empire at a time of wars and unrest. Enemies were penetrating several of its borders and there was also internal unrest. In AD 259 something unheard of happened: a Roman emperor was taken prisoner by the enemy. Emperor Valerian, who came to the throne in 253, was defeated by the Parthians and had to spend the rest of his life in captivity. An early Christian writer, Lactantius, wishing to put Valerian in the worst possible light after his persecution of the Christians, claimed that Valerian's body was stuffed and exhibited in a temple. The fate of the emperor was a huge humiliation for Rome, adding to the immense strain on the empire that the Plague of Cyprian caused during this period of crisis.[21]

The epidemic has been named after Cyprian, bishop of Carthage in North Africa, who was one of the most prominent Fathers of the early Church. He wrote the most complete account of the epidemic in his work *De mortalitate* (On Mortality). The common view was that the epidemic had started south of Egypt in Ethiopia, from where it spread northwards and westwards. All the countries round the Mediterranean were affected within a couple of years, and the epidemic probably also spread elsewhere in the empire. Town and country, young and old – all were under attack.[22]

Even though Cyprian lacks the precision of Thucydides or Galen's vast knowledge of medicine, he provides us with a graphic description of the symptoms of the disease, which must have been highly dramatic. It began with acute fever and severe, sometimes bloody, vomiting and diarrhoea, with bleeding from the eyes. The patients' legs often developed inflammation and became paralysed, or 'cut off', as Cyprian writes. Some people went blind or lost their hearing.

The mortality rate was extremely high: in Athens 5,000 people died on one day, according to a contemporary historian. We lack reliable mortality figures for the entire empire, but they must have been considerable. Cyprian suggests that the epidemic could be interpreted as a sign of the end of the world. Two emperors, Hostilian and Claudius II, probably died of the disease.

Among non-Christians, this disaster – as with former epidemics – was viewed as having supernatural, divine causes. There are also indications, however, that many thought some form of person-to-person transmission was involved. A contemporary historian wrote that the disease could be transmitted via clothing and even by exchanging

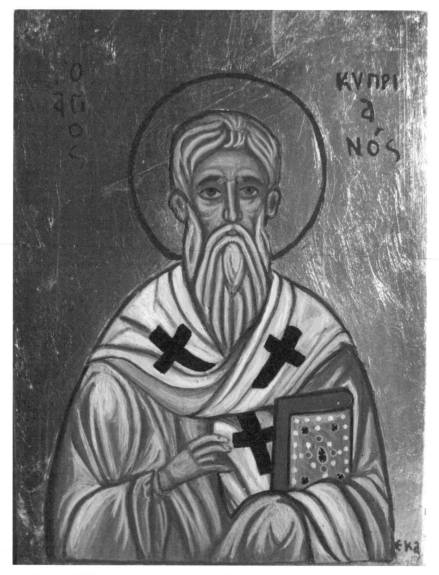

Cyprian was bishop in Carthage in North Africa during the extensive epidemic ravaging the Roman Empire in AD 249–70 – the Plague of Cyprian, named after him.

glances.[23] In 2014 Italian archaeologists in Luxor in Egypt discovered a mass grave with bodies that had been partially doused in bleach and burned, probably to prevent contagion.[24]

The cause of the epidemic, which perhaps deserves the term 'pandemic', is still unclear. Many microbes have been proposed, including the smallpox virus. This diagnosis is somewhat improbable, for it is striking that Cyprian and the few other sources we have do not mention anything about a rash and subsequent scars, which are such conspicuous signs of smallpox. An influenza epidemic similar to Spanish Flu in the twentieth century has also been suggested. This, too, is unlikely since we have no information about life-threatening lung failure, which was so characteristic of Spanish Flu.

An American historian has recently suggested that the cause of the epidemic may have been the Ebola virus.[25] Many of the symptoms described by Cyprian could possibly fit a fever with much bleeding and high mortality, which this particular virus causes. Even so, I find it highly unlikely that this virus could strike Europe in such a widespread fashion as early as the third century AD, since until now we have only seen outbreaks in the second half of the twentieth century in equatorial Africa, where the animal reservoir is probably located. The Ebola virus has never spread to other parts of the world, except in isolated cases via air travel. We probably have to accept that the cause of the epidemic is unknown and may well remain so. The mass grave in Luxor can unfortunately not be used for molecular-biological detective work, since genetic material from microbes is not likely to have been preserved in the remains of the corpses.

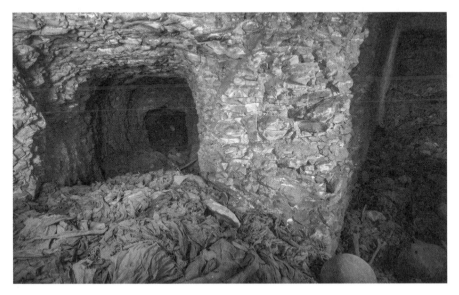

In 2014 Italian archaeologists outside Luxor found remains of a large number of victims of the Plague of Cyprian. The corpses had clearly been burned in haste and without religious ceremonies, after which they had been doused with bleach.

During the Plague of Cyprian, Christianity was presumably consolidating its position in the Roman empire.[26] With their belief in eternal life, the Christians feared death from the plague less than the rest of the population. Many Christians made great efforts to take care of the sick, something that must have made quite an impression. Despite this, Christians were sometimes made scapegoats for the horrendous epidemic and Cyprian himself died a martyr, beheaded in AD 258.

English Sweating Sickness

From the Plague of Cyprian we jump more than 1,000 years forwards to the next great challenge for historians of epidemics: English sweating sickness. The microbe responsible remains a mystery to this day.

This epidemic took place during a period of extreme unrest in British history.[27] The Wars of the Roses, a civil war between two royal families which had ravaged England for thirty years, ended with the Battle of Bosworth on 29 August 1485, where Richard III died after having offered his kingdom for a horse, at least according to Shakespeare's play about the hunchbacked king. The victor, Henry Tudor, who was declared Henry VII, entered London a few days later. In his retinue there was possibly an invisible escort, the microbe that gave rise to the epidemic disease that was given the name 'English sweating sickness', known in Latin as *Sudor anglicus*. It broke out in London on 19 September and led to thousands of deaths, including two Lord Mayors. It did not only attack London, however: rural communities were hit even harder than towns – with the exception of the capital.[28]

The epidemic died down in the course of 1485, but it returned to England on four occasions: in 1508, 1517, 1528 and 1551. Ireland and Scotland were spared. These epidemics were limited to England, except in 1528, when the disease also spread to Germany and then eastwards to Poland and Russia (whereas France and Italy were spared). On that occasion the epidemic also spread to Scandinavia, where the number of deaths in southern Norway was allegedly so great that farmers had to import labour from the Faroe Islands. That epidemic died down in 1530.

This disease was dramatic. It began with acute headaches, chills, high temperatures and muscular pains, quickly progressing to stomach pains, vomiting, increasing headaches and often mental confusion. During the first hours the patient began to produce profuse, evil-smelling sweat – hence the name of the disease. It is impossible to determine the case fatality rate accurately, but it may have been between 30 and 50 per cent. Death very often took place within 24 hours. Those who survived were utterly exhausted for a long time afterwards.[29]

The sheer rapidity of the course of the disease naturally made a strong impression. Someone wrote at the time that 'people were healthy at lunchtime and dead by dinnertime.' The physician Thomas Forestier, who described the epidemic, wrote, 'We saw two priests standing chatting and saw both of them suddenly die,' and also that, 'Another young man walking down the street suddenly fell down.' Another tells of seven Londoners who 'ate dinner together in the evening, and by dawn cock-crow five of them were dead'.

The epidemic had a number of striking characteristics.[30] It tended to select men between the ages of twenty and forty and to a great extent spared children, the elderly and women. It was also striking that it attacked members of the social and economic upper class, and far less

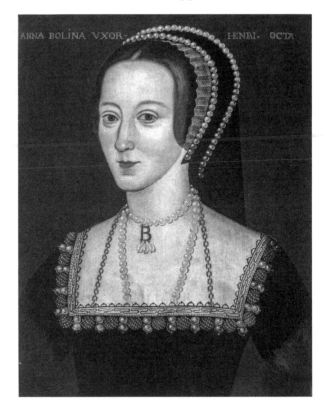

Anne Boleyn, late 16th century (based on a work of *c.* 1533–6), oil on panel. Anne, who became Henry VIII's second wife, contracted English sweating sickness in 1528, but survived. She did not, however, escape the executioner's axe in 1536.

those of the poor lower class. Monasteries and the universities of Oxford and Cambridge, where practically all the students died, were hard hit. During the epidemic of 1528 the court was also attacked and Henry VIII fled to the country. His mistress, Anne Boleyn, contracted the disease, but survived to marry Henry in 1533, only to lose her head three years later at the executioner's sword.[31]

The epidemic raged across the country for a few weeks at a time and then was gone. Each of the epidemics in England started in August and disappeared in September, but this seasonal pattern was not as pronounced on the continent.

Mortality was high and the disease instilled great fear. It says something that half a century later William Shakespeare mentioned it in his play *Measure for Measure* (even though it nominally takes place in Vienna). Despite this, the total number of deaths was far lower than the other great epidemics that ravaged Europe at the time, such as plague and typhus.

What microbe was behind this disease? The matter has still to be resolved, but a number of candidates with varying credentials have been presented in the years since the bacteriological revolution. With the exception of anthrax, which has been advanced but more or less dismissed, there are various possible viruses. Some of the symptoms, and the seasonal pattern, indicate that the microbe in question could have had an animal reservoir; in other words, it was a zoonosis. If this is the case, it was most likely down to various types of rodent, the population of which tends to be highest in late summer and autumn, particularly after a rainy spring and summer.

Some prefer to plump for a virus that is transmitted by bites from insects, such as mosquitoes or ticks.[32] The problem is that such viruses are nearly all found in other parts of the globe. A representative of this group, Crimean-Congo haemorrhagic fever (CCHF), which is transmitted by ticks, is admittedly found in Eastern Europe and has been advanced as the cause of sweating sickness.[33] I remain unconvinced by the arguments. First, the accounts of the course of the disease in England do not provide any arguments for a haemorrhagic fever. Second, the virus has not been found in England. In addition, the existing accounts of the epidemic strongly suggest person-to-person infection: entire families and large households were often hard hit.[34] This is not typical of CCHF.

We also have several viruses with reservoirs among small rodents that can cause infection in humans where this is not dependent on insects. Such a virus group is the so-called hantavirus, which is found in various parts of the world. The representatives of this group known in Europe do not produce such a dramatic pathological picture as sweating sickness, but in 1993 a new hantavirus was discovered in the southern USA – the *Sin Nombre* virus – which has a very serious pathological picture, with a high case fatality rate. The disease is called Hantavirus Pulmonary Syndrome (HPS). Recently this virus, or a possible medieval precursor of it, was proposed in a discussion of English sweating sickness, but there are weighty arguments against this. The descriptions of the disease do not give the impression of severe pulmonary failure, as is a feature of HPS.[35] Nor is the development of *Sin Nombre* infection as rapid as with sweating sickness. This virus, which gives rise to a few dozen infections every year in the USA, does not transmit infection from person to person either, even though there are a few isolated reports of this from Argentina.[36] Last but not least, hantavirus of this type has not been detected in Europe.

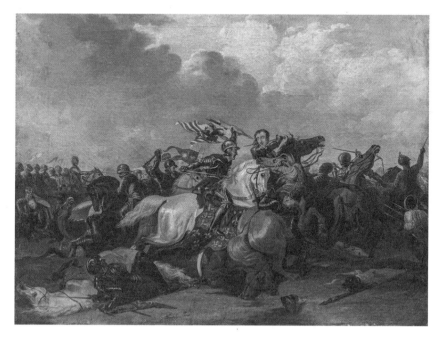

The Battle of Bosworth in 1485, in which Richard III fell, marked the end of the Wars of the Roses. The English sweating sickness broke out shortly after the battle. Painting by Abraham Cooper, 1790.

Where did this epidemic come from? Did it start in England? It was a widely held view in 1485 that it came with the mercenaries that Henry Tudor brought home with him from France to fight Richard III. These mercenaries, who at the time made up a large part of the opposing armies, came from many different countries, and they had a highly dubious reputation, which extended to the epidemics they often brought along with them (we have seen earlier that the spread of syphilis was to a great extent caused by the travels of such mercenaries through Europe). In this connection, however, they are perhaps innocent, for there are grounds for claiming that the epidemic already existed in the north of England before the Battle of Bosworth.[37] In the weeks before this decisive battle, one of the king's most important vassals, Lord Stanley, used sweating sickness as an excuse for not joining the king's army, choosing instead to station his forces separate from the rival armies at Bosworth and wait to see which was winning before joining in.[38] Did the epidemic

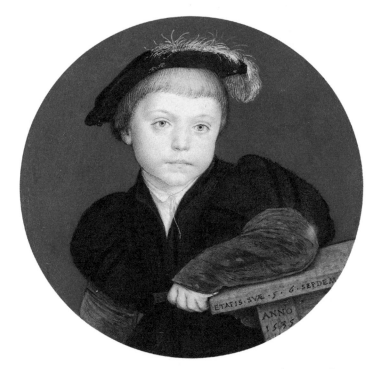

Henry Brandon, 2nd Duke of Suffolk, died of the English sweating sickness at the age of fifteen in 1551, followed a few hours later by his brother Charles. In this instance, the epidemic struck down those of the social and economic upper class more than the lower class – something that was not the case for most earlier epidemics. Painting by Hans Holbein the Younger, *c.* 1541.

perhaps contribute in this way to Richard III's fall and the ascent of the Tudor dynasty to the throne?

Several historians have suggested that the epidemic may have come from Scandinavia, possibly Norway, via the trade in furs containing infected rodents or insects.[39] But these theories are also highly speculative. I think we must reconcile ourselves to the idea that we will never find out which microbe caused English sweating sickness, or where it came from.

Rade Disease (*Radesyke*): The Tragedy that Stimulated the Norwegian Health Service

An epidemic that deserves its place in this list of mysteries hit Norway just over three hundred years ago: *radesyke*. A Russian vessel dropped anchor off Stavanger in 1709 and stayed there for the winter. Not surprisingly, this visit led to considerable contact between the crew and the young women of the area, as Professor Carl Wilhelm Boeck wrote in 1860: 'On board this ship there had been a number of dissolute crew who had sought intercourse with the Norwegian females in the harbour area and the surrounding farms.'

This was to mark the beginning of an epidemic tragedy that took a severe toll in southwest Norway, in particular, over the next 150 years. The crew would seem to have given their female acquaintances a sexually transmitted infection that was regarded at the time as new to Norway, or, as Boeck describes it: 'The Russians had shared with our Norwegian womenfolk their venereal fruits.' This infection spread rapidly during the succeeding years and was given the name *radesyke*, initially in the oral tradition and then extended to medicine as well. *Rada* is an old dialect word that means 'nasty, grim.'[40] The word *syke* means 'illness, disease'.

What was *radesyke* and what caused it? These questions have led to a long-lasting debate that has not yet come to a definite conclusion.[41] First, however, we will look at the disease and trace how the epidemic spread through society.

What was clear from the outset was that *radesyke* nearly always struck down the poor, who lived in wretched conditions with regard to both hygiene and nutrition. All age groups were affected (it was also

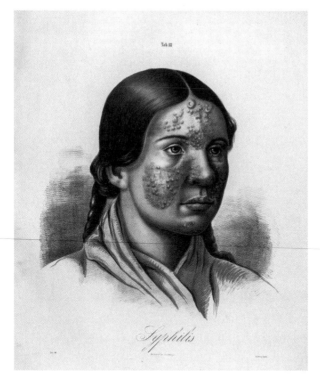

Patient with *radesyke*, drawn by Johan Ludvig Losting, and published in Carl Wilhelm Boeck and Daniel Cornelius Danielssen, *Hudens sygdomme* (1855–62). Boeck has written 'Syphilis' under the illustration, since in his opinion *radesyke* was a form of syphilis. He may have been right.

common among children). It normally began with painless sores in the skin and mucous membranes. These sores gradually became deeper, infected and evil-smelling. Very often the cartilage and external parts of the nose were attacked, causing the bridge to collapse and leaving a feature known as 'saddle nose'. Many victims had a characteristic symptom, described as an 'ant-crawling feeling', in their nose. The cartilage of the larynx was also attacked, giving victims a particularly hoarse voice. Sores in the throat could become so serious that they prevented the victim from eating and led to malnutrition. In far-advanced stages, the skeleton could also be affected, as a Danish doctor wrote in 1801, 'It wastes away its victims slowly, and often maltreats them in such a way that they look like living carcasses, and they steal around like frightful parodies of their fellow-humans.' The repulsive appearance of many of the patients often led to a stigmatization of those affected.[42]

The disease reached epidemic proportions in the eighteenth century in southern Norway and numbers gradually rose in western Norway as well. Cases also occurred in other parts of the country. It is difficult to assess just how many people were affected, but in the former Lister and Mandal county there were about 30,000 patients. The clergy were obliged to report cases of *radesyke*. It is probable, however, that there was considerable under-reporting, both because of stigmatization and because treatment included brutal mercury cures that were often regarded as just as terrible as the disease. For these reasons, many victims tried to avoid being registered by the authorities.

There was considerable disagreement among doctors as to the cause of *radesyke*. Such diagnoses as scurvy and leprosy were suggested, while others believed it to be a separate disease. The discussion of the disease led to an upsurge in the number of medical publications. It was also the topic of the first doctorate in Norway, awarded to the physician Frederik Holst in 1817. Some of those listening to the discussion of the subject at the dissertation found it a bit strong. A clergyman present wrote afterwards: 'All that talk about abscesses and lumps and scales and scabs I found revolting.'[43]

It is extremely likely that the diagnostic label *radesyke* was also used for patients with other diseases that attack the skin, such as leprosy, tuberculosis and certain skin diseases. Even so, it was definitely a separate disease that was the nucleus of the *radesyke* epidemic. Professor Boeck threw himself energetically into the debate, maintaining in a long work on the disease that it had to be a form of syphilis. This was also the prevalent view later on.[44]

In my opinion Boeck was definitely correct. It is highly likely that *radesyke* was a chronic infection with the bacterium *Treponema pallidum*. But there are still a number of unanswered questions. First, how was the disease transmitted? If we accept that the epidemic was imported by the Russians in 1709, transmission was presumably sexual to begin with. The further development of the epidemic, on the other hand, indicates that non-sexual transmission was extremely common, since all age groups, including children, could contract the disease. The clustering of cases within families was an important pattern. Extremely close contact in cramped housing and wretched hygienic conditions were probably important. At the same time, the disease was often transmitted sexually in what was a parallel development. That was also the opinion of doctors at the time.

As we have seen in connection with syphilis, there are *Treponema* bacteria very closely related to the 'classic' syphilis bacterium that also result in chronic diseases, which can infect non-sexually via close physical contact or by sharing eating utensils, glasses and the like. This applies for example to endemic syphilis, also known as bejel, which is found in the Middle East and the southwestern Sahara, areas with an extremely dry and hot climate. The syphilis bacterium has possibly developed at some point with several mutations from the other *Treponema* bacteria, which have changed its characteristics somewhat. It is conceivable that syphilis bacteria imported in 1709, under the influence of special environmental factors in Norway, could have changed slightly, including the ways in which transmission took place. In that case it would just be an illustration of the microbes' ability to adapt to external conditions.

And second, what is the explanation for the rapid spread of the epidemic in Norway during the eighteenth century? It is reminiscent of the rapid spread of syphilis in Europe in the sixteenth century, where part of the explanation may be the lack of immunity to the bacterium in the population. Could this also have been the case in the Norwegian population of the eighteenth century? Syphilis admittedly appeared in Norway as early as the sixteenth century, but the occurrence during the next couple of centuries could have been so sporadic that immunity in the population was low.[45] The disappearance of *radesyke* in the middle of the nineteenth century might have been the result of improved living conditions for the poor when it came to hygiene, housing and nutrition.[46]

These considerations are speculative. We will perhaps never get a complete answer to the nature of *radesyke*. Nevertheless, it ought to be possible to advance via further research, since we can now carry out experiments on material from the many graves of *radesyke* patients that exist. Modern molecular-biological methods could perhaps shed light on the mystery surrounding *radesyke*, since it has recently proved possible to detect *Treponema* bacteria in archaeological material. Furthermore, examining skeletons could be another way to gain greater clarity. It definitely ought to be possible to acquire suitable material for this.

It would be wrong to believe that *radesyke* is exclusively a Norwegian phenomenon, even though Norway was particularly hard hit. It has become clear that similar pathological pictures under similar social and environmental conditions were common in other peripheral European regions, including Bosnia, under the name *skerljevo*, and Scotland, where the disease was called 'sibbens'.[47]

The *radesyke* epidemic had a positive effect on the emergence of a Norwegian health service. The authorities in Denmark and Norway made great efforts to combat the epidemic. Special *radesyke* doctors were appointed and about fifteen hospitals established with a special responsibility to treat and isolate *radesyke* patients and not simply park them on a side-line, as had been done in earlier hospitals. A number of these hospitals were later converted for conventional use. Despite the many tragedies this disease caused in the 150 years it was active, something positive nevertheless emerged from *radesyke*.

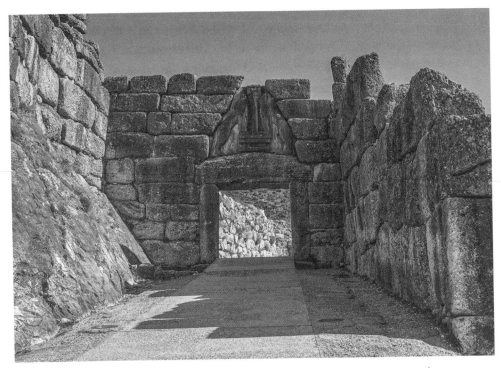

The Lion Gate in Mycenae in the Peloponnese, the city that gave its name to the Mycenaean civilization which flourished between 1600 and 1200 BC. It is still unclear what brought about the fall of this civilization.

SIX

The Contribution Made by Epidemics to the Fall of Empires

A recurrent feature of world history is how all empires and civilizations grow, flourish and, apparently inevitably, decline. Historians have always been extremely interested in finding the underlying causes or mechanisms of this process. Philosophers of history have advanced learned hypotheses about laws that govern this path of development, even though such theories are not considered to be completely *comme il faut* in present-day historical research. The German Oswald Spengler claimed that civilizations could be compared to organisms that pass through a cycle of growth, ageing and death. The English historian Arnold Toynbee, on the other hand, placed great emphasis on non-material factors in the development of civilizations from growth to decline and fall.

In particular, the causes of the decline and fall of empires have been the subject of in-depth studies. Such analyses are extremely demanding, for the nature of the causes will doubtless be extremely complex and our comprehension of them incomplete. Nor are there any examples from history of one single factor being able to explain the rise and fall of civilizations. This only takes place in the world of myth. The classic example here is the legendary island of Atlantis, referred to by Plato in his dialogues *Timaeus* and *Critias*. The mighty Atlantis sank into the sea in the space of a single night in connection with a terrible natural disaster. The basis for this legend is still unclear. In the real world, historians have to consider a great many possible individual factors in their more or less speculative explanations of the fall of empires, which, unlike the sinking of Atlantis, do not take place in one night.

Historians have placed special emphasis in their work on the importance of economic conditions, external enemies, internal unrest and civil war, as well as psychological and religious factors. Far less interest has been shown in the possible significance of extensive epidemics and climatic and ecological changes. William H. McNeill broke down some sort of barrier with his book *Plagues and Peoples*, but there are still only a few historians who seem to ascribe any great importance to epidemics in connection with the destabilization and fall of states and civilizations.[1] I believe that this will change, since the circumstantial evidence for the importance of epidemics is increasing, partly because new scientific research findings have supplemented historical knowledge and archaeology to a considerable extent.

We have already looked at several examples of this in new finds using molecular-biological methods, as in the study of major plague pandemics. Several of the following examples, in my opinion, show that epidemic diseases have often played a considerable role in the decline and fall of powerful empires and civilizations.

Were the Conquerors of Troy Struck Down by the Plague?

The late Bronze Age civilization that flourished in Greece between about 1600 and 1200 BC has been named after Mycenae in the Peloponnese, where impressive ruins with the famous Lion Gate can still be seen. It was based on a number of fortified city states governed by monarchs and an upper warrior caste. The generally accepted view today is that Homer's *Iliad* and *Odyssey* reflect the conditions of the Mycenaean era, and that Agamemnon, Achilles and Odysseus were warrior chieftains in Mycenaean city states. About 1450 BC the Mycenaean conquerors subjugated the Minoan civilization on Crete. The Mycenaean states engaged in widespread trade in the eastern Mediterranean. While this culture was apparently at its height, relatively sudden and dramatic events took place that led to its collapse over the following 150 years. Archaeological finds show that a number of the Mycenaean centres were plundered and burned, in some cases more than once.[2]

Earlier historians believed that immigrants from the north, the so-called Dorians, were responsible for the fall of Mycenaean culture, but this is no longer regarded as being probable. Large-scale civil war between the individual warrior states has also been proposed as an explanation, as have attacks from warring seafaring peoples that harried the Mediterranean at the time.

Could large-scale, deadly epidemics also have played an important role? One hypothesis that has been advanced is that an epidemic of bubonic plague caused by *Yersinia pestis* could have swept through Mycenaean society and brought it down.[3] Recent finds indicate that the plague bacterium already existed in Eurasia during the Bronze Age.[4] The extensive Mycenaean sea trade would undoubtedly have facilitated the import of new epidemics. The problem is simply that there is a complete lack of concrete facts that make the plague theory plausible.

There are no references to any epidemic in the Mycenaean sources on clay tablets written in the script known as Linear B, the oldest form of Greek that has been deciphered. Nor are there any archaeological finds that could imply the existence of either the plague bacterium or other microbes. Even if *Yersinia pestis* probably already existed, we have no tangible evidence of any major plague epidemic before the Plague of Justinian in the mid-sixth century AD. It is highly improbable that the bacterium would disappear from the scene after having destroyed Mycenaean society and remain absent for more than 1,500 years. New epidemics would undoubtedly have occurred at various intervals during this long period. So what happened to Agamemnon's descendants remains an unsolved mystery.

The Collapse of the Indus Valley Civilization

At school we hear about the first great civilizations in Egypt and Meso-potamia, but scarcely anything about another that flourished at the same time, one that developed over a wide territory that comprised Pakistan and adjacent regions of today's India, Afghanistan and Iran. It arose around 3000 BC and reached its peak between 2600 and 1900 BC. It is usually referred to as either the Indus Valley civilization, after the river that flows through its core, or the Harappan culture, after one of its largest cities.

A considerable proportion of the population lived in towns, which were laid out according to a regular plan and included large brick-built houses. A striking feature is the highly developed drainage system for sewage and waste, the most sophisticated system at the time. Advanced handicraft and agriculture were an essential basis of this civilization, which also had comprehensive shipping and trade with lands in the

Middle East and Southeast Asia. It had a well-developed written culture, but as yet the Indus or Harappan script has not been deciphered.[5]

Decline set in relatively swiftly in the early second millennium BC, although at various rates in different parts of the empire. In most areas it can be seen that the towns became dilapidated and the populations dwindled.

What was the cause of the end of the Indus Valley civilization? Most scholars have stressed the comprehensive climatic and ecological changes that took place around the end of the third millennium BC.[6] Some areas were exposed to major floods, others to lasting periods of drought. This led to large-scale economic and social changes, leading to a final collapse around 1900 BC. This is probably a good example of climate change having fatal consequences for a civilization's capacity to survive. It can take place in several ways. As far as the Indus Valley civilization is concerned, it is reasonable to assume that the climate changes, among other things, led to serious problems for agriculture that weakened all of society.

New research has shown that the climate changes probably also had biological consequences for the unfortunate people of this civilization. Extensive examination of skeletons from graves in Harappa reveals that the infection load on the inhabitants increased considerably during the final phase of the town's decline.[7] Tuberculosis and leprosy were

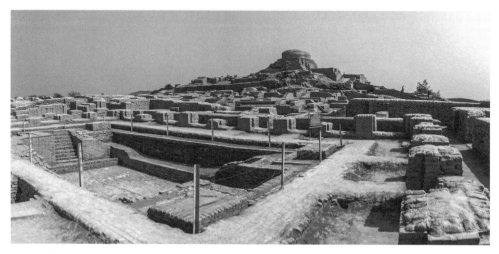

The ruins of the city of Harappa, one of the two largest cities in the Indus Valley civilization, which arose around 3000 BC and culminated around 2600–1900 BC. This civilization is also known as the Harappan culture, after the city.

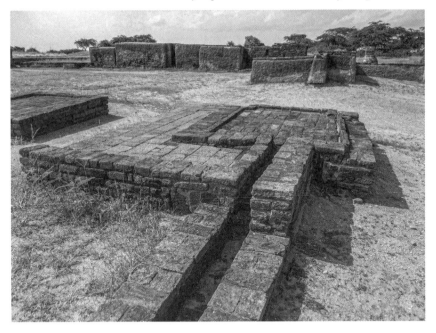

Archaeologists who have studied the Indus civilization have particularly admired the well-developed draining system for sewage and waste, which was the most advanced at the time. However, this drainage and waste-pipe system with its many wells was constructed in such a way that the well-water could easily become polluted with sewage if the drainage pipes were overloaded. And this may have led to a considerable risk of epidemics with waterborne microbes.

clearly commonplace, in addition to skeletal changes that imply other bacterial infections. The inhabitants were also possibly hit by more acute, serious epidemics. The American evolutional biologist Paul W. Ewald has advanced the interesting hypothesis that it was precisely the advanced waste-disposal system of the Harappan culture that made the town extremely vulnerable to waterborne epidemics such as cholera.[8] The numerous wells that characterized the town could very easily have become polluted with the contents of the sewage system and nearby drainage pipes, causing the town to be hit by regular waterborne epidemics. We do not know how old the cholera bacterium is, but a disease resembling cholera is mentioned in Sanskrit writings as far back as 500 BC. Other waterborne microbes may also have played a role.

If one day the writings of the Indus culture are deciphered, we will perhaps be able to read accounts of widespread epidemics. Will future molecular-biological examinations of skeletons from Harappa and other towns perhaps provide answers about the possible contribution of microbes to the fall of the Indus Valley civilization? Such finds would not only be of significance to researchers interested in this civilization, but perhaps also shed light on the role microbes doubtless played in human history.

The Decline and Fall of the Athenian Empire

After the Graeco-Persian wars came to an end in 479 BC, Athens took the initiative of establishing a league of more than 250 Greek city states on the coasts and islands of the Aegean Sea. This alliance was known as the Delian League after the island of Delos, where its treasury lay and where meetings were held. The league had a considerable fleet. Athens was the undisputed leader of the league. Its position at the forefront of Greek political life was regarded as a threat by its rival, Sparta, which led its own alliance of city states, and this led to the outbreak of the Peloponnesian War in 431 BC. The plague that hit Athens with terrifying strength shortly after the outbreak of war has already been discussed in Chapter Five.

Historians generally agree that the immediate consequences for the Athenian population were considerable. There is less agreement, however, regarding the long-term consequences of the epidemic. Sparta and its allies were to a great extent spared the epidemic. Did Athens manage to completely recover after the first epidemic shock? Did the epidemic play an important role in the defeat of Athens in the war? In that case, it was also an important factor in Athens's loss of its dominant position as leader of the Delian League, which disintegrated after the war was over.

The arguments in favour of major long-term consequences of the epidemic are quite strong.[9] There is no doubt that Athens's military striking force rapidly weakened after the outbreak. Thucydides relates that already by the winter of 427 BC some 4,400 heavily armed infantrymen known as hoplites and three hundred cavalrymen had died from the epidemic, about a quarter of Athens's elite troops.

Even so, the fact is that Athens apparently managed to recover militarily and was able to fight on until its eventual defeat in 404 BC. The mysterious microbe behind the Athenian Plague did not directly reduce Athens's military striking force in the long run, but it might have played a crucial role in another way, for in 429 BC the city's greatest statesman, Pericles, died – probably a victim of the epidemic. This was a blow that may well have proved decisive for the later defeat. Pericles, who enjoyed great authority and was highly respected by his citizens, was followed by a series of politicians who were often demagogues and charlatans. They completely lacked Pericles' statesmanship and noble qualities, which even his enemies admired. Through a series of unfortunate decisions and hasty military operations, the chance of making a peace favourable to Athens was wasted, leading to defeat and a humiliating peace. Athens was economically exhausted and had to raze its walls, give up its fleet and pay tribute to Sparta, which now became the dominant state in Greece.

It is claimed that no one is indispensable, but there are good reasons to believe that the Peloponnesian War would have ended differently if Pericles had not been laid low by the epidemic and had continued to lead Athens.[10] In that case, Athens might possibly have continued to have a leading position in a Greece that would have had a different political development from the fragmentation that finally left the country prey to Philip II of Macedon and his son, Alexander the Great. But writing counterfactual history is, of course, uncertain and dangerous.

Certain historians have also blamed the Athenian Plague for what is perceived as a lasting deterioration of the social and political climate in Athens. Thucydides points out early in his account of the epidemic that it led to a brutalization of the Athenians' attitude towards social norms and seemly behaviour. A weakened public spirit, cynicism and the prioritizing of personal interests rather than those of society were probably typical of Athens in the years after the epidemic as well as later. It is difficult to determine just how much of this can be ascribed to the epidemic and how much is due to the inevitable psychological consequences of a long period of almost total war.[11]

The Decline and Fall of the Roman Empire: An Eternal Problem for Historians

The Roman empire was one of the most impressive in all history. The Romans claimed that the city itself was founded by Romulus in 753 BC and some form of Roman political power continued for more than 2,200 years until the Ottoman conquest of Constantinople in 1453. For several centuries historians have discussed the reasons why the empire fell. The extent of this discussion can be illustrated in the words of the nineteenth-century French historian and philosopher Ernest Renan: 'The two great problems of history are to explain why Rome came into existence and why it fell.' A German historian has tallied no fewer than two hundred different causes that have been advanced over the ages to explain the fall of the Roman empire.[12] Military, economic, social and cultural causes are among those proposed – and even the harmful effects of lead poisoning from water pipes. No one has any ready answer here, but a number of different factors in all probability contributed to the Roman giant eventually being brought down.

To a medical man, however, it is striking that medical factors are often conspicuous by their absence in the many theories advanced by capable, highly specialized historians. This I find unfortunate, since medical-historical research in recent years has provided us with new information about important epidemics at various periods of the Roman empire.

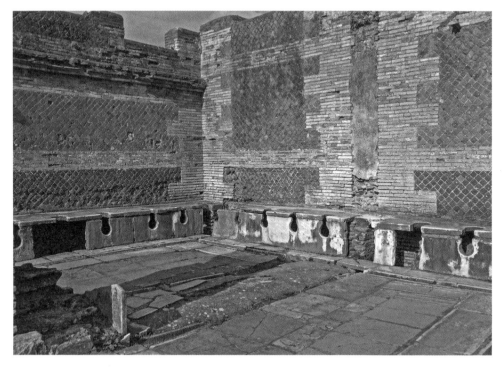

Public toilet, Ostia Antica, Province of Rome. Roman towns had public toilets that could cater for twenty people at a time.

To understand the development of the Roman empire, and its fall in particular, it is therefore necessary to study the considerable problems with infection faced by the Romans. Certain features of Roman society created a major, persistent infection load on its citizens. The average life expectancy was less than thirty years and the most frequent cause of death was infectious disease.

The towns in particular were a paradise for microbes. Even though a city such as Rome is justly famous for its well-organized water supply via a series of aqueducts and its many public baths, sanitary conditions were nevertheless so bad that inhabitants were infested with microbes, including bacteria and intestinal worms, which are transmitted by food and water polluted by faeces. Human faeces were often used as fertilizer in agriculture, with the risk of infection that this involved. A new and useful, though not particularly choice, branch of archaeology is the study of latrines and toilets in former times, where such facilities existed. Investigations of fossilized excrement in a public latrine under the Palatine Hill in Rome have revealed that its users were infected with various kinds of intestinal worms.[13] These public toilets involved a certain risk of infectious diseases, particularly because the Roman version of toilet paper was a stick with a sponge that was shared by users. It was not without good reason that a depiction of the goddess Fortuna was often found on the walls of toilets as a kind of protection.

As we have seen, malaria gradually became a large problem in the Roman empire, including Rome itself. Chronic malaria can constitute a serious health risk in a population, as is still seen in Africa. Every year malaria caused a considerable number of deaths among the inhabitants. The success of the Pax Romana formed the basis for extensive trade by sea across the widespread empire, but provided ideal conditions for the dissemination of microbes, both within the empire and from its outside trading partners. Tuberculosis and leprosy are examples of chronic infections that contributed to the Romans' problems.

With this constant burden of infection, it is perhaps not surprising that the average Roman was not very tall, since stunted growth is a well-known consequence of constant infections during childhood.[14] This makes it all the more impressive that the short Roman legionaries were so often victorious when fighting huge Germanic warriors. This was first and foremost due to their iron discipline and training, as well as their superior tactics and strategy. The legionaries were also exposed to infection, but as long as sick and dead legionaries could be replaced without any difficulty, this did not create problems for the military striking power of the empire.

What did probably have serious consequences for the whole of Roman society in both the short and the long term were the major epidemics with high mortality that hit the empire from the middle of the second century AD.[15] We have already seen that the first of these major epidemics, the Antonine Plague, had a total mortality of at least 10 per cent of the population over the twenty years it raged in various waves across the Roman empire. The great loss of human life caused by the epidemic can be seen from the fact that it proved necessary to recruit slaves, gladiators and even condemned criminals to fill the ranks in the legions. The Roman army now increasingly began to recruit German mercenaries. The epidemic also led to problems in filling positions in public administration. Shortages of agricultural workers in the wake of the epidemic led to the price of land soaring and to farmland lying uncultivated. Agricultural production declined, the tax base in the population shrank, and the state began to have major economic problems. Marcus Aurelius was once obliged to sell valuable objects from the palace to raise money. In several peace agreements Germanic tribes were allowed to settle in the border provinces that had been laid waste by epidemics and war, and this led to an increasing Germanic presence in the empire.

The Roman empire recovered after the Antonine Plague, but it was never the same again. As early as the 1820s the Danish-German historian Barthold Georg Niebuhr stated: 'The Antique world never recovered after the battle fought against the epidemic that raged during the reign of Marcus Aurelius.' Even though some later historians felt that Niebuhr exaggerated the long-term consequences of the Antonine Plague, they must have nevertheless been serious. The population was considerably reduced. From then on, there was no talk of expanding the empire but of maintaining the borders against constant barbarian attacks.

Then came the Plague of Cyprian in, or shortly before, AD 250, which raged for a further twenty years.[16] Here too mortality was high. Agriculture was hit, partly because of a decline in the labour force as a result of the plague and partly because of the flight of the rural population to the towns. This was also, in different ways, a time of crises, with much internal unrest and signs of potential civil war. A weakened political and military leadership, combined with increased mortality among the legionaries because of the epidemic, made it extremely difficult to defend the borders of the empire against the constant attacks from outside.

Christianity flourished during the Plague of Cyprian despite persecution, because the Christians' belief in a life after death led them to display a distinct fearlessness in the face of the epidemic. This was evident in their devoted care of those affected by the plague. The epidemic probably contributed to the spread of Christianity. If Edward Gibbon's view that the emergence of Christianity really was an important cause of the decline and fall of the Roman empire, the Plague of Cyprian definitely contributed to this, if only indirectly.

After the Roman empire recovered from this twenty-year epidemic it apparently flourished once again in the fourth century, but this was an empire unlike that under Marcus Aurelius. It was now governed by soldier emperors, and the old Roman upper class lost its power and military influence. Army recruitment problems meant that an increasing number of 'barbarians', particularly from Germanic tribes, were enrolled and even gained positions as senior officers. The Romans still had to repulse attacks from various outside ethnic groups, including Germanic tribes, Parthians and later the Huns, who poured in from the central Asian steppes, driving other peoples ahead of them.[17]

The climate had gradually changed from a stable, warm and humid period known as the Roman 'climate optimum' which lasted from about 300 BC to AD 400 and probably contributed to the former growth of empire. It now became less stable, with consequences for agriculture and perhaps also ecology-related infection problems. During this period the infection load on the Romans was perhaps even heavier than before. Infection-related mortality in Rome seems to have increased around AD 400. The problems with malaria in Italy had worsened, as we have seen, and may well have contributed to weakening the empire.[18]

At the beginning of the fourth century AD the Roman empire was administratively divided into a western and an eastern part, the latter with Constantinople as its capital. The fall of the western part is often regarded as having taken place in AD 476, when Odoacer, a military leader of East Germanic descent, deposed Romulus Augustus and assumed power, formally as a king subject to the emperor in Constantinople. The entire Western Roman empire was at that time dissolved and replaced by a number of states based on various Germanic tribes. With our present knowledge of the history of infection in the empire, it is difficult to ignore the contribution made by microbes when discussing the gradual decline and eventual fall of the Western Roman empire.

The Eastern Roman empire, which is often referred to as the Byzantine empire, lived on after 476. This had also come to feel the effect of attacks from epidemics and external enemies, but gained increased vitality during the sixth century, especially under Justinian, who was undoubtedly one of the greatest statesmen of antiquity, even though his contemporaries felt that he lacked both charisma and physical courage. Justinian's great plan was to re-establish the former Roman empire and for a while it looked as if he might succeed. His generals reconquered large sections of North Africa, Spain and Italy, and fortune seemed to smile on the Romans once more. Then the Plague of Justinian struck, greatly changing the subsequent path of history.[19]

Mortality during the two hundred years struck by repeated waves of plague is difficult to estimate with any certainty, but it is not unlikely that between 25 and 50 per cent of the population of the Eastern Roman empire perished. This greatly affected the empire's economy, especially with regard to its military strength. During the first attack of the epidemic, the army was reduced to a third of its size. At the same time, the borders still had to be defended against external enemies. Justinian's plan to re-establish the Roman empire had to be abandoned. The plague, which he himself had survived, seemed to have deprived him of all vitality and vigour. After his death in 565 his successors attempted, with reduced resources and mixed fortunes, to maintain the weakened empire.

Then a new actor came onto the stage of Mediterranean politics. In the 630s the armies of the new Islamic religion swept in from Arabia with an unshakeable belief in their prophet, one which often led to victories. In a very short time they overran the Persian empire and conquered large parts of the Byzantine provinces in the Middle East.[20] Many historians believe that this would not have happened at such speed if both empires had not already been greatly weakened by the Plague of Justinian. In the centuries after the plague, a continued, gradual reduction of the Byzantine empire took place under constant pressure from new attacks by external enemies. When Constantinople finally fell to the Ottoman Turks on 29 May 1453, and the young sultan Mehmed II, who was given the epithet 'Fatih' (The Conqueror), marched into the city, the Roman empire was finally consigned to history after more than two thousand years. Gibbon had been right when he wrote that it was more appropriate to ask why the empire had lasted so long than why it declined and fell.

Among the many factors discussed over the centuries by historians to account for the fall of the Roman empire, external enemies – Germanic tribes, Huns, Persians and slaves – have often had a secure place. But in my opinion it is now impossible to ignore the invisible enemies of the Roman empire: microbes. They attacked partly from the outside, in the form of new epidemics and pandemics, and partly from within in the form of a constant infection load linked to a series of special conditions in the Roman world.

The Fall of the Aztec and Inca Empires

In the New World, too, major epidemics contributed to deciding the fate of empires. In the centuries before the arrival of the Europeans, empires had flourished and fallen in Central and South America, but we know little about the causes and the possible role of epidemics.

After Columbus arrived in the Americas in 1492, there came what I have called the second epidemiological transition in the history of human infection, the exchange of microbes between the Old and the New World that is part of what the historian Alfred Crosby has called the 'Columbian exchange'.[21] As we have seen, this was not to the advantage of the indigenous population. The Europeans brought with them a great many microbes to which the American population had never been exposed and therefore to which they had no immunity. This importation of deadly microbes continued for several centuries, but its consequences became evident shortly after the Europeans' arrival.

The Aztec empire and the invisible attackers
When dealing with the history of the smallpox virus, we saw how Hernán Cortés, with a force of just four hundred men, was able to subjugate the

mighty Aztec empire of approximately 30 million inhabitants. Despite the courage, armour and weaponry of the conquistadors, they would hardly have stood a chance against thousands of well-trained Aztec warriors had Cortés not had an invisible ally: the smallpox virus. If this virus had not struck the Aztecs in the capital, Tenochtitlan, when Cortés and his men, under dramatic circumstances, had been forced to retire from the city, the Aztec soldiers would, without a shadow of doubt, have pursued and crushed them. But this did not happen.

No one who has studied the history of Mexico in the sixteenth century doubts that the smallpox virus was of decisive importance for Cortés's success. Without this ally from the world of microbes, his life, along with that of his men, would indisputably have ended on the sacrificial slab in the pyramid temple of Huitzilopochtli, the god of war, where his still-beating heart would have been torn out by the blood-bespattered priests of the god.[22]

The smallpox epidemic continued to ravage the indigenous population in the years following the conquest of Tenochtitlan and the victory over the Aztecs.[23] It is estimated that the population was reduced from between 25 and 30 million at the arrival of the Europeans to 6.5 million a decade later. After a while, the smallpox virus was well assisted by epidemics of other microbes from the Old World, including measles, influenza, typhus and scarlet fever.[24]

In addition to the direct and indirect effect of the smallpox virus and the other newly imported microbes on the Aztecs, the psychological effect of the epidemics was also of great importance. Since the Spaniards were clearly invulnerable during the epidemics, they must have support from supernatural powers. It was precisely the fact that the Aztec empire was so well organized with a good administration that, paradoxically, made it relatively easy for the Spaniards to seize the reins. It was also important that many of the peoples who had been subjugated by the Aztecs hated them and became allies of the Europeans in the struggle.

The fall of the Inca empire: smallpox virus and civil war

When the Spaniards came to the New World, the second major civilization on the continent was at the height of its power, controlling an empire that comprised what is now Ecuador, Peru, Bolivia and parts of

Chile and Argentina. There was a population of more than 30 million. The empire had a highly efficient administration and a considerable army, and was led by an absolutist monarch who was regarded as the son of the sun.[25] The mighty empire also collapsed like a house of cards when it was attacked by the Spaniard Francisco Pizarro at the head of only 180 men. How was that possible?

First, the Incas were totally unprepared for the attack. The Aztecs and the Incas do not seem to have had any contact with each other, so the Incas knew nothing about the tragedy that had hit the Aztec empire. There were admittedly rumours about foreign ships that had been seen along the coast, but no one knew what that signified. So when the small-pox virus struck in 1525 with terrifying force, and its victims included the mighty ruler of the Incas, Huayna Capac, this unleashed a destructive civil war between several pretenders to his throne, which, along with the ravages of the smallpox virus, paved the way for the arrival of Pizarro in 1532.[26]

The great empire of the Incas was conquered by the combination of Spanish conquistadors and the smallpox virus. As in Mexico, the well-organized administration of the empire made it easier for the Spaniards to seize power.

Microbes and Empires: Some Reflections

On the previous pages I have given some examples to illustrate the fact that the world of microbes can sometimes be a powerful player in histor-ical events and lead to the decline and fall of empires. Some people are probably suspicious that as a specialist in infectious diseases I have tended to overplay the importance of epidemics in the course of history. To this I would object that I naturally admit that the mechanisms under-lying the fall of civilizations are extremely complex and cannot derive from any single factor, including microbes or epidemics. Often our knowledge about the past is so deficient that we cannot count on any one foolproof answer. This also applies to the examples I have selected, though to varying degrees. We know extremely little about some of the empires I have mentioned, notably the Mycenaean and Indus Valley civilizations. On the other hand we know quite a lot more about the Roman and Aztec empires, without having the full answers.

What to my mind is important is that one does not ignore the possible significance of microbes and epidemics throughout history, as some historians have done earlier, and perhaps still have a tendency to do. This is seen all too often in textbooks and more popular presentations of history. One of the reasons for this could be that we know far too little about the epidemics of earlier ages and which microbes were responsible for them. The situation has changed somewhat over the past few decades since the advent of molecular-biological methods, which can provide valuable information about microbes in the event of archaeological finds. Archaeology and history must in the future be based to a far greater extent on scientific methods and expertise, which will undoubtedly offer us new opportunities to understand the past.

But it is just as important to have increased insight into the influence of microbes and epidemics on social, economic and political relations, since they are of crucial significance in enabling us to meet the infection problems of the future. The same mechanisms that throughout history have influenced the interaction between microbes, humans and ecological factors are still highly active and are sure to influence us in the future as well. In the following chapter we shall take a look at a number of new challenges from the world of microbes that illustrate how the rules of the game in the history of human infection are unchangeable.

SEVEN

New Infections, New Challenges

During the first decades after the Second World War there was a widespread belief that the days of infectious diseases as one of the great threats to *Homo sapiens* were numbered. People were convinced that the age of major epidemics was over. During those years, new, effective antibiotics were being produced that saved countless human lives. A series of vaccines had proved that they offered good protection against many infections. Great improvements in hygiene and sanitary conditions during the twentieth century had contributed to a high degree to the successful fight against such diseases, particularly in the Western world.

The future therefore seemed rosy when it came to the microbe menace. It was not only people in general who held this view but prominent politicians, health experts, specialists in infectious diseases and scientists.[1] The u.s. Surgeon General William H. Stewart is reported, perhaps incorrectly, to have stated in 1967: 'It is time to close the book on infectious diseases and declare the struggle against pestilence won.' The Australian Nobel Prize-winner Frank McFarlane Burnet wrote in 1962: 'One can think of the middle of the twentieth century as the end of one of the most important social revolutions in history, the virtual elimination of the infectious diseases as a significant factor in social life.'[2]

The Microbes Strike Back

The gods must have laughed heartily at this new demonstration of hubris, against which the Greeks of antiquity had warned so long ago. The microbes had by no means played out their role. In the first fifty years after the bacteriological revolution it had admittedly been possible, using steadily improving methods, to detect the cause of most of the well-known infectious diseases that were still relevant. But then people gradually discovered that completely new infectious diseases were appearing in increasing numbers. In the period from 1940 to 2004, no fewer than 335 new microbes were discovered as causes of disease in humans, some of them extremely serious.[3] Even so, it took many decades before this started to weaken the optimistic belief that the age of infectious diseases was over. The few voices in the medical world that warned against such a view were not listened to.

The great watershed was the AIDS epidemic, which broke out in the early 1980s and made a profound impression on both the public at large and the medical world. The radical change of mentality this prompted led to the introduction in the USA of a completely novel concept when faced with the new infectious diseases that had appeared: 'emerging infectious diseases', often abbreviated as EIDS. This concept applies to infections with microbes that were either not known earlier or have become far more widespread in recent years. The microbe in question can in some cases be new in the world, for example as the result of a mutation with evolutionary advantages, but this does not have to be the case. In most instances the microbe is hardly new, just formerly unknown to humanity, as was the Ebola virus, discovered in 1976. Other factors than changes to the microbe itself can be the cause of it emerging and acquiring increased importance – normally changes to ecological conditions. The latter is certainly the most common reason.

Experiences with EIDS have convincingly shown that the majority of the key factors that have promoted their appearance are linked to human activities, including man-made changes to the environment and ecology as well as new patterns of behaviour. Such changes have taken place at an accelerating rate and on a larger scale during the past 150 years and really mushroomed during the twentieth century. It is, among other things, this recognition that underlies the new concept of Anthropocene, the term used for the era in which we now live, one when *Homo sapiens* to an alarming extent is changing the environment and nature of the planet.

This change of mindset regarding EIDS and their underlying causes represented a new understanding of the duel between man and microbe, with far greater emphasis on ecological and environmental factors than previously. But this new way of looking at things ought not only to be applied to the EIDs of the twentieth century. A retrospective look at human history shows that ecology and the environment have played an important role in the duel between man and microbe for thousands of years. It is just that formerly people were unaware of this. An examination of the major pandemics and epidemics illustrates this motif with great clarity. There was a strongly increasing interest in EIDs from the 1990s onwards, which represented a breakthrough for the new mindset.

The new perceptions were brought centre stage by the U.S. health authorities in comprehensive, bulky reports that had strong media coverage, and at meetings and international conventions.[4] A special journal was launched, *Emerging Infectious Diseases*, which still prints new publications within the field. Such major book successes as Laurie Garrett's *The Coming Plague* and Richard Preston's *The Hot Zone*, which featured dramatic popular descriptions of the newly arrived infectious diseases, conveyed the message to the public at large.[5]

The microbes of the EIDs are found in all the main groups – bacteria, viruses, protozoa, intestinal worms, fungi and prions – but the most common are bacteria and viruses. More than 70 per cent of these infections are zoonoses, microbes that are mainly found in various animals, but can also attack human beings. The majority of these zoonoses have species of wild animal as their preferred hosts. The microbes do not normally cause a serious disease in the species that is the actual reservoir.

EIDs represent a large, varied spectrum of infectious diseases. Some are particularly found in exotic regions of the world, such as the dramatic epidemics with the Ebola virus in Africa and the Nipah virus in Asia. It is particularly these that are favourites with the mass media that specializes in 'grisly and gruesome' reporting. It is far less known that there is also a large number of EIDs in the Western world, some of which have just as dramatic pathological pictures as the Ebola virus and an even higher case fatality rate. An example of this is infections with the mould fungus *Aspergillus*.

Let us take a look at a small selection of EIDs as examples of the challenges they represent, and at the environment-related and ecological factors that underlie their appearance on the scene.

Immune Deficiency: The Price of Progress

'Each hour of happiness on earth with sorrow must be paid' is the somewhat gloomy conclusion of an old Norwegian hymn. This is actually a poetic way of describing certain serious problems we face in modern, hi-tech medicine, as it has developed in Western countries.

Medical treatment: a double-edged sword

We are justly proud of the impressive advances we have seen in Western medicine during the latter half of the twentieth century and up to the present day. Major steps forward have been taken, for example in organ transplantation and cancer treatment. However, it is an uncomfortable fact that a number of the forms of treatment we have successfully made use of lead to considerable weakening of the patient's immune system. With our eyes wide open, medical professionals may potentially cause a failure of the immune system's ability to respond adequately, which quite often leads to serious, sometimes even life-threatening, infectious diseases. It is precisely in such patients that we see demonstrated just how vital a role the immune system plays in normal life. In many cases, it is the unfortunate effect of the treatment on the patient's immune system that limits how strong the possible treatment can be.

Transplantation medicine has celebrated great triumphs during the past decades. Today, the transplantation of kidneys, liver, heart, lungs and bone marrow is a routine operation. A vital precondition for successful transplantation is that the transplanted organ is not rejected because of the immune system's natural reaction to alien tissue with foreign antigens. For this reason, the patient is prescribed immunosuppressive medication, which subdues the immunological reaction. In this way we also suppress 'useful' reactions and weaken the patient's immune system, increasing the susceptibility to serious infections from common and uncommon microbes.[6]

Cancer treatment is also one of the flagships of modern medicine. Many cancerous diseases can now be cured using a large number of medicines that include cell toxins, cytostatic drugs that kill the cancer cells. The majority of such medicines unfortunately affect not only the cancer cells but those of the immune system. Once again, this can result in a severe weakening of the system during and in a period after treatment, when the patient is extremely susceptible to infection.[7]

We also now use immuno-suppressive medicines to control immunological reactions in diseases where the patient's immune system attacks its own tissues and organs, including what we call autoimmune diseases. Many rheumatological diseases belong to this category, such as rheumatoid arthritis. But here too the treatment often has harmful effects on the useful parts of the immune system, which can lead to weakening of the system and infectious complications.[8]

The treatment of those patients who are most ill and need intensive treatment now takes place in highly specialized wards within hospitals' intensive-care units. As a result of treatment and monitoring routines, these patients too can experience a weakening of the immune system and problems of infection.

A large proportion of the infectious diseases that affect patients with immune deficiency are quite uncommon in the rest of the population.[9] Here, special microbes are involved that are called opportunists. The opportunist microbes lack the necessary characteristics to be able to cause serious infection in humans with a normally functioning immune system. But those with a weakened system can be attacked by them, often with life-threatening infections as a result.

During the past fifty years these opportunist infections have become increasingly common in Western countries and constitute an important

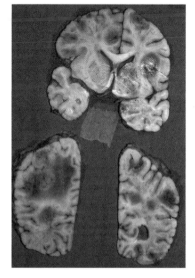
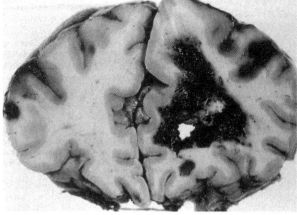

The mould fungus *Aspergillus* can produce life-threatening infections, including brain haemorrhages (*right*) and brain abscesses (*left*).

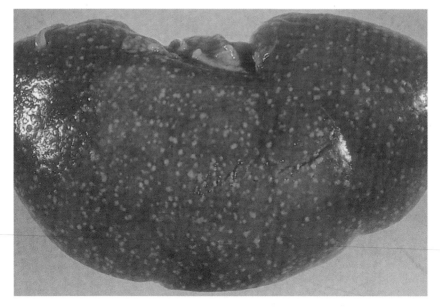

The yeast fungus *Candida* can pepper all the organs with tiny abscesses, including the kidneys, as seen in this photograph.

part of emerging infections. They represent a varied mix of microbes: fungi, viruses, bacteria, protozoa and even intestinal worms. The pathological pictures are similarly extremely different. The diagnosis of these infections can be difficult, and treatment can require special medicines. This has therefore become an important new specialist field in modern infection medicine.

The infection panorama in the event of immune deficiency

Infections involving a great many species of fungus illustrate the problems of patients with deficient immune systems. There are two forms of fungus that are a special threat to patients: the mould fungus known as *Aspergillus* and the yeast *Candida*.

Aspergillus, to which all of us are constantly exposed in our surroundings because of the omnipresent fungus spores, infects humans via the air passages. In patients with a deficient immune system, it most often attacks the lungs, where it can cause serious illness. The fungus can also spread via the bloodstream to other parts of the body. *Aspergillus* infection of the brain is greatly feared. It can result in abscesses or conditions resembling either a brain tumour or a common stroke, something that can confuse doctors and delay a correct diagnosis. The case fatality rate for *Aspergillus* infections is high, particularly with a cerebral infection, where it is more than 90 per cent. This is partly due to the diagnosis being made too late, and partly because the immune system of the patient is often badly weakened. In addition to this, our antifungal medicines are not as effective as we would like, even though considerable progress has been made within this field.

Candida means 'gleaming, white'. This might convey an impression of innocence and harmlessness, but there is no such innocence about this fungus once it has broken through the patient's immune system and spread via the bloodstream to most of the body's organs and tissues, as we see most dramatically in *Candida* infection. This type of fungus is also widespread in our surroundings. The sinister thing about this infection is that for a long time it only produces vague symptoms and signs, apart from a fever and general signs of a serious disease. Even though doctors make use of their most advanced methods of diagnosis, these do not always show what is taking place: that the fungus is peppering all tissues and organs with tiny abscesses that remain undetected. All too often the *Candida* diagnosis is not made until autopsy, for the infection is nearly always fatal without the proper treatment being administered as quickly as possible.

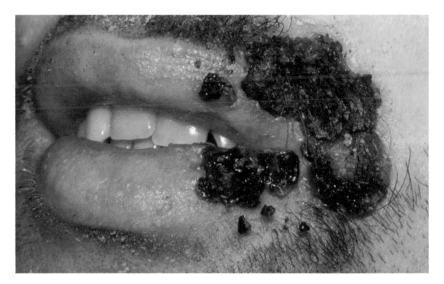

In the event of serious weakening of the immune system, the *Herpes simplex* virus, which normally only causes small cold sores in otherwise healthy individuals, can give rise to serious inflammatory conditions of the lips and round the mouth. Similar painful sores can also be seen round the anal orifice.

A third important fungal infection in patients with immune deficiency is the special pneumonia caused by *Pneumocystis jirovecii*, which also exists in our surroundings. It can be quite acute or develop stealthily over a period of time. If the diagnosis is not made early enough, something that requires special methods, a fatal outcome is the rule. There has actually been a striking increase in this otherwise uncommon form of pneumonia, which led to the discovery of the emerging AIDS epidemic in 1981.

Toxoplasma gondii, a special protozoon found in cats, can cause infection in humans with a normally functioning immune system, but normally without symptoms or in a mild form. In patients with a badly deficient immune system, however, it is a serious threat. Here it can cause many forms of serious infection, including encephalitis, which can resemble a brain tumour. Without treatment, this cerebral infection is fatal. Because of the risk of infection with *Toxoplasma*, patients with a badly functioning immune system should not keep cats.

Many viruses that are not normally a threat to humans with a healthy immune system can produce dramatic disease pictures if the system is working badly. This applies, for example, to the chickenpox virus, which normally causes a fairly harmless childhood disease with an itchy rash, but in the event of a deficient immune system can affect all organs and prove fatal. The related *herpes simplex* virus, which normally causes innocuous cold sores on the lips, or similar sores on the genitals, can in the event of a failure of the immune system produce deep sores that resemble cancer. Such sores are often seen around the anal orifice and in the oral cavity and throat. A relation, the CMV virus, infects most of us before adulthood, mostly without symptoms. If the immune system is not functioning properly, we see serious disease pictures, including inflammation with the formation of sores and bleeding in the intestines, pneumonia and inflammation of the retina that can lead to blindness.

These are just a few examples of the type of EIDs that have changed from rare curiosities of medicine a few decades ago to common challenges for the increasing number of patients with immune deficiency and for the doctors responsible for them. It is unnecessary to look to Africa and other developing regions to find dramatic and fatal infectious diseases. Our knowledge of these EIDs, however, has also increased considerably, so that to a much greater extent than before we are able to prevent, diagnose and treat them. Yet they still represent a considerable problem from both a medical point of view, since they are difficult to diagnose and treat, and an economic one, since many of the required forms of drug treatment are expensive.

Deadly Filament-like Viruses: Marburg and Ebola

In modern research laboratories monkeys are often used as experimental animals. That this is not hazard-free was graphically illustrated in 1967 at laboratories in Marburg (then in West Germany) and Belgrade (then in Yugoslavia).[10] These laboratories had just imported a number of monkeys from Uganda for experiments that were to include vaccines. Several of the monkeys died from an infection caused by a then unknown virus. The virus also attacked 25 humans who had been in contact with the monkeys, and these people infected a further six via direct contact. Seven of those infected died. The new virus was given the name Marburg virus. In the following years a couple of minor epidemics occurred, as well as several isolated cases of this infection in sub-Saharan Africa. The victims included both Africans and European and American tourists, who contracted a serious infection that has a case fatality rate of between 23 and 90 per cent. There are no effective drugs against the Marburg virus.

Many of those who were infected had been in caves with bats or had worked in gold mines. Intensive investigation of bats in these caves and mines revealed that in all probability a species of fruit-eating bat is the carrier of the virus, and that humans and monkeys are infected via direct contact with these bats or their excrement. Person-to-person infection can take place via blood and other body fluids, but in practice requires close physical contact.

The Marburg virus belongs to a special family of viruses that have a threadlike shape and are therefore known as filoviruses, from the Latin word for thread – *filum*. In this group we find a very close relative of the Marburg virus – the Ebola virus – which has many points of similarity as well as the same high mortality rate. This virus has been quite heavily publicized in recent years.

The Ebola virus has created considerably larger problems than its relative, despite being discovered nine years later.[11] In 1976 two epidemics broke out involving the virus in the northern part of Zaire (now Democratic Republic of the Congo) and in South Sudan, 850 kilometres away. In the first epidemic, 88 per cent of the 318 proven cases died, and in the second 54 per cent out of 284 cases. Blood from the patients was sent in a hurry to Western laboratories, which were quickly able to show that this was a new filovirus that strongly resembled the Marburg virus.

In the forty years or so that have passed since the discovery of the Ebola virus, which comes in several variants, we have seen more than twenty epidemic-like outbreaks in sub-Saharan Africa, particularly in Sudan, Uganda, the Congo and Gabon. Then a really major epidemic broke out in the West African countries of Guinea, Sierra Leone and Liberia in 2014. While the earlier epidemics had particularly hit the rural districts, the virus now also struck the major towns. More than 28,000 cases and over 11,000 deaths resulted before the epidemic died down in 2016. There were also sporadic cases in such neighbouring countries as Senegal, Nigeria and Mali. In 2018 a new epidemic broke out in the Congo, which has only recently been possible to stop. It also spread to the neighbouring country of Uganda.[12]

The epidemic of 2014–16 had serious consequences for a number of sectors, including agriculture, which almost came to a halt. The health service, which is not very highly developed in the countries involved, was paralysed, since most of the resources went to combatting the Ebola epidemic. This meant that almost as many patients died of such diseases as diabetes, tuberculosis and AIDS as of the Ebola virus.

The disease pictures of infection with Ebola and Marburg are quite similar.[13] Initially there is a high fever, nausea, muscular and stomach pains, vomiting and diarrhoea. After a few days a rash breaks out. After about a week many patients enter a state of shock, with a fall in blood pressure, and often with a tendency to bleed. From this stage the patient can either gradually recover or develop a fatal shutdown of all vital organs. The pathological picture is dramatic, but is also reminiscent of many other serious infectious diseases, such as malaria. At present we have no effective medication, although several promising medicines are being tested.

It is quite certain that the Ebola virus infection is also a zoonosis, but as yet we do not know for sure which animal species is the reservoir.

The Ebola virus seen through an electron microscope. The virus is filament-like in form and belongs to the filovirus group (*filum* = thread), to which its close relative the Marburg virus also belongs.

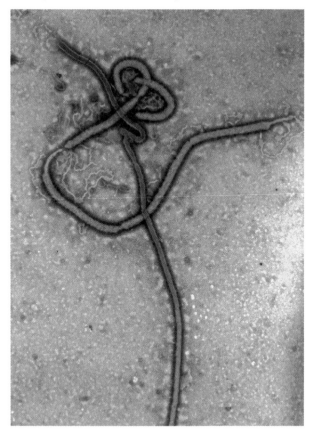

High up on the list of suspects is, however, the bat, although there is no direct evidence from any species of bat in nature to verify this.[14]

It has been shown that extensive deforestation has taken place in the two years preceding the majority of the epidemics in Central and West Africa.[15] Humans, monkeys and certain types of antelope can be attacked by the virus. In the time immediately prior to the outbreak of an epidemic, a large number of dead monkeys and gorillas, and occasionally also antelopes, have been found. This can be a useful warning of an imminent outbreak. An epidemic starts when humans come into contact with dead or sick animals, particularly monkeys, which are on the 'bush-meat' menu in Central Africa, or via contact with the host animal of the virus, probably bats. The virus then spreads from person to person via direct contact, when blood and other body fluids from patients come into contact with mucous membranes and sores in the skin of other individuals. Close physical contact is necessary for this to occur.

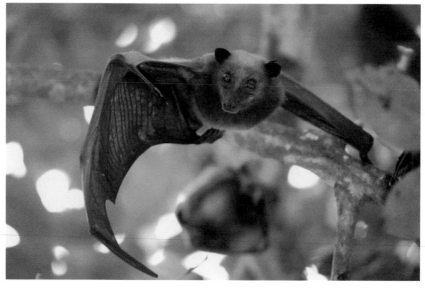

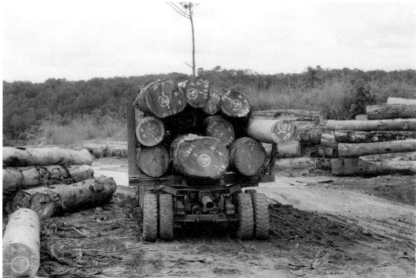

Top: Fruit-eating bats of the Pteropodidae family are assumed to be the reservoir of the Ebola virus. *Bottom*: Extensive felling of trees and deforestation have preceded most of the outbreaks of Ebola in Central and West Africa.

In the event of an epidemic, it is first and foremost family members and health personnel who have been exposed to infection, usually in cases where ordinary measures to prevent contagion have not been observed. Many African village communities have special burial rituals that require close contact between the deceased and members of the family, and this has resulted in a considerable risk of infection. The Ebola virus also continues to live for quite a long while in the semen of men who have recovered from the infection, and can then be transmitted via sexual contact. It has recently been shown that the virus can also stay alive for a long time in the eyes of survivors.[16]

Epidemics due to the Ebola virus have so far only been seen in Africa. The dramatic disease picture and high case fatality rate, however, have given rise to considerable fear that the virus could spread via international jet travel to other parts of the world. This has occurred in a few isolated cases in certain Western countries, including the USA, Spain and Norway. In Spain, a patient infected a nurse before the diagnosis had been made and measures were put in place to stop a further spread of the disease.

Fortunately, patients infected with the Ebola virus cannot infect others before the disease has broken out, and symptom-free patients

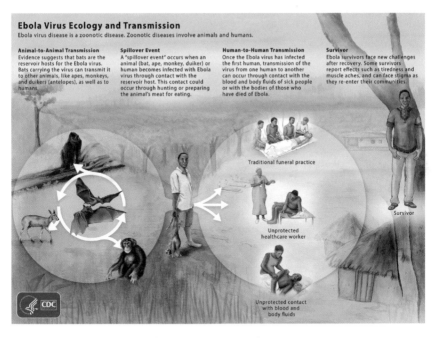

Ebola Virus Ecology and Transmission
Ebola virus disease is a zoonotic disease. Zoonotic diseases involve animals and humans.

Animal-to-Animal Transmission
Evidence suggests that bats are the reservoir hosts for the Ebola virus. Bats carrying the virus can transmit it to other animals, like apes, monkeys, and duikers (antelopes), as well as to humans.

Spillover Event
A "spillover event" occurs when an animal (bat, ape, monkey, duiker) or human becomes infected with Ebola virus through contact with the reservoir host. This contact could occur through hunting or preparing the animal's meat for eating.

Human-to-Human Transmission
Once the Ebola virus has infected the first human, transmission of the virus from one human to another can occur through contact with the blood and body fluids of sick people or with the bodies of those who have died of Ebola.

Survivor
Ebola survivors face new challenges after recovery. Some survivors report effects such as tiredness and muscle aches, and can face stigma as they re-enter their communities.

Traditional funeral practice

Survivor

Unprotected healthcare worker

Unprotected contact with blood and body fluids

CDC

The Ebola virus's paths of infection. The virus is found in a species of fruit-eating bat in Africa, and can also be transmitted to other animals, especially monkeys and gorillas and less frequently species of antelope. Humans can be infected via close contact with infected animals, for example, when hunting, preparing and consuming the meat ('bushmeat'). Person-to-person infection is possible via close contact. It has also taken place when injecting with infected syringes.

will thus not spread the infection, for example to other passengers on a flight. An infectious Ebola patient would be seriously ill and swift action would be taken to counter this. It is also obvious that regularly used measures to avoid contagion, such as isolating patients and using gloves and protective clothing, are extremely effective against the

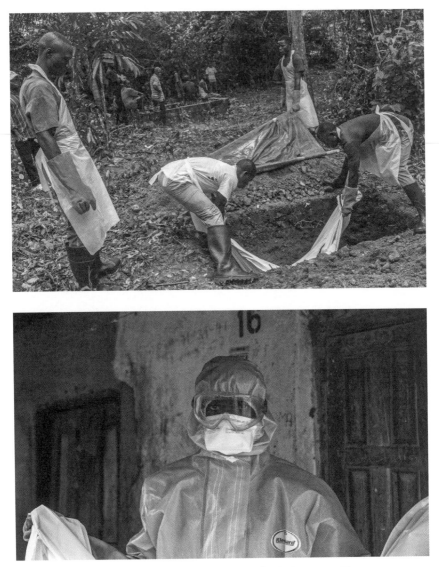

Top: Burial of a victim of the Ebola epidemic in Liberia in 2014, with necessary infection countermeasures observed. Traditional burials in the infected areas involve a considerable risk of infection, since direct physical contact with the deceased is part of the ritual. *Bottom*: Clothing worn to spray disinfectant outside the home of a victim of the Ebola virus in Sierra Leone in 2014.

virus, which therefore ought not to create major infection problems in a modern hospital.

The horrific disease picture of many of these infections has created fear and conspiracy theories both in the heart of Africa, where the epidemics have raged, and in Western countries, where the media have eagerly seized on the dramatic nature of the disease. In the areas of the epidemics, such reactions have led to stigmatization and discrimination against survivors of the infection, and, paradoxically, even physical attacks on health personnel involved in combatting the disease. The latter caused serious problems in the most recent epidemic. Irrational reactions, known as 'Ebolanoia', have also been seen in the USA towards people with links to West Africa in the wake of the 2014–16 epidemic. Grotesque examples of completely unmotivated fears of infection were seen.[17]

The Water Bacterium that Defeated Legionnaires

Hardly had the medical world recovered from the discovery of the Ebola virus than a new epidemic involving an unknown microbe created headlines in Western media. This time the outbreak was not deep in the jungle in a distant, exotic country but in the metropolis of Philadelphia in the USA.

In July 1976 Americans were celebrating the bicentenary of the Declaration of Independence. Military veterans of the American Legion organization, who called themselves legionnaires, had gathered for their annual meeting at four hotels in Philadelphia. An epidemic involving a severe form of pneumonia then broke out among the legionnaires and a number of other people in the same surroundings. A total of 221 people were affected, of which 34 died. It was soon clear that the epidemic was not due to any known causes of pneumonia.[18]

The epidemic in Philadelphia created quite a stir, including among politicians, leading to Congress setting up its own commission to deal with the problem. A group of researchers at the state-run Centers for Disease Control (CDC) hastily set about trying to find the cause of the disease. Conspiracy theories were rife in the media. Was some sort of poisoning involved? Was it perhaps a terrorist attack? After six months of intensive detective work, the researchers managed to identify the cause. It proved to be a previously unknown bacterium, given the name *Legionella pneumophila*, after the American Legion. The discovery of this bacterium also shed light on a number of former unexplained epidemics involving pneumonia that stretched all the way back to the 1950s. Examinations of preserved samples of blood and tissue from these epidemics revealed Legionella bacteria.[19]

Legionella pneumophila belongs to a family with many other Legionella species, of which at least thirty can also cause pneumonia, with *L. pneumophila* the most usual cause. Occasionally these bacteria also cause epidemics resulting in a fairly harmless high temperature that lasts a few days, known as Pontiac fever.[20]

The Legionella disease is an example of an infection that has become a problem as a result of human technological advances, in this instance modern hydro-technology. The bacteria exist in water, and are widespread in the fresh water of lakes and rivers. They thrive best at temperatures between 25°C and 40°C. It is hardly surprising that they have invaded the many forms of water systems of modern hydro-technology: cooling towers that are part of air-conditioning systems, hot-water cisterns, humidifiers and many other devices. Humans become infected with Legionella bacteria when conditions suit the formation of aerosols of polluted water in the air. This can take place with cooling towers and jacuzzis, when taking a shower, tapping spring water and with indoor fountains. Infection is due to the inhalation of Legionella-carrying aerosol particles that settle in the lungs. Patients with chronic pulmonary illnesses, smokers and elderly people are particularly susceptible, as are patients with weakened immune systems because of treatment with immuno-suppressive drugs.

The risk of Legionella infection has led to clear regulations for preventative measures and maintenance of the various water systems on which modern societies are utterly dependent, with purification and control of the water temperature. In spite of this, Legionella infections would seem to be on the increase in Western countries.[21]

The Most Frightening Pandemic of Recent Times: HIV

In December 1980 a young man was admitted to the UCLA Medical Center in Los Angeles with a strange disease. His oesophagus was almost completely blocked by an inflammation caused by the yeast fungus *Candida*, and in the course of the next few days he contracted a violent double pneumonia from the fungus *Pneumocystis jirovecii*, followed by other serious infection-related complications. He died the following March. The striking thing was that the infections that struck him down were so-called opportunist infections, which are normally only seen in patients with a serious weakening of the immune system. But this patient had been completely healthy, without any disease or treatment that can lead to immune deficiency.

During the following months, increasing numbers of similar patients appeared, both on the West Coast of the USA and the East.[22] All of them had been healthy before developing signs of immune deficiency. They did, however, have one thing in common: they were either homosexuals or bisexuals who moved in circles where widespread sexual activity

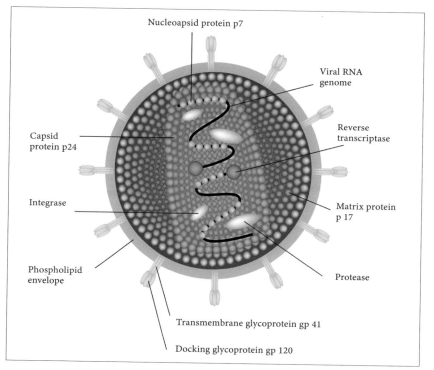

Nucleoapsid protein p7

Viral RNA genome

Capsid protein p24

Reverse transcriptase

Integrase

Matrix protein p 17

Phospholipid envelope

Protease

Transmembrane glycoprotein gp 41

Docking glycoprotein gp 120

The structure of the HIV virus (highly simplified). The virus has a surface membrane of lipids with 'spikes' of glycoprotein (gp 120), which stick out and are necessary for the virus to be able to penetrate the CD4⁺ T cells. The virus also has a sort of nucleus – the capsid – which contains the genetic material in the form of two strands of RNA. In the capsid there are also enzymes that are essential for the capacity of the virus to infect the CD4⁺ T cells.

was the rule, often with a great many partners over a relatively short period of time.

This strange and frightening epidemic naturally caused a considerable stir. The media announced, with its usual predilection for sensational headlines, that a 'gay plague' was now spreading across the USA. This was the beginning of what was to develop into the most serious and most extensive pandemic of recent times.

It quickly became obvious that the term 'gay plague' was not broad enough. In just a short time it was apparent that the disease did not only affect homosexual and bisexual men but patients with serious congenital bleeding disorders (haemophilia), immigrants to the USA from Haiti, drug addicts and female partners of men with the new disease. Even young children were affected.

American researchers quickly confirmed that patients with the new disease really had a serious weakening of the immune system, one that had a special pattern. The patients had developed a failure of the immune system's T-lymphocytes, mainly because a great many of the CD4$^+$ T lymphocytes had been destroyed, the central type of cell in the defence against infection.[23]

The disease was given the name AIDS, an acronym for 'acquired immuno-deficiency syndrome', since it had emerged in formerly healthy people and was not congenital. In fact, AIDS was an umbrella term for the most serious forms of the new disease. These cases had certain serious immuno-deficiency complications, which were laid out on an official list containing both a number of infectious diseases that mainly affect patients with immuno-deficiency and also special cancers that are often seen in such patients.

It was soon evident that the disease picture called AIDS was only the tip of the iceberg. A number of milder pictures existed in the same groups affected by the new epidemic and they were probably related to AIDS. These conditions very often subsequently developed into AIDS.

Why had this immune deficiency arisen in these groups of patients? What had affected precisely the CD4$^+$ T lymphocytes, the very conductor of the immunological orchestra? Uncertainty concerning the cause of this horrific new disease led to an enormous fear in large sections of the population, and to an extreme degree in the special risk groups it singled out. A great many theories about the cause of AIDS were advanced, from quite rational, medical hypotheses to the most absurd conspiracy theories.

Was it a microbe from outer space, such as the Andromeda virus in the disaster film *The Andromeda Strain* (1971, dir. Robert Wise), based on a thriller by the American author Michael Crichton?[24] Was it a microbe that had 'leaked' from a military medical laboratory working on biological weapons? Supporters of this theory believed in an American or a Soviet source, depending on their political views. In the sensational press, the focus was on the occurrence of AIDS in immigrants from Haiti, the implication being that there was some sort of connection with secret voodoo rituals.

Some people thought that the special, emancipated lifestyle of homosexual environments was the explanation, either as a form of divine punishment for leading a sinful life, or perhaps because intensive sexual activity, partly in unusual forms, and with the very frequent appearance of sexual diseases, quite simply exhausted the immune system. Some researchers believed that special sexually stimulating substances, so-called poppers which were popular in homosexual environments, were the cause of immuno-deficiency in the case of AIDS.[25]

The serious debate was, however, dominated by the belief that AIDS had to be an infectious disease. Some people suggested that the cause could be an already known virus that had mutated and become more 'malign'. Gradually an increasing number of researchers, however, became convinced that the cause of AIDS had to be a previously unknown microbe, probably a virus.

American health authorities during this period carried out intensive work with an expert team of 'infection detectives', who mapped out all factors of possible importance in patients and the groups particularly affected. These efforts led to a strong suspicion developing as early as the end of 1982 that it was a question of an infectious disease that was transmitted via sexual contact or via blood.

But what kind of microbe could it be? After intensive work in both American and French laboratories, the breakthrough came in 1983–4. It turned out that the cause of AIDS was a previously unknown virus that belonged to a special group of viruses, the so-called retroviruses, which are strongly represented in the animal world.[26] The means of infection for this virus were quickly mapped:

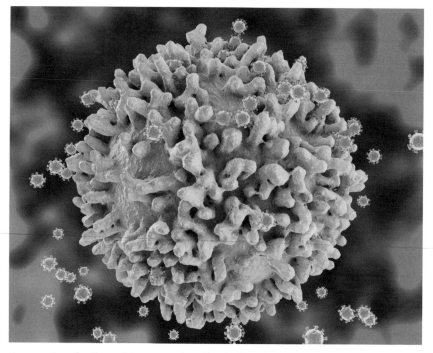

An HIV virus (red) attacking a CD4⁺ T cell, which is the central coordinator cell in the immune system. This is the starting point of an HIV infection and its later possible development of full-blown AIDS.

- Transmission via sexual contact, with intercourse in one or other form
- Transmission via blood or blood products, including the sharing of syringes
- Transmission from mother to child, either before birth or via breast milk

A virus can only live and reproduce inside living cells. To be able to penetrate cells, a virus must first latch on to a molecule on the cell surface that can function as a 'door-opener' for the virus.[27] These molecular 'door-openers' vary from virus to virus. The tragedy with the AIDS virus is that the 'door-opener' happens to be a molecule that is special for perhaps the most important cell in the immune system: the CD4⁺ T lymphocyte. When the AIDS virus penetrates this cell and reproduces, the cell dies. More and more of these cells are gradually destroyed, and the immune system is unable to manage to replace them. This results in a life-threatening breakdown of the immune system that normally takes several years to develop. For a long time the patient is without symptoms or has only very mild signs of disease, such as various forms of rash and swollen lymph nodes, but they are infectious from the outset.

The story behind the dramatic appearance of the AIDS virus in 1981 and its later spread to the entire world illustrates a great many of the ecological and environment-related factors that are so important in the duel between man and microbe. The AIDS virus was originally the result of a zoonosis, the origins being various species of Central African apes: monkeys, gorillas and the less common sooty mangabey. These ape species are carriers of retrovirus types that are closely related to the human AIDS virus. We estimate that contact between humans and apes has led to the original virus 'jumping across' to humans. This has particularly occurred when monkey meat is hunted as 'bushmeat', which leads to close contact with the blood of these animals. After probably many unsuccessful attempts, an ape virus managed to adapt to its new human host and changed into the AIDS virus, which is specific to humans. Molecular-biological examinations of various viruses indicate that this process probably took place on several occasions between 1900

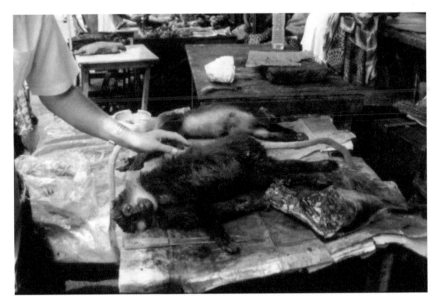

'Bushmeat', the meat of wild animals, is popular in many African countries. The animals can be carriers of dangerous microbes that can cause zoonoses. Such meat, from such animals as monkeys and bats, can represent an infection risk for both hunters who prepare the meat and those who eat it.

and 1910 and over the succeeding decades. AIDS is actually a quite new virus in the world.[28]

In fact, we are not dealing with just one virus, as there are two main forms that are quite dissimilar: HIV-1, which is the overwhelming cause of the AIDS pandemic, and HIV-2, which is almost completely confined to West Africa and would seem to be on the retreat. This virus produces a course of the disease that is slower and less serious than that we see with HIV-1. The latter derives from a chimpanzee or gorilla, whereas HIV-2 derives from the smaller monkey, the sooty mangabey. In the following, the term 'AIDS virus' refers to HIV-1.[29]

AIDS arose in the western part of Central Africa, in Cameroon and the neighbouring countries. From there it spread via heterosexual contact in the 1970s, first to countries in East Africa and then on to southern Africa and West Africa. Crucial to the rapid spread of the disease were the major socio-cultural and political upheavals that took place in Africa after the withdrawal of the colonial powers. This resulted in large migrations and considerable immigration to the rapidly growing cities, with a marked increase in prostitution, which led to many women being infected with AIDS. Much of the spread of the virus took place in groups of mobile men, seasonal labourers who commuted between urban societies and their homes out in the rural villages, long-distance drivers on the newly laid-out highways and military personnel who moved during the many wars that flourished in Africa during this period. Other cultural conditions also contributed to the spread of the virus: widespread promiscuity among many men, the subordinate role of the women in sexual relations, limited use of condoms and a great frequency of various sexual diseases that we know increase both infectiousness and susceptibility to HIV infection.[30]

When did the AIDS virus spread beyond Africa? This probably happened on several occasions via individual virus carriers (and also some from Western countries who had been infected in Africa) without this starting further dissemination. The first well-documented case of AIDS that I have personally described was that of a young Norwegian sailor who was sexually infected in Cameroon during the first half of the 1960s. He brought the virus home with him to Norway, where he transmitted it to his wife, who in turn infected a daughter. All three died of AIDS in 1976.[31] As far as we know, the virus did not spread outside the family. The virus in these cases was the HIV-1 variety, but a rare group mostly found in Cameroon.[32]

Another case of the export of HIV from Africa in the 1960s, however, did have serious consequences and probably set in motion the global epidemic. Comprehensive epidemiological detective work strongly suggests that a person from Haiti who had visited Africa brought HIV with him back to Haiti, where it quickly spread, first via sexual contact, but perhaps also in some other way. The Canadian researcher Jacques Pépin thinks there are reasons to believe that the spread of the virus in Haiti was also via the commercial production of blood plasma for export, under the regime of Haiti's brutal dictator François Duvalier ('Papa Doc'). Either way, the HIV epidemic was in full swing on Haiti by the 1970s.[33]

With its tropical climate and idyllic nature, Haiti was a favourite holiday destination for homosexual men, particularly from the USA. This led to a mushrooming of homosexual prostitution on the poverty-stricken island. Sex tourism brought the virus home to the gay environments in the USA, where the HIV epidemic then exploded and was 'discovered' by the health authorities in 1981. The intermediate station on Haiti on the path from Africa naturally explains the appearance of the virus among immigrants to the USA from this island – it was not sinister voodoo rituals that underlay the HIV frequency among these immigrants.

The virus rapidly spread from the USA to Europe and the other inhabited parts of the world. This also applied to Scandinavia. I was personally called on to make the diagnosis of Norway's first AIDS patient in my ward at the State Hospital in January 1983. This was a young homosexual man who had been infected in Copenhagen, where he had lived for a number of years. He was hit by serious complications resulting from a breakdown of the immune system and died in November that same year.[34] The virus was also directly imported from Africa to European countries such as France and Belgium by Africans from their former colonies.

In addition to sexual transmission (both homosexual and heterosexual), infection of the blood from syringes shared by drug addicts played an important role in Western countries. During the first few years, the virus also spread in the health service via transfusion of blood and plasma and the treatment with blood products of patients with congenital haemophilia. From the mid-1980s onwards all Western countries had almost completely eradicated this form of transmission through various measures, mainly by thoroughly testing all blood donors for HIV.

After the HIV virus had been discovered and the transmission mechanisms fairly rapidly detected, one might perhaps think that the enormous uncertainty and fear that had previously characterized people's attitudes to the AIDS epidemic would diminish. However, there now arose a widespread, often extreme, fear of being infected, which, both inside and outside the health service, could assume quite grotesque dimensions. In some cases health staff refused to shake hands with AIDS patients and dressed up in almost astronaut-like costumes when it was necessary to have contact with patients. This fear of being infected, ably assisted by hysteria in the media, whipped up a heated debate throughout the Western world about the measures that ought to be adopted to combat the epidemic, which had now become a pandemic. Doomsday prophets announced that this pandemic would bring about the end of human civilization.

Most Western countries have long since managed to stop the explosive spread of the HIV virus that was typical of the first years of the pandemic. This, unfortunately, does not apply to all parts of the world. The virus still rages in sub-Saharan Africa. There are also considerable problems in certain countries of Eastern Europe and Asia. Until now, 35 million people have lost their lives as a result of HIV infection, and almost 1 million still die annually. It is estimated that 37 million people in the world live with the infection.

This pandemic has had considerable consequences for social life, medical research and ethical thinking. And there can be no doubt that it was the AIDS epidemic that put an end to the far too widely held conviction that infectious diseases and epidemics no longer threaten present-day humanity.

Bats: Nocturnal Virus Carriers

The majority of the EIDS are zoonoses, like the HIV infection, where monkeys were the source. A much greater number of the new infections, however, originally come from other animals, including bats.[35]

Bats have always had a sinister reputation in popular superstition and literature. These soundless, nocturnal creatures often appear in such accounts in the company of witches, magicians and demons. The fact that blood-sucking bats exist in certain locations in the world also creates disturbing associations with vampires and the Dracula legend.

But are bats, of which there are more than 1,200 species in the world, generally speaking harmless creatures? Have they been given bad press? Well, we ought to disregard any connection between them and super-natural powers. Nevertheless, recent research has revealed that it is precisely bats that seem to play an important role as reservoirs for a whole range of viruses. Many of these can attack human beings and give rise to life-threatening diseases if the conditions for infection are present. A number of the EIDs have illustrated quite convincingly the important role the bat can play as a carrier of virus.

It has been known for many years that blood-sucking bats, which are admittedly not found in Europe, can carry the virus that can cause the terrible disease rabies, and that they can infect humans by sucking their blood. We have no effective treatment against this infection. The well-known rabies virus that belongs to a group called lyssa viruses has not been detected in bats outside the Americas, but there are other types of lyssa virus that *can* produce infection in humans.[36] This also

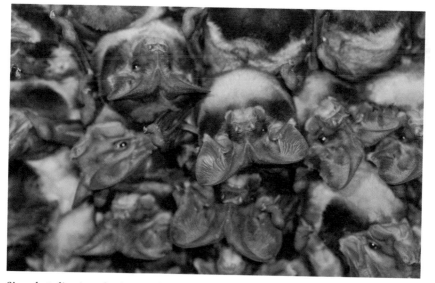

Since bats live in colonies numbering in the millions, the conditions for the spread of a virus to all the individuals in such a colony are highly favourable.

applies to Europe. Until now, we know of only two cases in Europe of humans being infected by these lyssa viruses: both proved fatal.

As mentioned earlier, the bat is the reservoir for the Marburg virus, and this is probably also true of the Ebola virus. Even though epidemics with Ebola virus have, until now, only occurred in Africa, there are reasons to be worried, since viruses similar to Ebola have recently been discovered in bats in Europe. Bats are also the reservoir for several recently discovered viruses that have caused serious infections, and even epidemics – the Hendra, Nipah, SARS and MERS viruses – which we shall look at presently.[37]

We do not yet know why bats are so well suited to be reservoirs for viruses, since they are difficult to study in the laboratory. In most cases where they are carriers of a virus, they do not fall sick themselves. This may be an example of 'peaceful coexistence', the result of millions of years of evolutionary adaptation, one that does not make the immune system of bats attack and destroy the viruses.[38] The relatively long lifespan of bats (up to thirty years), along with their special social life, also makes them highly effective reservoirs. They are very sociable animals that live close together in large colonies, which can comprise several million individuals in such habitats as caves and mine galleries. The conditions for the spread of a virus to all these individuals in such a colony are therefore highly favourable. Bats can also move with their virus stowaways over large distances and spread infection in that way. How does the transmission of a virus from a bat to a human take place? Experience gained from EIDS, among other diseases, has shed some light on this.

Hendra virus, horses and flying foxes

In autumn 1994 something broke out that looked like the start of an epidemic in a stable for race horses in Hendra, a suburb of Brisbane in Queensland, Australia. Within a short time, 21 horses died after being ill for a few days. Two people who cared for the horses were also struck down: one of them died, the other survived. At the autopsy of the horses, a previously unknown virus was discovered. Since it had certain points of similarity with the well-known measles virus, it was initially known as equine morbilli virus (equine measles virus). The name was quickly changed to Hendra virus after the place of origin. The two people were probably infected by the horses, but how had the horses been infected, and where had the virus come from?[39]

After a thorough examination of a number of suspected animals in the local area, it was discovered that the virus probably came from flying foxes, large fruit bats with a wingspan of approximately 1 metre. The horses had probably been infected when they sought shade from the strong sun under particular trees where the flying foxes roosted. Urine and excrement containing the virus had dripped down onto the grass, which was subsequently eaten by the horses. The humans had then been infected from the saliva and other body fluids from the sick horses.

There have since then been more than fifty outbreaks of Hendra virus among horses, with a case fatality rate of 75 per cent. To date there have been only seven cases among humans, all of them infected by horses: about half of them died. So this is a very rare infection indeed, but it illustrates how bats can infect humans via an intermediary host (in this case, horses).

Nipah virus, pigs and flying foxes

In 1998 a new virus struck that proved to be related to the Hendra virus. Known as the Nipah virus, this has proved to be considerably more problematic than its Australian cousin.[40]

The Nipah virus first appeared in western Malaysia, where an epidemic broke out on Chinese pig farms. Of the 257 people who fell acutely ill with a high temperature and signs of encephalitis and, in certain cases, pneumonia, 105 died. At the same time an epidemic with the same virus raged among the pigs, who developed a respiratory tract infection with a high mortality.

Apparently the humans had been infected by the pigs. Malays and Chinese are the most important ethnic groups in Malaysia. It was striking that there were no cases of the disease in neighbouring Malay villages. The explanation for this is that the Malays, who are Muslims, do not have any contact with pigs or pig products. Shortly afterwards there were several cases in Singapore among slaughterhouse workers who were in contact with pigs imported from Malaysia. The pigs had clearly brought the virus with them. This first epidemic led to the slaughter of a million pigs on the affected pig farms in Malaysia, which was a severe blow to the industry.

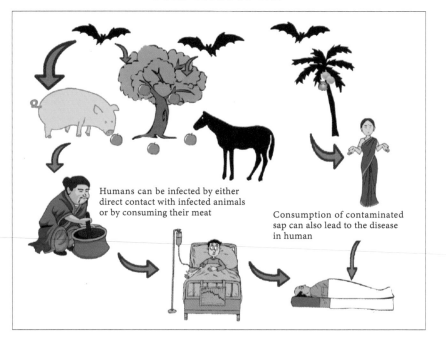

Humans can be infected by either direct contact with infected animals or by consuming their meat

Consumption of contaminated sap can also lead to the disease in human

Humans can be infected either by direct contact with infected animals, or by eating infected animals. The consumption of polluted fruit juice can also lead to humans contracting the disease. The Nipah virus is found in certain species of large fruit bats in Asia. Several other species of animals can be infected from bats. Humans can then be infected from these animals, or directly from bats via polluted fruit juice. Person-to-person infection also takes place, probably as a droplet infection.

As early as March 1999 the virus responsible was discovered and given the name Nipah virus, after the place where the actual patient test samples were from. Later on, new epidemics caused by the virus broke out in Malaysia, Bangladesh, India and the Philippines. The case fatality rate has stayed around 50 per cent, mainly caused by encephalitis, which is the most serious form of the disease.

It was quite quickly demonstrated that the reservoir for this newly discovered virus, as with its cousin the Hendra virus, was among flying foxes. These fruit bats are dogged flyers and can cover distances of hundreds of kilometres. On the basis of the first epidemic in Malaysia, it is believed that it was extensive changes to the climate in Indonesia, linked to El Niño disturbances, that made it impossible for the animals to stay in their accustomed habitat. The bats moved to Malaysia, where they often settled in clusters of trees close to pig farms. The pigs then became contaminated via urine, excrement and spit from the infected bats, which dripped down onto their food. But the virus can also be transmitted to humans from bats in other ways. A favourite drink in Bangladesh is a juice made from date palm bark, which is also popular with bats. The transmission of infection to humans has often taken place when half-eaten bark, polluted by bats, has been used in the production of juice.[41]

A disturbing characteristic of the Nipah virus is that it can infect other animals apart from pigs and humans, including dogs, cats and horses. In the epidemic in the Philippines, it is believed that transmission of the virus to humans came via horses, either through direct contact or from eating horse meat. We must therefore assume that various species of animals, apart from bats, can play a role in infecting humans. Most disturbing of all, however, is that this virus can also be transmitted from person to person, probably by droplets from the air passages. In some of the epidemics, up to half of the cases of infection took place in this way. So it is possible that we can get large-scale epidemics caused by the Nipah virus, mainly in countries with a poorly developed health service where conditions are ideal for the virus.[42]

So far, we have not seen any signs of an imminent pandemic from the Nipah virus. But we have experienced a threat from another formerly unknown virus, the SARS virus.

SARS: *the first pandemic threat of the twenty-first century*

This global epidemic broke out in the Guangdong province of China in autumn 2002. The first person to realize that a new epidemic was in progress was the Italian microbiologist Carlo Urbani, who was working in Hanoi, Vietnam, at the local division of WHO. He had formerly worked for the organization Médecins Sans Frontières, and was among the members who received the Nobel Peace Prize awarded to the organization in Oslo in 1999. In early 2003 Urbani was called in to a local hospital to assess a patient who seemed to be suffering from 'serious influenza'. Special symptoms caused him to suspect that he was looking at a new infectious disease, and he began a series of countermeasures and warned the WHO. The infection, however, had already spread to other health workers within the hospital environment. The patient died, and Urbani himself became infected and died shortly afterwards.[43]

Urbani's patient was a Chinese-American businessman who had recently stayed at a hotel in Hong Kong, where he had been infected by a Chinese doctor on the same floor. This doctor had recently treated patients with pneumonia in Guangdong in China. In the space of 24 hours, he infected sixteen other patients before falling ill and being admitted to hospital. These other patients, oblivious to what had happened, boarded various planes and spread the new microbe to Canada, Vietnam, Singapore and Taiwan. In addition to Guangdong province, these were the areas worst affected, but a total of 26 countries made the acquaintance of the new infectious disease, a frightening demonstration of how easily infectious diseases can spread via modern air traffic.[44] It was especially hospital staff treating patients who were hit. This was partly because the patients were not infectious until serious illness led them to the health service, and partly because the necessary measures against infection by droplets and aerosols were not applied quickly enough. The staff then spread the infection further to others. Pneumonia was the key disease found with SARS.

The SARS epidemic is actually an excellent example of how a coordinated international effort of preventative measures and research efforts can be crucial to halting the menace of a pandemic. The WHO, under Gro Harlem Brundtland's leadership, played an important role here. As early as March 2003 the WHO issued an international warning about the threat, followed shortly afterwards by concrete travel advice for international travellers. The WHO very rarely provides such advice in the event of epidemics.[45]

By the end of March 2003 the WHO was able to announce that the cause of the epidemic had been found, a new virus that gave rise to life-threatening pneumonia to which the name SARS (severe acute respiratory syndrome) had been given. The virus that is the cause of the disease belongs to a group of viruses known as coronaviruses, several other members of which can cause infection in humans. The SARS virus is now correctly called SARS-CoV-1.

The international effort that followed, which included introducing ways of swiftly identifying new cases and isolating patients, led to no new cases occurring after July 2003: the epidemic, which could have turned into a serious pandemic, had been halted. By then 8,096 cases of SARS had been discovered and 774 of these patients (nearly 10 per cent) had died.[46]

Where did the SARS virus come from? The Chinese, compared to Europeans, are unusually omnivorous when it comes to animals. A great many animal species are on the menu, and at Chinese markets there is also a wide selection of wild species that end up in restaurants and private households. Many of the early cases of SARS in Guangdong province were among workers at the animal markets and restaurants, which made people suspect that the virus could come from the many species of animals on offer. And the virus was indeed discovered in a number of the species at the markets. Quickly, however, interest began to focus on the civet, a small predator that looks like a long-nosed cat.

These animals are extremely popular as food and are richly represented at the markets and on restaurant menus. At first it was believed that this species was the reservoir of the SARS virus, and widespread culling of the animals was initiated. Then doubts arose and interest was concentrated on bats, in which many newly discovered viral infections had been detected. It turned out that bats were also a reservoir of the SARS virus. The civets and other species had probably been infected via urine and excrement from the bats. In addition, the animals at the markets were able to infect each other.[47]

Humans mainly infect each other with this virus via droplet infection, but transmission via airborne aerosols can also occur, especially in hospitals.[48] A few cases of SARS were later reported in China, but there has been no known epidemic. The reservoir in the bats, however, continues to exist and new epidemic outbreaks of the virus are absolutely a possibility.

MERS, camels and bats

In 2012 a man in Saudi Arabia died from a respiratory infection caused by a then unknown microbe. This was to prove the beginning of a new epidemic, with the infectious disease being given the name MERS, an acronym for Middle East Respiratory Syndrome. It was often fatal and proved to have been caused by an unknown virus of the coronavirus group, to which SARS also belongs. The two viruses produce similar disease pictures, with a serious pulmonary disease, and both are zoonoses.[49]

So far 2,494 cases of MERS have been confirmed, of which 858 (35 per cent) had a fatal outcome. The case fatality rate is probably lower, for there could have been cases of infection that are either without or with fairly mild symptoms of a respiratory disease. The great majority of cases of MERS have been in Saudi Arabia, with some cases in the neighbouring states in the Arabian Peninsula. Several countries in the world have had individual cases, resulting from travellers from these countries.[50]

Transmission of the MERS virus requires quite close contact. Some of the cases have been within families, but infection has mainly taken place in hospitals where adequate measures against transmission from patients have not been observed. Both health personnel and other hospital patients have been infected. Imported cases in other countries have not given rise to epidemics, with the exception of a MERS epidemic that broke out in South Korea in 2015, with 186 cases and 36 deaths. The virus had been imported from the Middle East. The epidemic was almost completely confined to patients in hospital.[51]

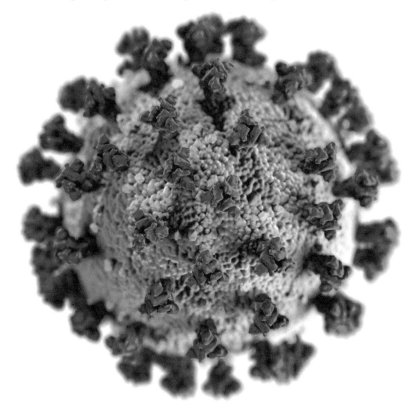

The large number of viruses known as coronaviruses includes SARS virus and MERS virus as well as the recently discovered SARS-CoV-2, shown here. The term 'coronavirus' is used since the virus particles under the electron microscope seem to have a kind of fringed edge around them that is reminiscent of what astronomers call the sun's corona (crown).

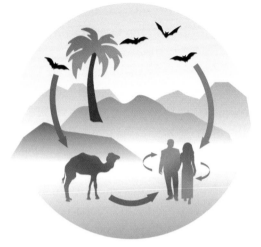

The paths of transmission of the newly discovered MERS virus, which probably comes from bats, which are the original reservoir. Dromedaries are then infected by the bats and become a new reservoir for the virus. Humans are in turn infected by the dromedaries. Interhuman infection is also possible to a certain extent.

It has been proved that dromedaries are the animal reservoir for the MERS virus. Infection with the virus is common in dromedaries both in the Arabian Peninsula and Africa. The animals display no or only light symptoms of a respiratory infection. People in close contact with these animals become infected and spread the disease further. How can dromedaries have been infected? Once again it would seem that bats are in the dock. In various species of bat coronavirus has been detected that is extremely similar to the MERS virus. Although conclusive proof is still lacking, we can therefore assume that the virus at some point has jumped from bats to dromedaries, which have become the main reservoir.[52]

MERS, then, is not particularly infectious. Apart from preferably avoiding too close contact with dromedaries, this disease therefore does not have to lead to special travel restrictions for the Arabian Peninsula. Even so, one cannot completely exclude the possibility that the virus might mutate, making person-to-person contamination more efficient. In that case, a situation could arise similar to the SARS epidemic.

Of Mice and Men

While bats have only recently come into focus as reservoirs for viruses that threaten humans, rodents of various kinds have been recognized as carriers of microbes for many years, including a fairly large number of viruses that have rather sinister characteristics. A number of them have given rise to new or recently discovered infectious diseases in human beings and in some cases also to major epidemics.

In 1969 three female nurses at Adam Mission Hospital in Nigeria developed a serious disease, one after the other. The third patient was transported to the USA, where it was discovered that the cause of the disease was a then unknown virus, which was given the name Lassa virus after the place where the first patients had fallen ill.[53]

The Lassa virus had probably been active in West Africa for many years before it was discovered. Infections with the virus are quite common in Nigeria, Liberia, Sierra Leone and Guinea and also occur in neighbouring countries. We do not have any reliable statistics, but certain surveys indicate that there may be several hundred thousand cases every year and perhaps 5,000 deaths.[54] The incidence of infection has steadily increased in recent years. In 2018 Lassa fever caused an extensive epidemic in Nigeria, and the health authorities declared a state of emergency with various quarantine measures.[55]

The virus can cause a wide spectrum of disease pictures, ranging from fairly mild fever to a life-threatening disease attacking many organs and causing pronounced haemorrhages, as with other conditions to which we give the overall name haemorrhagic fevers. For those with serious conditions who become hospitalized, the case fatality rate with Lassa fever is at least 20 per cent and can even reach 50 per cent during epidemics. In total, it is estimated that the case fatality rate is only 1 per cent for all types of infection. Some of those who survive develop chronic deafness.

Lassa fever is also a zoonosis. The animal reservoir for this virus is a particular species of mouse, *Mastomys natalensis*, which is extremely common in West Africa and likes to be close to humans and inside houses. Humans become infected by contact with food or objects polluted by excrement or urine from the mice. The size of the mouse population varies a great deal according to changes in climate, and plays an important role in the frequency of Lassa fever. Person-to-person infection by direct contact can also occur. This has often taken place in hospitals with the infection of health personnel when countermeasures have not been used.[56]

Since the discovery of the Lassa virus, there has been a constant fear of it spreading to areas outside Africa as a result of today's worldwide flight connections. So far this has not taken place to any extent that has given cause for concern, but the possibility is always present.

The Lassa virus belongs to a major group of viruses known as Arena viruses. In this group we also find other representatives that can cause serious infections in humans. This includes viruses that cause South American haemorrhagic fever. The best known of these are the Argentinian Junin virus, the Bolivian Machupo virus and the Venezuelan Guanarito virus, discovered in 1955, 1959 and 1989, respectively. All these have species of mice as the animal reservoir, and humans are infected via contact with the urine or excrement of the animals or via direct contact. These forms of haemorrhagic fever are examples of infection problems that follow human-made changes to nature by deforestation and the expansion of agriculture, which leads to increased contact with animals and the risk of new zoonoses.

These viruses mainly create local problems and have not displayed any tendencies to spread widely outside the core areas.[57]

Viruses and Mosquitoes: An Increasing Threat

Yellow fever was the first viral infection where it was discovered that the virus made use of mosquitoes as carriers from animals to humans. This has later proved to be quite common in the world of viruses. A number of viruses that today are worldwide threats to health are transmitted in this way, among others two viruses related to the yellow fever virus: the West Nile fever virus and Zika virus. Both have been very much on the advance in the world in recent years and they illustrate many factors behind EIDs.

West Nile fever: transmitted via mosquitoes and birds

This virus was discovered for the first time in Uganda in 1937. During the following decades there were certain individual cases of infection, and some small-scale epidemics in Africa and parts of Western Asia and Southern Europe. On the whole, it was a fairly mild fever that lasted for a few days. From the mid-1990s the virus caused outbreaks in which a number of patients also developed encephalitis with a certain mortality.[58]

It caused quite a stir in 1999 when New York was hit by an epidemic with several instances of encephalitis. The cause was West Nile fever after the virus had reached the Americas. Since then the virus has gained a stronghold in North America and has given rise to several major epidemics there.

West Nile fever is also a zoonosis. The reservoir of the virus in Africa is a large number of bird species, where the virus is effectively spread via certain types of mosquito that are not all that choosy about where they get their blood from. Some of these species get their blood from infected birds, after which they begin to suck blood from humans and thereby transmit the virus. For the virus humans represent a blind alley, for it cannot then be spread from person to person since the amount of virus in the blood is too small for further transportation via mosquito after blood-sucking.

About 80 per cent of infected humans remain completely without symptoms after being infected with the West Nile fever virus, while 20 per cent have a light fever that lasts for a few days. But in just under 1 per cent of cases the virus attacks the brain and the spinal cord. This results in cerebrospinal meningitis, encephalitis or a disease resembling poliomyelitis with paralysis. In such cases the mortality is approximately 15 per cent, and half of the survivors will have chronic neurological symptoms, such as paralysis.[59]

How does the virus spread, even managing to cross the world's oceans? Here birds play an important role as carriers of the virus. The West Nile fever virus is now a common disease in southern Europe, where we have seen a number of major epidemics in recent years. Migratory birds from Africa probably continue to import the virus to Europe, where local species of mosquito infect the bird population, as in Africa. Other local species of mosquito form a bridge between infected birds and humans.[60]

This virus is highly adaptable and does not only depend on mosquitoes. It can also be transmitted via blood transfusions and organ transplants, and even via breast milk.[61]

The virus may have come to New York in 1999 with a single bird from the Old World that had perhaps been blown off course by a storm. Alternatively, an infected mosquito may have been a stowaway on a plane, something we know has happened with other mosquito-borne infections such as malaria. Several hundred species of American mosquito received the virus with what might be called open arms after its arrival in North America, and a whole series of species of bird were subsequently also infected by the virus. These bird species then became a permanent reservoir for the virus, and certain ones become ill and die. This applies for example to crows, which often die in great numbers in the period leading up to an epidemic, something which can provide an important advance warning. Occasionally the birds simply fall down dead from the sky at such a time.[62]

Landscape conditions and climate play an important role in the spread of the West Nile virus. Inside Europe, large wetland areas with teeming birdlife and mosquitoes are a common habitat and starting point for epidemics involving this virus. This applies, for example, to the popular tourist area of the Camargue at the estuary of the Rhône, along the Lower Danube and in the delta areas of the Volga. Densely populated urban areas where mosquitoes thrive, however, can also form a basis for West Nile fever. This has been very obvious in the USA, where not only New York but other big cities such as Chicago have been hit by epidemics.[63]

Such climate factors as temperature, humidity and precipitation also influence the activity of the West Nile fever virus. Conditions are extremely complex, but it is clear that higher temperatures increase the potential of the virus to infect human beings. That is probably the explanation why northern Europe has so far not been affected. It may also mean that the feared climate changes with higher temperatures will increase the spread of the virus to Europe's northern regions.

Zika virus: from long-lasting anonymity to global threat

The Zika virus was first detected in a monkey in Uganda in 1947, but did not cause much of a stir at the time. For more than fifty years it was thought to be completely harmless. The majority of human infections caused no symptoms, while a few people had a mild illness with a high temperature, headache, rash and aches in muscles and limbs. Like so many other EIDs, this is also a zoonosis. The behaviour of the Zika virus is similar to that of yellow fever. In Africa monkeys are the reservoir, with infection between monkeys being spread via mosquitoes. Occasionally mosquitoes will also transmit the virus to humans.[64]

For a long time the virus spread extremely slowly in Africa and also in Asia, where it was detected as early as the middle of the twentieth century. The first major epidemic outbreak came in 2007 on the small island community of Yap in Micronesia in the Western Pacific. Here more than half of the 7,000 inhabitants became infected. The virus then spread eastwards across the Pacific to Polynesia and via Easter Island to South America, where the epidemic almost exploded in Brazil in 2015 and spread to other countries in South and Central America. At that point, the Zika virus gained wide publicity over the whole world.

Admittedly the great majority of those who become infected, approximately 80 per cent, experience no symptoms. But the epidemic in Brazil showed that the Zika virus can have far more serious consequences, since pregnant women often infect their embryos. This can result in congenital deformities, for example microcephaly, in which the head is much smaller than normal, and in serious disturbances in the development of the brain. Blindness can also occur. Even though just under 10 per cent of the children of affected mothers experience such deformities, at least 3,000 such cases have already been reported, the great majority of them in Brazil.[65] In adults the virus can also cause a serious neurological disease, Guillain-Barré syndrome, which may result in paralysis and even lead to death.

The commonest form of infection in the New World is transmission via various species of mosquito. This especially takes place in cities where these species are well established. So far there is no evidence that the Zika virus has managed to establish itself as a permanent reservoir in wild monkeys, as its relation the yellow fever virus has managed to do in the Americas. If this were to happen, and recently there have been disconcerting reports that would seem to suggest this, the Zika virus, like yellow fever virus, would be impossible to eradicate from the continent.[66]

Experiences with the Zika virus in recent years have also revealed other unpleasant news. The virus can also be transmitted sexually – between men and women and between men. We must therefore also consider this to be a sexually transmissible infection. It is possible that the virus can be transmitted via blood transfusion.[67]

It is not without good reason that the WHO declared this once-neglected virus to be a public health emergency in 2016. That year the Summer Olympic Games were to be held in Rio de Janeiro and the Zika

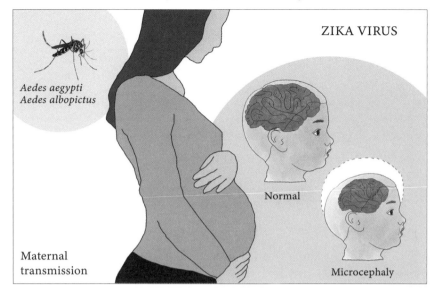

When a pregnant woman becomes infected with Zika virus after having been bitten by a mosquito, the child can be born with brain deformities, especially microcephaly – a head much smaller than normal size.

virus threat caused some to insist that the Olympics ought to be cancelled. Contingents from individual countries such as Kenya initially wished to stay away. Eventually the Olympics did take place, but both participants and public doubtless took extra precautions against mosquito bites.

What lay behind the sudden arrival of the Zika virus as a global health threat? Environmental and ecology-related factors must have played a role. Both international travel and the adaptation by various species of mosquitoes to urban environments have clearly contributed to the spread of the virus. But the intensive research in the field after 2015 has also provided a firm basis for assuming that the virus changed via several mutations on its way from Asia to America. Some of these mutations have made the transmission of the virus via mosquitoes more effective, while others may have increased its capacity to damage the brain cells of a human embryo, with brain malformations as a result.[68]

Cannibalism and Modern Meat Production

Prions are the smallest constituents in nature that can cause infectious diseases. It is extremely doubtful, however, that they can strictly be said to be alive and considered part of the world of microbes. They consist of a single protein molecule and lack genetic material that is linked to RNA or DNA. The diseases that they cause affect the brain, and are incurable and ultimately fatal.[69]

Scrapie, a disease in sheep that we now know is caused by prions, has been known for hundreds of years by sheep farmers. Prion diseases, however, can also affect humans. The special characteristics of these diseases can be illustrated by two that have arisen in regions that are far apart and with different external conditions. One of them has probably disappeared.

Kuru: an intellectual challenge in New Guinea's jungle

Around 1930 increasing numbers of the Fore tribe, which lives in the highlands of the Okapa district in the southeastern part of Papua New Guinea, were hit by a horrible disease.[70] It began almost imperceptibly, with headaches and muscle pains, but after several months there were increasing signs of a disease in the nervous system, making walking troublesome and causing shaking and unintentional movements. These symptoms always developed inexorably, with increasing dementia. The disease always proved fatal due to malnutrition and pneumonia after a maximum of two years. It was normally women and children who were affected, and the decline in the female population became a problem in a number of villages.

The Fore tribe called the disease *kuru*, which in their language means 'shaking' – either from fear or cold. The local view was that the disease was caused by magic and evil people were responsible for it.

In the years after the Second World War, when Papua New Guinea was under Australian administration, Australian health personnel began to notice this special disease, which was previously unknown. They began to study it in collaboration with a research institute in Melbourne. The almost self-appointed leader of this research project was the dynamic young American paediatrician Carleton Gajdusek, who had come to Papua almost by chance and became fascinated by the challenges offered by the rare disease. Gajdusek and a second doctor, Vincent Zigas, single-handedly established a small hospital with a laboratory where they studied kuru patients.

Working intensively and comprehensively, the two doctors examined everything that they thought could be the cause of the disease:

earlier known infections, toxic substances in food and the surroundings, vitamin deficiencies and the lack of trace elements in the food. All in vain. At first Gajdusek was working on the theory that kuru had to be a special hereditary disease that had hit the Fore tribe.

Then a reader's letter about the disease was published in the medical journal *The Lancet* by a veterinary researcher, William J. Hadlow, which moved kuru research onto a new path.[71] He pointed out that there was a great similarity between the cerebral changes caused by kuru and those found in sheep with scrapie, which has long been known to sheep farmers. Scrapie also causes brain disease. Could this new disease have the same underlying cause as scrapie?

It was of course impossible to carry out experiments on humans, so Gajdusek chose chimpanzees as experimental animals. He injected them with cerebral tissue from kuru patients in order to see if the disease was due to a microbe. For a long time, nothing happened to the chimpanzees. But after two and a half years the chimpanzees started to develop a disease that greatly resembled kuru. It was, then, an infection, but what was the microbe responsible? Perhaps it was a special type of virus where the incubation period – the time from infection to disease – was particularly long?

And how did infections occur? Here it was anthropologists who found a solution that was quite surprising and very bizarre. The kuru patients had been infected through religious burial rituals during which relations ate parts of the body of the deceased person, including the brain. After a few days of decay, the remains were boiled and consumed. It was nearly always the women and children who took part in these cannibalistic rituals, whereas the men often did not. If the dead person had been infected with kuru, the disease was transmitted in this way.[72]

At the end of the 1950s all forms of cannibalism were forbidden by the Australian authorities, and it is estimated that no humans have been infected since 1960. The incubation time of kuru is normally ten to fifteen years, but it can be up to fifty. As a result there were regular new cases of the disease throughout the second half of the twentieth century; the last known case was in 2005.

Part of the story is that Gajdusek also studied another quite rare disease that affects humans, Creutzfeldt-Jakob disease, normally abbreviated as CJD. This is also a fatal brain disease resulting in dementia, with

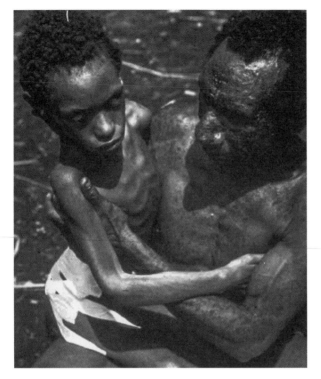

Young girl of the Fore tribe in New Guinea in 1959, who is suffering from kuru.

changes in the brain that resemble those of kuru and scrapie. Gajdusek managed to cause this disease in chimpanzees after injecting them with brain tissue from patients with CJD. He concluded that kuru, scrapie and CJD must be due to a particularly slowly developing virus. For his work on these diseases, he was awarded the Nobel Prize in 1976. In his later years he worked for a time in Tromsø, Norway, where he died in 2008, far away from the jungle of New Guinea where he had celebrated his first triumphs.

Gajdusek was to be proved not completely correct when it came to the cause of the special diseases he had studied. It was not a question of a special form of virus, but a formerly unknown infectious agent. It was to be another researcher, Stanley Prusiner, who made the epoch-making discovery that a very special type of protein molecule can both cause serious illness in the brain and be infectious. It is these prions, as Prusiner called them, that cause kuru, CJD and scrapie as well as a number of similar diseases in many animal species. After having faced massive criticism for his prion theory, Stanley Prusiner was awarded the Nobel Prize for his findings in 1997.[73] Kuru was the first prion disease in humans where it had been proved that infection can take place by ingesting food. It was not to be the last.

Mad cow disease and fear

In the mid-1980s an epidemic of a serious brain disease broke out in cattle in England. The epidemic spread rapidly and in the press was given the name 'mad cow disease', because of the abnormal behaviour of the animals, which had trouble walking. The official term used for the disease is bovine spongiform encephalopathy (BSE).

Autopsies carried out on the animals revealed that the disease was very much like the well-known sheep disease scrapie, which was now known to be infectious and due to prions. It turned out that mad cow disease had also been caused by a type of prion. Since the disease in cattle was clearly new, it was supposed that the prions had infected the cattle via modern methods of feeding, where measured amounts of meal including brain tissue are included from cattle and sheep that had probably had scrapie. Such feeding methods are therefore now forbidden.[74]

The epidemic of mad cow disease caused hardly any stir until 1990. Researchers and health authorities did not believe that human beings

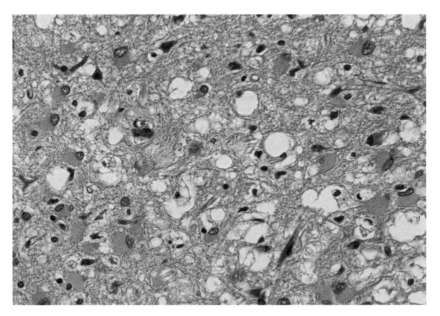

Creutzfeldt-Jakob disease is caused by prions. During this incurable brain disease, the brain tissue becomes spongelike, as shown in the picture. The prions can be transmitted via infected cattle meat, but the disease can also be inherited.

could be infected after eating infected beef. Scrapie in sheep had existed for hundreds of years without this having led to problems in human beings. But now instances of prion disease in zoos began to occur, in various species of animal that had been given the same food as the cows. This in turn demonstrated that the prions were able to jump from one species of animal to another. Fear in the population now began to increase. But the government stood firm, supported by the media, claiming that there was no risk to humans from eating beef. The minister for agriculture, fisheries and food demonstrated this by allowing his four-year-old daughter to eat a hamburger on TV.

Then everything exploded in 1995 with the discovery that many patients shared the same pathological picture seen in the now well-known disease CJD. These patients were nearly all quite young, whereas the previously known form of CJD affected people over fifty years of age. It was clearly caused, however, by prions – and the patients with this new and increasing form of CJD had in all probability been infected by meat from cattle. The British government was now forced to concede this, after having denied it for a number of years. This led to a political crisis as trust in politicians plummeted and a sense of fear developed in the population that sometimes bordered on hysteria. Many people expected there would be a huge epidemic of this horrible disease. This fortunately did not prove the case, and during recent years there have been fewer and fewer instances of the disease as a result of preventative measures taken in industrial meat production. A total of almost 250 cases are known, most of them in Great Britain, where the last recorded case was in 2016.

The prion epidemic demonstrates yet again how humans, through a change in their behaviour – in this case by adopting new forms of industrial meat production – can bring about completely new epidemics. Part of the picture, however, is that we now know that CJD can also be transmitted via various methods of medical treatment: treating people with growth hormone made using tissue from dead bodies, the transplantation of corneas and, perhaps, even common blood transfusions.[75]

The possibility that new prion diseases will be discovered in the future cannot be excluded. Such diseases occur in many species of animal, and the experiences gained from mad cow disease show that prions can occasionally jump to new species of animal, including humans. A present-day problem in North America and Scandinavia is the prion disease chronic wasting disease (CWD), which affects members of the deer family, including deer and elk. New research data perhaps implies that these prions have a certain tendency to change their characteristics over time, something which may well involve an increased risk for humans.[76]

The COVID-19 Pandemic: A New Greeting from Bats

On 31 December 2019 the authorities in the Chinese megalopolis of Wuhan, a city of 11 million inhabitants in the province of Hubei, announced that cases of a mysterious pneumonia had appeared and were increasing in number. Many of the patients had been in contact with the large wet market in the city, where the sale of a great many animal species, both tame and wild, took place. The suspicion was that the patients had been infected by animals there, in a repeat of the SARS epidemic. Initially it did not seem that person-to-person infection was taking place to any particular extent, but there is still a veil of uncertainty about what happened early on in Wuhan and rapidly developed into an epidemic.[77]

In the course of the first few weeks Chinese researchers were able to prove that the cause of this epidemic was a new coronavirus and to determine its structure. It transpired that the virus was quite closely related to the SARS virus of 2002. The World Health Organization (WHO) decided, for diplomatic reasons, to call the virus COVID-19, a neutral term that indicated neither the origin of the virus nor the connection with the former SARS virus, which it was felt could give rise to unfortunate associations, particularly in China. The correct virological term for the virus, however, is SARS-CoV-2 (the original SARS virus is now referred to as SARS-CoV-1). The term 'COVID-19' ought, strictly speaking, only be used about the disease caused by the virus. During January 2020 so-called PCR tests were developed in many laboratories to detect the virus in patients.

The epidemic in Wuhan spread rapidly, with a considerable number of serious instances of pneumonia that overloaded the health service and hospitals. The number of deaths gradually increased, but initially the Chinese authorities kept their cards close to their chests as regards both the number of deaths and the increasing suspicion of person-to-person infection. It was not until 21 January 2020 that the WHO officially confirmed that such transmission of the virus was taking place.

China, with its unfortunate experiences with the SARS virus in 2002–3, was now facing a new epidemic with a different coronavirus that was spreading almost explosively, also outside Wuhan. For as long as possible the rest of the world hoped that the epidemic would remain inside China, but already in mid-January the first cases began to appear in other countries. This was to mark the beginning of a pandemic that has since spread to every continent.[78]

Intensive research in many countries during the few months after the pandemic first appeared has given considerable insight into the new coronavirus, particularly as regards how transmission takes place and its pathogenic characteristics. Important research results have come more rapidly than for any former epidemic. Yet there is still a great deal we do not yet know.

When it comes to the ways of infection, there has been and still is some considerable debate. Most people now believe that the most important means of transmission in most situations is droplet infection. Infectious individuals expel virus-carrying droplets when they cough, sneeze or talk. These droplets can lead to infection if inhaled or if they land on mucous membranes in the nose, mouth or eyes. Droplet infection requires close contact (less than 1–2 metres) since the virus-carrying droplets quickly fall to the ground. In addition, infection can also take place if one comes into contact with objects that carry such droplets, although this form of infection is probably less important than direct droplet infection.[79]

A highly controversial question has been the role played by airborne infection (infection by aerosols that can stay in the air for some time and cover larger distances than droplet infection). As well as this possibly taking place in the health service during medical procedures that form aerosols, there is a great deal of evidence to suggest that this type of infection can also occur when several people are together for some time in an enclosed space with bad ventilation.[80]

The interval between infection and disease (the incubation period) is between two and ten days. Of great importance for combatting the pandemic is that infected individuals are infectious for two or three days before showing symptoms of the disease. Much of the spread of infection probably takes place during this period. Infectiousness decreases considerably during the first five or six days after the outbreak of the disease.[81]

There is also some uncertainty when it comes to the disease-causing capacity of the new coronavirus. In some cases, perhaps as high as 30 to 40 per cent, the infection is completely without symptoms. As already became clear from the first weeks of the pandemic in Wuhan, the virus mainly causes a respiratory tract infection, ranging from a quite mild infection with traits of a common cold to, in the worst instances, fatal pneumonia. The mildest cases often go undetected.

We now know why the SARS-CoV-2 virus first takes hold in the air passages. Like all other viruses, this coronavirus has to latch on to a receptor on the surface of cells that function as 'door-openers', enabling the virus to penetrate the cell. The receptor for this virus is a molecule called ACE2 (an abbreviation of angiotensin converting enzyme). On its surface, the coronavirus has many spikes with a protein that binds effectively to the ACE2 receptor.[82] This ACE2 molecule is found on the mucous membrane cells in both the nose and mouth, and there are plenty of such cells in the lungs. ACE2 normally has a number of important functions in the body. Among other things, it contributes to the regulation of the blood pressure, and counteracts inflammatory mechanisms. Infection with the coronavirus leads to a decreased functioning of ACE2, and this contributes to inflammation in the air passages. An important sign of infection that can occur early in the process is a loss of smell and taste, which is due to infection of cells in the nasal mucous membrane.

The ACE2 molecule is found not only in the air passages but in cells in many other organs, including the heart, kidneys, small intestine, liver and blood vessels. This can partially explain why patients with COVID-19 can also have complications from these organs. This is particularly the case with critically ill patients. An effect on the heart and kidneys is quite common in this group of patients, in addition to thrombosis and bleeding disturbances. Not infrequently the brain and nervous system also display symptoms – and occasionally there is serious encephalitis.[83] It also appears that long-term health consequences ('long Covid') after the acute infection may be a problem.[84]

The risk of serious illness and death after being infected with SARS-CoV-2 varies a great deal among different groups. Early on in the pandemic two main groups became obvious: elderly patients and those who had one or more other illnesses that may weaken the immune system.[85]

The risk of dying from the infection increases considerably from the age of sixty upwards, and the highest case fatality rate is seen in patients over eighty. This is not due to age alone: this patient group often has other complicating illnesses, which in themselves increase the risk in the event of a COVID-19 infection.

Important risk factors, apart from age, are a number of chronic diseases, including heart and lung diseases, cancer, transplantation, diabetes, obesity and forms of treatment that weaken the immune system.[86] The list is long, but new observations lead to regular changes. The first experiences with COVID-19 indicated, for example, that high blood pressure – hypertension – is a risk factor, but this is now regarded as uncertain. The importance of smoking, which makes people susceptible to many lung diseases, is not clear. For unknown reasons, men have a greater risk of developing serious infection than women. Most children who are infected are either without symptoms or only display light symptoms. Very rarely, a serious disease is seen in very young children, characterized by high temperature and inflammation of various organs, including the heart. This disease comes weeks or months after the acute COVID-19 infection. Recently the same condition has also been seen in adults.[87]

The risk factors mentioned earlier do not fully explain why some people display no symptoms when infected with SARS-CoV-2, while others, apparently with the same risk profile, fall seriously ill. Recently it has been discovered that certain genes that *Homo sapiens* inherited from the Neanderthals 40,000 to 60,000 years ago increase the risk of serious illness. These Neanderthal genes, which are inherited collectively, are unevenly dispersed around the globe. In Bangladesh they are found in no less than 63 per cent of the population, whereas the figure in Europe is only 8 per cent.[88] Other genes may also have some importance.

Naturally, the immune system, as with other infections, plays an important role in the outcome of coronavirus infection. Numerous studies have been carried out on the immune system in COVID-19 patients. Even though the picture is rather confused at the moment, a pattern appears to be emerging: a dysregulation of the immune response against the coronavirus.[89] The virus affects the so-called natural or innate defence of the immune system, which impairs its effectiveness as the first line of defence against the virus. At the same time a number of inflammation factors are also overproduced by T-cells. The antiviral functions of both T-cells and antibody-producing B-cells are at the same time impaired. The pattern described is especially pronounced in the most serious forms of the infection, where the immunologically triggered inflammation contributes to a great extent to both lung disease and other organ complications.

The pandemic has already resulted in a great many deaths. But just how lethal is this infection? The case fatality rate differs substantially from one country to another. This is not surprising, for the many factors that are of importance for how the pandemic progresses vary considerably in the world. This applies to the age of the patients and the presence of risk factors. In addition, the quality of the health services differs a great deal, as does the intensity of testing: the more patients without symptoms one discovers, the lower the calculated case fatality rate. Increased testing is probably an important reason why mortality has displayed a tendency to decrease in many countries, but treatment has also improved during the period of the pandemic. The way in which the deaths are registered also differs from one country to the next.

The published figures show that the total case fatality rate in the individual countries varies from less than 1 per cent to more than 10 per cent. Young people without risk factors have extremely low mortality, while the highest age groups and patients with risk factors can have a mortality rate well in excess of 10 per cent. Even so, a report in October 2020 showed that COVID-19 was then the most frequent cause of death among people between 19 and 44 in several American states.[90]

Infection with the SARS-CoV-2 virus has a higher case fatality rate than common seasonal influenza, which lies around 0.1–0.2 per cent: it is at least three to four times as high, possibly even ten times higher.[91] This coronavirus, however, is less dangerous than its related viruses SARS-CoV-1 and MERS, which have a case fatality rate of 10 and 34 per cent respectively. These viruses are, however, less infectious.

What is the origin of the new coronavirus? There is still no answer to this question after more than a year of the pandemic.[92] There is general agreement that the first cases of the disease arose in Wuhan, but where does the virus come from? The great majority of researchers believe that the virus originally comes from bats. We have already had two serious epidemics with coronavirus – the SARS and MERS epidemics – where the virus originally came from that source. There is proof of a coronavirus in bats in China that is clearly related to the SARS-CoV-2 virus. While it is reasonable to argue that the present pandemic virus has an ancestor in bats, how has it developed subsequently? A number of theories have been advanced, some more imaginative than others.

As with many earlier epidemics, including the AIDS pandemic, conspiracy theories soon surfaced. It was claimed on social media that the virus had been manipulated in a Chinese laboratory as a biological weapon, and that as the result of an accident it had leaked out of the laboratory and thereby started the pandemic. Early investigations of the structure of the virus in Western laboratories, however, concluded that this theory was highly unlikely, and that the virus had probably arisen naturally. It was claimed that if the virus had been 'fiddled with' in the laboratory, this would leave traces in its structure. Despite this, there is still no agreement in the research world that the leakage theory can be dismissed, for the SARS-CoV-2 virus displays characteristics of its having gone through a so-called recombination, that is, an exchange of gene segments from several virus variants. This can occur in nature, but it can also be the result of manipulation in laboratories as part of ongoing legitimate research.[93]

The Wuhan Institute of Virology has carried out advanced research on bats and coronaviruses for several years, including those related to today's pandemic virus. This laboratory has security measures that operate at the highest level. Even so, as has happened before in other laboratories of this standard, accidents can occur as a result of human failure, leading to microbes leaking into the surrounding area.

This leakage theory has gained considerable publicity, particularly because it had supporters among certain American top politicians in the Trump administration. This placed an extra strain on the already tense relation between the USA and China. Both the Chinese authorities and the researchers at the Wuhan laboratory indignantly reject the leakage theory. Several Western countries called for a commission of international experts to be allowed to examine the condition around the start of the pandemic in Wuhan, including the possibility of a laboratory leakage of the virus. China rejected the idea for a long time, but under pressure from the world community the Chinese authorities accepted such a commission in May 2020, to be appointed by the WHO. In January 2021 the commission visited Wuhan. In its later report it concluded that it was 'very unlikely' that the virus had leaked from the laboratory, and that this theory should not be explored further. The report has been strongly criticized by a number of researchers who demand further, extensive investigation, since the commission apparently did not get access to all relevant material in Wuhan.

In all probability the SARS-CoV-2 virus originated in bats, but it has hardly made a direct transition from bats to humans. An alternative to the laboratory leakage theory is that the virus had another animal species as an intermediate host before it attacked humans. This was after all the case with the related SARS and MERS viruses. The present pandemic virus probably also had such an intermediate stage where it underwent changes that enabled it to cause infection in humans with the characteristic symptoms we see today. Another possibility is that the virus was not fully developed when it infected humans for the first time, but that it acquired 'finishing touches' in the human body.

Several things suggest that the much discussed wet market in Wuhan can hardly have been the starting point for the virus, although this market could have possibly contributed later to the spread of the virus in the city.[94] No animal species has been identified as the intermediate host for the pandemic virus, in spite of extensive investigation. One candidate is the pangolin, a scaly anteater, which is highly prized in China, both for its delicious meat and for the assumed medical benefits attributed to parts of the animal in traditional medicines. A coronavirus has been found in the pangolin that is closely related to SARS-CoV-2. But there are other candidates, for the coronavirus can infect a wide range of species.[95]

An important reason why people wish to map the path of the pandemic virus from bats to humans, while also facing many other unsolved problems about the pandemic, is that such knowledge can be useful for preventing future zoonoses. If we know the host animals for the pandemic virus, we have a greater possibility of preventing the return of this virus in the future.

What particularly distinguishes the fifth transition in the history of human infection from earlier ones is that globalization via modern means of transport has led to an enormous increase in the possibility of an infectious microbe rapidly spreading over the entire world. We saw this, for example, with the AIDS pandemic and even more clearly with the SARS epidemic in 2002–3. The present pandemic illustrates this in a frightening way. After the epidemic had explosively spread outside Wuhan to all Chinese provinces, it rapidly found a path beyond China's borders and in the space of a few months had spread to the whole of the inhabited world.

The entire world has been profoundly affected by the pandemic that started in Wuhan in 2020. As early as 30 January the WHO declared the new epidemic outbreak a 'public health emergency', as a serious warning signal. On 11 March the WHO stated that we were facing a pandemic. By then more than 118,000 cases had been reported in 114 countries, with 4,231 deaths. Soon afterwards the pandemic was active worldwide. In the course of a few months, people's everyday lives had been totally altered and the world economy had experienced a serious setback, with social consequences across a wide range of areas.

There have been major differences between the strategies adopted by various countries against the pandemic. The individual elements of the strategies have been basically the same in most countries, but the emphasis has differed considerably. This also applied to the point when the most powerful measures were introduced, which made a strong impact on the course of the pandemic. Without going into detail, let us look at some important features of the combat measures and the course of the pandemic.[96]

On the basis of the incomplete information we have, it looks as if the authorities in Wuhan were initially paralysed to a certain extent when an increasing number of the inhabitants were hit by a new disease that undeniably was reminiscent of SARS. The hope apparently was that it did not involve person-to-person infection to any great extent. It was thought that the infection had come from the city's wet market, which was disinfected thoroughly and closed. In addition an attempt was made, using quite authoritarian measures, to cover up any publicity about the new epidemic.[97] One of those affected by this was the young eye special- ist Li Wenliang, who reported on the first hospitalized SARS-like cases on Sina Weibo, the Chinese variant of Twitter. The authorities accused him of illegally spreading rumours and disturbing public order, and he was pressurized by the police to sign a declaration that his Weibo message was incorrect. Subsequent developments revealed the absurdity of this, but tragically Li himself died of the coronavirus in early February.

The new coronavirus could not have hit China at a more unfortunate time. Officially the Chinese authorities did not admit that the new virus was infectious, at least not until 20 January. But by then China was already well into the holiday period known as Chunyun, around the time of the Chinese New Year, when there is extremely high travel activity. In recent years some 2 billion people have set out on journeys during this period, which in 2020 started on 10 January. Practically half of the inhabitants of Wuhan had left the city, some of them travelling to other countries, and some of them were certainly infected with the coronavirus. There is every reason to believe that this gave the virus a 'flying start' on its journey out into the world.[98]

The measures that China imposed against the epidemic on 23 January were so draconian that the rest of the world was initially shocked. At first Wuhan and soon all the cities in Hubei province were almost completely sealed off from the rest of the world, meaning that more than 50 million people were affected by the quarantine measures. All public transport was shut down. Most shops, except those selling food or medicine, were closed. Restrictions were imposed on the inhabitants leaving their homes and a strict quarantine of individuals was implemented, partly with the help of the police. Similar measures were introduced elsewhere in parts of China.

The world had not seen such strict measures for combatting an epidemic in modern times, and followed the situation in Wuhan with a mixture of horror and admiration. It gradually became obvious that the strict measures had actually produced the desired effect, as far as it was possible to judge from the official Chinese infection figures, which should, however, be taken with a pinch of salt. It was, at any rate, possible after a period of two months to discontinue practically all the imposed measures in March. Even though there have since been scattered cases of new infection, there can be no doubt that China has enjoyed success with its strategy against the pandemic after the initial unfortunate hesitancy.

The results of attempts to combat the pandemic, on the other hand, have varied greatly in the rest of the world.[99] Basic measures in most countries have involved testing for the virus, the isolation of those infected, quarantine for those exposed to infection, social distancing (at least 1 metre between people) and restricting the size of groups in various contexts. In addition, there has been an entire spectrum of more restrictive measures that have been applied to various extents: the closing of borders, of restaurants, shops, schools, various kinds of restrictions on free movement for citizens and, after a while, the use of masks. Although the effect of each of these individual measures is probably limited, the overall effect can be considerable. The use of the most restrictive measures has definitely been inspired by China's success, even though they were originally met with scepticism and are still controversial.

Despite the fact that important features of the course of the pandemic vary in different parts of the world, it is even so possible to point to certain basic factors that seem to be essential for successfully combatting the coronavirus.

An important prerequisite for success seems to be that the measures involved are introduced early and implemented consistently, according to plan, and have sufficient duration. This places heavy demands on society, especially the most restrictive measures, which require a high level of loyalty in the population.

An example in this connection is New Zealand, which has been internationally praised for its systematic combatting of the pandemic: the spread of the virus in the country was effectively stopped during the spring, and a few isolated cases of infection that occurred in August were dealt with by similar measures.

South Korea is another example that demonstrates the beneficial effect of imposing measures quickly. In February the pandemic spread rapidly throughout the country. In the course of a few months, however, it seemed as if this was under control. It is interesting that an important reason for this was not comprehensive, restrictive measures, with a total lockdown of society, but a sophisticated use of electronic monitoring and tracing of infection via, among other means, smartphones and the tracing of credit cards. These measures could be implemented because of new legislation that had been put in place after the MERS virus outbreak in 2015. In spite of this early success, South Korea shows that the virus is capable of retaliating when most of the measures are discontinued: in August there was once more a strong increase of new cases, which led to a new tightening of the measures that seems to have had an effect.

Vietnam is another example of an Asian country that has been effective at combatting the pandemic. Although its position next to China makes it highly exposed, in the first year of the pandemic this poor country, which has a population of almost 100 million, saw only about 1,100 cases of infection and 35 deaths. An important reason for this is probably the firm leadership in this quite authoritarian country, where the ruling Communist Party has imposed heavy-handed quarantine and other measures, with plenty of help from its military forces. The regime has also managed to incite the population to fight the coronavirus, playing the patriotic card by referring to earlier military invasions.

In Europe, unfortunately, very few countries can show similar results.[100] During the second half of February 2020, Italy was hit by the pandemic, which, in the space of just a few weeks, exploded in Lombardy and several other regions of northern Italy. When the Italian authorities introduced strict measures in a number of areas on 8 March and a few days later throughout Italy, the pandemic was already raging in the north. The number of deaths rose rapidly and the intensive-care wards of the hospitals became overloaded. The central and southern parts of Italy, including Rome, got off far more lightly from the pandemic.

On the heels of Italy came Spain, which from 12 March introduced a complete lockdown of the country, including the closing of ports, with new measures being introduced in the following weeks. The number of deaths rose, particularly among the elderly and medical personnel. In Madrid the mortuaries were so inundated with corpses that some temporarily had to be stored on a skating rink.

The Spanish government has had to put up with criticism for its measures being imposed too late. When they were imposed, strict measures were carried out with a heavy hand, with the aid of the police and the army. Infringing infection regulations meant large fines and, in some cases, even imprisonment. Drones were used for enforcement of measures.

The first three cases of COVID-19 in Europe were reported from France on 24 January, and France also had the first death, on 15 February. From the second half of February, cases began to increase. Measures were introduced by the authorities from 12 March that led to a lockdown in

France as well. Even so, there were still new cases and the number of deaths peaked in April. It was not until the end of May and early June that it was possible to discontinue most of the measures.

The countries that have been named carried out their measures quite systematically, even though in retrospect one can claim that they came a little too late. The picture for the United Kingdom is somewhat different. Here there was more hesitation in implementing strong measures than in Italy and France. This did not take place until the end of March. The country's strategy has been strongly criticized from various quarters. Many people claim that the government underestimated the seriousness of the situation and that the measures came several weeks too late. Others feel that the lockdown strategy has caused a disproportionally large amount of damage. It apparently had a braking effect on the spread of the virus, but the UK, even so, has the highest mortality rate in Europe.

Sweden stood out from the rest of Europe by adopting a strategy for combatting the pandemic that differed from the lockdown measures inspired by China and gradually taken over by a number of countries. Apart from partially closing schools and providing general advice to the population about social distancing, activities were not restricted and borders remained open.

At the core of the Swedish strategy was probably the belief in herd immunity: the conviction that an acute epidemic in a population without immunity will stop when a high enough percentage of the population has been infected and thereby acquired immunity.[101] Depending on the infectiousness of the microbe, it is estimated that herd immunity requires between 50 and 90 per cent of the population to have gained immunity. This, as we have seen, was the pattern of such herd infections as measles when they appeared for the first time after the second transition in the history of human infection. With a number of similar infections we can now attain herd immunity using vaccines. Until the end of 2020, however, there was no vaccine against SARS-CoV-2. Nor does the Swedish experience indicate that herd immunity has been achieved. On the contrary, the infection and mortality have simply increased and are much higher than the corresponding figures for the neighbouring countries in Scandinavia, which introduced strict lockdown measures as early as March. The high number of deaths is partly due to the fact that the protection of the elderly in institutions has failed. The prevalent view today is therefore that there is little reason to adopt Sweden's strategy when combatting the pandemic.

Most European countries did fairly well in halting the spread of the virus during the spring of 2020, so that society could open up once more before and during the summer. All those with any knowledge of combatting epidemics, however, reckoned on the possibility of the virus returning in a second wave. From August onwards, this fear proved justified.[102] The second wave hit large parts of Europe. In several countries, including France, the UK and Germany, there was a sharp increase in the numbers of people infected, and the number of deaths was not far behind. In certain countries, such as Belgium, it was feared that the hospital capacity would be insufficient, and help would have to be sought from neighbouring countries. The problems were made worse by the fact that health personnel are highly exposed to coronavirus infection. This led to many countries being forced to re-introduce lockdown measures that were as rigorous as the spring ones. Europe was in for a winter of discontent. One factor that probably contributed to this is that transmission of coronavirus and other respiratory tract infections increases during the dry and cold time of the year, when people tend to stay indoors and are in closer contact with each other. In the beginning of 2021 Europe was hit by a third wave of the epidemic. This wave is to a large extent driven by new mutations of the virus with increased infectiousness.

The situation outside Europe was also serious.[103] The USA has been the hardest hit country in the Americas. Since March 2020 there has been a constant rise in the number of those infected or dead as a result of the virus. New York was the epicentre of infection in March. In June 2021 more than 34 million of the population of the USA had been infected and more than 600,000 had died, the highest figures for any single country at the time.

It is surprising that the USA, which since the Second World War has led the world in biomedical research, did not manage to implement effective means to combat the pandemic. The underlying reasons for this are complex. At an early stage it became clear that President Donald Trump underestimated the threat from the SARS-CoV-2 virus and displayed no initiative in implementing strong measures, since they might have unfortunate consequences for economic development. Much of the task of combatting infection was left to the individual states, which introduced measures in different ways and of varying strength. In many states, measures were also discontinued too soon, before the local outbreak was under control. Active testing for the virus, which is essential for tracing infection, was insufficient. The lack of central coordination in combatting the pandemic that typified the Trump administration led to strong criticism from the medical world. This was undoubtedly a liability for Trump in the presidential election on 3 November.

The pandemic arrived somewhat later in Latin America than in the rest of the world, but then spread rapidly with an increasing death rate.[104] In October 2020 this region had suffered 35 per cent of all COVID-19 deaths in the world. The most populous country, Brazil, reported its first case on 25 February. Since then the figures for cases have constantly increased, with the country in third place in the world (after the USA and India) in June 2021 (almost 18 million) and second place (after the USA) in the number of deaths (almost 500,000).

A problem for combatting the pandemic in Brazil is that President Jair Bolsonaro, like his former colleague in the USA, consistently belittled the threat of a pandemic, and at the time of writing he still seemed indifferent to protective measures against infection. He, like Trump, also became infected. Much of the action against the infection in Brazil was left to the individual regions, which introduced certain measures that the president unsuccessfully sought to counteract. Contradictory information about the importance of protective measures undoubtedly created confusion in the population that led to the spread of infection. Another problem was the density of population among the 13 million who live in *favelas*, the slum areas in the major cities.

In several other countries in Latin America, such as Peru and Ecuador, not even an early lockdown managed to stop the spread of the virus. This was partly due to the economies of the poorer countries not being able to cope with robust lockdown measures of the type used in Europe.

While a number of Asian countries can point to their successful pandemic strategy, India, the most populous country in Asia alongside China, has major problems. Lockdown measures were introduced during March 2020 throughout the entire country, with its 1.3 billion inhabitants, but this did not result in any decline in the increase of infection. Everything favoured the virus spreading through the slum quarters of India's many megalopolises, and the economic consequences were also great. Millions of workers who had lost their jobs returned to their home areas, taking the virus with them. Many of the lockdown measures were concluded during May, but this took place at different levels in different places. The number of infections and deaths went on increasing, culminating in September. Then a decrease in the number of new cases appeared to occur. In March 2021 the pandemic then increased explosively. The reason for this is unclear, but large political meetings and religious festivals, as well as new virus mutations, have probably contributed. The strain on health services has been dramatic. In June 2021, 30 million people had been infected and there had been almost 400,000 deaths.

The presentation of the ongoing pandemic in the world's media and the many reactions in the population can occasionally give the impression that today's situation is unique in the history of human infection. This is not the case. The way in which the pandemic has developed so far, since the beginning of 2020, has a number of features that we recognize from earlier serious epidemics and pandemics, although they are perhaps even more evident in the present-day situation. This is partly

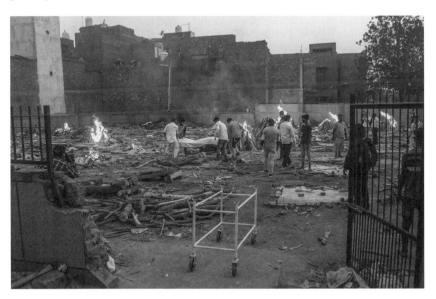

COVID-19 victims being cremated in Old Seemapuri crematorium in New Delhi, India, 8 May 2021. At that time India had more than 350,000 cases and more than 4,000 COVID-19 deaths per day, and in excess of 250,000 people had died in total.

due to extensive globalization, which provides particularly favourable conditions for the virus.

More than with any earlier epidemic, the eternal dilemma has been highlighted: how to achieve a balance between the positive benefits of measures adopted and their possible negative effects. This requires insight into both the medical aspects of the microbe involved – its pathogenic characteristics and infectiousness – and the harmful economic, social and psychological effects that the adopted measures can have.

In one country after the other we have seen examples of the negative effects of widespread measures that involve the lockdown of society to various degrees. Large sections of working life are hit by a loss of economic growth and increasing unemployment. International trade and travel are also hard hit. Closing schools and universities has major consequences for education and research. The harmful psychological effects resulting from restricting social contacts can be considerable. In addition to the medical consequences of being infected with the virus, treatment of other serious diseases may suffer as a result of the increased load on the health service.[105] This also affects other medical activities, such as vaccination campaigns, and the fight against serious infections such as AIDS, malaria and tuberculosis in many parts of the world.

Only the future will reveal the full picture of the negative effects of the pandemic. Let us content ourselves by stating that they are sure to be vast and long-lasting.

Until December 2020 measures against the pandemic were not able to rely on either vaccines against the virus or antiviral medications that have a convincing effect. Since then a number of vaccines have been rolled out which hopefully will change the situation. We will return to the present state of work with vaccines and drugs later.

Meanwhile, the many measures taken to combat the pandemic are viewed by sections of the population in many countries as a heavy burden. Questions have been raised about the necessity of all these measures that have so many unfortunate consequences for citizens. Many have expressed doubts as to whether the virus is as dangerous as the health authorities claim. In a number of countries this has led to demonstrations and unrest. Even more common, probably, is that many people ignore and sabotage the restrictions against infection that are in force. These problems will probably increase the longer lockdown measures last.

In addition to popular protests, we have recently also seen moves from the world of research questioning the expediency of the present pandemic strategy.[106] Once again, it is often the belief in herd immunity that underlies this. An alternative strategy has been proposed that, briefly, suggests that the virus should be let off the lead in society at large, without any restrictive measures, so that the majority of the population is infected and apparently will become immune, with herd immunity as the outcome. The pandemic will then grind to a halt. At the same time, the presupposition is that it will prove successful to protect the groups at risk of serious infection and death. In that way, one will avoid all the negative effects of lockdown measures.

Such a strategy may initially appear to be enticing. The problem is that it rests on an uncertain scientific foundation.[107] We do not yet know if infection with the SARS-CoV-2 virus results in lasting immunity, thereby making herd immunity possible. Without this, the pandemic will continue to rage. In practice, it will also be impossible to protect all those in groups at special risk. All in all, this probably involves between about 30 and 40 per cent of the population, partly in institutions, partly in their own homes. Such a strategy would therefore possibly involve an unacceptably high number of deaths.

It is at present unclear what the course of the virus will be in the next few years. There are a number of alternative scenarios, mainly depending on the effect of the many vaccines being rolled out. If the vaccines protect not only against serious disease, as seems to be the case, but to a large extent against infection, and the duration of immunity after vaccination is relatively long, it may be possible to achieve herd immunity. We will then have a situation similar to the one we have had for measles since the vaccine became available in the late 1960s – effective control of infection by the virus and a return to normal life.

If long-lasting immunity cannot be attained using vaccines, the situation will be quite a bit more difficult. Frequent revaccination may then be necessary, possibly annually, as with influenza. Possible new virus mutations with increased vaccine resistance may also make it necessary to revaccinate with modified vaccines. Many researchers today doubt that classical herd immunity against SARS-CoV-2 is a realistic target. The SARS-CoV-2 virus will probably be a part of our everyday lives in future. The virus will not disappear. Hopefully, however, we will be able to control its circulation effectively, making normal life possible. In this scenario drugs for the prevention and treatment of COVID-19 will be important to protect unvaccinated individuals and those in whom the vaccination has not been sufficiently protective. Our future coexistence with the virus will to a large extent depend on biomedical research, which has already supplied so many impressive results within the field of infection medicine.

Re-emerging Infections

In the wake of the newly introduced term 'emerging infections', it has also been necessary to launch the concept of 're-emerging infections'. The latter term refers to well-known infectious diseases that have formerly played an important role, but which for various reasons have declined sharply, only to increase once more as widespread, important diseases.

The reasons why these 'new-old' infections return can be found in the same mechanisms that underlie the emergence of EIDs. Once again, man-made conditions play an important role. A number of the microbes involved have already been mentioned as important causes of earlier epidemics and pandemics that many people believed had been consigned to history.

One example of such re-emerging infections is the formerly feared plague bacterium *Yersinia pestis*, which has recently led to epidemics in Madagascar and Central Africa.[108] Another is cholera, which has caused serious epidemics in the wake of the war in Yemen and on Haiti, in connection with the earthquake disaster there.[109]

While the Western world has gradually taken control of tuberculosis, this infectious disease has continued to ravage the poorer parts of the world. Even so, developments concerning tuberculosis in recent years have led to a dramatic worsening of the problems. This is due to two things. The explosive HIV/AIDS epidemic has created a large number of patients with an immune system so badly weakened against the TB bacterium that they have become easy prey to the disease, which has led to a sharp increase in the number of new cases. Furthermore, it has created a breeding ground for the emergence of multiresistant tuberculosis bacteria, which have developed a resistance to all the conventionally used drugs for this infection. This is partially due to the incorrect use of these drugs. It has resulted in a marked increased mortality of TB. In Western countries we are now also seeing cases of infection with multiresistant TB bacteria, nearly always as an import from the hardest hit parts of the world.

The problem with resistant TB bacteria fits in with what today must be called a heralded disaster, an increasing tendency for a whole series of common and less common bacteria, which until now we have been able to treat with good results, to become resistant to antibiotics.

Other important infectious diseases such as yellow fever and malaria are now also showing such serious signs of increasing in parts of the world that they must be included within the category of re-emerging infectious diseases.[110]

Further examples of such infections are those that had formerly been virtually eradicated from the developed parts of the world, partly due to effective vaccines, but are now re-emerging as a result of failures in vaccination coverage. This can occur if there is a breakdown in the health service during war conditions, as has been the case in Syria, where poliomyelitis has re-emerged, or in situations where the health service breaks down for other reasons, as was seen in Eastern Europe after the collapse of the Soviet Union, when such diseases as diphtheria flared up once more. Another reason for vaccination failure is the growing phenomenon of vaccine refusal for various reasons. This has led to a sharp increase in measles in a number of Western countries where this infection was regarded as eradicated.

The problems linked to returning infections illustrate with great clarity that *Homo sapiens* can never relax in the eternal duel against microbes.

Reflections

The new realistic perception of the lasting significance for humanity of infectious diseases, especially the discovery of one new infectious disease after the other, has had important consequences. One thing is that this has led to banner headlines in the media about lethal epidemics with horrific pathological pictures, along with films and novels with the same themes, creating a great deal of fear. It is far more important, however, that this has led to increased insight into the underlying factors and mechanisms that are vital in the duel between man and microbe.

Initially the interest was mainly in the background of the new infectious diseases. It was soon clear that the actual mechanisms gradually discovered were not in fact new. The same factors have always regulated the influence of the world of microbes on human health. These new experiences, therefore, represent a new angle of approach to studies of epidemics and problems with infections in former times. They have proved themselves to be a useful supplement to the conventional approach of historians to the past, from which the role of infectious diseases has often been glaringly absent.

Experiences with some of the new infectious diseases have also had profound consequences for areas other than medicine. This particularly applies to the HIV infection, which is not really surprising, since the HIV virus has caused the largest pandemic of modern times and still rages almost out of control in parts of the world.

The HIV pandemic has, among other things, increased understanding of the special problems experienced by exposed minority groups – homosexual men and drug addicts – both in the population in general and in the health service. Furthermore, the HIV issue has led to a greater awareness of the need to make blood transfusions and the treatment of blood products safe.

The often heated debate about strategy when combatting the HIV pandemic had consequences for medical ethics and led to a new discussion of the importance of human rights when faced with epidemics. The pressing need to develop effective HIV medication finally led to changes in the regulations for the testing of new medicines. This was in great part due to the activist efforts of patient groups and has created a pattern for similar activism with regard to other illnesses.

Unfortunately, increased knowledge is not always a blessing. In special cases, microbes can be used as weapons, even for acts of terror. We must be absolutely clear that some of the really dangerous microbes that have been discovered during the last decades, along with certain well-known microbes, can be relevant for people prepared to use them as weapons.

EIGHT

When Microbes
Are Used as Weapons

The significance of human behaviour and intervention in nature runs like a thread through most of the history of the duel between man and microbe. In the vast majority of cases where human behaviour has led to an increase in problems of infection, this has been unintentional, and the consequence of ignorance. Even so, it is a fact that throughout history we have had many examples of attempts to use microbes as weapons in various situations that may be referred to as biological warfare.

Biological Warfare

Thousands of years before the bacteriological revolution and the discovery of microbes as a cause of disease, humans must certainly have discovered that rotting bodies and excrement from humans and animals can be pathogenic. As far back as antiquity, the Greeks, Romans and Persians made use of this during warfare by using such material to poison wells and other sources of water in order to cause diseases in their enemies. This somewhat primitive strategy has been used right up until the present day. Herodotus, the father of written history, for example, relates that Scythian warriors in the area around the Black Sea used to dip their arrows in the rotting bodies of poisonous snakes, where both dangerous bacteria and venom could have contributed to military success.[1]

Perhaps the most discussed early example of biological warfare cited is the start of the Black Death – the second great pandemic. In Chapter Four we encountered the story of the Mongol Jani Beg Khan, who was laying siege to the city of Kaffa on the Crimea in 1346 without any particular success. When the plague broke out among the besiegers, the khan chose to let his catapults fling the corpses of soldiers who had died of the plague into the city, to weaken its defenders. Plague then also broke out inside the city and subsequently spread via ships to the rest of Europe. The story is without doubt a good one, but it has to be admitted that the plague probably reached the defenders of the city via the usual paths of infection and not by corpses being catapulted into it. Plague-infested fleas tend to leave cold dead bodies in order to find new living hosts, so it is unlikely that plague bacteria were spread from dead bodies.[2]

Let us move many centuries forwards in time to the Seven Years War between the French and the British in North America. In 1763 the British commander-in-chief, Sir Jeffrey Amherst, arranged that indigenous tribes hostile to the British were given woollen blankets that had been used by smallpox patients in the hope, as one of his officers wrote, that this 'would have the desired effect'. Smallpox did indeed break out among the recipients. At least one statue of the valiant Sir Jeffrey has been raised in the USA, presumably not for his attempts at biological warfare.[3]

It is difficult to estimate how effective attempts at biological warfare in former times actually were. It is highly probable that the many epidemics that always followed in the wake of war most often resulted from the usual channels of infection.

After the bacteriological revolution, the potential for really effective biological warfare was naturally completely changed, since it was now known what microbes were capable of. Germany, which had played an important role in the bacteriological revolution, was quick to realize the potential for using microbes as weapons of war. As early as the First World War Germany had established a programme to develop such weapons, which initially mainly focused on various animals of military importance to the enemy. Two bacteria were selected: the anthrax bacterium, which Robert Koch had studied with such great success, and *Burkholderia mallei*, which causes the serious disease known as glanders in horses, donkeys and mules. These bacteria were used, among other things, to infect Romanian sheep that were to be exported to Russia, and Argentinian cattle that were going to be exported to Germany's enemies. German saboteurs in France attempted to infect the cavalry horses of the French army, and German agents in the USA tried to incapacitate horses that were about to be sent to the arenas of war in Europe, since horses continued to play an important role during the First World War.

Only to a small extent were humans also a target group for German bacteriological warfare, which was overshadowed by the reaction to the horrific results of chemical warfare using poisonous gas during the First World War. The response led to the signing of the Geneva Protocol of 1925, which forbade the offensive use of both chemical and biological weapons, but it did not forbid research within this field or production of such weapons.

After 1925 a number of countries, many of which had signed the Geneva Protocol, actually started carrying out research with the aim of developing microbes that might be useful in war. The country that did so with the greatest enthusiasm was Japan, which in the period from 1932 to 1945 developed the most comprehensive programme for the development of biological weapons the world has ever seen. A series of special research institutions were established, with a major headquarters in northeastern China, the notorious Unit 731, as well as various smaller research centres. Unit 731 supported 3,000 researchers and its operations covered seventy buildings, including laboratories, crematoriums and its own airfield. Here, large-scale experiments were carried out on POWs and civilians, who were infected with various microbes, including plague, cholera and anthrax bacteria. Ten thousand people died in connection with these experiments, some from infections that had been inflicted on them, others as a result of executions after completed experiments.[4]

Japan's programme for biological warfare was led by General Shiro Ishii, a doctor well qualified in microbiology and a professor in immunology. The capable and ambitious Ishii was supported in his activities by the highest echelon of Japan's leaders, possibly even by Emperor Hirohito himself.

The Japanese did not content themselves with experimenting, but used bacteriological weapons during their ruthless campaigns in China as early as the late 1930s. At least eleven Chinese towns were attacked with such weapons, with the Japanese attempting to start epidemics by infecting drinking water and food. The Japanese air force was also involved. Fleas that had been infected in the laboratory with plague bacteria were released over Chinese towns, up to 15 million fleas per release. Despite the strong emphasis on biological weapons in China, it is uncertain just how effective this form of warfare was. There were a great many accidents in which up to 10,000 Japanese military personnel became infected as a result of poor control of their own bacteriological weapons, and 1,700 of them died.[5]

On the other hand, Japan's ally, Germany, made little effort to develop biological weapons during the Second World War. Adolf Hitler actually forbade the development of such weapons, for reasons that are somewhat unclear. It is possible that his own experiences as a victim of poisonous gas during the First World War made him a hardened opponent of both chemical and biological weapons.

The large-scale experiments in which prisoners in German concentration camps were given infections of various kinds were not carried out in order to develop bacteriological weapons. The Allies, however, did not know this and feared that Germany was going to use such weapons. As a result they started their own research and development programmes within the field.

At the beginning of the war, Britain began to develop the anthrax bacterium as a weapon. Comprehensive experiments of the effect of such bacteria on sheep were carried out on Gruinard Island, a tiny, uninhabited island off the west coast of Scotland. The experiments were

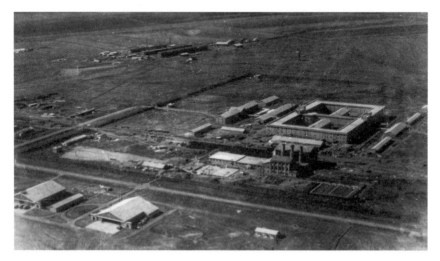

Unit 731 in northeastern China was the centre for the development of Japan's biological weapons. The centre had 3,000 researchers and its own laboratories, crematoriums and airfield. Here, large-scale experiments were carried out on POWs and civilian prisoners.

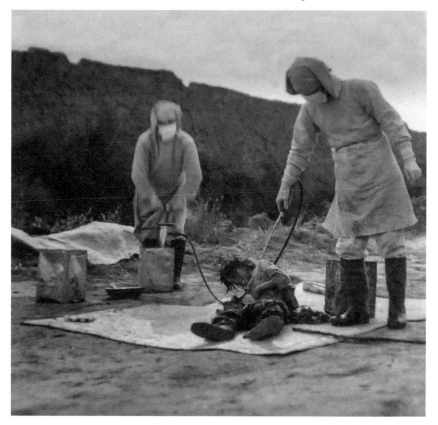

Bacteriological experiment carried out on a child in General Shiro Ishii's programme for biological warfare, 1940s.

regarded as successful, but it proved impossible to clear up afterwards. Gruinard Island was so saturated with anthrax bacteria that it was quite uninhabitable until 1990. In cooperation with the USA, Winston Churchill chose to invest in bombs with anthrax spores, but they were never put to use.

The USA started to develop bacteriological weapons in the first years of the Second World War. It gradually became known that the Americans, despite their knowledge of the horrific experiments the Japanese had carried out on humans, chose to offer the research leaders responsible immunity in exchange for their research results. The Americans began negotiations with Shiro Ishii and a number of his associates in 1947. At the same time, they understood that if news of this leaked out, it would show the USA in an extremely bad light, so the negotiations were kept top secret. In documents that later became accessible, there is not a single sentence in which ethical reservations are expressed about this horse-dealing. The decision must have been approved at the highest level, possibly by President Harry S. Truman himself.[6]

Experiments on animals involving various microbes (both bacteria and viruses) were carried out by the Americans at the project's head-quarters, Fort Detrick in Maryland, in distant desert areas and on rafts in the Pacific. Experiments were also carried out on volunteers, both military and civilian. In order to study the conditions for the spread of microbes in the air, clouds of bacteria believed to be non-dangerous were also released over American cities, including San Francisco. When this became publicly known in 1976, it led to strong criticism, partly because several cases of infection with one of the bacteria that had been used, *Serratia marcescens*, which is known to cause serious infection in people with weakened immune systems, occurred in San Francisco at the same time as these experiments with airborne bacteria. Similar experiments with other bacteria were later carried out in the New York subway.

American work within this area was intensified in connection with the Korean War of 1950–53. North Korea and China then accused the USA of having used bacteriological weapons, but these accusations have never been documented. Even so, by the end of the 1960s the USA had a considerable arsenal of microbes for military use.

During the 1970s interest in biological warfare using microbes diminished. President Richard Nixon issued a decree prohibiting the development and use of microbial weapons in 1969. In 1972 the Biological Weapons Convention (BWC) also forbade the development and use of all biological weapons and ordered the destruction of all stockpiles of such weapons. It was hardly just ethical considerations that lay behind this move. The perception in military and political circles was now that biological weapons had too many disadvantages to be regarded as militarily useful. It was thought that the effects are unpre-dictable and can affect the users as much as the opponents. Experiences gained from Japan's large-scale usage of such weapons supported this view.[7]

We know that several of the countries that signed the BWC in 1972 have nevertheless continued their work on developing biological weap-ons. This applies, for example, to the former Soviet Union, which started an active development programme for such weapons back in the 1930s. After 1972 it secretly continued this work at a number of research and production establishments that involved almost 55,000 researchers and technicians during the Cold War. The risk involved in this work became evident in 1979 when an anthrax epidemic broke out among those living and working up to 4 kilometres away from one of the research laboratories in Sverdlovsk (now Yekaterinburg). At least 77 people became infected, and 66 of them died. Animals also died of anthrax up to 50 kilometres away from the supposed source of infection. In the West it was assumed that the epidemic was due to the wind spreading anthrax spores from the research laboratory. The Soviet Union denied this for years until Boris Yeltsin admitted the connection in 1992.[8]

Terrorism and Microbes

Until the end of the twentieth century the focus of interest was mainly in the use of microbes as weapons in war. This is also evident from the international agreements made within this area, from the Geneva Protocol of 1925 to the BWC in 1972. Over the last few decades, however, it nevertheless became clear that such weapons are also of interest to players other than states at war. The phenomenon of bioterrorism has become an increasing threat. Both criminal individuals and terrorist groups of various sizes are capable of employing biological weapons. One of the aims of the terrorists, as the term implies, is to create fear, and deadly microbes are a way of doing so. Bioterrorism is a gruesome reality: there were 185 documented cases of it during the twentieth century.

In 1984 members of the Rajneeshee religious sect poisoned the food in a number of salad bars in Oregon with the bacterium *Salmonella typhimurium*. This bacterium causes acute intestinal infection that can be serious: in this case 751 people were infected, 45 were hospitalized, but no one died.[9] This sect was founded by the Indian philosopher Bhagwan Shree Rajneesh, who allowed himself to be worshipped like a guru and lived in considerable luxury, allegedly owning 93 Rolls-Royce limousines. The sect acquired a considerable number of members, first in India, but later also in Western countries. Its teaching was a mixture of Hinduism, Buddhism and Western philosophy and psychology, as well as the cultivation of sexual activity as a means of spiritual development.

In the 1980s the Rajneeshees moved to the USA, where they wished to establish a community close to the small town of Antelope, Oregon. They came into conflict with the local populace and attempted to take over the town, partly by criminal methods that included arson and assassination attempts on local officials. The terror attack with bacteria was an attempt to influence an election. Two members of the sect were given prison sentences, while the leader was deported.

In 1985 another religious sect, Aum Shinrikyo, struck in Tokyo with an attack on the metro system using the toxic gas sarin.[10] Twelve people died and more than a thousand needed treatment. This sect, which had started in Japan but gradually acquired members in many countries, had a kind of theology that was a strange syncretism of Tibetan Buddhism, yoga, Nostradamus' prophecies and Hinduism, including the worship of Shiva, the Hindu god of destruction. Their teaching proclaimed an imminent Day of Judgement, when the sect members would survive and found a new world. Terrorist attacks were intended to help bring about this judgement day.

In addition to a number of attacks with poisonous gas, it transpired that the sect had also been working on bacteriological weapons, including anthrax bacteria and the toxin from botulin bacteria, which were spread via drones – admittedly to no effect. They allegedly also had plans to try and use the Ebola virus for their terrorist ends. A number of the members were condemned to death, and seven of them were executed in 2018, including the founder of the sect, Shoko Asahara.

About a month after the terrorist attack on the World Trade Center on 11 September 2001, seven or eight letters containing anthrax spores were posted to various newspapers and radio stations as well as to two Democratic senators: 22 people were infected with anthrax and five died. It turned out that the anthrax spores in the letters had been produced in a way that indicated the source was the research laboratories of the American armed forces at Fort Detrick. A number of researchers therefore came under suspicion, but nothing could be proved. The pressure, however, led to one of the researchers at Fort Detrick committing suicide. The perpetrator behind the terrorist attack was never found.[11]

This example illustrates the consequences of even a limited terrorist attack on the population, in addition to deaths, the damage to health and the massive sense of fear it creates. The economic consequences in this case amounted to at least $300 million to disinfect all the buildings that had perhaps been affected. Between twenty and thirty federal agents worked on the case for seven years. In addition, one of the original suspects at Fort Detrick was paid several million dollars in compensation by the authorities.

Today, bioterrorism is a real threat. We will take a closer look at this problem later.

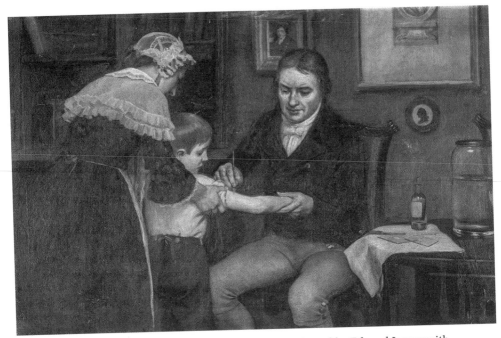

Eight-year-old James Phipps was the first to be vaccinated by Edward Jenner with his new vaccine on 14 May 1796; the scene is depicted here in a painting by Ernest Board from *c.* 1912.

NINE

Homo sapiens Strikes Back

Ll living organisms – from bacteria to *Homo sapiens* – are threatened by infection from microbes. That is why we find forms of defence against infection in even the simplest of organisms. As we move higher up the world of animals, we gradually see an increasingly complex immune system, which is the result of millions of years of perfecting via the evolutionary selection mechanisms – and with constant pressure from the world of microbes.

Behaviour as a Defence against Infection

The immune response against infection is often extremely effective and leads to the suppression of the microbe, but this comes at a price. The response calls for quite a lot of energy that could have been used for other important bodily functions, and it often involves symptoms such as a high temperature, feeling ill and fatigue, which, for a shorter or longer period, can be debilitating. So it is not surprising that patterns of behaviour have evolved by which individuals actively seek to avoid any encounter with pathogenic microbes, as this has obvious advantages for the survival of the species. We know of a great many examples of such mechanisms from the world of animals.[1]

The roundworm *Caenorhabditis elegans* has been much used in biological research. This small worm has only 302 nerve cells, yet it is capable of discovering and avoiding pathogenic bacteria in its surroundings. A certain species of lobster has been found to avoid other lobster individuals with viral infections. Studies of frogs have revealed that tadpoles, which apparently do not display any especially clever form of behaviour as they swim around, avoid other tadpoles with fungal infections.[2]

In insects we find similar examples of behaviour that prevents problems with infection. Bees remove sick and dead individuals from the hive, excrete outdoors and even make use of a kind of antibacterial agent. Birds and mammals also take care to keep their nests and lairs free of faeces, and many mammals have their own latrines. Sheep will not graze where excrement is lying, and it is believed that the migration of reindeer is partly due to the wish to avoid grazing areas with much excrement. All these forms of behaviour have probably developed because it is important to avoid excrement that contains pathogenic microbes. During the strict selection process of evolution, individuals whose genes have too little control over such behaviour simply go under, and individuals with stronger infection-preventative behaviour reproduce and pass on their genes.

These forms of genetically controlled behaviour, which prevent infections and, via evolution, have become an important supplement to the development of an actual immune defence system, are given the name 'the behavioural immune system'.[3] There are very strong indications that *Homo sapiens* also has a genetic legacy of this type. This is hardly surprising, and there have been many signs of this down through human history.

Loathing and revulsion as defence mechanisms

Only 130 years have passed since the bacteriological revolution and knowledge of the role of microbes in diseases. Even so, we find early on in the history of all human cultures special rules of conduct and patterns of behaviour that contribute to avoiding infection. Such patterns are based on long experience, but apparently also partly have a genetic background. These patterns of reaction are probably the expression of the same mechanism we see in many lower species of animal: infection-preventative patterns of behaviour that evolution has then cultivated.

Recent research suggests that psychological mechanisms linked to loathing and revulsion play an important role in our relation to threats from microbes.[4] Such emotions are often linked to a real risk of infection in certain areas. Human faeces, for example, contain amounts of possibly pathogenic microbes and give rise to strong loathing and an unwillingness to come into contact with it. The same applies to other human body fluids, rotting food and such animals as rats, mice and various insects that are possible threats as carriers of microbes. Smell and taste are involved in such mechanisms of revulsion, but so is a sense impression such as revulsion at the sight of sick individuals, and attempts are often made to avoid them or exclude them from the company of healthy people. An aversion to strangers who do not belong to one's own 'tribe' may also be an ancient protective mechanism against infections, since strangers can be carriers of new infectious diseases against which one's own group does not have any immunity.

Many of these ways of reacting to possible threats of infection gradually became formulated in religious writings, for example in India and the Middle East. The Vedas, from 200 BC, mention the so-called Manus laws, which tell one to avoid 'bodily impurities', including faeces, urine, semen, blood and nasal mucus. In both the Old Testament and the Koran we find passages where there is a linkage between impurity and sin and a call for purgation.[5]

Through the ages, views that diseases can be spread via contagion certainly lived alongside the 'official' medical teaching about the great importance of miasmas. Both views accord well with the ancient patterns of reaction to diseases based on loathing and revulsion and the desire to avoid illness. The miasma theories were, after all, especially based on the importance of dirt, waste and rotting, evil-smelling materials that are disgusting and give rise to revulsion. The sanitary movement that triumphed in European cities in the nineteenth century was probably inspired not only by the established miasma theories but by ancient reactions based on loathing and revulsion. The highly developed sewage and waste disposal systems of the Indus Valley and Roman civilizations were naturally not constructed because of any knowledge about microbes and infectious diseases, but were probably also based on the ancient revulsion to faeces, dirt and rotting waste.

Cultural and religious influences, however, can sometimes steamroller more or less natural, inherited patterns of reaction. That could well be the explanation why bodily dirt was for centuries seen as a sign of holiness among monks and hermits in the Middle Ages. The Byzantine-Greek concept of 'alousia', the state of being unwashed, was seen by certain theologians as a morally praiseworthy rejection of vanity and secularity. Such attitudes, however, are not found in Islam.

Nowadays, with every school pupil having heard about bacteria and viruses, most of them will probably assume that our disgust at dirt, faeces, rats and the like is based on a rational fear of microbes. Most likely, the truth of the matter is that we are still influenced by the ancient ways of reacting that have proved useful throughout human history.

Legislation and Microbes

From both the Old and the New Testaments it is clear that anyone with leprosy in biblical times was excluded from society and had to live in isolation, as has been the case ever since. It was not until after the Black Death struck in the mid-fourteenth century that public authorities started to take responsibility with regard to other epidemic diseases. Experiences from the ravages of the plague initially led to the introduction of the system we now know as quarantine.

Quarantine regulations sought to prevent the plague from entering a country via ships arriving at the country's ports, and it meant that all vessels coming from what were considered plague-infected areas had to lie at anchor for forty days before passengers, crew and cargo could be landed. In the course of the fifteenth century most Christian ports in the Mediterranean area began to use the quarantine system. This is not all that surprising, as it was these ports that were mostly in direct trading contact with the countries where the plague was still common.[6]

The various ports competed with each other to have the optimum quarantine system. In a number of towns, small hospitals called *lazaretti* (singular *lazaretto*) were built for people in quarantine. The word 'lasarett', variously spelled, is still used in certain languages as the word for a hospital. The implementation of quarantine varied from town to town and there was no standardization of the regulations. Quarantine could result in considerable commercial loss since it introduced obstacles to trade, and there are many examples of powerful trading companies and individuals attempting to influence the quarantine measures of authorities. It could often have major economic consequences for a city or an area if it was declared a plague location. There are examples of competing trading towns spreading false plague rumours in order to damage rivals.

Gradually quarantine measures were also introduced for other diseases, especially cholera and yellow fever. Inside a country, quarantine measures were also introduced outside the harbour towns in the event of an epidemic. Entire towns could be placed in quarantine if they were regarded as sources of infection.

Forms of quarantine measures were also used against individuals or groups of people suspected of being carriers of the plague. They were often forcibly placed in special plague houses where the quality of the care provided varied considerably. It was particularly the poor who were subjected to such measures, and their possessions could in certain cases be burned.

Did quarantine help combat epidemics? It is not easy to answer that question, since the effect depended on the manner of infection in the epidemic in question. Infections that are spread via mosquitoes, fleas and rats are not necessarily susceptible to quarantine measures. Furthermore, the effect will depend on how consistently the measures are applied. An example of strictly applied quarantine that might have worked is the measures adopted by the Habsburg empire against plague along the borders of the Ottoman empire, where the plague continued to exist right up until modern times. Over approximately 1,600 kilometres of borders, the Habsburg monarchy employed watch-towers and soldiers to maintain a cordon sanitaire against the Ottoman empire from the beginning of the eighteenth century until the end of the nineteenth. The soldiers had orders to shoot all travellers who did not comply with the 48-day quarantine. Woollen goods that could conceivably spread the plague were placed in a warehouse along with a number of low-status individuals. If these guinea pigs became infected, they were mercilessly shot and the wares burned. This strict quarantine policy is probably the reason plague did not occur in the Habsburg empire after 1716, while there were fresh outbreaks on the Ottoman side of the border.

Both in ports and on land, however, quarantine measures gave rise to major problems for trade and became increasingly unpopular, particularly during the nineteenth century.[7] More and more, people started to doubt if they were effective. A number of international conferences were held on this issue, and certain countries dispensed with the quarantine measures, while others retained them for quite some time. During the nineteenth century most Western countries introduced new legislation within the field of epidemics, in which quarantine, generally speaking, played a much more modest role than before. A modern state still has to be able to implement restrictive measures against epidemics that can also restrict the lives and activities of its citizens, but attention paid to human rights and the interests of private individuals are now emphasized in a completely different way than in former times.

Vaccination: The Great Step Forward

In the human struggle against microbes, no single measure has been as effective as vaccination. A systematic use of vaccines means that today we have gained control over a number of diseases that formerly led to serious illness and even death, diseases which the population resignedly regarded as unavoidable misfortunes.

We now know the basic principle of vaccination: by stimulating the immune system with a suitable vaccine against a microbe, we increase the strength of the system against further infection by the same microbe and thereby the chance of avoiding a recurrence. This is due to the capacity of the immune system to remember. Once the cells have reacted to an antigen – special, alien molecules – a memory of this is stored in special memory cells, which leads to a considerably stronger immune response if there is contact with the same antigen at a later stage.

We have only had this knowledge of how vaccination works for just over a hundred years. The first forms of vaccination, on the other hand, were introduced long before this. The history of vaccinations is long and both colourful and fascinating, with strong personalities in important roles.

Smallpox, society ladies and milkmaids

The first infectious disease against which vaccination was used in an early form was smallpox, which has ravaged civilizations down through the ages in the Old World, with constant epidemics and millions of deaths. From as early as the beginning of the Christian era, the Chinese used a form of vaccination, with powdered scabs from the rashes of smallpox patients being inserted in various ways up the nose of the person being vaccinated. This often led to a mild infection and gave immunity against smallpox.[8] It is unclear what lay behind this early form of vaccination, which was hardly the result of any scientific testing. Can it have been magic conceptions about the nature of the infection that lay behind the first experiments, or was it based on the experience that those who survived smallpox did not contract it at a later stage? Either way, this form of vaccination gradually spread westwards from China. In the sixteenth century we know that the Brahmins, the highest caste among Hindus in India, used the technique. It then spread to Persia and Turkey. As an alternative to the nose technique, after a while people began to rub the content of smallpox patients' blisters into small scratches in the skin.

The common history of vaccination in Europe begins in Turkey. The main character in this often highly oversimplified story is the intelligent and determined Lady Mary Wortley Montagu, who was married to the British ambassador in Turkey and lived in Constantinople. She had been a popular belle of society and had a greater interest than others in smallpox, since before her marriage she had contracted this infection. She survived, but without eyelashes and with considerable facial scarring. Just over a year before this, her younger brother had died of smallpox. She discovered that it was extremely common in Turkey for children to be inoculated with smallpox material from patients in small scratches made in the skin, which later protected them against this infection.[9]

In 1717 she described her experiences in Constantinople in a letter to her good friend Sarah Chiswell, who was to die from smallpox a few years later. In the letter Lady Mary states that she wishes to introduce the technique in England, even though she feared resistance from doctors, since they would lose a good source of income from the lengthy treatment of smallpox that had become usual. She started by allowing the embassy doctor to vaccinate her five-year-old son, first making sure that her husband, who opposed the method, was absent on a journey.

After returning to London, Lady Mary also had her young daughter vaccinated in 1721 as the first person in England, and she invited a number of people to see the result, including the prominent physician Sir Hans Sloane, who had treated Lady Mary for her smallpox infection and was the physician-in-ordinary to the king. The royal family became interested, particularly Princess Caroline, who was married to the Prince of Wales, later George II, and was a friend of Lady Mary. The princess had nearly lost a daughter to smallpox and now wished to vaccinate two other daughters. She gained the king's permission for this, but only after the method, for safety's sake, had been tried out in Newgate Prison on six condemned prisoners, who were promised their freedom if they survived. The experiment, which was watched over by more than 25 prominent physicians, was successful. The prisoners were released and later proved to be immune to smallpox. Children at an orphanage were also vaccinated. When that too was a success, the princesses were vaccinated.

In this account Lady Mary is portrayed as the heroine who must take the main credit for the new method being introduced in England, and later in other countries. Her role has probably been somewhat exaggerated. There is good reason to believe that Sir Hans Sloane played a more important role in introducing vaccination and has unjustifiably been overshadowed by the enterprising lady. (I dare to write this since the view has in fact been advanced by a female historian, Genevieve Miller.[10]) Nor is it completely true that it was Lady Mary who first sent news of the Turkish method of vaccination to England. European doctors in Constantinople had known of this method from the beginning of the eighteenth century. England's active scientific academy, the Royal Society, of which Sir Hans was incidentally president, had received notice of this as early as 1713, and other physicians on the continent had also been informed. Charles XII of Sweden, during his years of exile in Turkey after the defeat at Poltava in 1709, was able to purchase the 'secret' of the Turkish vaccination method for 100 ducats.[11] He did not, however, undertake anything as a result after returning to Sweden. Tragically enough, his sister Ulrika Eleonora, who succeeded Charles after he was killed when laying siege to the fortress of Fredriksten in Norway in 1718, died of smallpox in 1741.

The extent to which this early form of vaccination was used was uneven during the eighteenth century. Even in England, its popularity came in waves. There were several reasons for this. For a long time there was a certain scepticism about the use of this measure against smallpox. This was probably partly because the amount of smallpox virus in the vaccine caused a few people (perhaps 1–2 per cent) to develop a serious smallpox infection that led to death, although a far greater proportion of those unvaccinated died of the natural infection. Another fact was that for a time those who had been vaccinated could spread the smallpox virus and cause small-scale epidemics, so it became usual to isolate them

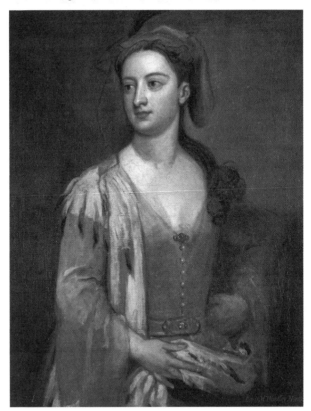

Lady Mary Wortley Montagu, as seen here in a painting by Sir Godfrey Kneller from 1715–20.

for a couple of weeks. Religious objections were voiced, particularly in Scotland, which was strictly Calvinist. Many regarded vaccination as an expression of a lack of trust in God's foresight.[12]

Attitudes also varied on the continent.[13] In France it took some time before vaccination caught on, despite the fact that the influential Voltaire, who had become acquainted with the method during a stay in England in the 1720s, was extremely positive and strongly recommended it to his fellow countrymen 'so that they can keep themselves alive and their women beautiful'. Then things eased in the 1750s. When the Duke of Orléans had his two daughters vaccinated, fashionable Paris rejoiced, and a new type of hat was introduced, the 'bonnet à l'inoculation', which had ribbons with spots that were intended to represent a smallpox rash. Then enthusiasm died down for a while, until Louis XV's horrific death from smallpox in 1774. When the new king, Louis XVI, was vaccinated without any problems that same year, his wife Marie Antoinette's hairdresser designed a new, bold hairstyle: the 'pouf à l'inoculation'. Smallpox vaccination also came to Scandinavia, where among others the Swedish crown prince, later King Gustav III, had himself vaccinated.

In the USA smallpox vaccination developed fairly independently of what was happening in Europe. The key figure here was the colourful, influential Puritan clergyman Cotton Mather. He is perhaps best known for his support of the notorious witch trials in Salem, Massachusetts, where two hundred people were accused and twenty executed. Mather, however, was also extremely interested in science. In 1706 he heard about smallpox vaccination from his Black slave Onesimus. Vaccination had been common in Africa for a long time and had possibly been introduced by Arab slave traders who, for economic reasons, wished to protect against smallpox the endless caravans of slaves that were still crossing Africa. Mather later read the reports to the Royal Society about such vaccination and he became an ardent advocate of the trials that started in Boston in 1721, the same year that Lady Mary Wortley Montagu had her daughter vaccinated in London. But the spread of vaccination in the USA was highly uneven, and this was to prove most unfortunate during the war of independence against Britain in the 1770s. The British soldiers had either been vaccinated or had had smallpox as children, whereas the Americans were unprotected. An outbreak of smallpox caused such serious problems for the American forces that George Washington, in 1777, ordered the entire American army to be vaccinated.[14]

Smallpox raged in Europe and North America throughout the eighteenth century, but even so it is usually agreed that vaccination with smallpox virus had a positive effect on public health and contributed to the population growth in the second half of the century, particularly where vaccination was carried out systematically on large groups.

This was, however, a quite primitive form of vaccine, since it made use of the common smallpox virus, with the elements of risk that this involved. Towards the end of the eighteenth century a sensational discovery by the British doctor Edward Jenner resulted in something that can be considered to mark the breakthrough of modern vaccination. The story of Jenner and his new smallpox vaccine is well known, but here too the traditional account is both simplified and partly based on myths. What actually lay behind the epoch-making discovery, which was to lead to the smallpox virus being eradicated two hundred years later?

Milkmaids play a certain role in the great majority of versions of the story. Jenner is said to have taken up a popular belief in rural England that milkmaids often became infected with cowpox, a fairly harmless infection, when milking cows. It was said that they never contracted smallpox and therefore had beautiful skin. In certain versions of the story Jenner picked this up while flirting with a young milkmaid at some point during the 1760s. It is impossible to ascertain today to what extent Jenner may have had a weakness for milkmaids, but in any case they played only a modest role in the history of vaccination. Recent research indicates that Jenner early on heard a rumour that people who had contracted cowpox previously could not be vaccinated in the 'old' way, as the vaccine would not produce the necessary skin reaction. He became interested in the idea, but did not follow it up for a number of years while he pursued his medical studies. One of his teachers in London was the Scottish surgeon John Hunter, whose motto was: 'Don't think! Carry out experiments!' Jenner probably made a mental note of this.[15]

As a qualified doctor, Jenner set up practice at home in Gloucester-shire, while also cultivating his strong interest in natural science. Among other things, he studied the cuckoo and was the first to describe the young cuckoo's uncongenial habit of pushing the host bird's own off-spring out of the nest. Thanks to his article, Jenner became a member of the prestigious Royal Society. All the while, however, he had been ruminating on the possible ability of cowpox to protect people against smallpox, and now he followed his former teacher's advice: he began to experiment.

First, Jenner attempted to vaccinate several people who had had cowpox against smallpox in the 'old way', and he was able to confirm that the vaccine refused to 'catch on' and produce the necessary skin reaction. In 1796 he took a small amount of fluid from a cowpox sore on the hand of a milkmaid by the name of Sara Nelmes and scratched it into the arm of a poor eight-year-old boy by the name of James Phipps. Six weeks later, when he scratched a small amount of pus from a smallpox patient into the boy's arm, there was no reaction at all. The boy, then, was now protected against the smallpox virus.[16]

Jenner sent a report of this to the Royal Society, but they refused to print it and warned him that he could lose his reputation as a scientist if he pursued the idea that cowpox could protect one against smallpox.

Despite this, Jenner carried out more experiments with the same result, and published his findings privately in 1798. He was convinced that his new vaccine ought to replace the old one – and large parts of the world agreed with him. His method quickly spread, first in England and then to other countries. It was both safer and cheaper than the old method, which soon ceased to be used. With the new method there was no risk of the vaccinated person developing smallpox or infecting others, as had been the case with the former technique.[17]

Edward Jenner became world-famous and received many honours, including from several royal houses who supported universal vaccination using his method in their respective countries. The Russian dowager empress sent him a diamond ring and decreed that the first person to be vaccinated in Russia – a child from a children's home – was to be given the name Vaccinov. Napoleon immediately realized the potential of this breakthrough and ordered the French army to be vaccinated as well as the civilian population. After an approach from Jenner concerning the release of some British prisoners of war, he agreed to this immediately with the words: 'Ah, Jenner, I cannot refuse him anything!'[18]

Not everyone was as positively inclined towards Edward Jenner and his discoveries. He also became the subject of considerable criticism. There were many, for example, who came forward and claimed (justifiably in some cases) that they had been vaccinating with material from cowpox before Jenner. Perhaps the best-documented case is the story of the English farmer Benjamin Jesty. As early as 1774 he vaccinated his wife and two children with cowpox in order to protect them during a smallpox epidemic, because he had heard the story that milkmaids seldom caught this infection. His neighbours laughed at him and he did not take it any further, although he did gain some recognition thirty years later, and after his death his widow made sure that an account of his efforts was fittingly inscribed on his gravestone in Worth Matravers, Dorset.

Jenner's vaccine was also attacked for other reasons. The English clergyman and social scientist Thomas Robert Malthus believed that smallpox epidemics were one of nature's ways of curbing population growth. There were also religious objections partly based on the idea that the vaccine interfered with God's plan for humanity, and partly on views about prohibitions in the Bible about 'the pollution of the blood'.

Professions that made lucrative gains from the rather expensive and complex 'old' form of vaccination, which included isolation under observation and special diets, were also among the critics. It is somewhat surprising that also the prominent scientist and evolutionary thinker Alfred Russel Wallace was a vociferous opponent of Jenner's vaccine.[19]

The story of Jenner and cowpox has a curious epilogue. New molecular-biological experiments have sown doubts about what was really in Jenner's vaccine. Did he vaccinate using cowpox virus? The virus used during the entire nineteenth century is not identical with present-day cowpox virus, but is more closely related to a virus that causes horsepox. Either the original variant of cowpox that Jenner used has become extinct, or the virus has changed its characteristics in the course of two centuries. Perhaps Jenner's original vaccine virus was horsepox. No matter the origins, though, this vaccine led to the eradication of smallpox in the world.[20]

The virus in Jenner's vaccine has been given the name *Vaccinia virus* and this is a reference to the fact that it originally came from a cow (*vacca* is the Latin word for cow). The term 'vaccination', which is also derived from *vacca*, started to be used after a suggestion from Pasteur, who wished to honour Jenner in this way. To be more precise, we ought therefore not, as I have done for the sake of simplicity, call the 'old' method introduced from China vaccination, but rather variolization or inoculation with the smallpox virus.

Jenner's smallpox vaccine was introduced quite rapidly in most Western countries and very often vaccination was compulsory. The occurrence of smallpox gradually declined in these parts of the world during the second half of the nineteenth century. Major epidemics still broke out at certain intervals because of uneven vaccination coverage. The value of smallpox vaccination was evidently clear during the Franco-Prussian War of 1870–71: in the German army of 800,000 men, practically all of whom had been vaccinated, only 459 soldiers died of smallpox. In the French army of a million men, more than 23,000 died of the disease, almost as many as the number of German soldiers killed in battle. In the wake of this war, the smallpox virus also quickly spread among the civilian population in a number of countries.

At the end of the Second World War, smallpox had more or less disappeared from Western countries. The virus did, however, continue to cause problems in developing countries and was therefore still a threat to those that, in practice, had eradicated smallpox within their own borders. In 1967 the WHO therefore began a large-scale campaign against smallpox, which involved monitoring the smallpox situation, isolating cases and promoting systematic smallpox vaccination. This led to the WHO being able to claim in 1979 that smallpox had been eradicated. Jenner had finally gained the ultimate triumph.

Rabies and anthrax: Pasteur makes his mark

After Louis Pasteur's first triumphs, in which he had demonstrated the importance of bacteria both in fermentation processes and in diseases in silkworms, he became increasingly interested in the possible importance of bacteria in diseases of higher species of animal, including humans. He started by studying the disease known as chicken cholera, even though it has nothing to do with ordinary cholera. This disease, due to the bacterium *Pasteurella multocida*, can give rise to epidemics with a high mortality rate in poultry. Pasteur had no problem detecting the bacterium and then carried out experiments to study the course of infection in chickens. He discovered that some chickens survived the acute infection and became healthy carriers of the bacterium. Pasteur could not understand why these animals survived while others did not. Was it the bacterium that had changed in those who survived, or had something happened to the animals themselves?[21]

Then something occurred by chance that would lay the foundation for all of modern vaccination medicine. Pasteur's holiday in the summer of 1879 led to his experiments needing to be discontinued for a while. Some of the test tubes with chicken cholera bacteria were left standing unused for several weeks. When he resumed his experiments on his return, the bacteria turned out to be still alive, but they no longer caused any disease in chickens. What was even more interesting was that when Pasteur gave fresh bacteria to the birds that had already been given the 'old' ones, they practically all survived, while the same bacteria given to freshly bought chickens gave them a deadly infection, as in the earlier experiments.

Pasteur realized that this demonstrated a phenomenon that was strongly reminiscent of Jenner's vaccination with cowpox virus. He reasoned that the 'old' chicken cholera bacteria, which had been left standing for several weeks, had become weaker and made innocuous because of the access to air, and in particular oxygen, in the test tube. Instead, these weakened bacteria had produced a resistance in chickens against infection with 'fresh' bacteria. For the first time Pasteur had detected what we now call immunological memory, which is the basis of all vaccination. He also realized the potential for demonstrating that the same applied to other infectious diseases and for exploiting this phenomenon, which he decided to call vaccination, in honour of Jenner.

The next infectious disease that Pasteur worked on to develop a vaccine, using the same principle as with chicken cholera, was anthrax.[22] It was through his epoch-making studies of anthrax that Pasteur's great rival, Robert Koch, had started his brilliant career by demonstrating that anthrax was definitely due to the anthrax bacterium. Some people had continued to doubt this, but Pasteur had already carried out a series of new experiments that clearly confirmed Koch's findings.

Now Pasteur envisaged the possibility of developing a vaccine against anthrax, which caused agriculture serious economic problems because of its high mortality rate in cattle, sheep and goats. Encouraged by his discoveries about chicken cholera, he started to weaken the anthrax bacteria in the laboratory using a series of different manipulations, and to experiment on various laboratory animals. Once again he was able to demonstrate a protective effect of the vaccine he had made.

Scepticism about Pasteur's results with the anthrax vaccine was considerable among both doctors and veterinary surgeons, and he was challenged by his opponents to demonstrate the effect of the anthrax vaccine in full publicity. This took place in 1881 at a dramatic and memorable event in Pouilly-le-Fort, south of Paris. Pasteur and his assistants vaccinated 24 sheep with two doses at ten-day intervals. After two weeks the animals were given a further injection with what would normally be a lethal dose of anthrax bacteria. Two days later, the spectators, who comprised a number of foreign journalists, were able to confirm that all the vaccinated sheep were healthy, whereas 21 of the 24 unvaccinated sheep that had also been given the bacterial injection had died. Two more of these unvaccinated animals died while the observers were watching, and the final sheep died the following day. Those watching gave Pasteur warm applause.

It has subsequently become obvious that Pasteur, with his usual flair for PR, to a certain extent 'doctored' the facts about the vaccine used at the dramatic demonstration in Pouilly-le-Fort.[23] The vaccine used was not the one Pasteur himself had worked on, but a variant developed by one of his assistants. However that may be, anthrax vaccine had now become a fact, and it soon became widespread. The economic gain for France of this vaccine was so great that it contributed to paying the country's war reparations to Germany, amounting to 5 billion gold francs, after its crushing defeat in the Franco-Prussian War.

The viral disease rabies, which today is no longer a problem in the Western world, was in the 1880s a feared threat in both France and the rest of Europe. Pasteur was convinced that the disease, which normally was the result of having been bitten by an infected dog, must be due to a microbe.[24] Viruses were unknown at the time, and Pasteur could not

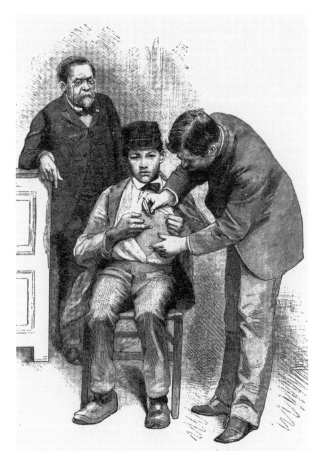

Nine-year-old Joseph Meister is vaccinated against rabies by one of Pasteur's assistants in July 1885, depicted here in the French newspaper *L'Illustration*, 7 November 1885. Before then, the vaccine had been given only to dogs.

manage to detect the microbe that caused rabies. On the other hand, he did succeed in cultivating it by injecting saliva from infected dogs directly into the brains of other dogs. When he removed spinal tissue from dead, infected dogs, he was able to transmit the disease by injecting it into new animals. Then Pasteur once more had a brilliant idea. Perhaps it would prove possible to weaken the unknown microbe in the cerebral tissue and make a vaccine against rabies in the same way as he had done with such success with chicken cholera and anthrax? After laborious work, he succeeded and was able to demonstrate that the vaccine protected the dogs against rabies. The great challenge now was to find out if the vaccine was also effective in humans.

Both Pasteur, who was not a medical doctor, and his medical assistants, especially, were extremely wary of trying out the vaccines on humans, until Pasteur suddenly found himself facing a dramatic challenge. A nine-year-old boy named Joseph Meister, who had been badly savaged by a dog with rabies a couple of days earlier, was brought to him. Pasteur hesitated, but then decided to vaccinate, despite the fact that his closest colleague, the doctor Émile Roux, protested strongly and left Pasteur for some time.

Pasteur began a series of vaccinations on the boy on 7 July 1885. The young patient did not contract rabies and experienced no complications from the vaccine. Over the following months several thousand people were vaccinated, but large sections of the medical world were in uproar at what they regarded as Pasteur's irresponsible behaviour with experiments on human beings. The criticism, which was printed in newspapers as well as medical journals, took its toll on Pasteur, who had already been ailing for a number of years.

Gradually, however, the rabies vaccine was also accepted as a real step forward in dealing with a fatal illness. Part of the story is that Joseph Meister as an adult became a caretaker at the Pasteur Institute in Paris. When an officer in the German occupying forces in 1940 commanded him to open Pasteur's grave, which lies in the basement of the institute, it has been claimed that the 64-year-old Meister chose to commit suicide rather than desecrate the grave of his hero.[25]

A cascade of new vaccines

Pasteur's vaccine triumphs triggered the constant development of new vaccines. Today we have vaccines against a great many infectious diseases that are caused by bacteria and viruses. Researchers into vaccines followed one of two paths: they either practised using live but weakened (attenuated) microbes, as Pasteur had done, or using whole, killed (inactivated) microbes as a basis for a vaccine. Both methods have been used up to the present day.[26]

In the former group we find such vaccines as those against tuberculosis (BCG vaccine), measles, mumps and German measles. In the latter group are vaccines against plague, cholera, typhoid fever, typhus, yellow fever, hepatitis A and meningococci. Against certain infections, such as influenza and polio, we have both types of vaccine. With certain infections, such as tetanus and diphtheria, it is toxins – bacteria-produced toxic proteins – that are the main problem when the disease develops. These toxins can be weakened so that they can be used in vaccines. This is the basis for vaccines against tetanus and diphtheria, which we have had for many years.

Vaccination science has to a great extent profited from the major advances made in molecular biology and genetics during the second half of the twentieth century. In addition to the classic types of vaccines mentioned, we now have effective so-called subunit vaccines based on particularly important parts of the microbes involved. This applies, for example, to vaccines against pneumococci, which are an important cause of pneumonia and meningitis. Gene technology has revolutionized the production of many vaccines of the type mentioned, which can now be produced from yeast cells or bacteria that have been modified for such a purpose.

An important future step is the development of a completely new group of vaccines: gene vaccines or nucleic-acid vaccines.[27] The principle here is that the vaccine does not consist of whole microbes or parts of them, but contains genetic information in the form of DNA or RNA coding for the microbe antigen against which one wants to have immune protection. After vaccination, this genetic material will be absorbed by the body's cells and instruct them to produce this antigen.

There are three main types of gene vaccine: virus vector-based vaccines, DNA vaccines and RNA vaccines. In the first of these forms the

13ᵉ ANNÉE. — N° 612. PARIS ET DÉPARTEMENTS 15 CENTIMES 13 MARS 1886

LE DON QUICHOTTE

Rédacteur en Chef: Ch. GILBERT-MARTIN.

BORDEAUX
Bureaux : RUE CABIROL, 7
ABONNEMENTS
UN AN...... 16 fr.
SIX MOIS..... 8 »
ÉTRANGER LE PORT EN SUS
PARIS
DÉPÔT GÉNÉRAL ET VENTE
17, Rue Saint-Mar
Distribution dans les kiosques
Chez les libraires et les marchands
de journaux.

ANNONCES
LES ANNONCES SONT REÇUES
« L'AGENCE HAVAS
POUR LA PUBLICITÉ DE BORDEAUX
Péristyle du Grand-Théâtre
côté est.
la ligne
Annonces sur 6 colonnes 25 c.
Réclames sur 5 colonnes 40 c.

L'ANGE DE L'INOCULATION (M. PASTEUR), par GILBERT-MARTIN.

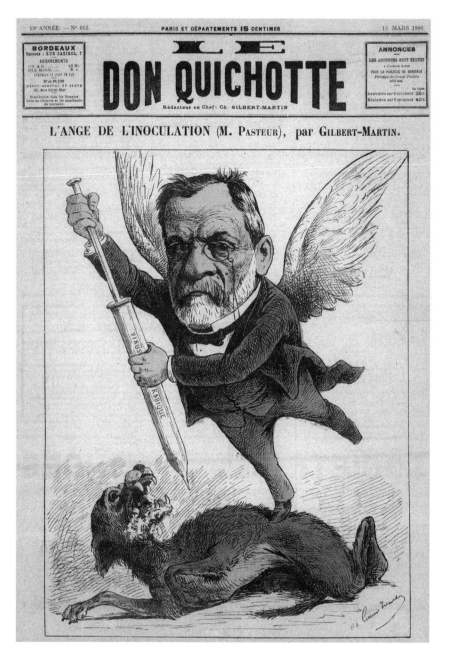

Caricature of Pasteur's fight against rabies, with his vaccine as weapon, in *Le Don Quichotte*, 13 March 1886.

genetic material is built into a harmless virus; in the other two DNA or RNA is given more directly. Only one of these types of vaccine had been approved for use on humans until late 2020, a virus-vector vaccine against the Ebola virus, but several messenger RNA (mRNA) vaccines against the SARS-CoV-2 virus have been developed, and are now being rolled out, as we will see later. In the future such vaccines will probably be employed against a number of other microbes as well.

Over recent decades the development of new vaccines has also become more rational than the old ways of making them. The explosive increase in our knowledge of details in the immunological defence system has meant that when developing new vaccines we can target them to deal with precisely the sections of the complex immune response that it is particularly important to strengthen in the infection involved. The 'classic' vaccines specially trigger the production of antibodies from the B cells, which are important in the defence against many acute infections. It has been more difficult to stimulate the T-cell system effectively against infection. This is highly important when dealing with microbes that cause such chronic infections as malaria, HIV and tuberculosis, diseases which are still a formidable challenge on the vaccine front.

Since the time of Pasteur a vast amount of work has been carried out in vaccine research, and the gains in preventing illness and death have also been enormous. These efforts have been characterized to a great extent by ongoing, patient hard work and by trial and error, which has brought about dramatic and at times bizarre episodes in the struggle to develop new vaccines. One such example is worth focusing on: work on typhus vaccines in Eastern Europe during the Second World War.

Typhus vaccination and sabotage

When Germany attacked the Soviet Union in Operation Barbarossa in 1941, it was not only the Red Army that the Germans feared. Typhus epidemics had raged in Eastern Europe during and after the First World War, affecting both soldiers and civilians. Now typhus was breaking out once more in war zones and Jewish ghettoes. Production of an effective vaccine was therefore a top German priority, mainly in order to protect military personnel.

One of the world's leading centres for typhus research in the inter-war years lay in the city of Lwów in Poland (now Lviv, Ukraine). The laboratory was led by the Polish biologist Rudolf Weigl, who had already developed a typhus vaccine that was fairly effective. The German army now seized control of the laboratory in order to ensure continued vaccine production under Weigl's leadership.[28]

It was not easy to produce a vaccine against typhus. One of the main reasons for this was that the bacterium, *Rickettsia prowazekii*, could not be cultivated in the laboratory. Weigl's method of vaccine production was extremely time-consuming – and also indelicate. Infection is transmitted via lice, and Weigl cultivated the bacterium in lice, which he infected through the rectum. Then the infected lice had to be fed a special diet: human blood. This Weigl did by installing a large number of people in his laboratory as 'louse-feeders'. Small cages were attached to their legs containing infected lice, so that the lice could suck blood through a kind of net. When the lice had been sufficiently fattened up, they were harvested and killed, and their intestines – containing a host of bacteria – were then used in the vaccine.

This procedure was not completely without risk to the louse-feeders. They were admittedly vaccinated in advance, had to have healthy skin and were given strict instructions not to scratch themselves, so that

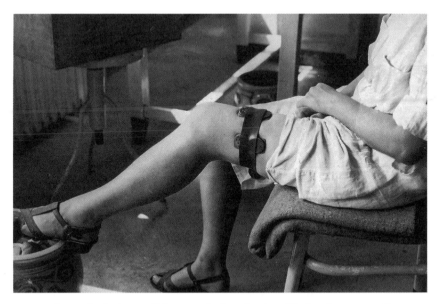

Human 'louse-feeder', a small box attached to the skin filled with 400–800 lice infected with typhus. The infected lice suck the human's blood through a net wall next to the skin. After a few days, the lice can be harvested to make a typhus vaccine.

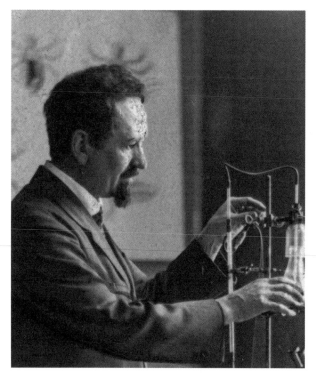

Polish biologist Rudolf Weigl (1883–1957) saved many intellectuals, Jews and resistance fighters from the Germans by using them as 'louse-feeders' in producing a typhus vaccine in his laboratory in the city of Lwów during the Second World War.

the bacteria could not penetrate the skin. Despite this, a few of them contracted typhus. Even so, the position of louse-feeder was in great demand, for Weigl recruited from the city's intellectual elite, members of the resistance and Jews, who were given a protected status in his laboratory. These were groups threatened with liquidation by the occupying power, but the German authorities interfered only rarely in activities that were regarded as important for the war effort. While the lice sucked their blood, the 'louse-feeders' could engage in a stimulating intellectual exchange of opinions in a way that in more peaceful times had taken place in the city's many cafés. During the interwar years, the city of Lwów had the reputation of being a 'mini-Vienna'.

As a scientist and expert in typhus, Weigl was naturally interested in producing an effective vaccine. On the other hand, this vaccine could promote the German enemy's war effort, a cause that his staff of louse-feeders were hardly likely to support. This led to some supplies of the vaccine intended for the Wehrmacht being intentionally of poor quality. Such sabotage, however, could not be exaggerated if discovery were to be avoided, leading perhaps to production being discontinued and maybe even worse consequences. Weigl also made sure that large supplies of effective vaccine ended up in the Jewish ghettoes in Lwów and Warsaw, thereby doubtless saving many lives.[29]

After the war Weigl was suspected of being a Nazi sympathizer. He was not given any recognition for his anti-Nazi activities until 2003, almost fifty years after his death. The Yad Vashem historical research institute in Israel then declared that Weigl was among the 'Righteous among the Nations' who had saved Jews from the Holocaust.

Weigl's laboratory, however, was not the only one working on the production of a typhus vaccine in Poland under the control of the occupying power.[30] A talented young Jewish doctor, Ludwig Fleck, was one of Weigl's assistants for a time before being placed in the Jewish ghetto in Lwów by the Nazis. There he continued to work on the typhus vaccine. The Nazis subsequently moved him to the Buchenwald concentration camp, where he was placed in a hotch-potch group of prisoners without particular forms of special knowledge of vaccines – including a baker, an upper secondary teacher and a politician – who were given orders to develop a typhus vaccine under the leadership of a German Nazi doctor who had greater ambition than scientific talent. The aim was to produce a vaccine from lung tissue in rabbits that had been infected with typhus bacteria.

Fleck, who was the only person with specialist knowledge, quickly realized that the vaccine produced by the group so far was completely unusable, and he had an idea why. The team decided to keep quiet about this and started to produce this ineffective vaccine, which was sent in large quantities to German soldiers. Under Fleck's leadership, however, the group also secretly managed to produce an effective vaccine, which they gave exclusively to needy fellow prisoners at the concentration camp.

Fleck and his assistants managed to carry out this bold sabotage for 18 months, right up until Buchenwald was liberated by the Americans in 1945. It was not until the Nuremberg trials in 1947, when prominent Nazi doctors were in the dock, that the ss doctors among the accused heard the truth about the typhus vaccine in Buchenwald. When one of them reacted with indignation about what he called a fundamental breach of medical ethics by Fleck's group, he was met by laughter from the gallery. This doctor had, after all, been responsible for deliveries of the deadly Zyklon B gas to the gas chambers and for a great many gruesome medical experiments on prisoners.

Part of the story is also that the Allies gained access to an effective typhus vaccine produced by the Americans in 1940, even before the USA entered the war.[31] It was particularly useful during the battles in North Africa, where typhus was a serious problem for both soldiers and civilians.

No roses without thorns: side-effects of vaccines

It is beyond doubt that vaccination medicine has saved countless lives through the ages, and new vaccines will in all probability lead to further progress in the prevention of infectious diseases. Even so, one must always remember that no vaccine is absolutely free of side-effects. Serious side-effects, however, are extremely rare with the common vaccines if the guidelines for use are properly observed.

With a vaccination it is not uncommon for there to be a slight inflammatory reaction at the injection site and possibly a slightly elevated temperature for the first 24 hours. Very rarely, serious allergic reactions to certain substances in the vaccine may occur, causing breathing difficulties and a fall in blood pressure.

Vaccination has in practice eradicated many acute infectious diseases from Western countries. This applies, for example, to childhood diseases such as measles, which was once extremely common. Paradoxically enough, the success of the vaccines has led to many people now focusing far more on possible side-effects than on the problems linked to the original infection. The large number of people still vaccinated also means that other illnesses in society are occasionally – in most cases unjustly – viewed as side-effects of vaccination. One example of this is stubborn assertions that the MMR vaccine against measles, mumps and German measles can cause autism. This has long since been thoroughly disproved.

On very rare occasions an unexpected side-effect of a new vaccine that has not been tested for long enough is discovered. One such is the slightly increased occurrence of the rare disease narcolepsy in children and young people after the use of a special vaccine developed to counter the swine flu epidemic in 2009.[32]

Broadly speaking, serious side-effects are extremely rare in connection with vaccinations, assuming the vaccines are used correctly. An important measure against serious side-effects is that live vaccines, that is those where the microbe in the vaccine is live but attenuated, are not given to individuals with a seriously weakened immune system. In such instances, even the weakened microbe, which cannot cause disease in people with a normally functioning immune system, can lead to serious infection.[33] Rare cases of this occurred with the BCG vaccine against TB and with the smallpox vaccine, both of which contained live but attenuated microbes. Another example is the admittedly rare occurrence of polio with paralysis, which can be seen in countries that use live polio vaccine. In such cases the attenuated polio virus has spontaneously changed inside the vaccinated person and become more dangerous.[34]

Important new challenges for vaccination medicine

The major technological advances in developing vaccines and ever-increasing knowledge about the immune system's response to infections will undoubtedly lead to new vaccines in the coming years.[35] Many existing vaccines will probably be replaced by better variants. There will also be a need for completely new vaccines against new microbes that regularly appear on the scene. In the event of new pandemics, it will be very important to develop effective vaccines as quickly as possible, in addition to other measures. While the development of vaccines used to take many years, present-day vaccine technology allows a much faster tempo.[36]

Some of the greatest challenges on the vaccine front today are related to a number of important and well-known infections against which we either have no vaccine or ones that have only a partial effect.[37]

Malaria still causes more than 400,000 deaths a year in developing countries, mostly children. An effective malaria vaccine would be of very great importance in combatting this infection. Despite many years of work on just such a project, however, we still do not have a vaccine. The reason for this is that the defence against infection by malaria plasmodia is far more complex than against ordinary bacteria and viral infections, for which we have long since had effective vaccines.

The malaria plasmodia, as we have seen, have a complicated life cycle, appearing in mosquitoes and humans in very different forms, some inside cells, others outside. Hundreds of different antigens exist on the various life forms, and we do not know which of them are important to focus on in a vaccine. This is also because we have insufficient knowledge about which parts of the immune system are important in the defence against malaria plasmodia. An effective vaccine probably ought to strengthen the immune response against several of the various life forms in which the plasmodia appear. In addition to these problems, the individual main forms of malaria also appear in different variants that have various antigens, something that further complicates the development of a vaccine.

Of the vaccine candidates for malaria that have been assessed so far, the so-called RTS,S vaccine is the one that has proved the most promising, even though the first trials have given only 40 per cent protection. In spring 2019 tests of this vaccine started in three African countries that aim to vaccinate several hundred thousand children.

The HIV virus is at least as awe-inspiring an opponent as the malaria plasmodia within the field of vaccination. There is reason to believe that we will hardly gain control over the HIV epidemic that still rages in some of the developing countries without a vaccine as a supplement to the other measures being employed.[38]

Already by the mid-1980s the first attempts were being made to develop a vaccine against the HIV virus. While the construction of this virus is far simpler than that of the malaria plasmodia, with far fewer antigens, it turned out that the problems in developing a vaccine were at least as formidable as with malaria, though in completely different ways.

Over the years, a series of extensive trials of various HIV vaccines have been carried out in various parts of the world. These attempts, which have cost millions of dollars, have not yet proved successful. Belief in the possibility of developing a vaccine against HIV infection has followed a roller-coaster pattern, with periods of great enthusiasm alternating with deep pessimism.

The reasons for the lack of success are many. First, we do not know for sure which parts of the immune system are the most important in combatting the HIV virus. Furthermore, it is a fact that the immune system does not normally manage to eliminate the HIV infection, which always becomes chronic. A particular problem is that the virus attacks the most central cells in the immune system, the $CD4^+$ T lymphocytes, which coordinate the immune response. Another problem is that the virus exists in so many variants that one vaccine would be hard put to protect a patient against all of them.

It is still uncertain whether we will manage to get an effective vaccine against the HIV virus. New attempts are being planned that involve exploiting the experience gained so far. It may be that a vaccine that is not as effective as the well-tested vaccines employed against other infections will, even so, be a valuable supplement to the other measures used against the HIV pandemic.

Tuberculosis is also high on the list of important infections for which an effective vaccine is necessary.[39] This is perhaps surprising to all those who are old enough to recall that they were given the BCG vaccine at around the age of fourteen. This vaccine was developed by Albert Calmette and Camille Guérin about a hundred years ago and has been named after them (**B**acille **C**almette **G**uérin). They were inspired by Pasteur's discovery of weakened vaccines, and their vaccine is a weakened form of the bacterium that causes tuberculosis in cattle (*Mycobacterium bovis*). In 1921 it was successfully given to humans for the first time and was then rapidly used in both Europe and on other continents. For many years the BCG vaccine was the most used vaccine in the world.

Comprehensive studies of the results of the BCG vaccine has, nevertheless, come to very different conclusions. There is agreement that it probably protects children against the most acute and life-threatening forms of TB. On the other hand, the protection against pulmonary tuberculosis in adults varies a great deal around the world. In those parts of the world worst hit by the HIV pandemic, where tuberculosis is also widespread, it is also a problem that the BCG vaccine, which is a live vaccine, can cause serious complications in patients with a weakened immune system, including those with an HIV infection.

In present-day vaccine research there is agreement that the development of a new and more effective vaccine against tuberculosis ought to have high priority. One can either improve the BCG vaccine or produce a completely new vaccine using modern principles. Either way, it will take some considerable time before the hundred-year-old BCG vaccine finds its successor.

For a number of years the world has waited for a new pandemic of an influenza A virus, and it will inevitably materialize. Such a pandemic will be able to spread throughout the globe before researchers have managed to manufacture a vaccine against the virus using present-day principles. So there is wide agreement that the world needs a more effective influenza vaccine – a so-called universal vaccine – that gives far broader immunity against most types of the influenza A virus. Such a vaccine will radically change the possibilities for preventing both new pandemics and seasonal influenza.[40]

When it became clear that the new pandemic virus SARS-CoV-2 represented a serious global threat, a number of vaccine producers and research institutes rapidly started intensive work on developing vaccines against the virus. According to the WHO, there were 173 registered candidate vaccines on 28 August 2020. Of these, 31 were already at the clinical trial stage. Several of these have completed what is known as phase 3 testing, which includes extensive studies of their efficiency and safety in several thousand people. Of the four vaccines authorized by the EU for use as of July 2021, two are RNA vaccines, while the other two are virus vector-based vaccines.

A number of other vaccine producers will undoubtedly have carried out their clinical testing in the near future. All the various principles of vaccine development will be represented.[41] Several of these vaccines have already been rolled out in many countries, particularly vaccines produced in China and Russia. It is quite likely that the various vaccines have different characteristics and roles to play in combatting the pandemic and will supplement each other.

The tempo of the vaccine development is impressive. There are various reasons why it has proved possible to develop apparently effective vaccines over the course of a few months. Effective alliances have been formed between the vaccine producers, governmental and academic institutions together with large economic resources. Furthermore, there has been considerably increased efficiency in the actual testing of the vaccines. An advantage of RNA vaccines is that such vaccines can be developed much more quickly than traditional vaccines.[42]

While the tempo of the rollout of vaccines varies, it has been impressive in many countries. There are therefore grounds for optimism. We know already that the first vaccines protect against serious disease, and probably also to a considerable extent against infection. Even so, a certain degree of sober-mindedness is called for. There are still many unanswered questions regarding the vaccines.[43] How long will a protective effect last? Will frequent revaccination be necessary? Will it be possible to create effective herd immunity? Will the vaccines prove to be as effective on the risk groups involved as on the rest of the population? It is, for instance, well known that vaccines, generally speaking, achieve less immune response in the elderly with weakened immunity. Precisely these groups are often poorly represented when trying out new vaccines. An additional problem is the challenge from the new virus mutations that appeared in 2021. If the current vaccines are not fully effective against mutations, it may be necessary to modify them at intervals. With the new vaccine technology this can be done quickly. Even though the vaccine has been tested on thousands of people without any serious side-effects, one can never completely exclude these when dealing with new vaccines. This will probably lead to sections of the population refusing to be vaccinated. The problem with serious but rare side-effects has already materialized with the two virus vector-based vaccines in use.

An important problem is that the capacity for vaccine production is limited in the foreseeable future. It will call for carefully planned prioritization of vaccination among various groups in the individual countries, based on both relative risks and their importance for society. It is also urgent to ensure a fair global distribution of vaccines.[44]

Even though effective COVID-19 vaccines will lessen the pressure on society from the virus, it will take some time before the full effect can be attained.

The stepchild of vaccine research: neglected tropical infections

Progress with regard to vaccines against global infectious diseases such as malaria, HIV and tuberculosis will, of course, also benefit poor developing countries. Even so, it is a fact that the great advances in vaccine research over the past hundred years have first and foremost benefitted Western countries, where a number of infectious diseases that once played a large role have now been eradicated as a result of systematically implemented vaccination programmes. Considerable work that calls for large resources is still required to make it possible for developing countries to gain the same advantages from the many effective vaccines we now have.

The developing countries also have a number of other special challenges in the form of tropical infections, which to a great extent have been neglected when it comes to developing both medicines and vaccines.[45] The majority of these infections are chronic and can lead to serious illness or even death. Examples of such are a number of infections involving intestinal worms, where various forms of schistosomiasis (bilharzia) play a major role, with more than 200 million patients spread over various continents. An effective vaccine against this disease would be of great importance.[46] Other examples are various infections with protozoa, including Chagas disease in Latin America. Together, these neglected diseases have considerable medical, social and economic consequences.

There are several reasons why these diseases have become the stepchildren of vaccination medicine. One important reason is that the mechanisms of these diseases are extremely complex and we still know too little about the interaction between microbes and immune response. Further studies and the development of vaccines would require considerable resources. Since this is mainly viewed as a problem for the poorer regions of the world, it also means that the major pharmaceutical companies have shown little desire to concentrate on this field, on the basis of sober economic considerations. An important challenge within the field of vaccine development for the neglected tropical diseases is therefore procuring the resources necessary for the large-scale efforts needed, both within further basic research and vaccine development. Such efforts would be a highly important contribution to the poorer countries.

'Blood is a very special fluid': The Era of Serum Therapy

After the fundamental initial discoveries by Robert Koch and Louis Pasteur, which can be said to have triggered the bacteriological revolution, there came a string of new reports of bacteria as a cause of disease. Even so, these epoch-making finds did not have any immediate consequences for the treatment of infections. Koch was undoubtedly distracted by his mistaken gambling on tuberculin as a treatment for tuberculosis, while Pasteur, with far greater success, threw himself into the field of vaccines, focusing on the prevention of infections. At the end of the nineteenth century there was still only one medicine known to have an effect on an infectious disease: the quinine treatment of malaria.

It was almost by chance that someone stumbled on the first effective treatment of other serious infections.[47] One of the many young, talented and ambitious researchers who gathered around Koch in Berlin was the

German Emil Behring, who studied diphtheria in guinea pigs. At that time diphtheria was an extremely common infectious children's disease, with a high mortality: 50,000 German children contracted diphtheria in 1892, and half of them died.

A few years earlier two other researchers in Koch's group, Friedrich Löffler and Edwin Krebs, had detected the bacterial cause of diphtheria, *Corynebacterium diphtheriae*.[48] In diphtheria, this bacterium causes an inflammation of the throat, with a greyish white layer forming on the mucous membrane, which can completely block the windpipe and lead to suffocation. Nevertheless, the most usual cause of death with diphtheria was acute damage to the heart and nervous system, which can result in heart failure and paralysis, including the muscles used for breathing. It was unclear how these 'long-range' effects took place, for the bacterium was only found in the trachea. It was two researchers from Pasteur's group, Émile Roux and Alexandre Yersin, who found the explanation. They discovered that the diphtheria bacterium in the throat membranes secreted a very powerful toxin that got into the blood and caused life-threatening damage to the heart and nervous system.[49]

In his experiments with guinea pigs, Behring injected the diphtheria bacterium and then attempted to treat the infection with the disinfectant iodine trichloride. This proved completely unsuccessful. Most of the guinea pigs died, some from diphtheria, others from the treatment received, which is quite toxic. A few animals did, however, survive, albeit in a fairly sorry state. When Behring then injected a normally lethal dose of diphtheria toxin into these animals, they survived, surprisingly enough. He then carried out the key experiment that led to the first effective treatment of infectious diseases: he took serum, the cell-free fluid in the blood, from these animals and gave it to healthy guinea pigs, who were simultaneously given a dose of toxin that would normally have proved fatal. These animals also survived. Behring was thus able to conclude that the animals that had survived diphtheria and become immune had acquired a substance in the blood that neutralized the diphtheria toxin. He called this substance an antitoxin.[50]

At the same time as Behring was studying diphtheria, the Japanese researcher Shibasaburo Kitasato was working in Koch's laboratory on the life-threatening infection tetanus. He detected the bacterial cause, *Clostridium tetani,* and demonstrated that this bacterium also secreted a powerful toxin, which, like the diphtheria bacterium, can lead to the production of a protective antitoxin in animals that survive.

Behring realized the treatment potential opened up by the detection of antitoxins. But it was not until he cooperated with Paul Ehrlich, another of the pioneers of the bacteriological revolution, that serum treatment of diphtheria became a reality. Ehrlich, who was also working in Koch's laboratory at that time, managed via meticulous attempts to standardize the dosage of antitoxins, so that reliable use on humans became possible. Behring and Ehrlich then started mass production of serum containing antitoxin from cows and horses by injecting them with diphtheria toxin.

In the early 1890s an anti-serum against diphtheria was first used on children's wards in Berlin, with convincing results. Behring was internationally celebrated and named 'The Children's Saviour'. In 1901, together with Kitasato, he was awarded the very first Nobel Prize in medicine for the discovery of serum treatment. In his acceptance speech he cited Mephistopheles' famous words from Goethe's *Faust*: 'Blut ist ein ganz besonderer Saft' ('Blood is a very special fluid'). That same year he was raised to the Prussian nobility by Kaiser Wilhelm II and became entitled to call himself Emil von Behring.

Behring was not a saint, however. He had an extremely well-developed flair for making money out of his discoveries, in a way that was somewhat reminiscent of the increasing present-day tendencies to commercialize research results, including a dogged fight to gain patents for them. He considerably understated Ehrlich's invaluable contribution to serum treatment, and he also managed to outmanoeuvre Ehrlich when it came to the economic gains resulting from their collaboration.[51]

Serum therapy for diphtheria spread to all Western countries and this breakthrough led to a similar treatment being developed for a number of other important bacterial infections. Good results were achieved with treatment of tetanus, pneumonia caused by pneumococci and the common forms of bacterial meningitis. Even though the results varied considerably and the official statistics were not completely reliable, there is no doubt that the mortality rate for these common infections was considerably reduced.[52]

Serum treatment, however, also had its drawbacks. Since the anti-serum came from species other than humans, especially horses, serious

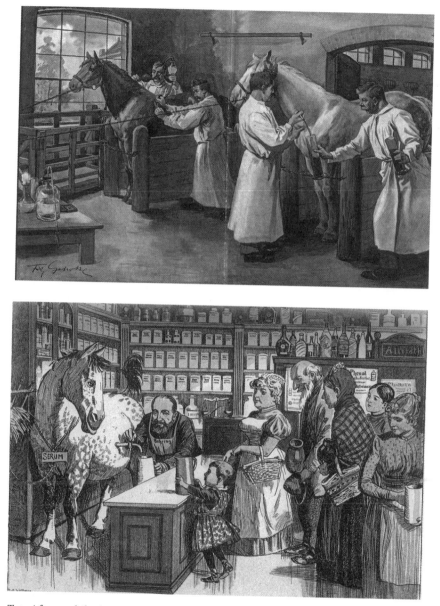

Top: After a while, it was mainly horses that were used as a source of serum for the treatment of infections, after the animals had first been injected with the microbial substance involved, for example, diphtheria or tetanus toxin. *Bottom*: This is how a cartoonist in a German newspaper envisaged future treatment of infections would be after Emil von Behring's development of serum therapy. Serum could be fetched from the chemist's, where von Behring himself draws off the life-giving medication directly from horses.

allergic reactions were a threat. Such side-effects could be acute, including even life-threatening reactions, or could assume the form of a so-called serum sickness that developed after a few days, with a high temperature, aching limbs and often nephritis (inflammation of the kidneys). Serum treatment was also complicated and quite expensive. It required a very precise bacterial diagnosis before the treatment could be given. As more experience was gradually gained, however, the treatment became safer.

Serum therapy was in common use for many decades, right up until 1940, when it was replaced by sulfonamides and after a while by penicillin and other antibiotics. This form of treatment, which is now largely forgotten, was for almost 50 years the only effective treatment that existed for serious bacteriological infections. Goethe really did have a point.

Malaria Against Syphilis: Desperate Diseases Call for Desperate Remedies

When I claim that serum treatment was the only effective treatment for bacterial infections during the first decades of the twentieth century, I have to admit that I am ignoring an interesting parenthesis in modern infection medicine: using malaria against syphilis.

A feared late complication of syphilis was *paralysis generalis* (general paralysis), the most serious complication from the nervous system in the final stage of the disease. Between 10 and 45 per cent of patients in mental hospitals during the first part of the twentieth century had this diagnosis, which normally led to death within five years. The Austrian psychiatrist Julius Wagner-Jauregg discovered that patients with this disease who developed a fever often recovered, for some reason or other. In the laboratory, it had also been detected that the syphilis bacterium (*Treponema pallidum*) died at temperatures corresponding to a high fever in human beings. Wagner-Jauregg therefore carried out a series of experiments by giving patients who had general paralysis an injection of malaria plasmodia. He was able to observe with the first experiments that more than a third of the patients clearly improved.[53] This treatment caused quite a stir, spread rapidly and during the interwar years was the standard method of treatment of general paralysis in syphilis patients. The most 'benign' of the malaria plasmodia, *Plasmodium vivax*, was used.

Experience gained in other countries confirmed Wagner-Jauregg's findings. Almost a third of the patients became considerably better, and others showed at least some improvement. The treatment, however, did introduce a certain level of mortality because of the inflicted malaria, even though the infection was normally easily brought under control using quinine. Nonetheless the malaria treatment was considered to mark a great advance in the treatment of general paralysis, and Wagner-Jauregg was awarded the Nobel Prize in medicine in 1927. His malaria treatment was used until penicillin became available.

We still do not know how the malaria treatment worked. It is not improbable that the increased body temperature in the patients led to an activation of the immune system against the syphilis bacterium, in addition to the fever directly damaging the bacteria. In later years, forms of fever treatment have also been attempted against infection with HIV and the *Borrelia* bacterium. This has not produced any convincing results.

Even though the treatment of syphilis with malaria is now only a historical curiosity, it led to increased knowledge about malaria infection in humans, since it was possible to follow precisely the development of the disease after infection.

Paul Ehrlich and Salvarsan: The Rewards of Patience

When Robert Koch presented his anthrax findings for the first time in 1876 at the university in Breslau (now Wrocław in Poland), he was introduced to a student by the name of Paul Ehrlich.[54] The young Ehrlich was extremely interested in trying out new methods of staining sections of tissue, but had not been able to impress his teachers. Koch's host afterwards described Ehrlich somewhat dismissively as 'That's little Ehrlich. He's very good at staining, but will hardly manage to pass his exams.' 'Little Ehrlich' was to prove one of the most prominent pioneers of the bacteriological revolution, with fundamental discoveries within both infection medicine and immunology, in addition to important contributions to other areas of medicine. In my view, he is just as fascinating a figure as Pasteur and Koch – and probably much more engaging as a person.

It is correct that Ehrlich was good at staining. His fascination with dyeing methods when examining cells and tissue was to be significant for several of his great medical discoveries.[55] An area of German industry that was very much to the fore internationally was precisely the development of new dyes, particularly aniline dyes, which were a by-product of the production of coal tar. These dyes were used not only in the textile industry but in medicine for staining cells and tissue, and Ehrlich had been keenly interested in this since he started on his studies. Using his staining methods, he was able to detect the so-called mast cell, which is a key cell in allergic reactions. Later he managed, via continued experiments, to detect several of the important types of white blood cell, and thus contributed to the basis of haematology, the study of the causes of diseases of the blood.

Ehrlich, however, explored the matter in greater depth, wondering _why_ different cells had different staining properties. Could the explanation perhaps be that the individual cell types have special superficial chemical structures – receptors or receiver-molecules – which react specifically to one single dye, so that these structures fit the dye as a key does a lock? He transferred this idea to the experiments with antitoxins and toxins that he had carried out with Behring. Ehrlich wondered if, for example, the diphtheria toxin reacted like a dye with a special cell product, which was then produced in such quantities that it entered the blood as what he called antibodies. With this Ehrlich laid the foundation for the view of antibodies in immunology, which react very specifically to a single antigen.

Ehrlich's contribution to serum treatment was considerable, but even if he saw this was a possible method of treatment, he also soon realized its limitations. He recognized that the treatment had to be given early in the course of the infection to have its full effect, and also found that it could only be used for certain infectious diseases.

Ehrlich's dream was to arrive at chemical substances that could be used for treating infectious diseases, what he called chemotherapy.[56] Once again, he used his theories about staining specific cells and tissues. Perhaps it was possible to find chemical substances that reacted specifically to certain molecules on bacteria and thereby damaged them, without reacting to other cells in the body? Ehrlich wished to arrive at what he referred to as a _Zauberkugel_ (magic bullet), which with unfailing accuracy would only hit what it was aimed at, as one finds in folk tales. For a long time Ehrlich was very much on his own within this area, for the majority of the medical world was intoxicated by serum therapy, based on the body's own defence mechanisms. It was not eager to consider introducing alien chemical substances for internal use when treating infections. Later, however, Ehrlich had plenty of opportunity to work on his dreams of chemotherapy at two different research laboratories that he led in Frankfurt.

Without a doubt, Ehrlich was what today one would call a workaholic. He spent hardly any time eating, but was very fond of cigars. He paid hurdy-gurdy men handsomely to play popular music outside his laboratory every week, claiming that he thought best when they did so.[57]

He started his work on chemotherapy by investigating whether dyes had any effect on mice infected by trypanosomes, protozoa that produce sleeping sickness in humans. He found a few substances that had a certain effect on this infection in mice, but they had no effect on humans. Then he heard that British researchers had discovered that the arsenic compound atoxyl had an effect on trypanosomiasis. This substance proved to be too toxic to use on human beings, since among other things it could result in blindness. Ehrlich and his chemists, however, started to produce a whole series of variants of atoxyl, which they thoroughly tested on animals with a trypanosoma infection. After a great deal of trial and error, they finally arrived at a promising substance. Then they temporarily called a halt to their work.[58]

In 1908 Ehrlich was distracted for a time by the award of the Nobel Prize, which he shared with a Russian researcher from Pasteur's group, Ilya Mechnikov (or, as he was known in France, Élie Metchnikoff). Mechnikov was first and foremost interested in the macrophages (the 'eating cells') and their role in the response to infection. Ehrlich was awarded his prize for his immunological theories about antibodies, which actually only interested a smallish circle of specialists. The discovery that was to make him an international celebrity still lay a few years ahead.

Ehrlich had not abandoned his idea of a magic bullet, and he now focused on syphilis. The syphilis bacterium had been discovered in 1905. Ehrlich, among others, believed, albeit mistakenly, that it was related to trypanosomes, an area he had studied extremely thoroughly. He wished to see if any of the arsenic combinations he had investigated in connection with trypanosomiasis could have an effect on syphilis. A young Japanese researcher, Sahachiro Hata, had just arrived from Japan to work with Ehrlich. Hata had successfully made a model for syphilis by infecting rabbits with the bacterium. Ehrlich now set Hata to work on testing all the arsenic combinations they had studied for trypanosome infections. It was an enormous task, as each single substance was tested in a series of experiments. But patience was finally rewarded. The substance, which had the label 'no. 606' and was the chemical compound arsphenamine, had a convincing effect on syphilis in rabbits. Ehrlich had finally found his magic bullet. The substance was given the name Salvarsan, and the pharmaceutical company Hoechst began production.[59]

At first Ehrlich generously shared Salvarsan with clinical departments all over the world. The positive experiences with Salvarsan were quickly confirmed. The effect on syphilis was clearly best in the early stage of the disease, but a certain effect could be seen even in the later stages. Ehrlich and several of his colleagues first published their results at a large medical convention in Germany in 1910. His findings were well covered in the world's press and he became an overnight celebrity.

While the great majority of people were enthusiastic about this first effective treatment for syphilis, which at the time was a widespread disease that affected up to 10 per cent of the population in several countries, there were also some negative reactions. Salvarsan definitely had side-effects that could be serious, but many of them were due to incorrect use of the medication, which called for special treatment when used. Ehrlich and his colleagues continued to experiment and in 1912 arrived at a somewhat altered and improved version of Salvarsan, which they called Neosalvarsan. This was to become the standard drug for the following 40 years.

Certain reactionary critics believed that Ehrlich's discovery would lead to a collapse of social morals, since syphilis was no longer a threat. Others accused Ehrlich of profiting inordinately from the sale of Salvarsan. These accusations were troubling for Ehrlich, who, in addition to his vast consumption of cigars, was under enormous pressure from his responsibilities organizing the Salvarsan treatment.[60]

The city of Frankfurt am Main paid tribute to Paul Ehrlich by naming the street outside one of his laboratories after him. After the Nazi takeover in 1933, however, the street was renamed and all of Ehrlich's writings were burned – because he was Jewish.

Paul Ehrlich looms large in the history of infection medicine. Not only did he discover the first effective drug against a bacterial disease

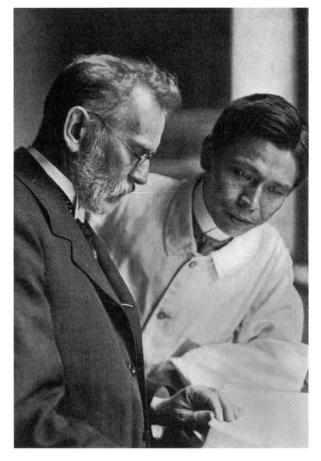

Paul Ehrlich and his young Japanese colleague Sahachiro Hata. Under Ehrlich's leadership, Hata carried out a daunting task of investigating the effect on syphilis in experimental animals of a long series of arsenic combinations that Ehrlich and his colleagues had prepared. The work resulted in the first really effective treatment of syphilis – Salvarsan.

in humans, but his work on Salvarsan also laid the foundation for the modern testing of pharmaceuticals, with step-by-step, meticulous studies of effect, safety and side-effects. His deep insight into the conditions for successful research is summed up by what he called his 'four Gs', referring to the German words: *Geduld* (patience), *Geld* (money), *Geschick* (proficiency) and *Glück* (luck). Ehrlich had all four of these.

Ehrlich's Legacy: Sulfonamides

In the first decades of the twentieth century bacterial infections still claimed many lives. Common infections with streptococci and pneumococci, for example, still had a high mortality rate. Although Salvarsan and Neosalvarsan had proved a success with syphilis, there were not many in the medical world who believed that other bacterial infections could be treated using chemical means. Serum therapy dominated people's thoughts, but, as we have seen, it had its limitations.

There were still those, however, who remembered Ehrlich's idea about the 'magic bullet' and the possibilities of using dyes in the treatment of infection. Not surprisingly perhaps, these ideas had taken root in a chemical company that had specialized in the production of dyes, Bayer AG. By following Ehrlich's guidelines, with systematic, patient testing of new substances that had been altered chemically, the chemists at Bayer managed to find an effective medication against trypanosomiasis, as well as a completely new medicine for malaria. But would this also work for bacterial infections? This was the dream of the young doctor Gerhard Domagk, who had become one of the infection experts in a team at Bayer.[61]

Domagk first wanted to find a medicine against streptococci. He used mice for his experiments. Along with some extremely proficient chemists who produced a series of dye variants, Domagk systematically tested the effect of each individual substance on streptococcal infection in mice. This was a laborious task in which more than three hundred chemical substances were tested. After these produced only negative results, some of Domagk's colleagues lost faith in the project. Success finally came in 1932, when a substance was found that could cure streptococcal infection in mice. It was a red dye that was given the name Prontosil.

The new 'magic bullet' was first used in early 1933 to tackle streptococcal infection in a patient at a hospital close to Domagk's laboratory. This was an eighteen-year-old girl who was treated for a severe streptococcal infection with abscesses in her throat. The infection gradually spread and became life-threatening. Since the patient was almost dying, treatment with Prontosil was started and four weeks later she could be discharged from hospital. During the following years, increasing numbers of patients were treated with Prontosil, with similarly positive results. Among the first patients was Domagk's own six-year-old daughter, Hildegard, who had a serious streptococcal infection. She too recovered.

Domagk did not publish his sensational news until 1935. Many have wondered why he waited such a long time, and some have suspected that it had something to do with the company's commercial interests and patent rights. Most probably, the delay had to do with the admirable thoroughness and caution of Domagk and his colleagues. After the dramatic results had been published, Prontosil triumphed worldwide and the new treatment inspired great enthusiasm. The fact that President Franklin D. Roosevelt's son was cured of a life-threatening streptococcal infection of the throat undoubtedly enhanced the publicity. Sulfonamides may also have had a major impact on world events, since Winston Churchill contracted pneumonia after visiting the troops in North Africa in December 1943, but recovered with the aid of sulfonamides.[62]

In 1939 Gerhard Domagk was awarded the Nobel Prize in medicine. The Gestapo then arrived at his house and forced him to write a letter in which he declined to accept the prize. The reason for this was that Adolf Hitler had forbidden all German citizens to accept this prize, since he believed that the Nobel Committee had insulted him and Germany by awarding the 1935 Peace Prize to the journalist Carl von Ossietzky, who had been arrested and sent to a series of concentration camps for exposing information about Germany's rearmament programme. In 1947 Domagk was finally awarded the Nobel Prize medal and diploma, although not the sum of money that usually accompanies them. The prize was greatly deserved. Domagk's discovery of Prontosil marked the beginning of a new era in the treatment of infections. For the first time there was an effective treatment available for a number of bacterial infections that had previously often been fatal.

From the outset it was clear that Prontosil only worked on bacteria inside the bodies of humans and animals, not on bacteria in a test tube. The explanation for this, which was discovered by researchers at the Pasteur Institute in Paris, was that the Prontosil molecule had to split inside the body, so that the active half (sulfanilamide) was released and could start to work. Sulfanilamide was rapidly introduced in the treatment of infections and was actually just as active as Prontosil. The substance could also be produced at a reasonable cost and became the cornerstone of a whole series of so-called sulfonamides that were gradually introduced.[63]

The introduction of sulfonamides in the treatment of infections marked a milestone in the history of medicine. During a ten-year period, until penicillin became available, they led to a considerable decrease in the fatality of infections that included pneumonia caused by pneumococci and such common streptococcal infections as childbed fever, scarlet fever, erysipelas and wound infections. In the case of child-bed fever, the effect was so striking that some people talked of 'a new Semmelweis effect'.

It is somewhat unjust that the sulfonamide era has now been forgotten by many, probably because these medications were overshadowed by the introduction of penicillin in the early 1940s. It must, however, be admitted that the sulfonamides had certain disadvantages, some of which could be serious, such as violent skin reactions and damage to the kidneys. Nor were they effective against all types of bacteria, with many bacteria developing a resistance to them. In this, however, the sulfonamides did not in fact differ from most other antibacterial medicines that came later, including penicillin.

The Discovery of Penicillin: Myths and Facts

Gerhard Domagk and his colleagues at the Bayer laboratories in Germany were not the only ones who dreamed of finding medicine. A Scottish bacteriologist working at St Mary's Hospital in London probably shared this dream, inspired, in part at least, by his experiences of serious war wounds at a field hospital close to the front in France during the First World War. His name was Alexander Fleming, and this name was to become immortal in the history of medicine.[64]

Fleming may well have believed that he was close to his goal when, in 1921, he discovered a substance in nasal secretion that had a devastating effect on certain bacteria. He called the substance lysozyme and over the next few years he also found it in other body fluids. Lysozyme, however, was not very effective against pathogenic bacteria, and Fleming realized that this substance was not the answer to his dreams.[65]

The advantage of having an untidy laboratory

In 1928 Fleming made a discovery of historic proportions. Like so many such events, this one is shrouded in myth. The usual version, which all medical students get to hear, is that Fleming went off for a month's holiday at the end of July and left behind on his desk some culture dishes on which he had sprinkled staphylococci, a quite common bacterium. His laboratory desk was usually rather untidy. When Fleming came back to work he was about to throw away the dishes when he suddenly noticed something strange about one of them. 'That's funny', he said to his assistant, who was never to forget this moment.[66]

What Fleming saw was that many colonies of staphylococci had sprung up in the dish, but so had a large, greyish colony of mould. And what was funny about this was that no staphylococci grew in an area around the mould, only elsewhere in the dish. A reasonable explanation of this was that some substance or other had leaked out from the mould colony and stopped the growth of the bacteria. The mould in the culture dish had probably come as airborne fungal spores from a laboratory on the floor below, where another bacteriologist was working on fungi.

There are several reasons for doubting that this story is absolutely correct. It was first printed in 1944, and Fleming's notes from 1928 provide no valuable information. It is possible that Fleming's first reaction was simply that this was a new example of the effect of his well-known lysozyme and that he did not at first understand that he was dealing with an entirely new phenomenon. Even so, he continued to cultivate the mould and discovered that it secreted a completely different substance from lysozyme: a substance that also killed pathogenic bacteria, which lysozyme did not. He called this bactericidal substance penicillin, after the name of the mould (*Penicillium notatum*).

Fleming proved by experiments on mice and rabbits that penicillin was hardly toxic at all. For reasons that nobody has quite understood, however, he did not carry out animal experiments to investigate the effect of penicillin on infections with, for example, staphylococci, even though such experiments would have been the obvious course of action. He did not manage to purify the substance, and made only half-hearted attempts to get help from professional chemists. After a while, he clearly lost interest in penicillin and started to work on sulfonamides instead.

It was to be twelve years before work really started on the development of penicillin treatment in medicine. One important reason for this delay was probably Fleming himself.[67] He lacked the ability to 'sell' his discovery in a convincing way. When he presented his findings at a scientific meeting in London in 1929, he did so in such a soporific and half-hearted way that it was easy to get the impression that he hardly believed in it himself: there was a deafening silence after his lecture, without a single question from the audience. Fleming was incidentally

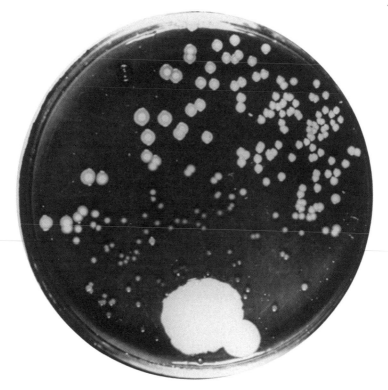

The original culture dish which led to Alexander Fleming discovering penicillin. Across the dish small colonies can be seen of the bacterium *Staphylococcus aureus* (yellow staphylococci), but they are completely lacking in a zone around the large single colony of the mould *Penicillium notatum* at the bottom. Fleming deduced from this that the mould must secrete a bactericidal substance. This proved to be penicillin.

known by the students to be a hopeless, mumbling lecturer. He published an article about his findings in 1929 in the important medical journal *The Lancet*, but this too was completely uninspiring and did not arouse any interest for many years. Today, however, it is regarded as one of the most important publications in the history of medicine.

Could it be that Fleming himself did not have a strong belief in the potential of penicillin? He later implied that those around him had not supported him. This explanation is unconvincing. It is probably true that his powerful and authoritarian superior, Sir Almroth Wright (known by his opponents as 'Sir Almost Right' or 'Sir Always Wrong'), mostly believed in the potential of vaccines in infection medicine, but even so he gave Fleming quite a lot of support.

Penicillin is retrieved from oblivion

The story of penicillin could have ended there if it had not been for Howard Florey, a dynamic Australian pharmacologist, who took the baton from Fleming's somewhat limp hand.[68] Florey was Professor of Pathology at Oxford University, where he had established a group of researchers to study bactericidal substances produced by other micro-organisms. He also appointed a gifted but temperamental biochemist, Ernest Chain, who was a Jewish refugee from Germany, and the bacteriologist Norman Heatley.

Florey had encountered Fleming's old article about lysozyme, and the group began by studying this substance. Then, in 1938, Chain discovered Fleming's forgotten article about penicillin, which the group eagerly began to study, probably in 1939. Their interest was purely scientific and theoretical. In a famous later remark, Florey candidly stated: 'People sometimes think that I and the others worked on penicillin because we were interested in suffering humanity. I don't think it ever crossed our minds about suffering humanity.'

The research group got hold of the fungal mould *Penicillium notatum*, which Fleming had used as a source of penicillin. It was, however, extremely difficult to produce sufficient penicillin from the mould to carry out meaningful experiments, which delayed their work.

On Saturday 25 May 1939 Florey and his colleagues carried out a historic experiment. They infected eight mice with streptococci and gave penicillin to four of them. On Sunday morning all the untreated mice were dead, but those who had received penicillin were in the pink of health. Even Florey, who usually contained his emotions, displayed signs of enthusiasm. The findings were confirmed by further experiments and they published the results in 1940, without causing a stir of any kind. The Second World War was in full swing and Britain feared an imminent German invasion. To be on the safe side, Florey, Chain and two of their assistants smeared spores of the invaluable mould into the lining of their jackets in case they had to flee the country.[69] The precious mould had to be saved at all costs!

In February 1941 penicillin was given to a patient for the first time. Albert Alexander, a policeman in Oxford, was dying from a staphylococcal infection. His condition rapidly improved after only 24 hours of treatment, and there was further dramatic improvement after a total of four days of penicillin injections. After ten days, however, the patient's condition gradually worsened; unfortunately there was no more penicillin available and Alexander died. Over the following weeks the group managed to produce enough penicillin to treat several patients with good results, and that same year they published again, once more with little effect.[70]

Florey now firmly believed in the potential of penicillin, but he realized that it was necessary to find methods of considerably increasing production. London during the Blitz was hardly the place for this, so he and Heatley went to the USA for assistance. Working with researchers in Peoria, Illinois, they found another variant of the mould on a rotten melon from a market, one that produced even more penicillin than Fleming's had done. Florey established cooperation between the U.S. government and a number of major pharmaceutical companies, and over the course of a year managed to overcome the production problem. He now returned home, but initially could not gain access to the American-produced penicillin. His group therefore had to continue producing its own penicillin for further experiments on patients. Since penicillin was excreted unaltered in the patients' urine, it was necessary to extract the precious substance once more from urine: Florey's wife, Ethel, who was also a doctor, was among those who cycled round to fetch urine from patients. In 1943 Florey and his colleagues were able to publish extremely good results from 170 patients treated with penicillin.[71]

As early as 1942 the press had got hold of information about the new wonder medicine and gave this news banner headlines. The journalists emphasized the efforts by Fleming and St Mary's Hospital, but said very little about Florey and the Oxford group. An important reason for this was probably that the journalists were welcomed with open arms by Fleming. Florey, on the other hand, was reserved towards the press, gave no interviews and also forbade his colleagues to do so. This may well have marked the beginning of what has been called the 'Fleming' myth: the story of penicillin in which Alexander Fleming is the key figure who donated his discovery to humanity, just as Prometheus in Greek mythology brought fire from the heavens to mankind. Fleming rapidly became an international celebrity, something that suited him down to the ground. He was received by the pope on three occasions and made an honorary chieftain of the Kiowa tribe in the USA. He has even had a crater on the moon named after him.[72]

Howard Florey never gained the same place in the public consciousness as Fleming, the darling of the media. He never spoke in public of the fact that he and his colleagues found the one-sided emphasis on Fleming's contribution highly frustrating. In the scientific world, on the other hand, people were aware of the invaluable contribution Florey and his colleagues had made to the development of penicillin treatment.

The collaboration between Florey and Chain came to nothing. An important reason for this was that Chain wanted to take out a patent on the production of penicillin, while Florey thought this was wrong, because their findings, in his opinion, belonged to humanity. Florey's stance I find laudable, and it forms a stark contrast to the attitude of present-day researchers, who queue up to get their findings patented, mainly for commercial reasons. The patent system can occasionally hinder free research and, at worst, slow down medical progress.

Fleming, Florey and Chain were awarded the Nobel Prize in medicine in 1945 for the discovery of penicillin. Fleming received half the prize, while Florey and Chain shared the other half. Norman Heatley, who had also been a central figure, did not receive a prize. Fleming and

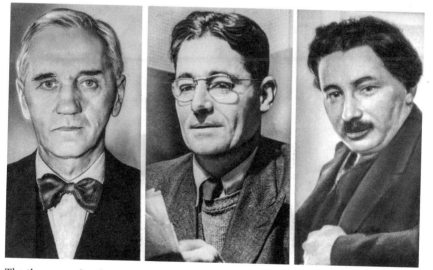

The three people who were awarded the Nobel Prize in 1945 for the discovery of penicillin. Fleming (left) received half of the prize, while Florey (centre) and Chain (right) shared the other half.

Florey were both knighted in 1944. When Fleming died in 1955, he was buried in the crypt of St Paul's Cathedral, London, alongside many other distinguished figures in British history. Florey continued to receive honours until his death in 1968, including a life peerage in 1965. His portrait later appeared on Australian $50 banknotes.

Penicillin began to be used by the Allied forces in 1943 and it proved to be an extremely valuable addition to the treatment of wound infections and sexually transmitted diseases, particularly gonorrhoea. Some people wanted patients with war wounds to take precedence over those who had inflicted sexually transmitted diseases on themselves. The matter was taken to the highest level, to Churchill, who made the Solomonic decision that only military considerations should be prioritized in the use of penicillin. In practice, this meant that most of the gonorrhoea patients were treated, so that the soldiers could swiftly return to the front. Without a doubt, penicillin gave the allies an advantage over the German forces.

The Third Man *and penicillin*

During the war penicillin was at first reserved mainly for military personnel, and it was not until 1944 that it gradually became available to civilians. In such countries as Germany and Austria, which were occupied by the Allies, who controlled the use of penicillin, it became a coveted item in short supply. Penicillin was stolen from military hospitals and sold on the black market. To increase profits, it was sometimes mixed with sugar and other substances, and such spiked and inactive penicillin was sold by criminals. This formed the basis of the classic film *The Third Man* (1949, dir. Carol Reed), with a screenplay by Graham Greene based on his own novella.[73] The action takes place in murky post-war Vienna, where the unscrupulous black market racketeer Harry Lime, played by Orson Welles, sells diluted, spiked penicillin to a hospital for children with meningitis, with terrible consequences for the sick children, some of whom die and others of whom survive with badly damaged brains. Greene's novella is based on real events: members of a criminal gang in Berlin were sentenced for such crimes.[74]

Penicillin was also used by the American CIA in Vienna as a means of payment for military secrets to Russian soldiers with sexually transmitted diseases, since they had no access to penicillin.

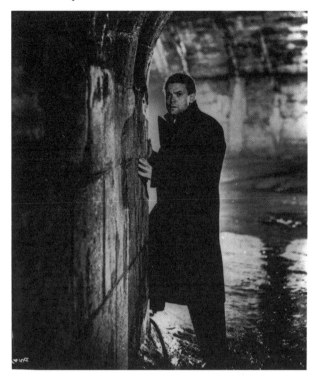

Orson Welles as the unscrupulous criminal Harry Lime in the British film *The Third Man* (1949).

The enthusiasm for the new miracle medicine knew no bounds during the early post-war years. Many people believed it could help cure most illnesses, not only bacterial infections. This led to a vast over-consumption, since early on it was available over the counter without any prescription.

The White Death Is Defeated

It quickly became obvious that penicillin, although it had an effect on many bacteria, did not affect tuberculosis, which was still a widespread disease with a high mortality rate. A number of experiments with sulfonamides had given a certain degree of hope that this infection could also be treated by medication, but sulfonamides ultimately proved ineffective against tuberculosis.

At a convention in New York in 1939, Alexander Fleming, who had not forgotten his early discovery of penicillin, met Selman Waksman, a Ukrainian-American microbiologist who for some years had been interested in microbes in the soil.[75] Fleming told him of his discovery of penicillin from mould, and Waksman became extremely interested. That same year a former research fellow under Waksman, the French-American René Dubos, had found a germicidal substance, tyrothricin, in a soil sample, but this had not been suitable for internal use as it was toxic. Waksman now returned to his laboratory and started an intensive search for other bactericidal substances in soil samples. It was in fact Waksman who introduced the term 'antibiotics' for antimicrobial substances produced by microorganisms.

This search for antibiotics in Waksman's laboratory was to lead to an important breakthrough, the discovery of streptomycin, the first effective drug against tuberculosis. A key figure in this story is Albert Schatz, a talented 23-year-old student under Waksman. After only a few months' work on his thesis, Schatz's intensive and creative research led to the discovery in 1943 of a substance that was given the name streptomycin, because it was produced by the soil bacterium *Streptomyces griseus*. This substance was effective against many bacteria, but Schatz was particularly interested in its striking effect on the tuberculosis bacterium.[76]

Waksman and Schatz started to collaborate with two tuberculosis researchers, William Feldman and Horton Corwin Hinshaw, who tested streptomycin on guinea pigs with astounding success. That same year, in 1944, the first TB patients were treated with streptomycin, and there was no doubt as to its effect. At last, a means of treating tuberculosis had been found.[77]

At around the same time as streptomycin was discovered, the Danish-Swedish doctor Jørgen Lehmann in Gothenburg demonstrated that the chemically simple drug para-aminosalicylic acid (PAS) also had a striking effect on tuberculosis in both guinea pigs and humans. The impressive thing was that Lehmann had arrived at this result via a purely theoretical, logical argument, without any previous experiments.

Even so, it soon became evident that treatment with just one of these two drugs, which had to be given for several months, often lost its effect after a while since the TB bacteria became resistant. This was not the case, however, if one combined streptomycin and PAS. One of the first people to benefit from such combination therapy was William Feldman, who had contracted a life-threatening pulmonary tuberculosis during his experiments with tuberculous guinea pigs.

In 1952 Selman Waksman was awarded the Nobel Prize in medicine for the discovery of streptomycin. He was the sole prize-winner, even though the majority opinion, which even included that of Waksman himself, was that Lehmann fully deserved to be included. It has been claimed that Lehmann was omitted because of strong resistance from a single member of the committee, allegedly motivated by rivalry and jealousy, emotions that, alas, are not uncommon in research circles. Schatz, for his part, was extremely bitter that he had not shared in the prize. He even wrote a letter to the Swedish king. Schatz's claim was supported by a number of researchers, but others felt that Waksman, as the leader of the research group, was the natural candidate for the Nobel Prize.[78]

During the following years several new drugs against TB were found that are used in special combinations. But all of this was not enough to finish off the fight against tuberculosis. This infection, which has ravaged humanity for thousands of years, has recently been on the increase, especially because TB bacteria have appeared that are resistant to the usual forms of medication.[79] The HIV pandemic has contributed to a serious increase in the number of TB cases in the world. After a period of many

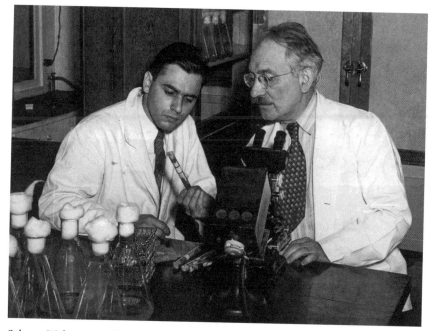

Selman Waksman and his 23-year-old student Albert Schatz – the discoverers of streptomycin, the first really effective medication against tuberculosis. Waksman was awarded the Nobel Prize for this in 1952.

years when TB research had low priority, there is now considerable activity within the field, particularly with regard to developing new medicines.[80]

The Golden Age of the Antibiotic Era

Penicillin revolutionized the treatment of a whole range of common and less common bacterial infections, since it had obvious advantages over the sulfonamides. It had far fewer side-effects and any allergic reactions were, on the whole, rarely life-threatening. Sulfonamides had also become less effective after many injections, since the microbes to a great extent had developed resistance to them.

Penicillin was an example of what Waksman had called antibiotics, antimicrobial drugs that are produced by microorganisms such as bacteria and types of mould. The ability to produce antibiotics has developed over millions of years and they are a weapon in the struggle for existence by the microbes in competition with other microbes. Antibiotics are just one of many examples of the ability of microbes to adapt through evolution. *Homo sapiens* has exploited this over the past 75 years in the human struggle against pathogenic microbes.

The introduction of penicillin to infection medicine set in motion a global hunt for new microbicidal agents produced by microbes other than Fleming's famous *Penicillium notatum*. Some people believed, as did Waksman, that many microorganisms in the soil could be an important source of new antibiotics. The discovery in 1943 of the next significant antibiotic, streptomycin, inspired an intensive search for new antibiotics, mainly using soil samples. Every possible method was explored: the pharmaceutical company Eli Lilly, for example, asked Christian missionaries to send back soil samples from all the exotic locations in which they found themselves.[81]

This search produced a rich crop of antibiotics. During the 1950s and '60s many completely new antibiotics were discovered. Some of these were chemically related to penicillin, such as the cephalosporins, while others, such as chloramphenicol and the tetracyclines, differed completely. To some extent the properties that these new substances demonstrated set them apart from penicillin, with an effect on different bacteria and with other side-effects.[82]

Not only naturally occurring antibiotics were of interest. The pharmaceutical industry gradually developed new variants by chemically altering them, which led to drugs that had useful new properties. This was done, for example, with penicillin, which became the 'progenitor' of a whole range of other penicillin variants. Gradually it also became possible to manufacture new, completely synthetic groups of bactericidals, such as the valuable quinolones.

The term 'antibiotics', which was originally reserved for substances produced by microorganisms, is now used, although imprecisely, to cover all antibacterial agents.

This development led gradually to the accumulation of a large number of bactericidals that offered possible treatment for a broad spectrum of infections. For a few decades it seemed as if *Homo sapiens* had gained the upper hand in the duel with bacteria, partly by secretly stealing the enemy's own weapons. Not unexpectedly, however, the microbes, as the formidable opponents they are, have struck back by developing resistance to an increasing number of our microbicidal medicines. At the same time, access to completely new antibiotics has dried up. The never-ending duel still rages back and forth.

The Treatment of Viral Infections

As early as the end of the nineteenth century people were aware of the existence of viruses, microbes that were far smaller than bacteria and could cause disease. But it was not until around 1930, after the development of electron microscopes capable of far higher magnification than ordinary microscopes, that it became possible to study viruses directly. Knowledge about their composition and 'lifestyle' gradually increased. When it became clear that viruses can only live inside living cells and that they intimately interact with the metabolism of their host cells, this led to a certain degree of pessimism about the possibility of finding medicines to combat them. Would it ever be possible to find medications that inhibited or destroyed the virus particles without at the same time damaging the host cells? Such attitudes, as well as the fact that the detection of viruses became possible only 50 years after the bacteriological revolution, explains why we did not get effective drugs against viral infections until several decades after the sulfonamides and penicillin.

It was not until the 1960s that the first drug for internal use against viral infections, vidarabine, became available.[83] Vidarabine had to be injected in hospitals and was used to combat serious infections to do with the herpes virus, encephalitis in particular. Acyclovir, a highly effective drug against both mild and serious herpes infections as well as against the chickenpox virus, which can cause shingles, was introduced in the early 1980s and is still in use.[84]

Several years after acyclovir came ganciclovir, a related medication that is particularly valuable against infections with the CMV virus, which causes serious infections in patients with a weakened immune system, such as patients with AIDS or those who have received organ transplants. We now also have other drugs against the CMV virus. Both acyclovir and ganciclovir have become extremely important in transplantation medicine, where they are also used to prevent infections with the CMV virus.

The revolution in the treatment of HIV

AIDS, the most serious forms of infection with the HIV virus, was 'discovered' in the middle of 1981, while the HIV virus was not detected until 1983–4. During the following years HIV research made an impressive effort to map the properties of the virus and find out how it attacks the human immune system, particularly the vital $CD4^+$ T cells that control important parts of the immune response. A number of weak points in the HIV virus's armour were discovered that could be possible points of attack for drug treatment. Despite this, many years were to pass before there was an effective treatment for the HIV infection. During these difficult years, all one could do was to try treatments that might hold back the many life-threatening complications of a weakened immune system in HIV patients. This had a certain life-prolonging effect, but in the vast majority of cases the infection proved fatal.

A development that can be called a revolution in the treatment of the HIV infection came about in 1996.[85] This was the introduction of combination therapy, using new drugs – protease inhibitors – as well as the older nucleoside analogues. Together with new methods of measuring the amount of the virus in the blood, these proved to have a striking effect. With this treatment it became possible to stop the propagation of the virus, which is the most important cause of the destruction of the immune system in patients. With treatment the weakened immune system recovers to a large extent. Since then we have acquired more than thirty new drugs that are even more effective and have fewer side-effects. They attack the virus in different ways. When one uses drugs with various points of attack in combination, the effect is enhanced, and the virus has a much smaller chance of forming resistant mutants that can lead to resistance to the medicines and thus to treatment. As we have seen, this principle is also used in the treatment of tuberculosis.

After the treatment breakthrough in 1996, the mortality rate of HIV infection has drastically decreased in all Western countries where the treatment is accessible. Today, an HIV patient, with the right treatment, can lead a quite normal life and have an almost normal life expectancy. Modern HIV treatment also has an important bonus: a well-treated HIV patient will in practice no longer be contagious in a sexual context.

In the poorer parts of the world, particularly in Africa, the HIV virus is still an enormous problem. Even though the situation has gradually improved, there are still a great many patients who have not had access to the advances in treatment. This is a constant challenge for the richer countries to deal with.

Even though the advances in treatment have been impressive, it is both surprising and sad that some people, including some with a scientific background, have continued to deny that AIDS is due to an infection with the HIV virus. Despite the fact that their arguments have been disproved, they have nevertheless managed to persuade some patients to turn down modern drugs, with the inevitable result – a fatal collapse of the immune system.

The greatest tragedy resulting from this denial came in South Africa under President Thabo Mbeki.[86] When he succeeded Nelson Mandela in 1999, almost 20 per cent of the population was infected with HIV, and 300,000 had already died from AIDS. A further 2.7 million died during Mbeki's period in office up to 2008. The responsibility for a considerable number of these deaths lies with Mbeki and his political colleagues. For reasons that are still unknown, Mbeki chose to join the ranks of the HIV deniers and refused to allow his fellow countrymen to be treated with modern HIV medicines. Researchers at Harvard University have calculated that more than 330,000 deaths from AIDS and 35,000 cases of mother-to-child infection could have been avoided if he had not joined the deniers.

Even though present-day HIV treatment is highly effective, it does not eradicate the virus from the patient. Therefore, treatment has to be lifelong: if the patient stops taking anti-HIV drugs, the virus starts to reproduce once again and the disease resumes, resulting in a failure of the immune system. What we could call 'the Holy Grail' among HIV researchers is therefore to find a form of treatment that completely eradicates the virus from the patient, who can then stop medication. This is an enormous scientific challenge. Not all researchers believe that it will ever be possible.[87]

Fighting the hepatitis virus: the second-treatment revolution

Certain global infection problems are strikingly visible, with quite dramatic disease consequences, for example malaria and HIV infection. Viruses that attack the liver often have less obvious symptoms for a number of years before the inflammation of the liver (hepatitis) that they cause gives rise to severe problems. The two most important viruses are hepatitis B and hepatitis C, both of which are serious global challenges. In 2015 more than 250 million people were infected with the hepatitis B virus, resulting in 900,000 deaths. There were 70 million infections with hepatitis C, resulting in 400,000 deaths annually. The deaths are due to the development of cirrhosis of the liver, leading to liver failure and liver cancer.

For a number of years, we have only had one form of treatment for hepatitis C, a combination of the virus drug ribavirin and interferon, a cytokine that can be given as an injection. This treatment often has only a limited effect, does not work on all variants of the virus and can produce major side-effects. In recent years we have acquired new drugs to use against this virus, with considerably better results and far fewer side-effects than the former treatment.[88] Today, hepatitis C is the only chronic viral infection that can be cured, with complete eradication of the virus from the patient's body. In principle it ought now to be possible to eradicate the hepatitis C virus from Western countries, where the economy makes it possible to use these extremely expensive medications.[89] In the poorer parts of the world, such treatment is rarely accessible to most people.

In the case of hepatitis B, we also now have more drugs, but their effect is often less striking than the results of treatment against hepatitis C.[90]

Further challenges on the virus front

Despite the gratifying breakthroughs in the treatment of some of the major viral infections, we still have a whole series of viruses for which we have either no treatment or only drugs with a fairly moderate effect. In this latter group we find the influenza virus. The means at our disposal, the neuraminidase inhibitors, have only a limited effect and must be given within 48 hours of the patient falling ill. Two quite new drugs against influenza that act in a way unlike that of the neuraminidase inhibitors have recently been launched in certain countries, but are probably not all that superior to the existing medicines.[91] Every year some patients die from influenza, particularly those in high-risk groups, such as people with chronic heart and lung problems and ageing patients, and these are the patients who most need new and more effective drugs. Influenza vaccination is still our most important weapon against the disease.

We also need drugs for such well-known virus diseases as poliomyelitis, yellow fever and rabies, as well as for extremely frequent but undramatic infections caused by the many coughs-and-colds viruses that swirl around us. Likewise, we completely lack medicines for the new viral infections among the EIDs, including most forms of haemorrhagic fever, the Zika virus infection and, as mentioned, various types of coronavirus. Very recently two new drugs – so called monoclonal antibodies – against the Ebola virus have become available and have been used in the epidemic in the Congo.

When the COVID-19 pandemic broke out at the beginning of 2020 with an ever-increasing number of deaths, the development of drugs to fight this coronavirus was given very high priority. This started a veritable rush of medical experiments involving in excess of two thousand small and large studies in what has been called 'research chaos'.[92] Initially attempts were made to 'brush the dust off' older drugs used for other viral infections.[93] Many of these studies were of dubious quality and only a very few have provided us with valuable new information. The drugs tried out against COVID-19 fall into two main groups: drugs that directly attack the coronavirus and those that prevent immune responses and inflammation caused by the infection.

Two drugs belonging to the former group of antiviral drugs that have been a focus of interest are hydroxychloroquine and remdesivir.

Hydroxychloroquine is a malaria drug that is also used for rheumatic diseases. After an early, uncontrolled study claimed a distinct effect against serious COVID-19 infection, a number of trials were started using this agent, and many people started to take it on their own initiative to prevent coronavirus infection. Controlled trials have now shown that this drug has no useful effect on the COVID-19 infection and it is not recommended by the WHO.[94]

Remdesivir is a drug developed to combat the Ebola virus, where it was not a great success. There was a certain hope that this drug would be effective against the coronavirus. A large WHO-sponsored trial found that this drug does not have any effect on the mortality of serious COVID-19,[95] although a previous trial has found that treatment shortens the course of the disease to a certain extent.[96] This drug, which can also have serious side-effects, is apparently not the solution to COVID-19 treatment, at least not when used alone.

There is also considerable interest in using antibodies against the coronavirus, either blood plasma from patients who have been through infection, or laboratory-constructed monoclonal antibodies. The considerable challenges we are still facing regarding the treatment of serious viral infections have led to a renaissance of the principles underlying the classical serum therapy, which was so popular in the first half of the twentieth century. Major advances in medical technology mean that it is now possible to 'tailor' monoclonal antibodies that target specific microbes, including many viruses. Many people believe that such antibodies can play an important role in both treatment and prevention of the viral infections for which we do not yet have medicines available.[97]

Certain promising results against COVID-19 using monoclonal antibodies also gained publicity when President Donald Trump was given such treatment, in addition to remdesivir, when he was infected by the coronavirus. The results of plasma treatment are uncertain at present.[98]

The other main group of drugs for treatments that target harmful immune responses and inflammation has only had one breakthrough so far. For very serious COVID-19 infection, treatment with the corticosteroid drug dexametasone reduces mortality and is now standard.[99] Several trials are also being carried out with drugs that target cytokines, which are produced in increased amounts by the immune system and are thought to contribute to inflammation. No breakthrough has occurred as yet.[100]

The way forward to really effective drugs against the SARS-CoV-2 virus may well be long and difficult, as we have seen with many other viral infections. The major advances in molecular biology and immunology do, however, give us grounds for optimism when it comes to developing new virus drugs in the years ahead.

The Greatest Challenge: The Treatment of Life-threatening Fungal Infections

Among the newly arrived infections over the last few decades are a number of extremely serious fungal infections, mainly with the yeast fungus *Candida* and the mould fungus *Aspergillus*, but also with other types of fungus. These fungal infections did not become a serious challenge in Western countries until the major breakthroughs in transplantation medicine and cancer treatment. They are first and foremost dangerous for patients with badly weakened immune systems, where they can cause life-threatening infections and where diagnosis and treatment are problematic. This risk group is on the increase, since more and more people are being treated with medicines that weaken the immune system.

The use of modern cancer treatment is also increasing in the poorer parts of the world, with subsequent fungal infections that are a burden on health services with extremely limited resources. In addition, a number of serious fungal infections occur as part of the 'normal' infection load in tropical regions. The history behind the increasing problems with serious fungal infections explains why effective medicines within this area have been introduced only several decades after bactericidal agents.

The first effective drug against serious fungal infections became accessible in the late 1950s. This drug, amphotericin B, was originally found as a product of a bacterium. It had to be injected and caused many side-effects, some involving serious kidney damage. For that reason the treatment often failed. It is, however, still being used, mainly in countries with few resources, as it is inexpensive. In Western countries, chemically altered variants of this medication are used that have fewer side-effects, but cost a great deal more. Despite this, amphotericin B has not solved the major problems we have with fungal infections in present-day medicine.[101]

The next important step forward in the treatment of fungal infections came in the 1990s, with new medicines within the so-called azole group of drugs. New, improved variants came in the 2000s. During these years the first drugs in a completely different group, the echinocandins, also started to appear.

Today we have a number of effective drugs against fungal infections at our disposal, compared to a couple of decades ago.[102] In spite of this, fungal infections are one of the largest problems in infection medicine, with a high case fatality rate. One important reason for this is that these infections mainly attack patients with weakened immune systems that can only help combat infections to a limited extent. Furthermore, our diagnostic methods still leave a lot to be desired, and the symptoms of fungal infections are often misleading. This means that the infection has often become too well established by the time the diagnosis is made and treatment can be started. Better diagnosis and more effective new drugs are both needed. Work is also being carried out on ways to stimulate the patient's immune system, which it is hoped will then improve the effect of the fungal medicines.

The Curse of Poverty: The Neglected Tropical Diseases

Infectious diseases are an important cause of illness and death in the developing countries, which have been disproportionately hard hit by the 'major' infectious diseases known as the 'big three': malaria, TB and HIV/AIDS. These diseases have also received great attention in recent years. On the other hand, a great many infectious diseases that affect populations in poor countries get far less attention and little drug development takes place. These are known as NTDs (neglected tropical diseases).[103]

The NTDs are linked to poverty and special ecological conditions. Many of them are chronic and contribute to poverty by delaying children's physical and intellectual development and by reducing the adults' capacity for work. For the microbes involved we have no effective drugs for treatment, or those that exist have little effect, have serious side-effects or are simply too expensive for poor countries.[104]

There are a number of reasons why these infections have been neglected. Until now, at any rate, little research has been carried out on these diseases because the advanced research institutions are established in Western countries where the patients involved do not live. The major pharmaceutical companies, with their unsentimental business ethic, have not given the tropical infectious diseases high priority either, since there is little profit involved in developing drugs to combat them. Western aid has also been concentrated to a great extent on other important needs in these countries.

Since the NTDS contribute greatly to lasting poverty and social problems, it is necessary to give this field greater priority than it has received so far. The greatest obstacle to this is the weak economies of the poorer countries, which make it impossible to combat their infection problems effectively without outside assistance. This financing problem must probably be solved by Western countries through cooperation between governmental and private participants, as we have seen employed in vaccination assistance and action against AIDS.[105]

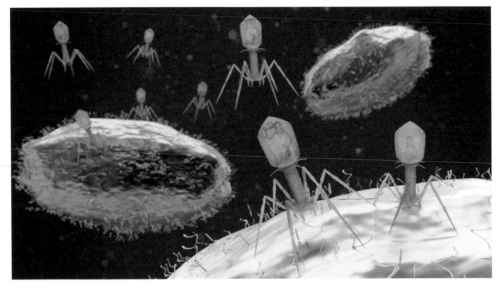

Bacteriophages on the surface of a bacterial cell. Bacteriophages are viruses that infect bacteria and can probably be used to treat bacterial infections. Like other viruses, they first attach themselves to special molecules on the bacterial cell they infect before injecting their genetic material into it. This can lead to the death of the bacterium.

TEN

New Challenges from the Microbes – and Possible Countermeasures

T he history of humanity is full of accounts of epidemics that at times have had the scale of pandemics. These are not just infection-caused disasters from a distant past. Over the last hundred years we have seen a number of pandemics that have sometimes had far-reaching consequences. Since the turn of this century alone, several new pandemics have struck: SARS, swine flu and the Zika virus, and in 2020 the COVID-19 pandemic.

The microbes that have caused these recent pandemics are examples of the many new microbial threats that have emerged in the present age, phenomena that characterize what I have chosen to call the fifth transition in the history of human infection. Typical of this latest period is that the many ecological changes that are increasingly due to *Homo sapiens*, as part of the Anthropocene era, have made it easy for formerly unknown microbes to invade humans and cause infection. In all probability, the basic mechanisms behind this will lead to new threats from the microbial world – and also unleash new pandemics.

Enthusiastic scientific optimists will probably shrug their shoulders at the probability of new pandemics and epidemics and the threats they involve. Are we not far better equipped than before to combat new microbes with the fantastic advances we have made in medicine and molecular biology? Will we not quickly be able to solve the problems by developing new vaccines and effective drugs? Despite all our scientific advances, however, we are in many ways even more vulnerable than earlier generations to large-scale epidemics and pandemics.

We have not only increasingly arranged conditions to enable new microbes to appear on the scene. Modern transport and means of travel also ensure the microbes are able to spread in a completely different manner than formerly.

We must regard it as a certainty that new threats of pandemics will occur. The great questions are *when* this will take place, and *which microbes* will be involved. The answers are vital if we are to be able to combat new pandemics effectively and, preferably, prevent them from happening.

Unfortunately, it should be noted that no experts have yet been able to predict any of the pandemics or epidemics that have occurred. In this respect, we still have a long way to go in spite of the extensive work carried out in recent years to develop reliable methods of advance warning.[1]

When it comes to which microbes are likely to be a cause of future pandemics, and where such pandemics will probably start, we can undoubtedly learn from former pandemics. Practically all the pandemics of recent years have been zoonoses, that is to say, they originally come from animals, and they have been caused by viruses. Furthermore, they have started in certain geographical areas around the globe where conditions are highly favourable for animal microbes to come into contact with humans and possibly start an epidemic. These hotspots normally have a particularly wide variety of wild animals and of microbes, particularly viruses. Often these areas have undergone considerable changes in nature and climate. Most hotspots lie in tropical regions.[2]

Can we say anything about which viruses we ought to fear? There are, after all, about 5,000 mammal species and 10,000 bird species on the earth, and each species is a carrier of several different viruses. So as a point of departure it may well seem hopeless to try to identify the most probable viral causes of new pandemics. One type of virus, however, does stand out, influenza A virus, which has caused pandemics at regular intervals for at least the past five hundred years.[3]

There is still a great deal we do not yet know about the influenza viruses, and experts also disagree in many areas. Everyone agrees, however, that we will at some point get a new influenza A pandemic – and it could come at any time, probably from wild or tame species of bird, or possibly from pigs. Which of the many types of influenza virus found in birds will cause the next pandemic can only be a wild guess. Such a virus must be capable of infecting humans and causing disease, as well as effectively infecting from person to person.

For several years people have particularly feared the bird influenza virus H5N1, and recently also H7N9.[4] In rare cases these viruses can cause disease in humans as well, and the case fatality rate is then high, but they do not spread all that easily – as yet. What is feared is that mutations of these viruses will suddenly enable them to infect effectively from person to person. It is uncertain whether this will occur. Perhaps completely different influenza viruses will turn up instead. The influenza viruses have many secrets and surprises in store for us.

Which other viruses are potential causes of new pandemics? It is natural to fear certain already known viruses that have appeared in recent years and created considerable problems, even though they have not all started pandemics.

The SARS virus, now called SARS-CoV-1, came in 2003 and showed how rapidly a virus can spread and create problems because of modern communications, mainly global air connections. After half-hearted initial efforts to contain it, especially because China withheld information about the seriousness of the epidemic in Guangdong province, the international community managed collectively to stop this epidemic, partly via information from the WHO, with travel advice, and partly by implementing routine measures against infection, including consistent isolation of patients suspected of having SARS. The SARS virus has not been eradicated and could reappear, possibly causing a pandemic if something goes wrong in the initial treatment of an outbreak.

The Ebola virus is also the subject of considerable attention. A new epidemic with this form of haemorrhagic fever broke out once more in Congo in 2018 and until recently has proved difficult to halt. This is mainly due to a series of local problems. Political unrest and military conflicts have placed great obstacles in the way of combatting the epidemic. Furthermore, there is a mistrust of both the authorities and aid organizations, with armed attacks on health centres and a number of deaths among aid workers. Considering the way this Ebola virus infects, a full-blown pandemic ought to be avoidable through fairly basic counter-measures, but the virus may increase its capacity to infect via mutations.

The Nipah virus, which some people have focused on as a possible pandemic threat, is probably not a very likely candidate. When it comes to the MERS virus, the future is uncertain. This coronavirus is already present in the camel population in not only the Arabian peninsula but in countries in the Horn of Africa. If an epidemic breaks out in Africa, it can become difficult to stop. If mutations lead to the virus spreading more easily from person to person, the possibility of a pandemic cannot be excluded.

The fact of the matter, however, is that a new pandemic may be due to a completely new virus among the thousands to be found in mammals and birds. Bats in particular, which constitute 20 per cent of all species of mammals, are carriers of a large number of viruses.[5] Some of them have already created epidemic problems such as the Hendra and Nipah viruses. Completely new bat viruses are also possible candidates for pandemics. This applies to relations of the Ebola virus and a number of coronaviruses other than the SARS and MERS viruses. The threat from the large family of coronaviruses has recently been realized by the pandemic caused by SARS-CoV-2, but this may not be the last one.

Possible scenarios for pandemics particularly focus on microbes, especially viruses, which are spread by droplet or aerial infection.[6] The potential spread of such microbes in modern big cities, with dense congregations of people in the streets and large residential areas, and on many forms of public transport, is frightening.

There has been far less emphasis on potential pandemics and widespread epidemics with microbes that infect via sexual contact. This is surprising if one considers the situation a few decades ago and recalls how effectively the HIV virus managed to spread. The almost explosive spread was not because HIV is particularly infectious, but because sexual behaviour in large sections of the public all over the world offered favourable conditions for a virus to spread. If a new, potentially deadly microbe that infects in this way were to strike again, I am afraid we would get a rerun of the HIV-AIDS scenario. Sexual behaviour has not taken a more puritanical direction in any way compared to the first years of the HIV pandemic. On the contrary, a sexually transmitted infectious agent would now probably have even better chances of spreading, particularly since the use of condoms among many risk groups is now regarded as unnecessary, due to the advances in HIV treatment. This has already led to a rapid increase in sexually transmitted infections among such groups. The HIV epidemic showed us how difficult it is to change sexual behaviour, even when deadly microbes are linked to sexual contact.

The consequences of pandemics in today's world

History reveals that the consequences of pandemics in former times have often been enormous for the societies involved.[7] We have to face the fact that also in today's world pandemics can have terrible consequences that are not only medical, but political, economic and social. To an increasing extent we have become aware that pandemics and large-scale epidemics can actually threaten the security of societies at both a national and a global level.[8]

When it comes to the medical consequences, they will naturally vary according to the virulence of the actual microbe. During the influenza pandemic of 1918–19 and the HIV pandemic prior to 1996, mortality was high and led to 10 million deaths. Even the swine flu pandemic of 2009, which is regarded as relatively mild when it comes to mortality, led to 6 million deaths, globally speaking. The Zika pandemic, on the other hand, had a far lower mortality rate – only twenty deaths in 2016 – but gave rise to other medical problems. If we get to experience a new, highly virulent pandemic virus, it is very likely that we will not have any effective drugs and no effective vaccine either – at least not during the first phase of the pandemic. We will therefore be forced to meet the crisis with traditional infection-preventative measures such as patient isolation, quarantine and travel restrictions. The SARS epidemic showed us that such measures can be effective if strongly implemented. Valuable experience will also be gained during the ongoing pandemic.

A large-scale pandemic with a virulent microbe would place a great burden on the health services, even in the richest countries. Victims of the pandemic would place heavy demands on hospital capacity, both as regards ordinary beds and beds in highly specialized intensive-care units, where the worst-hit patients would end up. A considerable proportion of health personnel would be involved in the treatment of pandemic patients. The provision of care for other serious diseases in developed countries may also suffer during a raging pandemic. Developing countries with poorly developed health services would inevitably be extra-vulnerable here. We saw this clearly during the Ebola epidemic in West Africa in 2014–15, when roughly 12,000 Ebola patients died. Almost as many patients with other illnesses died because of a failure to treat them as a result of the epidemic.

Much important medical equipment and many vital drugs are currently produced in only a few locations around the world. This applies, among other things, to many antibiotics. A possible serious consequence of a pandemic is that vital medical equipment will be scarce in the rest of the world if an important production country is paralysed by the pandemic or international trade is affected.

The experience gleaned from earlier pandemics and epidemics indicates that political and social unrest can easily be triggered under such conditions.[9] This is particularly a threat in countries where unrest and discontent with governments that lack the trust of the population are rife. Smouldering conflicts can flare up and result in a state of civil war when a society is hit by an epidemic. This was evident during the recent Ebola epidemic in Congo, where political and military unrest prevented the enforcement of measures against the epidemic.[10] Even in Western societies, a really violent pandemic would, at worst, be capable of resulting in social unrest and lack of trust in politicians and government. Several instances of this have already been seen during the SARS-CoV-2 pandemic.

Civil unrest might also increase because of the major economic consequences of a pandemic. Both nationally and internationally, trade and industry would be more vulnerable than before to its inevitable consequences and the measures it might lead to in today's world. Some of the measures that might be adopted would be reasonable enough within the context of infection, while others could be triggered by fear, which would be an important factor during a pandemic. International trade with particularly hard-hit countries would decline drastically. An example of the major economic losses that can arise is the SARS epidemic of 2003, which cost the world between $30 and $50 billion, even though it was halted relatively quickly.[11]

Industry can be paralysed in the individual hard-hit countries, as was evident during the Ebola epidemic of 2014–15 in Guinea, Sierra Leone and Liberia, where mining and agriculture, for example, were badly affected because of a labour shortage following both a fear of infection and travel restrictions imposed by the health authorities. Foreign investment would plummet in parts of the world that are especially under attack, something we saw in several African countries in the first years of the HIV pandemic. Tourism, on which many countries base their economy to a great extent, would, of course, be extremely sensitive to a fear of infection.

All in all, the economic consequences of future pandemics would definitely be extremely serious. Attempts to calculate the probable outcomes have arrived at quite frightening figures. An American commission has reckoned that the average annual expenditure caused by future epidemics would be $60 billion, and that is without taking into account the economic consequences of the considerable mortality that must be expected.[12] Another group of experts took this mortality into account and arrived at an annual expenditure of $490 billion as a result of future epidemics and pandemics.

All the factors I have mentioned explain why national and global security experts are extremely worried about the threat of future pandemics. One of these, the American Andrew T. Price-Smith, wrote a book in 2009 with the catchy title *Contagion and Chaos*, in which, citing examples from both early and recent history, he claimed that pandemics and large-scale epidemics can present a serious threat to security and stability in our societies.[13]

The role of international cooperation in combatting pandemics

The serious consequences of pandemics mean that the international community must devise effective plans to combat approaching pandemics and, preferably, seek to prevent them. The many measures that are necessary will be extremely expensive, but the cost of ignoring such planning will be far greater, possibly threatening millions of human lives.[14]

By the nineteenth century it was already obvious that international cooperation was necessary in dealing with such epidemics as cholera, yellow fever and plague. From the mid-nineteenth century onwards a number of international conferences were held to plan such work. This culminated in an international agreement, the International Health Regulations (IHR), to which 196 countries are now signatories. One of the issues agreed on is how the health services of the member countries are to contribute as soon as possible upon the discovery of an imminent epidemic, so that the necessary measures can be implemented without delay. Furthermore, member countries are to warn the WHO of epidemic outbreaks at once. In the event of outbreaks, the WHO is to provide the necessary advice about appropriate measures as quickly as possible, and lead and coordinate international cooperation to fight the epidemic.[15]

The organization of international measures to combat epidemics and pandemics is, then, a pyramid, with the individual countries at the base and the WHO at the top. Obviously, a great deal would depend on the efforts of the individual countries and on the quality and resources of their health services. All countries ought to have contingency plans ready in case of pandemics. Here, however, there are considerable deficiencies that must be improved. It is too late to make plans once the pandemic has broken out.

As mentioned earlier, a likely cause of future pandemics is the influenza virus. The WHO has established a well-organized global network here, made up of national centres and special laboratories that constantly monitor the influenza situation in the world, and also that of the feared bird influenza viruses.[16]

When it comes to microbes other than the influenza virus, international cooperation is less well organized. Experience of pandemics and large-scale epidemics over the past twenty years has revealed considerable deficiencies in the world's preparedness for pandemics. This is not only due to a lack of resources and knowledge in the health services of many countries. The WHO has also been criticized for a lack of leadership, for example during the Ebola epidemic in West Africa in 2014–15, when many felt that the organization acted too late. In addition, WHO has only limited resources.[17]

All this has led to a host of new international organizations springing up in recent years with the aim of improving pandemic readiness in the world. Such measures are normally based on cooperation between governments, universities, pharmaceutical companies and aid organizations.

An important aim is to strengthen the possibilities for early detection of pandemic threats at the local level, particularly in areas that are perceived as hotspots. This work consists partly of training personnel and partly of improving the standard of laboratories around the world, so that more reliable diagnosis will be able to make it easier to detect new threats from microbes as soon as they become evident.

A great challenge when it comes to pandemic readiness is that we have no idea which microbe will turn up next time. In order to stop a pandemic from the very start, it is not enough to discover that something is happening: it is important to identify the microbe responsible as quickly as possible and determine the means of transmission. Is it a known microbe or a completely unknown newcomer? To be able to answer this crucial question we must rely upon the most modern and advanced molecular-biological methods.[18] And in this respect, great progress has been made.[19] It took two years to detect the HIV virus as the cause of AIDS, which first appeared in 1981, while in 2013 it took only two weeks to detect the coronavirus that was given the name MERS, and in 2020 an even shorter time to determine the structure of the newly discovered coronavirus SARS-CoV-2. An important prerequisite for our being able to make use of such progress is that these methods are accessible globally, particularly in the poorer countries, where hotspots for the start of new pandemics are nearly always located.

If a completely new microbe, in all probability a virus, were to appear at the start of a pandemic, it would be of vital importance to develop a vaccine as quickly as possible. We know from experience that this takes a certain time. Can we prepare ourselves in some way to shorten the time if an outbreak comes? Here are some of the initiatives that have been launched.

The Coalition for Epidemic Preparedness Innovations (CEPI), founded in 2017, is an international organization that was established to develop vaccines in advance of pandemics that might arise in the years ahead, including Nipah, Lassa, SARS and MERS viruses.[20] Vaccines against these viruses would undoubtedly be useful, but are these the most probable potential causes of new pandemics? Not everyone agrees that they are.

Critics have claimed that it is vital for vaccine research to seek to arrive at certain basic principles for the development of new vaccines, since this will enable the faster production of vaccines than with traditional methods when completely new microbes appear on the scene.[21] CEPI seems now to have organized its work on the basis of such principles.

The ideal when combatting pandemics is, of course, to discover a possible cause before it has started to set even a local epidemic in motion. Certain enthusiasts of molecular biology therefore wish to take a step beyond investigating patients after an epidemic has broken out, as is the case today. They feel that modern molecular biology can be employed to map all threatening viruses in animal reservoirs, which would involve research into the tens of thousands of viruses that could possibly jump from animals to humans.[22] Others, however, regard this as almost science fiction and feel that the limited resources available for combatting pandemics could probably be put to better use, and definitely ought to be increased.[23]

It is unfortunately not only within the medical area that measures to combat epidemics encounter obstacles. There are many examples of measures that need to be implemented in an acute situation meeting with resistance in the population. Fear, delusion and a lack of trust in the authorities are often the cause. Earlier pandemics provide plenty of examples. In our own age we have seen this during both the Ebola pandemic in West Africa in 2014–15 and the most recent outbreak in Congo.[24] An important component of combatting epidemics is full and open information from the authorities, not just to prevent fear and conspiracy theories but to inform people about the correct behaviour to prevent infection in the individual citizen.

An acute pandemic will be an exceptional situation that often calls for extraordinary measures that are otherwise not employed. This can include various compulsory measures such as enforced isolation of possibly infectious patients, quarantine and travel restrictions.[25] All countries ought to have legislation on infectious diseases that makes such measures possible with due respect for human rights. It is crucial for such measures to be well explained to the population and not be characterized by more coercion than the situation necessitates. Of importance here is naturally an assessment of the seriousness of the microbe threat involved. How dangerous is the microbe? In what way and how easily does infection occur? During the pandemics of recent years we have seen a number of examples of enforced measures that have been exaggerated, inspired more by fear and panic than by knowledge of the actual infection situation.[26]

It is particularly challenging to establish measures that are sufficiently effective to combat an epidemic without the negative impact on society becoming too great. This responsibility ultimately rests with the politicians, who must naturally base their measures on advice from experts on epidemics. This has proved problematic in many countries that have introduced extensive measures against the ongoing SARS-CoV-2 pandemic.

The Paradise of Antibiotics after the Fall:
The Development of Resistance

As we have seen, the discovery of penicillin and subsequently strepto-mycin ushered in a golden age in the treatment of bacterial infections that was to last several decades. Enthusiasm for the new miracle medicines led to hubris in doctors, politicians and the population in general with regard to the threat from the world of microbes, which became much less immediate. Other medical issues were now considered a great deal more important and therefore given higher priority. In retrospect, we can see that this attitude was rather naïve. The duel between man and the microbes has been fought for tens of thousands of years, and the microbes have proved themselves worthy opponents with an impressive ability to adapt to new conditions. Could it not have been foreseen that the bacteria would retaliate against man's new weapon – antibiotics?

The slow tsunami

In Greek mythology Cassandra, the daughter of King Priam of Troy, was cursed by Apollo with the ability always to predict the future correctly, but that nobody would believe her. In a sense, Alexander Fleming, the discoverer of penicillin, had this role. He may not have predicted the future of penicillin correctly when he first made his discovery, but in his acceptance speech in Stockholm when he was awarded the Nobel Prize in 1945, he pronounced some prophetic words. He foresaw even at that early date that bacteria would develop resistance to penicillin if the drug was used incorrectly. Few people took note of Fleming's warning. Had Salvarsan not been used against syphilis for forty years without any resistance developing in the bacterium? Strangely enough, people ignored the fact that several bacteria had already become resistant to sulfonamides by the end of the 1930s.

Gradually it became an inescapable fact that many bacteria were developing resistance to penicillin and more recent antibiotics. This still did not make any real impression, for in this antibiotic golden age new antibiotics were constantly being added. The development of new antibiotics had high priority in the large pharmaceutical companies, which placed heavy emphasis on research and development of new antibacterial drugs that gave them a considerable income potential.

Shortly after new antibiotics had been introduced, however, the first resistant bacteria started to appear.[27] When, for example, methicillin appeared, a new penicillin that was effective against yellow staphylococci that were resistant to normal penicillin, it took only two years before resistant staphylococci appeared on the scene.

By the end of the twentieth century a great many bacteria had become resistant to at least one antibiotic, and very often to several. This also applied to a number of bacteria that quite often give rise to life-threatening infections, often in seriously ill patients in hospitals – so-called gram-negative intestinal bacteria. There now remained relatively few drugs effective against these bacteria. In recent years, bacteria have appeared that have also become resistant to the antibiotics we have had in reserve against resistant bacteria. The occurrence of these multi-resistant bacteria, often known as 'superbugs', varies considerably around the world, but in many localities the situation is starting to become precarious. This has meant that occasionally it has been necessary to start using older antibiotics that have previously been regarded as toxic if used internally, such as colistin. Reports are now coming in of resistance developing against even this antibiotic, which can in some cases be a last resort for certain infections.

What lies behind this frightening development of resistance, which has created serious problems for modern infection medicine? The cause is that the genetic characteristics of the bacteria have changed to an increasing extent after the introduction of antibiotics. Pressure from the extensive use of antibiotics in many regions means that the resistant bacteria now carry genes that code for resistance to one, several or even all accessible antibiotics.

Where do these resistance genes come from? Bacteria have a far higher propagation rate than *Homo sapiens*. A single *Staphylococcus aureus* bacterium can divide ten times in less than twelve hours and give rise to 1 million successors. At every division there is a possibility of a mutation taking place. Under the influence of an antibiotic, a mutation that leads to resistance towards precisely this medicine will give the bacterium a survival advantage. In certain cases, this is the basis for resistance development, but it is probably the exception rather than the rule.[28]

In most cases, the resistance genes have not come into being recently but have existed in the world of microbes since time immemorial.[29] In the permafrost of Alaska, bacteria with resistance genes have been found in the soil that are more than 30,000 years older than when penicillin started to be used. Similar finds have been made in subterranean cave systems that have been isolated from the rest of the world for 4 million years. In the 1960s, resistance genes were detected in bacteria from the faeces of bushmen in the Kalahari Desert who had never had contact with the outside world, let alone antibiotics. Similar finds have been made in other isolated population groups and in wild animals that have never been in touch with antibiotics.[30]

We know that antibiotics are produced by a whole series of microbes in nature, possibly as weapons in the struggle for survival against other species of microbe. It is natural, then, to suppose that genes providing resistance to antibiotics from other microbes are also part of the defence system of the world of microbes. It is also possible, however, that both antibiotics and resistance genes can have completely different functions in microbes, functions that we as yet know nothing about. One theory is that they are part of a system for signalling between the individual bacterium cells of a species.[31]

How do these genes cause resistance to antibiotics? Here a broad spectrum of effective mechanisms has been discovered. An extremely common one is that the resistant bacterium produces an enzyme that breaks down and deactivates the antibiotic substance involved. This is seen, for example, in resistance to penicillin and all penicillin-related antibiotics. Other resistance genes ensure that antibiotics do not penetrate the bacterium, or that antibiotics are actively 'thrown out' of the bacterium. Other genes lead to changes in the bacterial molecule that an antibiotic attacks. Nature and the ingenuity of the bacteria are overwhelming in this area.[32]

In the late 1950s Japanese researchers made a discovery that was both surprising and shocking. They found that genes for antibiotic resistance can be transferred from one species of bacterium to another. It turned out that these resistance genes were located on plasmids, small rings of DNA that many bacteria carry as an 'extra supply' of genes in addition to their one chromosome. The plasmids partially lead their own life and can roam from one bacterium to another, thereby bringing with them new genetic information to the next bacterium. Plasmids can then also carry resistance genes along with them. This is extremely common and has the highly unfortunate consequence that resistance can spread rapidly from one type of bacterium to another. Conditions in the intestines, with their enormously varied flora of bacteria in both humans and animals, are ideal for the exchange of resistance plasmids.

It is a depressing fact that the cause of the widespread resistance to antibiotics we are at present confronted with is due to humans' own behaviour. Just as man, according to the third chapter of Genesis, ate of the Tree of Knowledge and brought about the Fall, so our knowledge of the miraculous effect of antibiotics led to an abuse of these substances and to a similar 'Fall' in infection medicine.[33]

Initially, penicillin and other antibiotics were regarded as miracle medicines that could be used for many different diseases. This led to both over-use and incorrect use. One of the reasons for this was that many of the large antibiotics producers, following commercial considerations, 'pushed' their products directly and recklessly on the populations of many countries, at a time when there were no official regulation mechanisms in place. Gradually the authorities began to take over control, so that antibiotics needed a doctor's prescription, but such requirements still have not been introduced everywhere. It is possible to buy antibiotics over the counter in many places. And within the health services there has definitely been an over-consumption of antibiotics, both inside and outside the hospitals. They are, for example, wrongly used for banal throat and lung infections that are due to viruses – where antibiotics have no effect whatsoever. To a great extent our hospitals have seen too much use of so-called broad-spectrum antibiotics that are effective against many different bacteria, where more narrow-spectrum antibiotics would have solved the infection problem. This increases the risk of resistance developing. The many years of over-consumption of antibiotics for medical purposes, which still continues, has contributed significantly to the resistance problems we now face.

Human behaviour, however, has also contributed in a different way to the development of resistance to antibiotics, for there has been considerable use of these medicines for non-medical purposes. During the past decades, large amounts of antibiotics have been used in agriculture and animal husbandry. It probably comes as a surprise to many people that more antibiotics are actually used within these areas than for treating human infections. This started as early as the 1950s, when it became clear that low doses of antibiotics in farm animals' feed led to faster growth and a higher weight. This was discovered by chance in the USA, when anglers downstream from a pharmaceutical factory that produced a new antibiotic noticed that the trout there grew bigger and bigger. Today, antibiotics are used in animal husbandry in a great many countries, not only on land but in fish and shellfish farms. Antibiotics are also used when treating and preventing plant infections in agriculture.[34]

Not surprisingly, these non-medical ways of using antibiotics have created considerable problems of resistance in the animal world, which is then passed on to human beings. Many of the antibiotics that are used in animal husbandry are the same as those used for human beings. Resistant bacteria that have arisen in animals will then be capable of being transmitted to humans via contact with these animals and through foodstuffs from agriculture.

The exchange of resistant bacteria between humans and the environment, however, works both ways. Humans excrete resistant bacteria in faeces, which then pollutes water sources, and resistance genes can then be spread to bacteria in the environment. It has recently been discovered that a number of widely used antibiotics can also be detected in the world's rivers as a result of human and animal excretion. This too will contribute to the development of resistance in bacteria in nature.[35] It has just been shown that wild birds, particularly gulls and crows, which live close to humans, can be carriers of multi-resistant bacteria that they may transport over long distances.[36]

As long as the pharmaceutical industry continued to develop new antibiotics, the worrying issue of the development of resistance was on the whole confined to a few experts, since the consequences were not obvious. But gradually the rich supply of new antibiotics started to dry up. We have seen in recent years that fewer and fewer completely new antibiotics with original effect mechanisms are being produced. What we now see, generally speaking, are variants of old medicines, so-called me-too drugs which do not solve the resistance problems in the world.[37]

Why has the stream of new antibiotics dried up? There are several reasons. Today it is highly demanding for pharmaceutical companies to find new antibiotics. It takes many years to bring an antibiotic to the patient's bedside, and a great many initially promising drugs also fall by the wayside because of a lack of effect or too-serious side-effects. It is estimated that out of five or ten thousand medicines that start to be investigated, only five will end up being tested on humans – and only one of these five will end up as an approved drug. This process is extremely expensive. Unsentimental but realistic commercial analyses in industry have therefore concluded that developing new antibiotics is no longer profitable, as it was in the golden age of antibiotics. Antibiotics are quite cheap compared to many other drugs. Furthermore, they are most often used for a short time only, whereas medicines for chronic diseases are used over a long period of time and are therefore far more profitable for their producers.[38]

Today, the consequences of resistance to antibiotics are serious worldwide. Not only are resistance genes being effectively spread from one bacterium to another via plasmids, but the vast amount of present-day travel means that resistant bacteria are also being constantly spread from one corner of the earth to another. We are actually in the midst of a 'slow tsunami' of resistance development, as one American infection specialist has put it.

The result is that when we face serious, possibly life-threatening infections, we often have fewer antibiotics to choose between, even in the wealthy parts of the world. In many poorer countries, the access to reserve medicines will often be far worse, while the development of resistance will frequently have come further there. In these countries, the spread of resistant bacteria will occur especially rapidly because of bad sanitary conditions, high population density and open access to antibiotics in the shops. It is estimated that 700,000 people die annually from infections because of resistance to antibiotics. If this trend continues without our being able to turn it around, the WHO's gloomy prediction is that no fewer than 10 million people in the world will die annually by 2050 because of resistant bacteria. In just the rich Western countries, approximately 2.4 million will die in the period up to 2050 if we do not get the development of resistance under control.[39]

Increasing resistance will also have serious consequences for many key areas within modern medicine, such as transplantation and advanced surgery, where treatment with antibiotics is essential to prevent and deal with infections. Costs in the health services are increasing, partly because infection with resistant bacteria leads to longer hospitalization and more specialized and expensive treatment. Illness and death because of resistance reduce productivity in society. Calculations of the economic losses in the years ahead in the event of increasing resistance development have been made, and predictions involve enormous sums, although such calculations are uncertain. One report concluded that the global economic loss would be $100 billion by 2050.[40] Poor countries would be hardest hit, and it would lead to a further increase in poverty.

Without a doubt, resistance to antibiotics represents a real crisis in the world community, and the WHO has recently stated this, with the support of the governments of a number of countries. The situation has several similarities with the much-discussed climate crisis. In both instances, the negative development will continue to increase, with extremely serious consequences, if we do not take countermeasures. This fits in well with the pattern that characterizes the new geological period, the Anthropocene, in which humanity leaves its distinct impression on our planet.

Humanity Must Retaliate Against Resistance– But How?

If we do not respond to the problems of resistance with strong countermeasures, over the course of a few years we risk being thrown back almost a hundred years when it comes to the treatment of infection, to the time before sulfonamides were discovered. In such a scenario, a small, bacteria-infected abrasion could be fatal. But, just as *Homo sapiens* has successfully managed to withstand many threats from nature in the past, there is always the hope that we can hit back effectively against the microbes. There are actually many possible measures here, some of which are quite concrete and well established, while others are more or less on the drawing board.

To begin with, the world community must seek to correct all the human errors in the control and use of antibiotics that have led to the resistance problems. When it comes to the treatment of infection, misuse in illnesses that are not caused by bacteria must be avoided to a greater extent. This applies, for example, to a great many respiratory infections that are caused by viruses, where doctors far too frequently prescribe antibiotics, quite often under pressure from patients and relatives. In those cases where treatment with antibiotics is necessary, they ought not be given for too long.[41] In addition, more should be done to prevent infection in and outside hospitals to avoid the spread of resistant bacteria.

An increased use of vaccines could be extremely useful.[42] Vaccination against common bacteria would reduce the need for antibiotics and thereby the development of resistance. This has been demonstrated for vaccines against such bacteria as pneumococci and *Haemophilus influenzae*, which can cause serious infections. Today, work is going on to develop new vaccines against several other bacteria that can develop resistance, such as *Staphylococcus aureus*. A new and effective tuberculosis vaccine is also highly desirable on account of the spread of highly resistant TB bacteria that are a large problem in certain parts of the globe.

It is also crucial to drastically reduce the use of antibiotics in non-medical contexts such as agriculture, animal husbandry and fish farming. Both national and international measures have tried to do this, so far with varying degrees of success.

Even so, we must face the fact that all these measures will be far easier to implement in the rich Western countries than in the more impoverished parts of the world, which are hampered by poorly developed health services, lack of access to medical help and absence of control of the sale and use of antibiotics.

Although the access to new antibiotics has gradually decreased over the past decades, it is not impossible to turn this tendency around if the right measures are adopted. It is vital for basic research to be carried out within this field, which has been given less priority in recent years. There are still definitely great possibilities for finding completely new antibiotics in nature, using modern, advanced molecular-biological methods. The more research uncovers the resistance mechanisms of the bacteria, the greater the chance one will have of constructing new antibiotics in the laboratory.[43]

Many people have also proposed measures that seek to encourage the pharmaceutical industry to resume its interest in antibiotics, partly by means that would increase profitability. One can, for example, simplify the procedures for testing new medicines. Cooperation projects between government authorities, industry and university research environments have also been suggested, and perhaps also between pharmaceutical companies, as when penicillin was developed during the Second World War. The antibiotics crisis calls for extraordinary measures.[44]

Bacteriophages: my enemy's enemy is my friend

All living organisms on the earth can be infected by viruses. This also applies to bacteria.[45] Viruses that have specialized in bacteria are called bacteriophages ('bacteria eaters'). These are actually the most common organisms on earth and are found everywhere: on land, in the water, in the air and right up into the stratosphere. In 1989 Norwegian researchers showed that there are about 250 million bacteriophages per millilitre of seawater.[46]

Since bacteriophages attack bacteria, one could envisage *Homo sapiens* forming an alliance with these special viruses in the battle against bacteria. This might sound a bit like science fiction, but it is actually a reality.

Bacteriophages were discovered as far back as the late 1910s at the Pasteur Institute in Paris by the self-taught French-Canadian microbiologist Félix d'Herelle.[47] Certain bacteriophages, so-called lytic bacteriophages, kill the bacterial cells they invade. This is why d'Herelle and others were able to show that using bacteriophages in treatment can have a definite effect on serious bacterial intestinal infections, such as dysentery and cholera. Such treatment was therefore widely used in the 1920s and '30s. Bacteriophages were marketed widely for the treatment of infections, but many of the commercial products available were probably of dubious quality.[48]

When sulfonamides and later penicillin were discovered, researchers lost interest in bacteriophage treatment, which was consigned to oblivion in Western countries. Interest has, however, always been sustained in such countries as the former Soviet Union and Poland.[49] Many publications from these areas show sometimes convincing results from treatment with bacteriophages for a large number of infections. During the Winter War between the Soviet Union and Finland in 1939–40, thousands of Russian soldiers were treated with bacteriophages, probably preventing amputations and reducing deaths from gangrene by two-thirds. The German forces under Erwin Rommel in North Africa were given similar treatment during the Second World War against bacterial intestinal infections such as dysentery.

During the Cold War, the research environments behind the Iron Curtain were isolated from Western science. After the fall of the Soviet Union, certain Western researchers became interested in the experiences of bacteriophage treatment, which is still actively practised, particularly in Georgia and Poland. This interest has grown further in recent years because of increasing resistance to antibiotics in the world. Many people now believe that such treatment can be worth using on infections involving highly resistant bacteria, as we now have little left with which to combat them. It is widely held, however, that this interesting form of treatment has not been tested under strict controls that meet Western requirements, despite the long traditions and many publications from Eastern Europe about bacteriophages.[50]

Over the past few years, several controlled experiments have therefore been carried out on bacteriophages in Western Europe and the USA, in some cases with promising results. More trials are taking place. In addition, a number of thoroughly studied individual cases involving bacteriophage treatment seem to have proved successful when other forms of treatment failed.

Many researchers are now enthusiastic about the potential for using bacteriophages in treatment. They do not have any known side-effects, as is the case with antibiotics. A bacteriophage is super-specialized to attack only one type of bacterium. Injection treatment using bacteriophages must therefore be tailor-made to use those that attack a particular bacterium. Such treatment will not affect other, 'useful' bacteria in the patient, as antibiotics often do. Bacteriophages can be administered in different ways, without serious allergic reactions taking place. It is also possible to give 'cocktails' with various different bacteriophages in order to increase the treatment's effectiveness.

Even so, there is still much to be done in the way of further research before treatment with bacteriophages can be introduced. This is something that will inevitably take several years. Are there possibly side-effects that have not yet been discovered? Will the patient's immune system react to the bacteriophage and render it inactive? Will bacteriophages, which are far larger than many antibiotic molecules, manage to penetrate into all parts of the body where bacteria are possibly located?[51]

It is, of course, also a challenge that one has to make a speedy, highly precise bacterial diagnosis before the exact bacteriophage needed for treatment can be selected. Such tailor-made treatment will therefore require a 'bank' equipped with a large number of bacteriophages to deal with various bacteria and kinds of bacteria. Nature itself, however, is a particularly rich source of all kinds of such variants. Modern molecular biology can also be used to alter bacteriophages existing in nature in order to make treatments more effective. This has just been demonstrated in one successful treatment situation.[52] Whichever way you look at it, bacteriophage treatment is a fascinating prospect for the future.

Back to the future: immune therapy against bacteria

The first decades of the twentieth century were the golden age of serum therapy, an age that disappeared with the advent of the antibiotic era. The results, which were based on the discoveries of Behring, Kitasato and Ehrlich, were not at all bad, as we have seen. Today we know that the antibodies in serum on which this treatment was based are large protein molecules, immunoglobulins.

Great advances have been made within this field. Using modern technology, it is possible to produce tailor-made immunoglobulin medicines (so-called monoclonal antibodies) with an antibody effect against any desired bacterial antigen. One is no longer, as in the classic age of serum therapy, dependent on producing antibodies in horses, or any other animals. In this way it is also possible to avoid the sometimes serious side-effects of the earlier serum treatment, known as serum sickness, which are due to the reaction of the immune system to proteins from non-human sources.

It is natural to attempt to resume antibody treatment for infections with highly resistant bacteria, where antibiotic therapy is no longer possible. Work is at present being carried out to develop such treatments for a number of common bacteria. As with the classic serum treatment, it is necessary to have a highly precise and rapid diagnosis of the bacterium in the patient in order to produce a tailor-made treatment, but modern diagnostics are far more advanced than those in the time of

Behring and Ehrlich, and speedy diagnostics are sure to be considerably improved in the years to come.

With today's comprehensive knowledge about the role of the immune system in responding to infection, a great many other possibilities for new forms of immune therapy exist where one stimulates or strengthens important antibacterial defence mechanisms in the body. A number of such forms of treatment are being tested in laboratories, but it is still uncertain if they may be successfully used on humans. If this becomes possible, such treatment will probably be combined with antibiotics.[53]

Sir Almroth Wright, Alexander Fleming's superior at St Mary's Mart's Hospital, had an almost fanatical belief that future infection treatment would involve methods of stimulating the patient's immune system, and probably had more faith in this than in antibacterial drugs, such as penicillin. He was ridiculed for his theories, but perhaps one of his nicknames, 'Sir Almost Right', was more apt than people imagined. Treatment that stimulates the immune system is in fact a promising field.

Not only bacterial resistance

Not only bacteria have the capacity to adapt to changing external conditions and develop resistance to medicine. We see the same in the rest of the world of microbes: in fungi, viruses and protozoa. The increasing problems of resistance in these microbes have nevertheless been overshadowed by those of bacterial resistance.

Increasing resistance in types of fungus that can cause life-threatening disease, in particular the yeast fungus *Candida* and the mould fungus *Aspergillus*, is a cause of serious concern. Life-threatening infections with these species of fungus are mainly seen in patients with a weakened immune system. This group is increasing in number in Western countries, particularly because of the advances in transplantation medicine and cancer treatment. The case fatality rate is still high for the commonest fungal infections, also with treatment using the antifungal drugs we have acquired in recent years. It is all the more worrying that we are now witnessing an increasing resistance to these drugs, of which we still have only a few.

This is partially due to an increasing use of drugs against fungi, as it leads to mutations that cause resistance, and to an increase in species of fungi that are resistant from the outset to the medicines being used. A particular yeast fungus, *Candida auris*, which was discovered in Japan as recently as 2009, is often resistant to a number of common fungicides and is now creating infection problems in various parts of the world.[54]

Even greater problems arise with the mould fungus *Aspergillus*.[55] Infection with this fungus is one of the greatest threats that exist for patients with a weakened immune system, where mortality for patients with, for example, a brain infection is almost 100 per cent. In recent years an increasing resistance has been discovered to triazoles, which are some of the commonest drugs used against *Aspergillus*. An important cause of this, in most people's opinion, is that, as with antibacterial agents, there is also considerable non-medical use of antifungal drugs. Drugs closely related to those used on humans are widely used in agriculture to combat fungal infections in plants. Since *Aspergillus* is found everywhere, including in the soil, this fungus will therefore be able to develop resistance. Spores from resistant types of *Aspergillus* can be borne on the wind and breathed in by exposed patients. Antifungal drugs are also used for other non-medical purposes, such as protecting wood. It is human activities then that are the cause of resistance problems in the case of fungal infections, just as it was with bacterial infections.

At present, we have no vaccines against fungal infections. Both because of their high mortality and the possibility of growing resistance to our medications, work is proceeding on the development of fungal vaccines, though it is still uncertain if this will prove successful.

The development of resistance can also be a considerable problem for the relatively few but important viral infections for which we have effective drugs, since it can make treatment ineffective. This applies, for example, to HIV infections, where it is important for the patient to take medicine regularly and have scheduled check-ups with the health service. The development of resistance is then unlikely. Resistance was an especially serious problem in the early years of the HIV epidemic, when few medications were available and side-effects common, but this is still a threat if patients are careless about taking their medicine.[56] In sub-Saharan Africa the problems with resistance are considerable.

Resistance is already found against the new medicines that have revolutionized the treatment of the hepatitis C infection, and against the few influenza medicines that are available.

Protozoa infections make up a sizeable group, the majority of which are found in tropical or subtropical regions, and hence very often in the poorer parts of the world. Here too the threat of developing resistance to the medicines available, which are usually old and frequently not particularly effective, is considerable.

One of the largest problems when it comes to protozoa is probably the development of resistance to malaria drugs, which we can now observe in the most dangerous of the malaria parasites, *Plasmodium falciparum*.[57] For a number of years, treatment of this serious form of malaria has been based on a combination that contains the most recent malaria drug, artemisin. Resistance has now been detected against artemisin in several countries of South East Asia, including Cambodia, Thailand, Vietnam and Myanmar. If this resistance spreads, to Africa for example, the malaria situation will become extremely serious.

Opposition to Vaccination: A Considerable Challenge

A recurrent theme in the account of the duel between man and microbes has been that human behaviour has often given the microbes new opportunities, which they have quickly exploited. Opposition to vaccines – an old, but still topical phenomenon – is a notable example of this.

The introduction of vaccination has been one of the major medical advances that have led to a drastic decrease in the frequency of a number of infectious diseases and their complications and consequences. One of the great causes of pandemics down through the ages, the smallpox virus, has been eradicated from our planet through vaccination. Edward Jenner's smallpox vaccine ushered in modern infection medicine and quickly spread in the nineteenth century. While many people welcomed the vaccine as a major advance, there was also a certain resistance to it, and this created problems. In 1871 an independent organization of vaccine opponents, the Anti-Vaccination League, was set up in England, followed by the formation of a number of similar organizations.

Since the end of the nineteenth century, a large number of additional vaccines have been introduced and gained a central position in modern medicine, yet there remains in most countries a certain resistance to vaccines that can sometimes be quite stubborn. In recent years we have seen many examples of the consequences of such attitudes. A highly topical one is the outbreak of measles epidemics in certain locations around the world, which can be traced back to a lack of vaccination in particular groups in society.

In Western countries, vaccination over the past decades has practically eradicated measles. It was, therefore, a considerable backward step when the WHO reported that there has been a steady increase in Europe of measles cases in recent years, with 89,000 cases and 74 deaths in 2018, and 90,000 cases in the first six months of 2019. It has also been difficult to halt major outbreaks of measles in the eastern states of the USA. A lack of vaccine coverage because of resistance to vaccination underlies these outbreaks.

Opponents of vaccination are a mixed group, often with quite differing motives. Some of them we recognize from the opposition to vaccine in earlier periods. This applies, for example, to religious arguments, which we find in various religions and religious sects. In the USA, for instance, we find practising Catholics who are opposed to vaccination against German measles (rubella) because they mistakenly believe that tissue from aborted foetuses is used in manufacturing the vaccine. Even though the pope has given permission for this vaccine, it has not solved the problem. Other sets of religious beliefs are based on the idea that the body, and blood in particular, are holy and would be 'polluted' by vaccines. Others believe that vaccination represents a lack of faith in God's ability to heal.[58]

Special philosophical concepts of the body and soul can also form the basis of opposition to vaccines. This applies, for example, to anthroposophy and Rudolf Steiner's scepticism about vaccines, which he believed could interfere with human mental development. According to this perception, it is better for the human mind to undergo natural infections than be artificially protected by vaccination. Today, opposition to vaccines is not uncommon in anthroposophical environments: there have been outbreaks of measles linked to a lack of vaccination at a number of Steiner schools around Europe.

In recent years, anthroposophical ideas about the negative effects of vaccination have been given a new 'packaging' in the so-called hygiene hypothesis which has been the subject of much debate, including in scientific environments.[59] This, briefly, states that it is harmful for an individual to grow up in an environment that is 'too clean', so that one avoids natural infections. According to this hypothesis, this leads to an increase in allergies and autoimmune diseases. This is allegedly why such diseases are on the increase in modern Western environments, where there is great emphasis on cleanliness. This theory fits certain observations, but absolutely not all – and the hygiene hypothesis is at present controversial. It can hardly be used to justify opposition to vaccination.

An important cause of opposition to vaccination in recent years has been based on pseudo-scientific concepts. The British doctor Andrew Wakefield has done irreparable damage by claiming that the child vaccine MMR against measles, mumps and German measles can cause autism in children, which results in drastic developmental disturbance that, among other things, affects the ability to make human contacts and interact socially. Wakefield's findings, based on studies of twelve patients, were printed in the prestigious medical journal *The Lancet* in 1998, but were later withdrawn.[60] His results were based on false research, and he lost the right to practise medicine in Great Britain. His erroneous claims, however, led to a sharp decrease in the uptake of the MMR vaccine and, without a doubt, have led to outbreaks of measles and deaths. Despite this, Wakefield still has many supporters, who regard him as a kind of Semmelweis, a truth-seeking heretic who has been persecuted by a reactionary and authoritarian medical profession.

A number of other undocumented, pseudo-scientific arguments against vaccination are also circulating. Without a shred of evidence, it is, for example, claimed that measles vaccination can lead to cancer and heart disease.

A constantly recurring argument against vaccines is that they contain harmful additives. One such substance, the mercury compound thiomersal, has been the subject of considerable debate. Even though harmful effects due to thiomersal have never been documented, this substance was nevertheless removed from child vaccines some years ago. No other additives in present-day vaccines have been alleged to cause harmful effects.[61]

It is paradoxical that it is precisely the triumph of vaccination medicine that has contributed to resistance to vaccine. In Western countries, people no longer recall the problems that used to be linked to infectious diseases, and make light of their seriousness. Measles, for example, is regarded as a completely harmless infectious disease despite the various complications that can follow in its wake, although admittedly they are not often life-threatening. Recent research, however, has shown that the measles virus in the event of natural infection has a profound, hampering effect on the immune system that for two to three years can make patients susceptible to other infectious diseases.[62] This is because the virus destroys the memory cells of the immune system.[63] During this period mortality is clearly increased when compared to children who have not contracted measles. Measles cannot therefore be dismissed as a harmless infection, as vaccine opponents often assert.

There are then many different reasons for today's opposition to vaccination. In social media and on the Internet, where misunderstandings and conspiracy theories flourish, vaccination deniers find support for their views on a large number of websites.[64] Many of the views we find there are related to other irrational phenomena in present-day society, such as alternative medicine and an increased belief in astrology. Such ideas are often combined with anti-scientific attitudes and a distrust of experts. Postmodern scepticism about scientific findings may well have contributed to these ways of thinking, which we not infrequently also encounter in well-educated people.

No matter what the causes of opposition to vaccines may be, the consequences are extremely unfortunate. If these attitudes persist and spread, we will lose much of what we have gained through modern vaccination medicine. We will experience new epidemics with an increasing number of deaths, as we are now seeing in various parts of the world with respect to measles. The economic cost of new outbreaks of acute infectious diseases can be considerable. In the USA, for example, it has recently been estimated that one new case of measles, with the ensuing consequences, can cost up to $142,000.[65]

How is one to confront opposition to vaccination? The debate is quite heated in many countries. Many people feel that vaccinations ought to be compulsory by law. Some countries that have seen outbreaks of measles, such as Italy, have already introduced this measure. We see the same in certain states of the USA. Others feel that it should be possible to employ various measures such as denying places in nurseries and schools to unvaccinated children.[66]

Such a discussion brings us back to a fundamental question in modern societies: how to balance the rights of the individual against the interests of society. This issue is crucial to the combatting of epidemic infectious diseases and to the debate about opposition to vaccination. In my opinion, coercion and restrictive measures should always be considered only as a last resort, when the infection problem involved is really threatening the interests of society. To prevent a measles epidemic, for example, it is estimated that between 93 and 95 per cent would need to be vaccinated to reach herd immunity. Unfortunately, this is not the case in the majority of European countries, including France, the United Kingdom, Italy and Greece.

The imposition of enforced vaccination without the medical situation clearly indicating its necessity would possibly have unfortunate consequences, including the strengthening of attitudes towards vaccines that cite conspiracies, for example that the authorities are colluding with vaccine manufacturers in failing to disclose the serious side-effects of vaccines.

Vaccine deniers ought, initially, to be met with information and dialogue that may help persuade them to change their views. Their motives, as mentioned, can vary greatly. What I call pseudo-scientific arguments are probably easier to influence than religious opposition to vaccines.[67]

Even so, vociferous anti-vaccine activists who circulate blatant untruths and misunderstandings should be confronted in the public arena with strong counter-arguments. In certain cases, commercial interests underlie such tactics. It is possible that the medical profession has so far been too reticent in the vaccine debate.[68]

Bioterrorism: A Threat Easily Ignored

The possibility that terrorists may use microbes and microbial products as weapons is a reality for which society is obliged to prepare, even if this threat is hardly something most people think about. As we have seen, there are plenty of examples of such terrorist attacks having been carried out by single terrorists or terror groups. Formerly it was admittedly mainly states that concentrated on microbes as part of their arsenal of weapons, and in some cases used them on a large scale, such as Japan before and during the Second World War. The reason for this was that it was predominantly states that had the necessary resources to develop such weapons.

That is no longer the case. Today it is not difficult for non-state terrorists to acquire microbes for terrorist purposes. Many potentially lethal microbes can quite simply be bought on the Internet from commercial laboratories the whole world over, and it does not take all that much specialist competence to process such microbes for terrorist purposes. In addition, it is possible for disgruntled employees at specialized microbiological laboratories to be tempted to sell particular microbes to individuals or to organizations with terrorist intentions. As the Nobel Prize-winner Joshua Lederberg has said: 'Today, one man can wage war. A bio clown with luck can kill 400,000 people.' And states can still be behind bioterrorism directed against other countries.[69]

Many potentially lethal microbes are of interest to terrorists, both bacteria and viruses. This particularly applies to microbes that cause infection with a high case fatality rate and are easy to spread. It is, of course, also an advantage if the microbe can easily infect from person to person, but this is not absolutely necessary. Anthrax is high on the list of probable bioweapons, even though it is not contagious from person to person.[70]

Among the large number of bacteria and viruses that can conceivably be used for terrorist attacks, the focus in recent years has been on certain particularly topical ones that have the desired characteristics from the terrorists' point of view. It is also a fact that many common microbes can easily be modified in the laboratory using modern molecular-biological methods, so that their virulence can be increased as well as their infectiousness.[71] Modern medical technology also makes it possible to produce new microbes in the laboratory.

The microbe used in a terrorist attack can be spread in several ways, but it is air infection using microbes as aerosols that will affect the maximum number of people. Here, for example, the spores from the anthrax bacterium are ideal. They are robust and can cope with cold and heat, and they can be spread through the air over long distances. Furthermore, they can be produced in large quantities with only a modest amount of expertise and under simple laboratory conditions. In 2001 there was evidence in Washington, DC, of just how effective even a relatively modest anthrax attack can be (see Chapter Eight). In this instance, anthrax spores were sent through the post.

The smallpox virus, *Variola*, is feared as a potential terrorist weapon. Smallpox was admittedly eradicated from the planet in 1978, but the virus still exists in two laboratories approved by the WHO: one in Novosibirsk, Russia, and one in Atlanta in the USA. The possibility cannot be excluded that the virus also exists elsewhere. The smallpox virus can also be spread extremely effectively through the air and is highly infectious from person to person. Bioterrorism using this virus could therefore bring about a disaster on a par with the major smallpox epidemics of former times. Few people nowadays are protected by smallpox vaccination, which was discontinued in 1980, and we have no drugs against the virus. The world's stores of smallpox vaccine are also minimal and would be far from sufficient in the event of a widespread epidemic or pandemic.

The haemorrhagic fever viruses Ebola and Marburg are also high on the list of possible terrorist weapons. They are infectious in the event of direct contact and have a high case fatality rate. Except for two recently developed drugs against Ebola infection, there are no effective medicines. We have recently acquired a quite effective vaccine against the Ebola virus.

The plague bacterium *Yersinia pestis* still causes natural infections in some parts of the world and is also on the list of particularly feared weapons for terrorists. When the bacterium is spread through the air as an aerosol, it causes pneumonic plague, which develops rapidly, is often fatal and is highly infectious. Today we have no effective vaccine to protect against pneumonic plague.

A highly toxic bacterial product, botulin toxin, could create major problems in terrorist hands. It is quite easy to produce and is one of the most toxic agents we know of. Terrorists could use it to attack the drinking-water supplies of cities, since it would pass through the bacteria filters.

Until now, many people have counted on certain microbes, such as smallpox virus and Ebola virus, being too dangerous for the terrorists themselves, and therefore less likely to be used. This is not necessarily an obstacle for suicide terrorists. A possible new way of spreading disease is by self-infected people – a counterpart to suicide bombers – who can spread highly infectious microbes in large crowds or as air passengers. A smallpox-like virus would be extremely efficient here.

During the last two decades many resources have been earmarked for the prevention of bioterrorism, particularly in the USA after the terrorist attack with anthrax in 2001. These efforts have been so comprehensive that some people have sharply criticized what is felt to be an exaggerated focus on terrorism, which has drained resources away from other sections of the health service.[72] There may be something in this, but it is beyond doubt that bioterrorism represents a sinister threat in the volatile world we live in at present, where terrorist attacks frequently occur. Every state is therefore obliged to defend its inhabitants against such a threat. Furthermore, relevant research and various defensive measures against bioterrorism can also have a positive consequence on other areas of infection medicine. The challenges in combatting bioterrorism are related to those we have seen with new infectious diseases, EIDs, which emerge at regular intervals, sometimes as serious epidemics.[73]

We must face the fact that bioterrorism is difficult to completely prevent in an open, modern society that is extremely vulnerable to such threats, particularly in urban environments, where large gatherings of people are common. Terrorist attacks can, for example, hit underground railway stations, major sporting events and other venues where many people are present. It does not take much imagination to envisage frightening scenarios in such situations. Remote-controlled drones, which are now commercially available, could very well be used to release aerosols containing microbes. It is almost surprising that this has not already been attempted.

Microbes that could possibly be used for terrorist attacks will not necessarily be common types causing disease pictures that are easily recognizable by doctors. The challenges here are really the same as those faced in outbreaks of epidemics with new microbes. In the event of both 'naturally' occurring infections and bioterrorism arising, it is a question of discovering the threat as early as possible in order to implement the necessary countermeasures. Early warning will depend on health personnel being alert and quickly raising the alarm. Crisis plans for bioterrorism ought to exist, and to a great extent these should be capable of being incorporated into existing plans for pandemics.[74]

Microbes and 'Ordinary' Chronic Diseases

By the mid-twentieth century the microbial cause of the great majority of diseases that were regarded as infections had been identified, and in many cases they could be treated. In addition to infectious diseases, we are also afflicted by many chronic diseases: cardiovascular diseases, cancers, rheumatological diseases and those that attack the nervous system, including various dementias. These chronic diseases, some of which are referred to as 'lifestyle diseases', now play an ever-increasing role in society, partly because many of them are seen in the ageing population. And life expectancy has steadily increased in recent years.

The 'common' chronic diseases have complex causes, with genes interacting with environmental factors. Unlike these diseases, many infectious diseases have a distinct, acute start, but some of them can change into chronic, quite often lifelong conditions. Examples of this are tuberculosis and infections with the viruses hepatitis B and hepatitis C, both of which can cause chronic illness. So it is reasonable to ask whether some of the chronic diseases that we traditionally have not connected with infection are perhaps caused or triggered by microbes.[75] In the last few decades it has been demonstrated that this may be the case for a number of them.

Perhaps the most surprising discovery has been that gastric ulcers, which affect the stomach or the duodenum, are due to infection by the formerly unknown bacterium *Helicobacter pylori*.[76] This was proved by the Australian doctors Robin Warren and Barry Marshall in 1982. Most people doubted their findings, which were also partially ridiculed, since it was assumed that gastric ulcers were mainly due to stress and lifestyle. In addition it was an almost undisputed fact that no bacteria could survive in the stomach because of the strong acidity there. But Marshall proved that a quite brief course of antibiotics, combined with acid-suppressing medication, could enable wounds in the stomach and duodenum to heal, whereas formerly one had to resort to endless, uninspiring diet cures and acid-suppressing medicines. He actually drank a solution containing *Helicobacter pylori* bacteria and showed that his resulting ulcer was convincingly cured by the use of antibiotics. Marshall and Warren were awarded the Nobel Prize for their findings in 2005.

Countless people with gastric ulcers have since improved their quality of life thanks to these two heretical researchers.

A myocardial infarction (heart attack) is a common affliction that is due to coronary arteries becoming blocked. Underlying this is a process of inflammation and fatty deposits in the walls of the arteries, known as atherosclerosis. Here too, lifestyle, genetic factors and stress play an important role. In recent years it has become clear that an inflammation in the walls of the arteries is an extremely important part of atherosclerosis.[77] What triggers this inflammation? Many researchers believe they have evidence suggesting that an infection may be playing an important role in this respect. Various microbes have been in focus, including the bacterium *Chlamydia pneumoniae*, which can cause acute respiratory tract infections. Might this bacterium also be a cause of cardiac disease?

Several researchers have found signs of *Chlamydia* infection in patients suffering from atherosclerosis.[78] In certain cases, bacteria have also been detected in the sick arterial walls. This is not proof of a causal relationship, since the bacterium could be there by chance. Trials with antibiotics against the bacterium have sometimes had a positive effect, whereas in other trials there has been none whatsoever. So the findings are difficult to interpret. Even though there are many indirect factors suggesting that *Chlamydia* plays a role in atherosclerosis, we cannot view this as having been proved. A number of other microbes have been linked to myocardial infarction, including *Helicobacter pylori* and the CMV virus, which also causes problems to patients with weakened immune systems.[79]

Since inflammation of the arterial walls is so important in atherosclerosis, it is also possible that anything that increases the inflammatory level in the body can play a role via the production of cytokines and other substances in the blood, which then cause inflammation, also of the heart. An infection somewhere far away from the heart can thus possibly have a long-range effect on the heart, without the microbe itself influencing the arterial walls. This may be why certain researchers have focused on active inflammation of the gums (periodontitis), where many naturally occurring oral-cavity bacteria produce a strong inflammatory reaction linked to an increased risk of atherosclerosis and myocardial infarction.[80]

A stroke can very often be the consequence of atherosclerosis in the arterial walls of the brain and the blocking of the arteries by a blood clot. Finnish researchers have recently found DNA from oral bacteria in blood clots in the event of strokes.[81] This may indicate that these bacteria contributed to the stroke, but it could also be a chance finding of no significance. Either way, these findings and the possible importance of oral-cavity bacteria for heart disease mean that periodontitis ought to be actively treated.

Cancers are an important and steadily increasing cause of sickness and death. For the vast majority of cancers, the causes are still unclear in spite of intensive research over many years. As early as 1911 the American doctor Peyton Rous was able to prove that a special form of cancer in chickens was due to a virus. This discovery too was initially ridiculed and doubted. It was to be more than fifty years before Rous was awarded the Nobel Prize in medicine for his findings, which marked a breakthrough in cancer research, in 1966.[82]

The EBV virus that causes the common infection mononucleosis ('kissing disease') can also cause special forms of lymphoma and cancer of the nasopharynx. This was the first virus to be linked to cancer in humans. A relation of the HIV virus, HTLV1, may cause leukaemia.

Cervical cancer is a quite common form of cancer in women. Here the German cancer researcher Harald zur Hausen showed that certain types of the common papilloma virus, HPV, which is transmitted sexually, cause this form of cancer. This discovery, for which zur Hausen was awarded the Nobel Prize in 2008, has led to very important cancer-preventative measures through the vaccination of young women against the HPV virus. Since then the virus has been linked to rectal cancer, and vaccination of young males could also become relevant.[83] Similarly it is known that the *Helicobacter pylori* bacterium causes gastric ulcers as well as chronic inflammation of the stomach, which can end up as cancer.

Cancer of the liver can result from infection with hepatitis B and hepatitis C viruses. In the case of the formerly rare *Kaposi sarcoma* form of cancer, which is an important complication of AIDS, a viral cause known as herpes virus 8 has been detected, which is a relation of the common herpes viruses that cause cold sores and chickenpox. The intestinal worm *Schistosoma haematobium*, which is extremely widespread in the world, can cause cancer of the bladder.

In the great majority of cancers, however, no microbial cause has yet been found, but in most cases no really active attempts have been made to do so. We cannot discount the possibility, however, that advanced molecular-biological methods in the years ahead will reveal causes of infection in more forms of cancer. Perhaps this will lead to new preventative measures, as it has for cervical cancer. Nor can we discount the possibility that the discovery of microbes that cause cancer could have consequences for its treatment.

The causes of most diseases of the nervous system and psychiatric disorders have not yet been discovered. This, among other things, applies to the special form of dementia known as Alzheimer's disease, which seems to be on the increase in Western countries. Investigations in recent years have particularly focused on the herpes 1 virus, which normally produces cold sores.[84] In some of these studies, a certain connection has been found between herpes infection and later dementia. Special genes possibly also play a role, combined with a virus. It is as yet still impossible to come to any final conclusion about infection in Alzheimer's, but further active research linked to possible microbial causes is important. It is interesting that spouses of patients with Alzheimer's disease are 60 per cent more likely to get the disease compared to others.[85] And neurosurgeons, who in their profession are in contact with brain tissue, have a risk 2.5 times higher.[86] Perhaps it will at some point become possible to prevent this disease by vaccination or by medication against microbes – or even perhaps to treat full-blown dementia in this way.

Infection as the cause of psychiatric disorders such as schizophrenia and bipolar disorder has also been advanced, but the documentation is weak. We should, however, recall that the cause of such brain diseases as Creuzfeldt-Jakob and kuru was also completely unknown before prions were discovered.

A considerable health problem that appears to be on the increase in Western societies is *Myalgic encephalomyelitis* (ME), also called Chronic Fatigue Syndrome (CFS). A heated debate is taking place about the cause of this condition, which is still completely unclear. There is, however, no doubt that a number of acute infectious diseases seem capable of triggering ME, without our knowing why. Mononucleosis, caused by the EBV virus, is one of the many examples of such a triggering infection. Not long ago, some researchers believed that they had detected a retrovirus, related to the HIV virus, in ME patients, but this turned out to be a dead end. So far there is no proof that ME is due to any ongoing infection.[87]

Not even the most enthusiastic microbiologists and infection specialists would claim that the great majority of human diseases are due to infection. There is nevertheless reason to believe that there are still many chronic diseases with unknown causes where future research will one day prove that a microbe plays an important role. Such surprising discoveries can have considerable practical consequences, as we have seen for example in the treatment of gastric ulcers.

The Frankenstein Scenario with Microbes in the Leading Role

In 1818 Mary Shelley published the novel *Frankenstein; or, The Modern Prometheus*, which has inspired many film adaptations that vary greatly in how closely they keep to the original. The book has characteristics of both science fiction and a horror novel. Shelley tells the story of the scientist Victor Frankenstein, who, while experimenting in his laboratory in an attempt to produce an improved type of human being, creates a sinister but intelligent monster. She does not describe the details of how Frankenstein creates the monster, but it is probable that animal parts were used. His experiments have terrible consequences. The monster becomes a killing machine, with Frankenstein's new bride as one of the victims on their wedding night. Frankenstein finally attempts to kill the sinister creature he has brought into the world, and pursues the monster all the way to the North Pole, but does not succeed. It escapes and drifts off on an ice floe.

Shelley's novel has often been interpreted as a warning against humanity going too far in the attempt to tamper with nature. This is an objection that is often raised against modern natural science and medicine, which attempt to change natural processes in favour of humanity. Where the boundaries ought to go for human intervention in nature, however, is extremely difficult to determine. Several similar issues in medicine have been the subject of debate in recent years. This applies, for example, to research where one attempts to increase the virulence of microbes (their pathogenic capacity) by modifying their genes, so-called gain of function experiments.

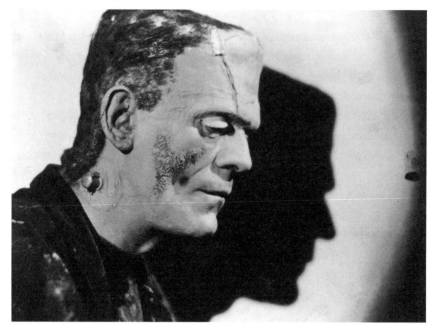

The intelligent monster created by the scientist Victor Frankenstein in Mary Shelley's book *Frankenstein; or, The Modern Prometheus* (1818). Boris Karloff here plays the monster in a film version of the book (1931, dir. James Whale).

It is of course absolutely necessary to carry out laboratory research on dangerous microbes, particularly in order to develop vaccines, drugs and new diagnostic tests. Laboratories that work on dangerous microbes must observe prescribed safety regulations that become stricter according to the danger level of the microbe. Despite this, we have to admit that sometimes glitches take place in safety precautions for either human or technical reasons. This may result in dangerous microbes infecting laboratory personnel, or escaping from the laboratory and infecting people in the local area, or, in the worst case, starting a widespread epidemic.

A tragic example of this risk is the last case of smallpox in the world in Birmingham in 1978.[88] A woman who worked as a photographer at the medical faculty was infected by the smallpox virus and died after a month. In the same building there was a laboratory where research into the virus was taking place. It is regarded as certain that the virus must have come from this laboratory, but it has never been ascertained how this came about. The head of the virus laboratory, an internationally recognized expert on the smallpox virus, was exposed to enormous pressure from the media and committed suicide, after a witch hunt instigated by the trade union of the infected photographer. Thanks to the health services' intensive efforts, using vaccination and isolation of those exposed to infection, further spread of the virus was avoided. But it could all have ended very differently, with a widespread smallpox epidemic.

In the USA alone a number of mishaps at state research laboratories working with particularly dangerous microbes have been reported. In 2014, for example, more than eighty laboratory employees were exposed to the anthrax bacterium, fortunately without any deaths resulting.[89]

For several years a pandemic with the bird flu virus H5N1 has been feared. Experiments with this virus some years ago triggered a major debate on the limits that should be permitted when conducting research into such dangerous microbes. This bird flu virus has a case fatality rate of 60 per cent when it infects humans, but the virus is practically non-infectious between humans. The fear remains, however, that by means of a spontaneous mutation the virus will acquire the capacity to infect through the air, with a horrific pandemic resulting.

Two laboratories, in the Netherlands and in the USA, made public in 2012 that they had managed to gene-manipulate the H5N1 virus in such a way that in experiments with ferrets it could now be effectively transmitted through the air. A heated debate in the research environment led to the public financing of such experiments by the USA coming to a halt for several years; the same measures applied to other viruses such as MERS and SARS.[90] If such a gene-modified bird flu virus were to leak out from laboratories, it could lead to a pandemic that infects and kills millions. After stricter safety precautions have been put in place, it has recently been decided to resume the financing of such experiments.[91]

Not everyone agrees that these experiments should be resumed. No matter what the safety precautions are, experiments of this kind always involve a certain risk. The possibility that they might lead to some improvement in our knowledge to employ in the duel with microbes must always be weighed against the risk. Thorough ethical research assessments are vitally important here. There have been calls from some researchers for an international set of regulations. Today, however, it is mainly the institutions financing the research that have the decisive influence. The problems with gain of function experiments and leakage of microbes from laboratories have become central to the discussion of the origin of the ongoing pandemic, as we have seen.

The Frankenstein motif is also present within another field of research: xeno-transplantation. This term is used to describe transplantation to humans of organs or cells from other species of animal. For a number of years this has been an active field of research, because the lack of human organs is a serious problem in modern transplantation medicine, while the demand is constantly increasing.[92]

Attempts to transplant animal organs into humans began in the early twentieth century, but they were unsuccessful for many reasons, mainly linked to the fundamental differences in species, which meant that the transplanted organs were not accepted by the human body. During the last decades, most experiments have concentrated on the pig as a donor of organs to apes, so as finally to pave the way for the later use of pig organs in humans. Many problems have gradually been solved, particularly because modern molecular biology has allowed genetic changes in pigs that facilitate transplantation to apes – and eventually, it is hoped, to human beings.

A problem that still gives cause for concern with xeno-transplantation is the possible risk of the transference of microbes from pig to human when transplanting pig organs.[93] Patients will be particularly vulnerable to infections, because, as with ordinary transplantations, they have to be treated with immuno-suppressive drugs. A number of viruses occur in pigs that can also cause disease in humans. Some of these viruses could probably be avoided by adopting various measures with the pigs used as donors. Even so, the worry is linked to special retroviruses that are part of the pig's DNA. Such viruses may cause problems in humans after transplantation of pig organs. A research group, however, recently made public that they have managed to remove such retroviruses from pig cells using the new method CRISPR. This makes it possible to 'edit' DNA in cells and has gone a long way towards revolutionizing molecular biology.

Despite this, the risk of transferring microbes will require comprehensive monitoring when the first attempts at xeno-transplanting pig organs to humans are launched, probably in the fairly near future. Will new, menacing microbes then emerge in the role of Frankenstein's monster?

Let us finally return to the subtitle of Mary Shelley's book, *The Modern Prometheus*. In Greek mythology Prometheus was a Titan who aroused the wrath of Zeus, god of the heavens, by creating men of clay and giving them fire, which he had stolen from Olympus. In one account of the story by Hesiod, Zeus attempted to punish him by sending the beautiful Pandora to him with a gift, a casket that Zeus had filled with all kinds of diseases and plagues.

Prometheus wisely refused to accept the gift, but the inquisitive and empty-headed Pandora opened the casket. Then all the plagues flew out into the world and descended on humanity. This was the result of Prometheus' well-meaning attempt to help mankind. Does a warning to modern science perhaps lie concealed in this myth?

Global Warming: A Gift to the World of Microbes?

A central topic of today's debate on society is the gradual increase in the average temperature on our planet and the consequences this will have for *Homo sapiens* and all other living organisms. There is no lack of gloomy predictions as to what might happen should we fail to halt this development. Increasing health problems have commanded great attention in the debate on global warming and there is a high level of agreement that, among other consequences, climate changes will influence the occurrence and frequency of many infectious diseases.[94]

Early in the history of humanity, people were undoubtedly already aware that there was a connection between climate and certain diseases. Hippocrates wrote a great deal about this in his book known in Latin as *De aere loci aquis* (On Air, Places and Water), and we find similar concepts advanced by physicians down through the centuries. But, naturally enough, they did not know *why* there were such connections. Today, we have clarified a great many of the ecological conditions that are important for the interaction between man and microbes.

As we have already seen, the connection between climate and infectious diseases is extremely complex. We must take a number of different climatic factors into account, such as temperature, precipitation, humidity and wind conditions, as well as the fact that these various factors affect the microbes, infection-carrying insects and species of animal that are reservoirs for microbes – and especially human beings, who often alter their behaviour when the climate changes. In practice, this means that it is extremely difficult to predict the consequences of global warming on many infectious diseases. Most professional climate researchers in this field are therefore cautious about advancing hefty claims about the future of infection medicine. It is highly complex to try and analyse the meaning of climate changes independently of the many other ecological and environmental factors that are also changing.[95]

Even so, we can just manage to make out patterns for what will happen to certain infectious diseases during the form of global warming that is taking place. This applies in particular to infections transmitted by insects, and certain waterborne infections.

Malaria, which is transmitted by the *Anopheles* mosquito, is a possible example. Both the mosquito and the malaria plasmodia like high temperatures to be active. The cooler highland areas of East Africa, which have been spared malaria up to now, have in recent years acquired increasing problems that, partially at least, could be due to an increase in temperature in these regions. It is therefore possible that a continued increase of the average temperatures in Africa will lead to a greater spread of malaria. On the other hand, neither the mosquito nor the malaria plasmodia like temperatures above 32°C. So some regions now ravaged by malaria will possibly become malaria-free, since the highest temperature increases in future years will probably hit these areas. Malaria will hardly become a problem in the northern hemisphere – and falling temperatures were not the cause of malaria disappearing from northern Europe.

Certain viruses transmitted by species of mosquito have increased their range in recent years, including the West Nile virus, which has recently gained a foothold in southern Europe. Average temperature increases may have contributed to this. It may be partly due also to an increase in the mosquito population and the length of the mosquito season, and also the biting activity level of the insects. Will this virus move inexorably northwards through Europe? It is difficult to say, and we must be cautious about ascribing the most important role to climate change.[96]

The same applies to another virus transmitted by ticks, which can cause encephalitis. Various investigations have shown that the species of tick that transmits this virus has moved further north in recent years, with an increase in the number of cases of viral infection, even in Scandinavia. This may be due to an rise in temperature, which has increased the range of the ticks and lengthened their season, but other factors may also have contributed.[97]

Waterborne microbes will possibly increase their range as a result of global warming. This applies, for example, to cholera. *Vibrio cholera*, the cholera bacterium, lives in water. If the temperature of the world's oceans rises, it may lead to an increased spread of the pathogenic cholera bacterium and possibly to epidemics. The cholera bacterium today is quite widespread in estuaries and brackish water in many locations around the world, not only in its original area in Bangladesh, but the water temperatures are often too low for the complicated ecological processes that lead to a significant increase of pathogenic bacteria. As we have seen, increased growth of special types of plankton in the sea is an important part of this scenario, something which a further rise in sea temperatures would make more likely.

Relatives of the cholera bacterium that can also produce other pathogenic pictures also thrive in relatively warm water and can affect northern latitudes during longish warm periods. An example of this is infections with *Vibrio vulnificus*, which can cause serious infections in bathers. Such infections could become more common in the years ahead.[98]

Life-threatening fungal infections have recently been linked to global warming.[99] Until now, such infections have affected patients with a weakened immune system. In nature, however, there exist a large number – probably several million – of types of fungus that until now have not been a threat to humans, mainly because they only thrive at considerably lower temperatures than the 37°C they encounter in the human body. So our body temperature has been an important part of our defence against such fungi. If these species adapt to a higher temperature by mutating, they could possibly cause serious infections in humans.

A possible example of this is the fungus *Candida auris*, which has appeared simultaneously during recent years as a serious infection threat on three continents. Researchers have found evidence that precisely this fungus has adapted itself to higher temperatures than its closest relatives and thus become able to cause infections that are often difficult to treat. Perhaps it is the first of many types of fungi that will increase the infection problems during global warming.

The development of antibiotic-resistant bacteria is an increasing problem, as we have seen. Researchers have recently shown that global warming contributes to this: with increasing temperatures in the environment, the bacteria reproduce more rapidly, leading to a greater frequency of mutations, including those that also increase resistance.[100]

History provides us with numerous examples of extreme, acute climatic occurrences, such as tropical storms and hurricanes, leading to outbreaks of epidemics. Many climate researchers believe that global warming will lead to such weather disasters increasing in both frequency and scope. In that case, it will also increase the infection problems in the world.

All in all, there can be little doubt that global warming will influence our relationship to the world of microbes and the pattern of infectious diseases we will encounter in the future. The picture, however, is highly complex and it is too early to draw any firm conclusions. As yet there is no need for prophecies of doom and sensational headlines, although certain observations can tempt one to indulge in them when it comes to the future of infection medicine during global warming. One example is the possible consequences of the thawing of the permafrost in the northern hemisphere.

Permafrost and Zombie Microbes

The term 'permafrost' is used to describe areas where the earth never thaws during the year. This is the case with more than 20 per cent of the land area of the northern hemisphere. The uppermost layers of the soil may thaw during the summer, but the lower layers are permanently frozen. In these frozen layers of earth there is also a rich selection of microbes – bacteria, viruses and fungi – but in an inactive, dormant state.[101]

The warming process we are now witnessing on the planet also influences the permafrost. A gradual thawing is taking place that will simply increase, resulting in many problems. If the profuse flora of microbes in the layers of permafrost wake up after thawing, there could be a massive release of gases such as carbon dioxide and methane from the large amounts of plant remains in these layers. This release of climate gases will, of course, contribute to climate problems and global warming. Will the microbes of the permafrost, when they awake from their enchanted sleep after thawing, be a threat to humanity? This has been much discussed in recent years and the possibility cannot simply be swept aside, since the layers of the permafrost can also contain pathogenic microbes. Since time immemorial, remains of both animals and humans that may have had infectious diseases have ended up in the frozen layers of soil. This also applies to earlier human species such as Neanderthals and Denisovans, who lived in Siberia where there are large expanses of permafrost.

Potential microbial threats from the permafrost could come from known pathogenic bacteria and viruses or from ancient microbes that are now extinct, but which might at some time have caused deadly epidemics. Today's humans would not have any immunity against such microbes, so could they cause epidemics?

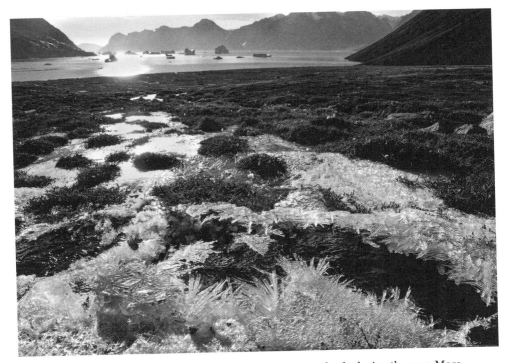

Permafrost – an area where the earth never thaws completely during the year. More than 20 per cent of the northern hemisphere is permafrost. There are now signs of increased thawing of these areas, and this will have various consequences, including for infectious diseases.

Such issues became highly relevant in 2016, when a twelve-year-old boy and more than 2,000 reindeer in Siberia died of anthrax. More than seventy people belonging to a nomadic tribe were hospitalized, and at least seven of them were confirmed to have anthrax. The probable cause was an intense heatwave in Siberia, which had melted a layer of permafrost containing the corpse of a reindeer that had died of anthrax in 1941.[102]

This event naturally commanded considerable interest. From the voodoo traditions on Haiti we know of the belief in zombies, the 'living dead', who return as some kind of monster at the invocation of voodoo priests. Bearing in mind the possible microbic threats of the permafrost, the press then launched the scary concept of 'zombie microbes', which could lead to a 'zombie apocalypse'.[103]

Is there really any evidence that thawed-out microbes from the permafrost are a real threat, apart from the anthrax episode in 2016? The anthrax bacterium is special in that its spores are extremely robust. Would other bacteria be able to survive for long in the permafrost? In 2005 researchers from the US space agency NASA claimed that they had revived a 32,000-year-old bacterium from the permafrost in Alaska. Some researchers admittedly cast doubt on this, and in any case the bacterium was not pathogenic to humans.

When it comes to viruses, there are in fact examples of viruses from the permafrost being revived and still capable of infecting. As yet, however, this has only been shown to apply to certain extremely special-ized viruses that can only infect single-celled organisms, amoebae, not humans.[104] These viruses had been frozen in the Siberian permafrost for 30,000 years. Other viruses still possessing their capabilities after thawing have not yet been detected, but the DNA of both the smallpox virus and the 1918 variant of the influenza virus have been found in the permafrost.

Broadly speaking, then, there is no basis for fearing what some jour-nalists have called a 'zombie apocalypse', but neither can one exclude the possibility that the continued thawing of the permafrost, in addition to other problems, will also involve threats from the world of microbes.

Microbes in Space: A New Threat?

In 1969 the American writer Michael Crichton enjoyed great success with his science-fiction thriller *The Andromeda Strain*, which was later turned into a film. In the book, the earth's population is hit by a pandemic caused by a horrific microbe from outer space. Later thriller writers have also taken up this theme.

Even very serious researchers have been highly interested in the possible existence of microbes in outer space. The best known of these is the English astronomer Fred Hoyle, who, along with his colleague Chandra Wickramasinghe, further developed the old theory of panspermia, which states that space is full of life spread in the form of microscopic life forms by cosmic dust and comets among the galaxies and solar systems. According to Hoyle and Wickramasinghe, life arose on earth not, as is usually assumed, from organic molecules in a 'primordial soup', but from living extraterrestrial organisms that settled on our planet. Since then, the earth has regularly received new contributions of life from outside, which have influenced the further development of life forms, 'topping up' regularly with new genetic material. The two astronomers also believed that some of the life forms from outer space occasionally caused epidemics on earth, including the influenza pandemic.[105]

The panspermia theory has been met with considerable scepticism and sometimes ridiculed, and it is absolutely not in line with the prevailing view of present-day science. Even so, Hoyle, who died in 2001, gained a kind of delayed recognition in 2009 when a bacterium was found in the uppermost stratosphere and named after him: *Janibacter hoylei*. It is also interesting that 33 researchers from serious universities and institutions published in 2018 a highly controversial article in the journal *Progress in Biophysics and Molecular Biology*, in which they list arguments in favour of the panspermia theory.[106] Perhaps Crichton's novel about the Andromeda microbe was more 'science' than 'fiction'.

I nevertheless think that it will require a great deal of evidence to reject the prevailing scientific view of life on earth in general and the origin of microbes in particular. Some researchers admittedly assert that fossil imprints of microorganisms have been found on meteorites – objects from other parts of our own galaxy, including Mars – that have landed on the earth. A research team from NASA believed it had found signs of this in 1996, and Hungarian researchers recently reported similar finds.[107] Microbes from outer space have, however, never been proved beyond doubt. When soil samples from Mars are brought back to earth as part of the Mars expedition now taking place, they will even so be treated with the same caution as, for example, the Ebola virus. The idea of alien microbes cannot be completely excluded.

But even if microbes perhaps do not exist outside our planet, microbes are of importance in space in a different way. For several decades, *Homo sapiens* has regularly travelled beyond the boundaries of the earth as space exploration has increased. Since 2000 the International Space Station (ISS) that orbits the earth has been continuously manned. Wherever humans move, microbes accompany them. Therefore it comes as no surprise that new investigations have shown that the astronauts are not completely alone in the ISS. A large number of species of bacteria and certain types of fungi have recently also been detected there.[108] Some of these bacteria are resistant to certain antibiotics, while some are closely related to bacteria that cause infection in humans, particularly those with a weakened immune system.[109] Why has it caused concern that such microbes have accompanied the astronauts out into space? There are several reasons for this.

First, we do not know for certain how microbes from the earth will behave under completely different conditions in space, where they are no longer influenced by gravity and are exposed to cosmic radiation that can conceivably lead to more mutations. Will the microbes perhaps become more dangerous – more virulent? There are also reasons to assume that they may react somewhat differently to antibiotics in space than on earth.

There is also the question of whether the astronauts themselves will change characteristics and become more vulnerable to microbe attacks in space. They are initially healthy and well trained, and have been carefully selected using medical and other criteria. But we know that medical changes take place in the human body under space conditions, as has been demonstrated by signs of osteoporosis and progressive muscular atrophy. In the context of infection it is extremely interesting that distinct changes alsotake place in the space travellers' immune system. Certain parts of the immune system function less well, other

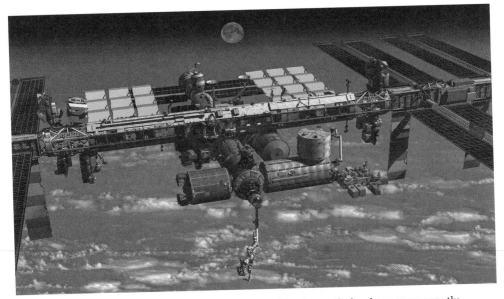

The International Space Station (ISS), which orbits the earth, has been permanently manned since 2000 by six people who live there for periods of up to six months. In the space station a considerable number of microbes have been detected, including antibiotic-resistant bacteria.

parts increase their function above what is normal, and the interaction between the various parts of the immune system is weakened.[110]

It is interesting that several studies have revealed a reduced function in astronauts of the special lymphocyte type NK cells. This type of cell is important both in the defence against viral infections and the combatting of cancer cells in the body. When we get an infection with one of the many types of herpes virus, the virus then remains in the body in an inactive, latent, state. It can later come out of its dormant state, be reactivated and cause new disease. The NK cells play an important role in preventing this. In space travellers we often see signs of such reactivation of the herpes virus, while the function of the NK cells is reduced. At the same time it has been shown that the ability of the NK cells to kill cancer cells is reduced by 50 per cent in astronauts.[111]

The effect on the astronauts' immune systems goes on increasing during their entire six-month period at the ISS.[112] Now lengthy space expeditions are being planned to the Moon and to Mars. An expedition to Mars will take about three years. Before such long expeditions are launched, it is crucial to clarify the importance of the immunological disturbances in the astronauts. Will they have increased problems with infections, perhaps with more virulent microbes that accompany them on their journey? Will these disturbances increase the risk of cancer, which already gives grounds for concern because of the increased radiation load the astronauts are exposed to in space?

At present, a series of measures is being planned to counteract harmful effects on the immune system of astronauts, such as special medicines, selected vaccines and what are assumed to be 'immuno-friendly' diets.[113]

Another concern, which so far is only theoretical, is the future risk that human exploration of space will lead to alien planets becoming polluted with earth microbes that also make the journeys. We do know of bacteria that are so robust that they might be able to survive on alien planets such as Mars, and perhaps further develop in unpredictable ways. 'Before Eden', a thought-provoking short story by one of the world's best-known science-fiction writers, Arthur C. Clarke, describes how bacteria brought from earth by astronauts not only survive on Mars but permanently annihilate the early beginnings of the planet's own life.[114]

All things considered, it is clear that man's exploration of space involves many challenges apart from the purely technological ones on which interest has previously focused. The duel between man and microbes will also continue out in space.

The Never-ending Duel

From the time when our human species, *Homo sapiens*, first appeared on the planet, we have been in extremely intimate contact with the world of microbes. Similarly, each and every one of us encounters microbes from the day of our birth, after normally having lived completely free of them in our mother's womb. The interaction between man and microbes is, for better or worse, very complex, and we are only in the early stages of mapping the importance of microbes for human development and health.

For a long time after the bacteriological revolution, with the discovery that microbes are important causes of disease, it was first and foremost the threat from the world of microbes that dominated people's minds. Until recently the description of our relation to microbes has therefore characterized by military terminology: battle and defence against opponents that exploit every opportunity to attack us and inflict disease and death. This is, of course, one important side of our relation to microbes. Early history, with its countless epidemics and pandemics, well illustrates that microbes can be merciless enemies. To a high degree we still have to protect ourselves from their threats.

It has not been clear until the last few decades that there are other, extremely important sides to man's relation to the world of microbes. Of the great number of microbes that exist, there are actually only very few that cause disease in humans.

One idea that has revolutionized our understanding of man's relation to the world of microbes is the human microbiome. This concept reflects the fact that a great many microbes have entered into an intimate coexistence with each one of us. Immediately after birth, they take up residence in our skin and mucous membranes, where they combine to make up our microbiome. The composition of the microbiome depends on various conditions, including our genes, diet and other factors from the outside world, such as antibiotics. We can see clear differences in the microbiome between different cultures with various lifestyles.

An important reason research within the field of the microbiome has increased so strongly during the last decade is that many findings suggest that changes to the intestinal microbiome are linked to various diseases.[1] With experiments on humans it is not easy to determine whether such changes constitute cause or effect. Much suggests even so that shifts in the composition of the microbiome play a role in the development of disease – among other things, inflammatory diseases of the intestines, autoimmune diseases, gross obesity, diabetes, asthma – and even mental states.

Recent research findings also suggest that the intestinal microbiome plays a role in the effectiveness of vaccines. Antibiotic influencing of the microbiome can actually weaken the desired immune response in the event of vaccination.[2]

Present-day theories about what is called dysbiosis, changes to the microbiome that influence the development of diseases, can in a way be seen as an echo of antique medicine and a modern version of the teaching of Hippocrates and Galen concerning the importance of a balance between body fluids for good health. Experiments are already being carried out in which attempts are made to change the microbiome as part of the treatment of disease. Perhaps the most drastic of these forms of treatment is so-called faecal transplantation, by which attempts are made to alter the patient's microbiome by inserting faeces from a healthy individual.[3] A new and promising way of altering the microbiome for therapeutic purposes is to use small-molecule drugs targeting microbes or microbe–host interactions.[4]

Within other areas as well, research into microbes has provided new inspiration in the treatment of disease, and not only with the discovery of antibiotics. Today, advanced molecular-biological methods make it possible to produce 'smart' bacteria via gene manipulation, so that they can be used for treating diseases. Examples of this are bacteria that, after having been inserted into the intestines, can produce useful medications. A number of such smart bacteria are now being tested on diseases such as diabetes, cancer and infectious diseases.[5] Viruses can also be used in treating cancer, since the injection of special viruses into cancerous tumours can lead to the death of cancer cells.

Microbes still have new secrets to reveal to us. An example of important knowledge we have gained from bacteria is the new CRISPR method, which has revolutionized molecular biology. The popular name for CRISPR is 'gene scissors', since the technique makes it possible to excise sections of DNA molecules in cells and bacteria and thereby 'edit' the genes and change cell characteristics. In nature, CRISPR is really part of the bacteria's own immune system in their defence against viruses. The potential uses of this in modern medicine are many, both in treatment and diagnosis. It was not unexpected when the Nobel Prize in chemistry in 2020 was awarded to Emmanuelle Charpentier and Jennifer Doudna for their research into CRISPR.

All in all, the traditional conception of microbes as being exclusively our enemies is only part of the large, detailed picture of the relationship between the world of microbes and humanity. However, certain microbes do cause disease when the conditions are propitious. And so it will also be in the future. As in former times, *Homo sapiens* will continue to be hit by infectious diseases, sometimes in the form of epidemics or pandemics.

Violent epidemics with deadly microbes that threaten humanity with extinction are a favourite theme of popular films and books. In reality, however, I believe that there is no basis for such pitch-black pessimism and fear of a Ragnarök triggered by microbes. Earlier pandemics naturally created enormous problems for the societies of the time. Even though today's world is more vulnerable to widespread epidemics in several ways, we are nevertheless better equipped to deal with threats from the world of microbes. Our knowledge of microbes has vastly increased since the bacteriological revolution at the end of the nineteenth century, and this has led to an impressive development in medical technology that has laid the foundation for major advances in the diagnostics, treatment and prevention of infectious diseases. This was demonstrated when tackling the epidemics of the SARS, Ebola, MERS and SARS-CoV-2 viruses. It took only a short time to identify the SARS and MERS viruses after they appeared on the scene, and in record time – a few weeks – the full structure of the SARS-CoV-2 virus was reported and diagnostic tests for the virus were developed. In a few months effective vaccines were developed.

Today we also know a great deal more than Koch and Pasteur and their immediate successors did about the ecological and environmental factors that are so important in the duel between man and microbes. Pasteur admittedly once said that, 'The microbe is nothing, the terrain is everything,' but he was probably thinking only of conditions within the individual patient. It was not until experience was gained from the EIDS, the many new infectious diseases that appeared in the second half of the twentieth century, that we acquired a deeper insight into the significance of the environment and ecology for human infectious diseases. An important part of this insight is the unpleasant but important recognition of the fact that it is human behaviour and the human impact on nature that very often play a decisive role – especially now, in the Anthropocene age. This knowledge is vital if one is to understand and, particularly, prevent new epidemics and pandemics.

It is realistic to hope that certain pathogenic microbes can be eradicated from our planet. This occurred with the smallpox virus after intensive efforts. Nor is it utopian to believe that it is possible to eradicate the polio and measles viruses. But, as far as the great majority of microbes that threaten us are concerned, eradication is not an option, first and foremost because these infections are zoonoses and always have an animal reservoir that it is unrealistic to think we can eliminate.

An optimistic view of our future with regard to infectious diseases, one for which there is a certain basis in my opinion, rests on particular assumptions. Our knowledge and our advanced medical technology will be of little use in combatting the threat from microbes if our societies are not reasonably well organized. There are numerous examples of lasting social and political unrest leading to dysfunctional societies where the quality of healthcare on offer is greatly impaired. This can have serious consequences for the fighting of infections in such countries, and it can also take place in formerly well-organized societies where the healthcare was originally at a high level.

The quality of the health service in poor countries has not approached that of Western countries. This results not only in a permanent and considerable infection load for the local population but a global threat, since the majority of the new infections and epidemics are expected to start in these parts of the world. This is where the hotspots are, the possible epicentres of new epidemics. Part of our common global defence against infection is to raise the quality of health services in poor countries, which will be a formidable assignment.

Another important precondition is well-organized, international cooperation within the field of infection. In today's globalized world – 'the global village' – nations must cooperate closely in combatting epidemics and pandemics. Experience of the most recent epidemics shows that further improvements are necessary here. No matter what one believes about globalization in other areas, the fighting of infection must be a global responsibility. The microbes themselves started the process of globalization thousands of years ago.

In the never-ending duel with *Homo sapiens*, microbes are undoubtedly dangerous opponents. Only quite recently has humanity really been on the offensive. This is mainly due to our having a crucial advantage that has ensured the survival of the species – our brain capacity. That is why I do not think we will buckle in the duel, which is sure to continue. Even so, we must face the fact that we will also meet serious infection problems in the future – epidemics and pandemics – which will place great strain on even well-prepared societies. The COVID-19 pandemic will not be the last. In the event of such crises, we must still expect there to be both serious medical consequences with considerable sickness and mortality, and huge material costs. But the consequences of such disasters will be far worse and more costly if we do not invest in plans for prevention and offensive action. If we fail to do this, the doomsday prophecies of the destruction of humanity by frightful pandemics will likely be proved correct.

At some point in time *Homo sapiens* will probably disappear from the planet. It may be that our species, like other animals through history, will become extinct, or that our descendants emigrate to extraterrestrial destinations, possibly because we ourselves have made the planet impossible to live on. One thing, however, is certain. When the last member of the human race disappears from our planet, microbes will still be here. The duel with humans on the earth, which has lasted some hundreds of thousands of years, will only be a brief interlude in the history of microbes, which has lasted for billions.

REFERENCES

Prologue: The Invisible Enemy

1 C. Renfrew, *Prehistory: The Making of the Human Mind* (London, 2007).
2 C. J. Bae, K. Douka and M. D. Petraglia, 'On the Origin of Modern Humans: Asian Perspectives', *Science*, 358 (8 December 2017).
3 M. N. Cohen and G. Crane-Kramer, 'The State and Future of Paleoepidemiology', in *Emerging Pathogens: Archaeology, Ecology and Evolution of Infectious Disease*, ed. C. Greenblatt and M. Spigelman (Oxford, 2003), pp. 79–81.

ONE The Duellists

1 R. Porter, *The Greatest Benefit to Mankind: A Medical History of Humanity from Antiquity to the Present* (London, 1999); C.-E. A. Winslow, *The Conquest of Epidemic Disease: A Chapter in the History of Ideas* (Madison, WI, 1980).
2 M. Karamanou et al., 'From Miasmas to Germs: A Historical Approach to Theories of Infectious Disease Transmission', *Infezioni in Medicina*, 20 (2012), pp. 58–62; J. Botero, *Mesopotamia: Writing, Reasoning and the Gods* (Chicago, IL, 1992).
3 W. H. McNeill, *Plagues and Peoples* (New York, 1976).
4 Karamanou et al., 'From Miasmas to Germs'.
5 V. Nutton, *Ancient Medicine* (London, 2004).
6 Homer, *The Iliad*, trans. Robert Fagles (London, 1996).
7 J. Jouanna, *Hippocrates* (Baltimore, MD, 1999).
8 I. Reichborn-Kjennerud, 'Vår eldste medisin til middelalderens slutt', in *Medisinens historie i Norge*, ed. I. Reichborn-Kjennerud, F. Grøn and I. Kobro (Oslo, 1936), pp. 1–97.
9 Porter, *The Greatest Benefit to Mankind*; Nutton, *Ancient Medicine*.
10 G.E.R. Lloyd, ed., 'Medicine', in *Hippocratic Writings*, trans. J. Chadwick and W. N. Mann, rev. edn (Harmondsworth, 1983).
11 Jouanna, *Hippocrates*.
12 S. P. Mattern, *The Prince of Medicine: Galen in the Roman Empire* (Oxford, 2013).
13 Thucydides, *The Peloponnesian War*, trans. Martin Hammond (Oxford, 2009).
14 Porter, *The Greatest Benefit to Mankind*.
15 M. M. Hudson and R. S. Morton, 'Fracastoro and Syphilis: 500 Years On', *The Lancet*, 348 (30 November 1996), pp. 1495–6.

16 V. Nutton, 'The Seeds of Disease: An Explanation of Contagion and Infection from the Greeks to the Renaissance', *Medical History*, 27 (1983), pp. 1–34.

17 V. Nutton, 'The Reception of Fracastoro's Theory of Contagion: The Seed that Fell among Thorns?', *Osiris*, 2nd ser., 6 (1990), pp. 196–234.

18 Porter, *The Greatest Benefit to Mankind*; R. P. Gaynes, *Germ Theory: Medical Pioneers in Infectious Diseases* (Washington, DC, 2011).

19 E. H. Ackerknecht, 'Anticontagionism between 1821 and 1867', *International Journal of Epidemiology*, 38 (February 2009), pp. 7–21.

20 Porter, *The Greatest Benefit to Mankind*; Karamanou et al., 'From Miasmas to Germs'.

21 Gaynes, *Germ Theory*.

22 Ackerknecht, 'Anticontagionism between 1821 and 1867'.

23 Porter, *The Greatest Benefit to Mankind*; Winslow, *The Conquest of Epidemic Disease*.

24 Gaynes, *Germ Theory*; Porter, *The Greatest Benefit to Mankind*.

25 J. Waller, *The Discovery of the Germ: Twenty Years that Transformed the Way We Think about Disease* (New York, 2002).

26 L. M. Irgens, 'Oppdagelsen av leprabasillen', *Tidsskriftet den Norske Legeforening*, 122 (2002), pp. 708–9.

27 B. Godøy, *Ti tusen skygger: en historie om Norge og de spedalske* (Oslo, 2014).

28 G. L. Geison, *The Private Science of Louis Pasteur* (Princeton, NJ, 1995); Gaynes, *Germ Theory*.

29 Ibid.

30 Ibid.

31 S. M. Blevins and M. S. Bronze, 'Robert Koch and the "Golden Age" of Bacteriology', *International Journal of Infectious Diseases*, 14 (September 2010), e744–51; Gaynes, *Germ Theory*.

32 C. Gradmann, *Laboratory Disease* (Baltimore, MD, 2009).

33 Waller, *The Discovery of the Germ*; Gradmann, *Laboratory Disease*.

34 Gaynes, *Germ Theory*; Waller, *The Discovery of the Germ*.

35 A. Morabia, 'Epidemiologic Interactions, Complexity, and the Lonesome Death of Max von Pettenkofer', *American Journal of Epidemiology*, 166 (2007), pp. 1233–8; Winslow, *The Conquest of Epidemic Disease*.

36 Gaynes, *Germ Theory*; Gradmann, *Laboratory Disease*.

37 Blevins and Bronze, 'Robert Koch and the "Golden Age" of Bacteriology'.

38 Waller, *The Discovery of the Germ*; Gaynes, *Germ Theory*.

39 B. Latour, *The Pasteurization of France* (Cambridge, MA, 1988).

40 N. P. Money, *Microbiology: A Very Short Introduction* (Oxford, 2014).

41 A. H. Knoll and M. A. Nowak, 'The Timetable of Evolution', *Science Advances*, 3 (2017), e1603076.

42 Money, *Microbiology: A Very Short Introduction*.

43 Ibid.

44 C. Zimmer, *A Planet of Viruses* (Chicago, IL, and London, 2011); Money, *Microbiology: A Very Short Introduction*.

45 J. Playfair and G. Bancroft, *Infection and Immunity*, 2nd edn (Oxford, 2004).

46 Ibid.

47 D. M. Dixon et al., 'Fungal Infections: A Growing Threat', *Public Health Reports*, 111 (1996), pp. 226–35.

48 Playfair and Bancroft, *Infection and Immunity*.

49 K. S. Maclea, 'What Makes A Prion: Infectious Proteins from Animals to Yeast', *International Review of Cell and Molecular Biology*, 329 (2016), pp. 227–76.

50 Money, *Microbiology: A Very Short Introduction*.

51 J. A. Gilbert et al., 'Current Understanding of the Human Microbiome', *Nature Medicine*, 24 (2018), pp. 392–400; V. B. Young, 'The Role of the Microbiome in Human Health and Disease: An Introduction for Clinicians', *British Medical Journal*, 356 (2017), J831.

52 R. L. Brown and T. B. Clarke, 'The Regulation of Host Defences by the Microbiota', *Immunology*, 150 (2016), pp. 1–6.

53 B. O. Schroeder and F. Bäckhed, 'Signals from the Gut Microbiota to Distant Organs in Physiology and Disease', *Nature Medicine*, 22 (2016), pp. 1079–89.

54 M. L. Wayne and B. M. Bolker, *Infectious Disease: A Very Short Introduction* (Oxford, 2015).

55 N. D. Wolfe et al., 'Origins of Major Human Infectious Diseases', *Nature*, 447 (2007), pp. 279–83.

56 Wayne and Bolker, *Infectious Disease: A Very Short Introduction*.

57 A. M. Silverstein, *A History of Immunology*, 2nd edn (London, 2009).

58 Playfair and Bancroft, *Infection and Immunity*.

59 S. S. Frøland and J. B. Natvig, 'Identification of Three Different Human Lymphocyte Populations by Surface Markers', *Immunological Reviews*, 16 (1973), pp. 3–217.

60 Playfair and Bancroft, *Infection and Immunity*.

61 A. Casadevall and L.-A. Pirofski, 'Benefits and Costs of Animal Virulence for Microbes', *mBio* (2019), e00863–19.

62 Wayne and Bolker, *Infectious Disease: A Very Short Introduction*.

63 Playfair and Bancroft, *Infection and Immunity*.

64 D. D. Richman, ed., *Human Immunodeficiency Virus* (London, 2003).

65 Playfair and Bancroft, *Infection and Immunity*.

66 Ibid.

67 Ibid.

68 P. W. Ewald, *Evolution of Infectious Disease* (Oxford, 1994); Wayne and Bolker, *Infectious Disease: A Very Short Introduction*.

69 Jouanna, *Hippocrates*; Nutton, 'The Seeds of Disease'.

70 Gradmann, *Laboratory Disease*.

71 J.-L. Casanova, 'Human Genetic Basis of Interindividual Variability in the Course of Infection', *Proceedings of the National Academy of Sciences*, 112 (2014), e7118–e71; E. K. Karlsson et al., 'Natural Selection and Infectious Disease in Human Populations', *Nature Reviews Genetics*, 15 (2014), pp. 379–93.

72 S. J. Chapman and A.V.S. Hill, 'Human Genetic Susceptibility to Infectious Disease', *Nature Reviews Genetics*, 13 (2012), pp. 175–88; Karlsson et al., 'Natural Selection and Infectious Disease in Human Populations'.

73 I. C. Withrock et al., 'Genetic Disease Conferring Resistance to Infectious Diseases', *Genes and Diseases*, 2 (2015), pp. 247–54.

74 Ibid.

75 Karlsson et al., 'Natural Selection and Infectious Disease in Human Populations'.

TWO **The Third Factor: Ecology and the Environment**

1 W. H. McNeill, *Plagues and Peoples* (New York, 1976).

2 Y. Hui-Yuan et al., 'Early Evidence for Travel with Infectious Diseases along the Silk Road: Intestinal Parasites from 2000-year-old Personal Hygiene Sticks in a Latrine at Xuanquanzhi Relay Station in China', *Journal of Archaeological Science: Reports*, 9 (2016), pp. 758–64; P. Frankopan, *The Silk Roads: A New History of the World* (London, 2015).

3 S. W. Lacey, 'Cholera: Calamitous Past, Ominous Future', *Clinical Infectious Diseases*, 20 (1995), pp. 1409–19.

4 M. E. Wilson, 'Ecological Disturbances and Emerging Infections: Travel, Dams, Shipment of Goods, and Vectors', in *Emerging Neurological Infections*, ed. C. Power and R. T. Johnson (Boca Raton, FL, 2005), pp. 35–57.

5 Ibid.

6 D. Otranto et al., 'Zoonotic Parasites of Sheltered and Stray Dogs in the Era of the Global Economic and Political Crisis', *Trends in Parasitology*, 33 (2017), pp. 813–25.

7 D. Steverding, 'The Spreading of Parasites by Human Migratory Activities', *Virulence*, 11 (2020), pp. 1177–91.

8 C. S. Bryan et al., 'Yellow Fever in the Americas', *Infectious Disease Clinics of North America*, 18 (2004), pp. 275–92.

9 A. Cliff and P. Haggett, 'Time, Travel and Infection', *British Medical Bulletin*, 69 (2004), pp. 87–99; A. J. Tatem, D. J. Rogers and S. I. Hay, 'Global Transport Networks and Infectious Disease Spread', *Advances in Parasitology*, 62 (2006), pp. 293–343.

10 A. Salmon-Rousseau et al., 'Hajj-associated Infections', *Médecine et Maladies Infectieuses*, 46 (2016), pp. 346–54.

11 M. S. Khan et al., 'Pathogens, Prejudice, and Politics: The Role of the Global Health Community in the European Refugee Crisis', *Lancet Infectious Diseases*, 16 (2016), e173–7.

12 Wilson, 'Ecological Disturbances and Emerging Infections'.

13 Ibid.

14 K. E. Jones et al., 'Global Trends in Emerging Infectious Diseases', *Nature*, 451 (2008), pp. 990–93.

15 H. Kruse, A.-M. Kirkemo and K. Handeland, 'Wildlife as Source of Zoonotic Infections', *Emerging Infectious Diseases*, 10 (2004), pp. 2067–72.

16 N. D. Wolfe, C. P. Dunavan and J. Diamond, 'Origins of Major Human Infectious Diseases', *Nature*, 447 (2007), pp. 279–83.

17 Ibid.

18 E. Dunay et al., 'Pathogen Transmission from Humans to Great Apes Is a Growing Threat to Primate Conservation', *Ecohealth*, 15 (2018), pp. 148–62.

19   A. J. McMichael, 'Environmental and Social Influences on Emerging
      Infectious Diseases: Past, Present and Future', *Philosophical Transactions
      of the Royal Society of London: Biological Sciences*, 359 (2004), pp. 1049–58.
20   K. M. Johnson, 'Emerging Viruses in Context: An Overview of Viral
      Hemorrhagic Fevers', in *Emerging Viruses*, ed. S. S. Morse (Oxford, 1993),
      pp. 46–7.
21   Wilson, 'Ecological Disturbances and Emerging Infections'.
22   Jones et al., 'Global Trends in Emerging Infectious Diseases'.
23   B. Roizman, ed., *Infectious Diseases in an Age of Change* (Washington,
      DC, 1995).
24   R. Porter, *The Greatest Benefit to Mankind: A Medical History of Humanity
      from Antiquity to the Present* (London, 1999); M. N. Cohen, *Health and
      the Rise of Civilization* (New Haven, CT, 1989).
25   P. W. Ewald, *Evolution of Infectious Disease* (Oxford, 1994).
26   S. P. Mattern, *The Prince of Medicine: Galen in the Roman Empire*
      (Oxford, 2013); M. Beard, SPQR: *A History of Ancient Rome* (London, 2015).
27   Roizman, ed., *Infectious Diseases in an Age of Change*.
28   McNeill, *Plagues and Peoples*.
29   D. L. Church, 'Major Factors Affecting the Emergence and Re-emergence
      of Infectious Diseases', *Clinics in Laboratory Medicine*, 24 (2004),
      pp. 559–86.
30   M. R. Smallman-Raynor and A. D. Cliff, 'Impact of Infectious Diseases on
      War', *Infectious Disease Clinics of North America*, 18 (2004), pp. 341–68.
31   A. Roberts, *Napoleon the Great* (London, 2015).
32   Smallman-Raynor and Cliff, 'Impact of Infectious Diseases on War'.
33   J. S. Sartin, 'Infectious Diseases during the Civil War: The Triumph
      of the "Third Army"', *Clinical Infectious Diseases*, 16 (1993), pp. 580–84.
34   Smallman-Raynor and Cliff, 'Impact of Infectious Diseases on War'.
35   Ibid.
36   Ibid.
37   A. T. Price-Smith, *Contagion and Chaos* (Cambridge, MA, 2009).
38   C. P. Dodge, 'Health Implications of War in Uganda and Sudan', *Social
      Science and Medicine*, 31 (1990), pp. 691–8.
39   S. L. Sharara and S. S. Kanj, 'War and Infectious Diseases: Challenges
      of the Syrian War', *PLoS Pathogens*, 10 (2014), e1004438.
40   McMichael, 'Environmental and Social Influences'; Church, 'Major
      Factors Affecting the Emergence and Re-emergence'.
41   Wilson, 'Ecological Disturbances and Emerging Infections'.
42   R. Rubin, 'Why Are Legionnaires Disease Diagnoses Becoming More
      Common in the United States?', *Journal of the American Medical
      Association*, 319 (2018), pp. 1753–4; B. A. Cunha et al., 'Legionnaires'
      Disease', *The Lancet*, 387 (2016), pp. 376–85.
43   S. S. Morse, 'Factors in the Emergence of Infectious Diseases', *Emerging
      Infectious Diseases*, 1 (1995), pp. 7–15.
44   Xiaoxu Wu et al., 'Impact of Climate Change on Human Infectious
      Diseases: Empirical Evidence and Human Adaptation', *Environment
      International*, 86 (2016), pp. 14–23; P. R. Epstein, 'Climate and Emerging
      Infectious Diseases', *Microbes and Infection*, 3 (2001), pp. 747–54.

45 Wu et al., 'Impact of Climate Change on Human Infectious Diseases'.

46 K. L. Gage et al., 'Climate and Vectorborne Diseases', *American Journal of Preventive Medicine*, 35 (2008), pp. 436–50.

47 A. J. McMichael, 'Insights from Past Millennia into Climatic Impacts on Human Health and Survival', *Proceedings of the National Academy of Sciences*, 109 (2012), pp. 4730–37.

48 Wu et al., 'Impact of Climate Change on Human Infectious Diseases'; A. J. McMichael, 'Extreme Weather Events and Infectious Disease Outbreaks', *Virulence*, 6 (2015), pp. 543–7.

49 Epstein, 'Climate and Emerging Infectious Diseases'; Wu et al., 'Impact of Climate Change on Human Infectious Diseases'.

50 A. Cheepsattayakorn and R. Cheepsattayakorn, 'Climate Changes and Human Infectious Diseases', EC *Microbiology*, XIV/6 (2018), pp. 299–311.

51 R. Monastersky, 'The Human Age', *Nature*, 519 (2015), pp. 144–7.

52 M. Subramanian, 'Anthopocene Now: Influential Panel Votes to Recognize Earth's New Epoch', *Nature*, 21 May 2019, www.nature.com.

THREE A Bird's-eye View of the History of Human Infection

1 R. Barrett and G. J. Armelagos, *An Unnatural History of Emerging Infections* (Oxford, 2013); M. N. Cohen, *Health and the Rise of Civilization* (New Haven, CT, 1989).

2 Barrett and Armelagos, *An Unnatural History of Emerging Infections*; Cohen, *Health and the Rise of Civilization*.

3 T. A. Cockburn, 'Infectious Disease in Ancient Populations', *Current Anthropology*, 12 (1971), pp. 45–62.

4 Barrett and Armelagos, *An Unnatural History of Emerging Infections*; Cohen, *Health and the Rise of Civilization*.

5 J. Diamond, *Guns, Germs, and Steel: The Fates of Human Societies* (New York, 1999); Barrett and Armelagos, *An Unnatural History of Emerging Infections*.

6 Cohen, *Health and the Rise of Civilization*; Barrett and Armelagos, *An Unnatural History of Emerging Infections*.

7 Cohen, *Health and the Rise of Civilization*.

8 Barrett and Armelagos, *An Unnatural History of Emerging Infections*; Cohen, *Health and the Rise of Civilization*.

9 N. D. Wolfe, C. P. Dunavan and J. Diamond, 'Origins of Major Human Infectious Diseases', *Nature*, 447 (2007), pp. 279–83.

10 R. J. Kim-Farley, 'Measles', in *The Cambridge Historical Dictionary of Disease*, ed. K. F. Kiple (Cambridge, 2003), pp. 211–14.

11 I. Glynn and J. Glynn, *The Life and Death of Smallpox* (London, 2004).

12 Diamond, *Guns, Germs, and Steel*.

13 W. H. McNeill, *Plagues and Peoples* (New York, 1976).

14 R. S. Bray, *Armies of Pestilence: The Impact of Disease on History* (Cambridge, 1996); McNeill, *Plagues and Peoples*.

15 Cockburn, 'Infectious Disease in Ancient Populations'.

16 R. Acuna-Soto, 'Megadrought and Megadeath in 16th Century Mexico', *Emerging Infectious Diseases*, 8 (2002), pp. 360–62.

17 Å. J. Vågene et al., 'Salmonella Enterica Genomes from Victims of a Major Sixteenth-century Epidemic in Mexico', Nature Ecology and Evolution, 2 (2018), pp. 520–28.

18 Barrett and Armelagos, An Unnatural History of Emerging Infections; Cohen, Health and the Rise of Civilization.

19 T. McKeown, The Role of Medicine: Dream, Mirage or Nemesis? (Oxford, 1979).

20 F. M. Snowden, 'Emerging and Reemerging Diseases: A Historical Perspective', Immunological Reviews, 225 (2008), pp. 9–26.

21 R. Monastersky, 'The Human Age', Nature, 519 (2015), pp. 144–7; M. Subramanian, 'Anthopocene Now: Influential Panel Votes to Recognize Earth's New Epoch', Nature, 21 May 2019, www.nature.com.

22 A. Cliff and P. Haggett, 'Time, Travel and Infection', British Medical Bulletin, 69 (2004), pp. 87–99.

23 L. Budd, M. Bell and T. Brown, 'Of Plagues, Planes and Politics: Controlling the Global Spread of Infectious Diseases by Air', Political Geography, 28 (2009), pp. 426–35.

24 S. S. Morse, 'Factors in the Emergence of Infectious Diseases', Emerging Infectious Diseases, 1 (1995), pp. 7–15.

FOUR **Major Epidemics and Pandemics: Examples from History**

1 Thucydides, The Peloponnesian War, trans. Martin Hammond (Oxford, 2009).

2 O. Dutour, 'Archaeology of Human Pathogens: Palaeopathological Appraisal of Palaeoepidemiology', in Palaeomicrobiology: Past Human Infections, ed. D. Raoult and M. Drancourt (Berlin and Heidelberg, 2008), pp. 125–44.

3 M. N. Cohen, Health and the Rise of Civilization (New Haven, CT, 1989); Dutour, 'Archaeology of Human Pathogens'.

4 M. Drancourt and D. Raoult, 'Molecular Detection of Past Infections', in Palaeomicrobiology: Past Human Infections, ed. Raoult and Drancourt, pp. 55–68.

5 P. Ziegler, The Black Death (London, 1997).

6 P. Slack, Plague: A Very Short Introduction (Oxford, 2012).

7 B. P. Zietz and H. Dunkelberg, 'The History of the Plague and the Research on the Causative Agent Yersinia pestis', International Journal of Environmental Health, 207 (2004), pp. 165–78.

8 Slack, Plague: A Very Short Introduction.

9 W. Rosen, Justinian's Flea: Plague, Empire and the Birth of Europe (London, 2008).

10 Procopius, The Secret History, trans. G. A. Williamson (London, 1990).

11 Rosen, Justinian's Flea; L. K. Little, ed., Plague and the End of Antiquity: The Pandemic of 541–750 (Cambridge, 2007).

12 Procopius, The Secret History; Little, ed., Plague and the End of Antiquity.

13 Ibid.

14 Zietz and Dunkelberg, 'The History of the Plague'.

15 Little, ed., Plague and the End of Antiquity.

16 Procopius, *The Secret History*.

17 Rosen, *Justinian's Flea*; Little, ed., *Plague and the End of Antiquity*.

18 L. Mordechai et al., 'The Justinianic Plague: An Inconsequential Pandemic?', *Proceedings of the National Academy of Sciences*, 2 December 2019, DOI:10.1073/Pnas.190.

19 M. Meier, 'The "Justinian Plague": The Economic Consequences of the Pandemic in the Eastern Roman Empire and its Cultural and Religious Effects', *Early Medieval Europe*, 24 (2016), pp. 267–92; Little, ed., *Plague and the End of Antiquity*.

20 Ibid.

21 O. J. Benedictow, *The Black Death, 1346–1353: The Complete History* (Woodbridge, 2004); Ziegler, *The Black Death*.

22 Slack, *Plague: A Very Short Introduction*.

23 Benedictow, *The Black Death, 1346–1353*.

24 Ziegler, *The Black Death*.

25 Benedictow, *The Black Death, 1346–1353*.

26 G. Boccaccio, *The Decameron*, vol. I, trans. Richard Aldington (London, 1972).

27 Ziegler, *The Black Death*.

28 Ibid.

29 Boccaccio, *The Decameron*, vol. I.

30 F. F. Cartwright, *Disease and History* (New York, 1972); Ziegler, *The Black Death*.

31 Ibid.

32 Ibid.

33 Slack, *Plague: A Very Short Introduction*; Cartwright, *Disease and History*; Ziegler, *The Black Death*.

34 Ziegler, *The Black Death*; Cartwright, *Disease and History*.

35 Ziegler, *The Black Death*; Cartwright, *Disease and History*.

36 D. Defoe, *A Journal of the Plague Year* (London, 2003).

37 Slack, *Plague: A Very Short Introduction*.

38 J. N. Hays, *Epidemics and Pandemics: Their Impacts on Human History* (Santa Barbara, CA, 2005); Zietz and Dunkelberg, 'The History of the Plague'.

39 L. Walløe, 'Medieval and Modern Bubonic Plague: Some Clinical Continuities', *Medical History Supplement*, 27 (2008), pp. 59–73.

40 I. W. Sherman, *The Power of Plagues* (Washington, DC, 2006).

41 Zietz and Dunkelberg, 'The History of the Plague'.

42 Hays, *Epidemics and Pandemics*.

43 Zietz and Dunkelberg, 'The History of the Plague'.

44 A. W. Bacot and C. J. Martin, 'Observations on the Mechanism of the Transmission of Plague by Fleas', *Journal of Hygiene*, XIII (Plague Suppl. III) (1914), pp. 423–39.

45 Hays, *Epidemics and Pandemics*; Zietz and Dunkelberg, 'The History of the Plague'.

46 B. Bramanti et al., 'Plague: A Disease Which Changed the Path of Human Civilization', in *Yersinia pestis: Retrospective and Perspective*, ed. R Yang and A. Anisimov (Dordrecht, 2016), pp. 1–26.

47 S. Ayyadurai et al., 'Long-term Persistence of Virulent *Yersinia pestis* in Soil', *Microbiology*. 154 (2008), pp. 2865–71.

48 Bramanti et al., 'Plague: A Disease Which Changed the Path of Human Civilization'.

49 R. E. Lerner, 'Fleas: Some Scratchy Issues Concerning the Black Death', *Journal of the Historical Society*, 8 (2008), pp. 205–28; Walløe, 'Medieval and Modern Bubonic Plague'.

50 M. Drancourt and D. Raoult, 'Molecular History of Plague', *Clinical Microbiology and Infection*, 22 (2016), pp. 911–15; M. Harbeck et al., '*Yersinia pestis* DNA from Skeletal Remains from the 6th Century AD Reveals Insights into Justinianic Plague', *PLoS Pathogens*, 9 (2013), e1003349; D. M. Wagner et al., '*Yersinia pestis* and the Plague of Justinian 541–543 AD: A Genomic Analysis', *Lancet Infectious Diseases*, 14 (2014), pp. 319–25.

51 Walløe, 'Medieval and Modern Bubonic Plague'; Bramanti et al., 'Plague: A Disease Which Changed the Path of Human Civilization'.

52 K. R. Dean et al., 'Human Ectoparasites and the Spread of Plague in Europe during the Second Pandemic', *Proceedings of the National Academy of Sciences*, 115 (2018), pp. 1304–9.

53 A. K. Hufthammer and L. Walløe, 'Rats Cannot Have Been Intermediate Hosts for *Yersinia pestis* during the Medieval Plague Epidemics in Northern Europe', *Journal of Archaeological Science*, 40 (2013), pp. 1752–9.

54 O. J. Benedictow, *What Disease Was Plague? On the Controversy over the Microbiological Identity of Plague Epidemics of the Past* (Leiden and Boston, MA, 2010).

55 N. C. Stenseth et al., 'Plague Dynamics Are Driven by Climate Variation', 203 (2011), pp. 13110–15.

56 B. V. Schmid et al., 'Climate-driven Introduction of the Black Death and Successive Plague Reintroductions into Europe', *Proceedings of the National Academy of Sciences*, 112 (2015), pp. 3020–25.

57 M. A. Spyrou et al., 'Analysis of 3800-year-old *Yersinia pestis* Genomes Suggests Bronze Age Origin for Bubonic Plague', *Nature Communications*, 9 (2018); S. Rasmussen et al., 'Early Divergent Strains of *Yersinia pestis* in Eurasia 5000 Years Ago', *Cell*, 163 (2015), pp. 571–82.

58 C. E. Demeure et al., '*Yersinia pestis* and Plague: An Updated Version on Evolution, Virulence Determinants, Immune Subversion, Vaccination, and Diagnostics', *Genes and Immunity*, 20 (2019), pp. 357–70.

59 Spyrou et al., 'Analysis of 3800-year-old *Yersinia pestis* Genomes'.

60 Rasmussen et al., 'Early Divergent Strains of *Yersinia pestis*'.

61 N. Barquet and P. Domingo, 'Smallpox: The Triumph over the Most Terrible of the Ministers of Death', *Annals of Internal Medicine*, 127 (1997), pp. 635–42.

62 D. R. Hopkins, *Princes and Peasants: Smallpox in History* (Chicago, IL, 1983).

63 Z. S. Moore et al., 'Smallpox', *The Lancet*, 367 (2006), pp. 425–35; A. M. Geddes, 'The History of Smallpox', *Clinics in Dermatology*, 24 (2006), pp. 152–7.

64 Moore et al., 'Smallpox'.

65 Hopkins, *Princes and Peasants.*
66 Geddes, 'The History of Smallpox'.
67 Moore et al., 'Smallpox'.
68 I. Glynn and J. Glynn, *The Life and Death of Smallpox* (London, 2004).
69 Hopkins, *Princes and Peasants.*
70 Geddes, 'The History of Smallpox'.
71 I. V. Babkin and I. N. Babkina, 'The Origin of the Variola Virus', *Viruses*, 7 (2015), pp. 1100–112.
72 W. H. McNeill, *Plagues and Peoples* (New York, 1976).
73 Hopkins, *Princes and Peasants.*
74 Ibid.
75 I. Reichborn-Kjennerud, 'Vår eldste medisin til middelalderens slutt', in *Medisinens historie i Norge*, ed. I. Reichborn-Kjennerud, F. Grøn and I. Kobro (Oslo, 1936), pp. 1–97.
76 McNeill, *Plagues and Peoples*; P. D. Curtin, 'Disease Exchange across the Tropical Atlantic', *History and Philosophy of the Life Sciences*, 15 (1993), pp. 329–56.
77 McNeill, *Plagues and Peoples*; R. S. Bray, *Armies of Pestilence: The Impact of Disease on History* (Cambridge, 1996); Hopkins, *Princes and Peasants.*
78 McNeill, *Plagues and Peoples.*
79 Bray, *Armies of Pestilence*; Hopkins, *Princes and Peasants.*
80 Ibid.
81 Ibid.
82 Bray, *Armies of Pestilence*; Hopkins, *Princes and Peasants.*
83 Ibid.
84 Hays, *Epidemics and Pandemics*; Bray, *Armies of Pestilence.*
85 J. O. Wertheim, 'Viral Evolution: Mummy Virus Challenges Presumed History of Smallpox', *Current Biology*, 27 (2017), pp. R103–R122.
86 A. M. Behbehani, 'The Smallpox Story: Life and Death of an Old Disease', *Microbiology Reviews*, 4 (1983), pp. 455–509.
87 Hopkins, *Princes and Peasants.*
88 Reichborn-Kjennerud, 'Vår eldste medisin til middelalderens slutt'.
89 Hopkins, *Princes and Peasants.*
90 B. A. Cunha, 'Smallpox and Measles: Historical Aspects and Clinical Differentiation', *Infectious Disease Clinics of North America*, 18 (2004), pp. 79–100.
91 Hopkins, *Princes and Peasants.*
92 Ibid.
93 Behbehani, 'The Smallpox Story'.
94 D. Raoult, T. Woodward and S. Dumler, 'The History of Epidemic Typhus', *Infectious Disease Clinics of North America*, 18 (2004), pp. 127–40.
95 Sherman, *The Power of Plagues.*
96 H. Zinsser, *Rats, Lice and History* (Boston, MA, 1934); Raoult, Woodward and Dumler, 'The History of Epidemic Typhus'.
97 Zinsser, *Rats, Lice and History.*
98 Raoult, Woodward and Dumler, 'The History of Epidemic Typhus'.
99 A. Zamoyski, *1812: Napoleon's Fatal March on Moscow* (London, 2004).
100 Bray, *Armies of Pestilence*; Sherman, *The Power of Plagues.*

101 Zamoyski, *1812: Napoleon's Fatal March on Moscow*.
102 D. Raoult et al., 'Evidence for Louse-transmitted Diseases in Soldiers of Napoleon's Grand Army in Vilnius', *Journal of Infectious Diseases*, 193 (2006), pp. 112–20.
103 Bray, *Armies of Pestilence*.
104 Sherman, *The Power of Plagues*.
105 Zinsser, *Rats, Lice and History*.
106 Bray, *Armies of Pestilence*; Hays, *Epidemics and Pandemics*.
107 Ibid.
108 Zinsser, *Rats, Lice and History*; Bray, *Armies of Pestilence*.
109 Raoult, Woodward and Dumler, 'The History of Epidemic Typhus'.
110 R. J. Lifton, *The Nazi Doctors: Medical Killing and the Psychology of Genocide* (New York, 1986).
111 Sherman, *The Power of Plagues*.
112 Ibid.
113 Raoult, Woodward and Dumler, 'The History of Epidemic Typhus'.
114 Zinsser, *Rats, Lice and History*; Raoult, Woodward and Dumler, 'The History of Epidemic Typhus'.
115 Sherman, *The Power of Plagues*; Zinsser, *Rats, Lice and History*.
116 Sherman, *The Power of Plagues*.
117 Y. Bechah et al., 'Epidemic Typhus, *Lancet Infectious Diseases*, 8 (2008), pp. 417–26; Raoult, Woodward and Dumler, 'The History of Epidemic Typhus'.
118 C. Somboonwit et al., 'Current Views and Challenges on Clinical Cholera', *Bioinformation*, 13 (2017), pp. 405–9.
119 D. A. Sack et al., 'Cholera', *The Lancet*, 363 (2004), pp. 223–33.
120 R. R. Colwell, 'Global Climate and Infectious Disease: The Cholera Paradigm', *Science*, 274 (1996), pp. 2025–31.
121 Ibid.
122 R. S. Speck, 'Cholera', in *The Cambridge Historical Dictionary of Disease*, ed. K. F. Kiple (Cambridge, 2003), pp. 74–9; Colwell, 'Global Climate and Infectious Disease'.
123 Sherman, *The Power of Plagues*.
124 A. Munthe, *The Story of San Michele* (London, 2004).
125 Hays, *Epidemics and Pandemics*; Sherman, *The Power of Plagues*.
126 Sack et al., 'Cholera'.
127 Somboonwit et al., 'Current Views and Challenges on Clinical Cholera'.
128 R. Porter, *The Greatest Benefit to Mankind: A Medical History of Humanity from Antiquity to the Present* (London, 1999).
129 E. H. Ackerknecht, 'Anticontagionism between 1821 and 1867', *International Journal of Epidemiology*, 38 (February 2009), pp. 7–21.
130 Ibid.
131 Porter, *The Greatest Benefit to Mankind*; Sherman, *The Power of Plagues*.
132 Hays, *Epidemics and Pandemics*.
133 R. J. Evans, 'Epidemics and Revolutions: Cholera in Nineteenth-century Europe', in *Epidemics and Ideas: Essays on the Historical Perception of Pestilence*, ed. T. Ranger and P. Slack (Cambridge, 1992), pp. 149–73.

134 Ibid.

135 Ibid.

136 Sack et al., 'Cholera'.

137 J. Reidl and K. E. Klose, '*Vibrio cholerae* and Cholera: Out of the Water and into the Host', FEMS *Microbiology Reviews*, 26 (2002), pp. 125–39; Colwell, 'Global Climate and Infectious Disease'.

138 J. G. Morris Jr, 'Cholera: Modern Pandemic Disease of Ancient Lineage', *Emerging Infectious Diseases*, 17 (2011), pp. 2099–104; Reidl and Klose, '*Vibrio cholerae* and Cholera'.

139 Colwell, 'Global Climate and Infectious Disease'.

140 Ibid.

141 Morris, 'Cholera: Modern Pandemic Disease of Ancient Lineage'.

142 Colwell, 'Global Climate and Infectious Disease'.

143 D. H. Crawford, *Deadly Companions: How Microbes Shaped Our History* (Oxford, 2007); M.B.A. Oldstone, *Viruses, Plagues and History* (Oxford, 1998).

144 J. Diamond, *Guns, Germs, and Steel: The Fates of Human Societies* (New York, 1999).

145 Crawford, *Deadly Companions*; Diamond, *Guns, Germs, and Steel*.

146 J. E. Drutz, 'Measles: Its History and Its Eventual Eradication', *Seminars in Pediatric Infectious Diseases*, 12 (2001), pp. 315–22; Oldstone, *Viruses, Plagues and History*.

147 Drutz, 'Measles: Its History and Its Eventual Eradication'.

148 Oldstone, *Viruses, Plagues and History*.

149 Ibid.

150 R. J. Kim-Farley, 'Measles', in *The Cambridge Historical Dictionary of Disease*, ed. Kiple, pp. 211–14; Oldstone, *Viruses, Plagues and History*.

151 Kim-Farley, 'Measles'.

152 Drutz, 'Measles: Its History and Its Eventual Eradication'.

153 McNeill, *Plagues and Peoples*.

154 Drutz, 'Measles: Its History and Its Eventual Eradication'; Kim-Farley, 'Measles'.

155 McNeill, *Plagues and Peoples*; Drutz, 'Measles: Its History and Its Eventual Eradication'.

156 Ibid.

157 Cunha, 'Smallpox and Measles'; Oldstone, *Viruses, Plagues and History*.

158 Cunha, 'Smallpox and Measles'.

159 Kim-Farley, 'Measles'.

160 Drutz, 'Measles: Its History and Its Eventual Eradication'.

161 Oldstone, *Viruses, Plagues and History*.

162 T. P. Monath and P.F.C. Vasconcelos, 'Yellow Fever', *Journal of Clinical Virology*, 64 (2015), pp. 160–73.

163 A.D.T. Barrett and S. Higgs, 'Yellow Fever: A Disease that Has Yet to Be Conquered', *Annual Review of Entomology*, 52 (2007), pp. 209–29.

164 D. B. Cooper and K. F. Kiple, 'Yellow Fever', in *The Cambridge Historical Dictionary of Disease*, ed. Kiple, pp. 365–70.

165 Barrett and Higgs, 'Yellow Fever: A Disease that Has Yet to Be Conquered'.

166 Ibid.

167 Cooper and Kiple, 'Yellow Fever'.

168 Barrett and Higgs, 'Yellow Fever: A Disease that Has Yet to Be Conquered'.

169 D. J. Gubler, 'The Changing Epidemiology of Yellow Fever and Dengue, 1900 to 2003: Full Circle?', *Comparative Immunology, Microbiology and Infectious Diseases*, 27 (2004), pp. 319–30.

170 J. E. Bryant, E. C. Holmes and A.D.T. Barrett, 'Out of Africa: A Molecular Perspective on the Introduction of Yellow Fever Virus into the Americas', *PLoS Pathogens*, 3 (2007), e75.

171 Crawford, *Deadly Companions*.

172 Barrett and Higgs, 'Yellow Fever: A Disease that Has Yet to Be Conquered'.

173 Cooper and Kiple, 'Yellow Fever'; Barrett and Higgs, 'Yellow Fever: A Disease that Has Yet to Be Conquered'.

174 Oldstone, *Viruses, Plagues and History*; Cooper and Kiple, 'Yellow Fever'.

175 Hays, *Epidemics and Pandemics*.

176 Oldstone, *Viruses, Plagues and History*.

177 Hays, *Epidemics and Pandemics*.

178 Ackerknecht, 'Anticontagionism between 1821 and 1867'.

179 Oldstone, *Viruses, Plagues and History*.

180 Ibid.

181 Ibid.

182 Ibid.

183 Porter, *The Greatest Benefit to Mankind*; Oldstone, *Viruses, Plagues and History*.

184 Cooper and Kiple, 'Yellow Fever'; Oldstone, *Viruses, Plagues and History*.

185 M. Espinosa, 'The Question of Racial Immunity to Yellow Fever in History and Historiography', *Social Science History*, 38 (2015), pp. 437–53.

186 Porter, *The Greatest Benefit to Mankind*.

187 Barrett and Higgs, 'Yellow Fever: A Disease that Has Yet to Be Conquered'.

188 Monath and Vasconcelos, 'Yellow Fever'.

189 C. Quétel, *History of Syphilis* (Oxford, 1990).

190 E. C. Tramont, 'The Impact of Syphilis on Humankind', *Infectious Disease Clinics of North America*, 18 (2004), pp. 101–10; E. W. Hook III, 'Syphilis', *The Lancet*, 389 (2017), pp. 1550–57.

191 E. G. Clark and N. Danbolt, 'The Oslo Study of the Natural History of Untreated Syphilis: An Epidemiologic Investigation Based on a Restudy of the Boeck-Bruusgaard Material: A Review and Appraisal', *Journal of Chronic Diseases*, 2 (1955), pp. 311–44.

192 Quétel, *History of Syphilis*.

193 Ibid.

194 R. J. Knell, 'Syphilis in Renaissance Europe: Rapid Evolution of an Introduced Sexually Transmitted Disease?', *Proceedings of the Royal Society of London: Biological Sciences*, 271, suppl. 4 (2004), pp. S174–6: E. Tognotti, 'The Rise and Fall of Syphilis in Renaissance Europe', *Journal of Medical Humanities*, 30 (2009), pp. 99–113.

195 L.A.P. Ferreira et al., 'Girolamo Fracastoro and the Origin of the Etymology of Syphilis', *Advances in Historical Studies*, 6 (2017), pp. 104–12.

196 Quétel, *History of Syphilis*.

197 Ibid.

198 Ibid.

199 M. Karamanou et al., 'Hallmarks in History of Syphilis Therapeutics', *Infezioni in Medicina*, 21 (2013), pp. 317–19; C. T. Ambrose, 'Pre-antibiotic Therapy of Syphilis', *Journal of Infectious Diseases and Immunology*, 1 (2016), pp. 1–20.

200 Quétel, *History of Syphilis*.

201 S. Bradford, *Cesare Borgia: His Life and Times* (London, 1976).

202 J. J. Norwich, *The Popes: A History* (London, 2012).

203 Quétel, *History of Syphilis*.

204 Ibid.

205 Ibid.

206 'Carl Wilhelm Boeck, 1808–1875', *International Journal of Leprosy*, XLI/2 (1973), p. 154.

207 Quétel, *History of Syphilis*.

208 R. E. Evans, 'Syphilis – The Great Scourge', 21 May 2013, *Microbiology Society*, https://microbiologysociety.org.

209 Ibid.

210 Ibid.

211 Quétel, *History of Syphilis*.

212 Ibid.

213 Norwich, *The Popes: A History*.

214 A. D. Wright, 'Venereal Disease and the Great', *British Journal of Venereal Diseases*, 47 (1971), pp. 295–306.

215 Cartwright, *Disease and History*; Tramont, 'The Impact of Syphilis on Humankind'.

216 F. Hackett, *Francis the First* (London, 1934).

217 Cartwright, *Disease and History*; Tramont, 'The Impact of Syphilis on Humankind'.

218 F. Hackett, *Henry the Eighth* (London, 1929).

219 Cartwright, *Disease and History*.

220 Ibid.

221 P. Stride and K. Lopes Floro, 'Henry VIII, McLeod Syndrome and Jacquetta's Curse', *Journal of the Royal College of Physicians of Edinburgh*, XLIII/4 (2013), pp. 353–60.

222 R. S. Morton, 'Did Catherine the Great of Russia Have Syphilis?', *Genitourinary Medicine*, 67 (1991), pp. 498–502.

223 Wright, 'Venereal Disease and the Great'.

224 V. Lerner, Y. Finkelstein and E. Witztum, 'The Enigma of Lenin's (1870–1924) Malady', *European Journal of Neurology*, 11 (2004), pp. 371–6.

225 R. M. Kaplan, 'Syphilis, Sex and Psychiatry, 1789–1925: Part 1', *Australasian Psychiatry*, 18 (2010), pp. 17–21; Quétel, *History of Syphilis*.

226 M. Worton, 'Of *Sapho* and Syphilis. Alphonse Daudet on and in Illness', *L'Esprit Créateur*, 37 (Fall 1997), pp. 38–49.

227 N. B. Nordlander, 'Heinrich Heine, plågad poet: "Ingen av mina läkare vet vad jag lider av"', *Läkartidningen*, CI/35 (2004), p. 2663.

228 Quétel, *History of Syphilis*.

229 Ibid.

230 M. Orth and M. R. Trimble, 'Friedrich Nietzsche's Mental Illness: General Paralysis of the Insane vs. Frontotemporal Dementia', *Acta Psychiatrica Scandinavica*, 114 (2006), pp. 439–45.

231 D. Hemelsoet, K. Hemelsoet and D. Devreese, 'The Neurological Illness of Friedrich Nietzsche', *Acta Neurologica Belgica*, 108 (2008), pp. 9–16; R. P. Henriques, 'Turin's Breakdown: Nietzsche's Pathographies and Medical Rationalities', *Ciência e Saúde Coletiva*, 23 (2018), pp. 3421–31.

232 Quétel, *History of Syphilis*.

233 H. Jedidi et al., 'Une petite histoire de la syphilis: La maladie à travers l'art et l'artiste', *Revue Médicale de Liège*, 73 (2018), pp. 363–9; C. Franzen, 'Syphilis in Composers and Musicians: Mozart, Beethoven, Paganini, Schubert, Schumann, Smetana', *European Journal of Clinical Microbiology and Infectious Diseases*, 27 (2008), pp. 1151–7; E. T. Rietschel, M. Rietschel and B. Beutler, 'How the Mighty Have Fallen: Fatal Infectious Diseases of Divine Composers', *Infectious Disease Clinics of North America*, 18 (2004), pp. 311–39.

234 Quétel, *History of Syphilis*.

235 K. N. Harper et al., 'The Origin and Antiquity of Syphilis Revisited: An Appraisal of Old World Pre-Columbian Evidence for Treponemal Infection', *Yearbook of Physical Anthropology*, 54 (2011), pp. 99–133.

236 D. Smajs, S. J. Norris and G. M. Weinstock, 'Genetic Diversity in *Treponema pallidum*: Implications for Pathogenesis, Evolution and Molecular Diagnostics of Syphilis and Yaws', *Infection, Genetics and Evolution*, 12 (2012), pp. 191–202.

237 B. M. Rothschild, 'History of Syphilis', *Clinical Infectious Diseases*, 40 (2005), pp. 1454–63.

238 V. J. Scheunemann et al., 'Historic *Treponema pallidum* Genomes from Colonial Mexico Retrieved from Archaeological Remains', *PLoS Neglected Tropical Diseases*, 21 June 2018, https://journals.plos.org.

239 W. G. Willeford and L. H. Bachmann, 'Syphilis Ascendant: A Brief History and Modern Trends', *Tropical Diseases, Travel Medicine and Vaccines*, 2 (2016).

240 A. Zumla et al., 'Tuberculosis', *New England Journal of Medicine*, 368 (2013), pp. 745–55.

241 P. L. Lin and J. L. Flynn, 'The End of the Binary Era: Revisiting the Spectrum of Tuberculosis', *Journal of Immunology*, 201 (2018), pp. 2541–8.

242 Zumla et al., 'Tuberculosis'.

243 S. Gagneux, 'Host-pathogen Coevolution in Human Tuberculosis', *Philosophical Transactions of the Royal Society of London: Biological Sciences*, 367 (2012), pp. 850–59.

244 F. Ayvazian, 'History of Tuberculosis', in *Tuberculosis: A Comprehensive International Approach*, ed. L. B. Reichman and E. S. Hershfield (New York, 1993), pp. 1–21.

245 J. Frith, 'History of Tuberculosis, Part 1: Phtisis, Consumption and the White Plague', *Journal of Military and Veterans' Health*, 22 (2014), pp. 29–35.

246 T. M. Daniel, *Captain of Death: The Story of Tuberculosis* (Rochester, NY, 1997).

247 Ibid.
248 Ayvazian, 'History of Tuberculosis'.
249 A. Sokal and J. Bricmont, *Intellectual Impostures: Postmodern Philosophers' Abuse of Science* (London, 1998).
250 I. Hershkovitz et al., 'Tuberculosis Origin: The Neolithic Scenario', *Tuberculosis*, 95, suppl. 1 (2015), pp. s122–6.
251 I. Comas et al., 'Out-of-Africa Migration and Neolithic Coexpansion of *Mycobacterium tuberculosis* with Modern Humans', *Nature Genetics*, 45 (2013), pp. 1176–82.
252 H. D. Donahue, 'Insights Gained from Ancient Biomolecules into Past and Present Tuberculosis: A Personal Perspective', *International Journal of Infectious Diseases*, 56 (2017), pp. 176–80.
253 Ibid.
254 J. J. Eddy, 'The Ancient City of Rome, Its Empire, and the Spread of Tuberculosis in Europe', *Tuberculosis*, 95 (2015), pp. 523–8; K. Harper, *The Fate of Rome* (Princeton, NJ, 2017).
255 Comas, 'Out-of-Africa Migration and Neolithic Coexpansion'.
256 K. I. Bos, K. M. Harkins and J. Krause, 'Pre-Columbian Mycobacterial Genomes Reveal Seals as a Source of New World Human Tuberculosis', *Nature*, 514 (2014), pp. 494–7.
257 Daniel, *Captain of Death*.
258 Ibid.
259 W. Shakespeare, *Macbeth*, IV.iii.168–78.
260 Daniel, *Captain of Death*.
261 Porter, *The Greatest Benefit to Mankind*.
262 Ibid.
263 Ayvazian, 'History of Tuberculosis'.
264 Porter, *The Greatest Benefit to Mankind*; Ayvazian, 'History of Tuberculosis'.
265 Porter, *The Greatest Benefit to Mankind*.
266 Daniel, *Captain of Death*.
267 B. Tallerud, *Skräckens Tid: Farsoternas kulturhistoria* (Stockholm, 1999); Daniel, *Captain of Death*.
268 Ibid.
269 Ibid.
270 Ibid.
271 Tallerud, *Skräckens Tid: Farsoternas kulturhistoria*.
272 Daniel, *Captain of Death*.
273 Ibid.
274 A. Stubhaug, *Et foranskutt lyn: Niels Henrik Abel og hans tid* (Oslo, 1996).
275 Daniel, *Captain of Death*.
276 Tallerud, *Skräckens Tid: Farsoternas kulturhistoria*.
277 D. Rayfield, *Anton Chekhov: A Life* (London, 1998).
278 Daniel, *Captain of Death*.
279 Tallerud, *Skräckens Tid: Farsoternas kulturhistoria*.
280 H. D. Chalke, 'The Impact of Tuberculosis on History, Literature and Art', *Medical History*, 6 (1962), pp. 301–18.

281 Ibid.
282 E. Bendiner, 'Baron von Pirquet: The Aristocrat Who Discovered and Defined Allergy', *Hospital Practice*, 16 (1981), pp. 137–41.
283 Porter, *The Greatest Benefit to Mankind*.
284 Daniel, *Captain of Death*.
285 T. Mann, *The Magic Mountain* (London, 1996).
286 A. E. Ellis. *The Rack* (Richmond, VA, 2014).
287 Daniel, *Captain of Death*.
288 Porter, *The Greatest Benefit to Mankind*.
289 F. Ryan, *The Forgotten Plague: How the Battle against Tuberculosis Was Won – and Lost* (Boston, MA, 1992).
290 Zumla et al., 'Tuberculosis'.
291 M. Pareek et al., 'Evaluation of Immigrant Tuberculosis Screening in Industrialized Countries', *Emerging Infectious Diseases*, 18 (2012), pp. 1422–9.
292 A. Zumla et al., 'Reflections on the White Plague', *Lancet Infectious Diseases*, 9 (2009), pp. 197–202; Daniel, *Captain of Death*.
293 T. M. Daniel, 'The Impact of Tuberculosis on Civilization', *Infectious Disease Clinics of North America*, 18 (2004), pp. 157–65.
294 A. S. Fauci, 'Addressing the Tuberculosis Epidemic: 21st Century Research for an Ancient Disease', *Journal of the American Medical Association*, 320 (2018), pp. 1315–16.
295 B. Godøy, *Ti tusen skygger: en historie om Norge og de spedalske* (Oslo, 2014).
296 R. R. Jacobson and J. L. Krahenbuhl, 'Leprosy', *The Lancet*, 353 (1999), pp. 655–60; F. Reibel, E. Cambau and A. Aubry, 'Update on the Epidemiology, Diagnosis, and Treatment of Leprosy', *Médecine et Maladies Infectieuses*, 45 (2015), pp. 383–93.
297 X. Y. Han et al., 'A New *Mycobacterium* Species Causing Diffuse Lepromatous', *American Journal of Clinical Pathology*, 130 (2008), pp. 856–64.
298 Jacobson and Krahenbuhl, 'Leprosy'; Reibel, Cambau and Aubry, 'Update on the Epidemiology, Diagnosis, and Treatment of Leprosy'.
299 A. G. Carmichael, 'Leprosy (Hansen's Disease)', in *The Cambridge Historical Dictionary of Disease*, ed. Kiple, pp. 192–4; A. G. Nerlich and A. R. Zink, 'Past Leprae', in *Palaeomicrobiology: Past Human Infections*, ed. D. Raoult and M. Drancourt (Berlin, 2008), pp. 99–123.
300 Jacobson and Krahenbuhl, 'Leprosy'.
301 Nerlich and Zink, 'Past Leprae'.
302 Ibid.
303 A. C. Stone et al., 'Tuberculosis and Leprosy in Perspective', *Yearbook of Physical Anthropology*, 52 (2009), pp. 66–94.
304 Reibel, Cambau and Aubry, 'Update on the Epidemiology, Diagnosis, and Treatment of Leprosy'.
305 X. Y. Han and F. J. Silva, 'On the Age of Leprosy', *PLoS Neglected Tropical Diseases*, 8 (2014), e2544.
306 Reibel, Cambau and Aubry, 'Update on the Epidemiology, Diagnosis, and Treatment of Leprosy'.

307 W. L. Washburn, 'Leprosy among Scandinavian Settlers in the Upper Mississippi Valley, 1864–1932', *Bulletin of the History of Medicine*, 24 (1950), pp. 123–48.

308 D. M. Scollard et al., 'The Continuing Challenges of Leprosy', *Clinical Microbiology Reviews*, 19 (2006), pp. 338–81.

309 A.-K. Schilling et al., 'British Red Squirrels Remain the Only Wild Rodent Host for Leprosy Bacilli', *Frontiers for Veterinary Science*, DOI: 10.3389/FVETS.2019.00008.

310 Nerlich and Zink, 'Past Leprae'.

311 B. Hamilton, *The Leper King and His Heirs: Baldwin IV and the Crusader Kingdom of Jerusalem* (Cambridge, 2000).

312 Nerlich and Zink, 'Past Leprae'.

313 Carmichael, 'Leprosy (Hansen's Disease)'.

314 Nerlich and Zink, 'Past Leprae'.

315 Carmichael, 'Leprosy (Hansen's Disease)'.

316 Ibid.

317 Nerlich and Zink, 'Past Leprae'.

318 Godøy, *Ti tusen skygger: en historie om Norge og de spedalske*.

319 Ibid.

320 O. Kazeem and T. Adegun, 'Leprosy Stigma: Ironing Out the Creases', *Leprosy Review*, 82 (2011), pp. 103–8.

321 A. J. Norheim and T. K. Norheim, 'Leprakolonien på Spinalonga', *Tidsskriftet den Norske Legeforening*, 132 (2012), p. 2646.

322 J. Pawlikowski et al., 'Damien de Veuster (1840–1889): A Life Devoted to Lepers', *Clinics in Dermatology*, 36 (2018), pp. 680–85.

323 A. F. Cowman et al., 'Malaria: Biology and Disease', *Cell*, 167 (2016), pp. 610–24; F. L. Dunn, 'Malaria', in *The Cambridge Historical Dictionary of Disease*, ed. Kiple, pp. 203–6.

324 R. Carter and K. N. Mendis, 'Evolutionary and Historical Aspects of the Burden of Malaria', *Clinical Microbiology Reviews*, 15 (2002), pp. 564–94.

325 Ibid.

326 Dunn, 'Malaria'; Carter and Mendis, 'Evolutionary and Historical Aspects of the Burden of Malaria'.

327 A. G. Nerlich, '*Plasmodium falciparum* in Ancient Egypt', *Emerging Infectious Diseases*, 14 (2008), pp. 1317–19.

328 Carter and Mendis, 'Evolutionary and Historical Aspects of the Burden of Malaria'.

329 Bray, *Armies of Pestilence*; McNeill, *Plagues and Peoples*.

330 S. P. Mattern, *The Prince of Medicine: Galen in the Roman Empire* (Oxford, 2013).

331 Hays, *Epidemics and Pandemics*.

332 L. J. Bruce-Chwatt and J. Zulueta, *The Rise and Fall of Malaria in Europe* (Oxford, 1980).

333 Bradford, *Cesare Borgia: His Life and Times*.

334 Bruce-Chwatt and Zulueta, *The Rise and Fall of Malaria in Europe*.

335 B. A. Cunha, 'The Death of Alexander the Great: Malaria or Typhoid Fever?', *Infectious Disease Clinics of North America*, 18 (2004), pp. 53–63.

336 Bruce-Chwatt and Zulueta, *The Rise and Fall of Malaria in Europe*.

337 M. R. Smallman-Raynor and A. D. Cliff, 'Impact of Infectious Diseases on War', *Infectious Disease Clinics of North America*, 18 (2004), pp. 341–68.

338 P. Schlagenhauf, 'Malaria: From Prehistory to Present', *Infectious Disease Clinics of North America*, 18 (2004), pp. 189–205.

339 Cohen, *Health and the Rise of Civilization*.

340 W. Liu et al., 'Origin of the Human Malaria Parasite *Plasmodium falciparum* in Gorillas', *Nature*, 467 (2010), pp. 420–25; D. E. Loy et al., 'Out of Africa: Origins and Evolution of the Human Malaria Parasites *Plasmodium falciparum* and *Plasmodium vivax*', *International Journal for Parasitology*, 47 (2017), pp. 87–97.

341 Carter and Mendis, 'Evolutionary and Historical Aspects of the Burden of Malaria'.

342 Ibid.

343 Ibid.

344 Dunn, 'Malaria'; Schlagenhauf, 'Malaria: From Prehistory to Present'.

345 Dunn, 'Malaria'.

346 Schlagenhauf, 'Malaria: From Prehistory to Present'.

347 Bruce-Chwatt and Zulueta, *The Rise and Fall of Malaria in Europe*.

348 Porter, *The Greatest Benefit to Mankind*; Sherman, *The Power of Plagues*.

349 Porter, *The Greatest Benefit to Mankind*; Sherman, *The Power of Plagues*.

350 Porter, *The Greatest Benefit to Mankind*.

351 Ibid.

352 Bruce-Chwatt and Zulueta, *The Rise and Fall of Malaria in Europe*.

353 McNeill, *Plagues and Peoples*.

354 Porter, *The Greatest Benefit to Mankind*; Carter and Mendis, 'Evolutionary and Historical Aspects of the Burden of Malaria'.

355 Bruce-Chwatt and Zulueta, *The Rise and Fall of Malaria in Europe*.

356 C. W. McMillen, *Pandemics: A Very Short Introduction* (Oxford, 2016).

357 A. Maxmen, 'The Enemy in Waiting', *Nature*, 559 (2018), pp. 458–65.

358 J. K. Taubenberger and J. C. Kash, 'Influenza Virus Evolution, Host Adaptation, and Pandemic Formation', *Cell Host and Microbe*, 7 (2010), pp. 440–51.

359 J. C. Kash and J. K. Taubenberger, 'The Role of Viral, Host, and Secondary Bacterial Factors in Influenza Pathogenesis', *American Journal of Pathology*, 185 (2015), pp. 1528–36.

360 Ibid.

361 Ibid.

362 Taubenberger and Kash, 'Influenza Virus Evolution, Host Adaptation, and Pandemic Formation'.

363 C. W. Potter, 'A History of Influenza', *Journal of Applied Microbiology*, 91 (2001), pp. 572–9; J. S. Long et al., 'Host and Viral Determinants of Influenza A Virus Species Specificity', *Nature Reviews Microbiology*, 17 (2019), pp. 67–81.

364 M. I. Nelson and M. Worobey, 'Origins of the 1918 Pandemic: Revisiting the Swine "Mixing Vessel" Hypothesis', *American Journal of Epidemiology*, 187 (2018), pp. 2498–502.

365 J. K. Taubenberger and D. M. Morens, 'Influenza Viruses: Breaking All the Rules', *mBio*, 16 July 2013, DOI: E00365–13; J. K. Taubenberger and

D. M. Morens, 'Pandemic Influenza – Including a Risk Assessment of H5N1', *Revue Scientifique et Technique*, 28 (2009), pp. 187–202.

366 Cohen, *Health and the Rise of Civilization*.

367 Taubenberger and Morens, 'Pandemic Influenza – Including a Risk Assessment of H5N1'.

368 A. W. Crosby, 'Influenza', in *The Cambridge Historical Dictionary of Disease*, ed. Kiple, pp. 178–80.

369 N.P.A.S. Johnson and J. Mueller, 'Updating the Accounts: Global Mortality of the 1918–1920 "Spanish" Influenza Pandemic', *Bulletin of the History of Medicine*, 76 (2002), pp. 105–15.

370 P. Spreeuwenberg, M. Kroneman and J. Paget, 'Reassessing the Global Mortality Burden of the 1918 Influenza Pandemic', *American Journal of Epidemiology*, 187 (2018), pp. 2561–7.

371 J. M. Barry, *The Great Influenza: The Epic Story of the Deadliest Plague in History* (New York, 2004).

372 Taubenberger and Morens, 'Pandemic Influenza – Including a Risk Assessment of H5N1'.

373 Barry, *The Great Influenza*.

374 J. S. Oxford and D. Gill, 'Unanswered Questions about the 1918 Influenza Pandemic: Origin, Pathology, and the Virus Itself', *Lancet Infectious Diseases*, 18 (2018), pp. e348–54.

375 M. E. Nickol and J. Kindrachuk, 'A Year of Terror and a Century of Reflection: Perspectives on the Great Influenza Pandemic of 1918–1919', BMC *Infectious Diseases*, 6 February 2019, https://bmcinfectdis.biomedcentral.com.

376 J. C. Kash et al., 'Genomic Analysis of Increased Host Immune and Cell Death Responses Induced by 1918 Influenza Virus', *Nature*, 443 (2006), pp. 578–81.

377 Ibid.

378 J. K. Taubenberger and D. M. Morens, '1918 Influenza: The Mother of All Pandemics', *Emerging Infectious Diseases*, 12 (2006), pp. 15–22.

379 Barry, *The Great Influenza*.

380 D. M. Morens and A. S. Fauci, 'The 1918 Influenza Pandemic: Insights for the 21st Century', *Journal of Infectious Diseases*, 195 (2007), pp. 1018–28; Oxford and Gill, 'Unanswered Questions about the 1918 Influenza Pandemic'.

381 Taubenberger and Morens, 'Pandemic Influenza – Including a Risk Assessment of H5N1'.

382 P. W. Ewald, *Evolution of Infectious Disease* (Oxford, 1994).

383 Morens and Fauci, 'The 1918 Influenza Pandemic'.

384 Hays, *Epidemics and Pandemics*.

385 L. Spinney, *Pale Rider: The Spanish Flu of 1918 and How It Changed the World* (New York, 2017); Oxford and Gill, 'Unanswered Questions about the 1918 Influenza Pandemic'.

386 Hays, *Epidemics and Pandemics*.

387 A. W. Crosby, *America's Forgotten Pandemic*, 2nd edn (Cambridge, 2003).

388 Hays, *Epidemics and Pandemics*.

389 Ewald, *Evolution of Infectious Disease*.

390 A. T. Price-Smith, *Contagion and Chaos* (Cambridge, MA, 2009).

391 Ibid.

392 Barry, *The Great Influenza.*

393 J. D. Mathews et al., 'Understanding Influenza Transmission, Immunity and Pandemic Threats', *Influenza and Other Respiratory Viruses*, 3 (2009), pp. 143–9.

394 Taubenberger and Kash, 'Influenza Virus Evolution, Host Adaptation, and Pandemic Formation'; Potter, 'A History of Influenza'; Long et al., 'Host and Viral Determinants of Influenza A Virus Species Specificity'.

395 Taubenberger and Kash, 'Influenza Virus Evolution, Host Adaptation, and Pandemic Formation'.

396 Ibid.

397 Crosby, *America's Forgotten Pandemic.*

398 M. M. Mehndiratta, P. Mehndiratta and R. Pande, 'Poliomyelitis: Historical Facts, Epidemiology, and Current Challenges in Eradication', *The Neurohospitalist*, 4 (2014), pp. 223–9; J. F. Modlin, 'Poliovirus', in *Principles and Practice of Infectious Diseases*, ed. G. L. Mandell, J. E. Bennett and R. Dolin (Philadelphia, PA, 2010), pp. 2345–51.

399 Mehndiratta, Mehndiratta and Pande, 'Poliomyelitis: Historical Facts'; Modlin, 'Poliovirus'.

400 N. Nathanson and J. R. Martin, The Epidemiology of Poliomyelitis: Enigmas Surrounding Its Appearance, Epidemicity, and Disappearance', *American Journal of Epidemiology*, 110 (1979), pp. 672–92; Mehndiratta, Mehndiratta and Pande, 'Poliomyelitis: Historical Facts'.

401 Cohen, *Health and the Rise of Civilization.*

402 Nathanson and Martin, 'The Epidemiology of Poliomyelitis'.

403 J. R. Paul, *A History of Poliomyelitis* (New Haven, CT, 1971).

404 Ibid.

405 H. J. Eggers, 'Milestones in Early Poliomyelitis Research (1840 to 1949)', *Journal of Virology*, 73 (1999), pp. 4533–5; T. Skern, '100 Years Poliovirus: From Discovery to Eradication. A Meeting Report', *Archives of Virology*, 155 (2010), pp. 1371–81.

406 Paul, *A History of Poliomyelitis.*

407 Oldstone, *Viruses, Plagues and History*; Paul, *A History of Poliomyelitis.*

408 Mehndiratta, Mehndiratta and Pande, 'Poliomyelitis: Historical Facts'.

409 Paul, *A History of Poliomyelitis.*

410 Nathanson and Martin, 'The Epidemiology of Poliomyelitis'.

411 N. Rogers, 'Dirt, Flies, and Immigrants: Explaining the Epidemiology of Poliomyelitis, 1900–1916', *Journal of the History of Medicine*, 44 (1989), pp. 486–505; Nathanson and Martin, 'The Epidemiology of Poliomyelitis'.

412 S. Bahl et al., 'Global Polio Eradication – Way Ahead', *Indian Journal of Pediatrics*, 85 (2018), pp. 124–31.

FIVE Mysterious Epidemics in History

1 C. B. Cunha and B. A. Cunha, 'Great Plagues of the Past and Remaining Questions', in *Palaeomicrobiology: Past Human Infections*, ed. D. Raoult and M. Drancourt (Berlin, 2008), pp. 1–19.

2 B. A. Cunha, 'The Cause of the Plague of Athens: Plague, Typhoid, Typhus, Smallpox, or Measles', *Infectious Disease Clinics of North America*, 18 (2004), pp. 29–43; M. A. Soupios, 'Impact of the Plague in Ancient Greece', *Infectious Disease Clinics of North America*, 18 (2004), pp. 45–51.

3 F. P. Retief and L. Cilliers, 'The Epidemic of Athens, 430–426 BC', *South African Medical Journal*, 88 (1998), pp. 50–53.

4 Cunha, 'The Cause of the Plague of Athens'; Soupios, 'Impact of the Plague in Ancient Greece'.

5 R. J. Littman 'The Plague of Athens: Epidemiology and Paleopathology', *Mount Sinai Journal of Medicine*, 76 (2009), pp. 456–67.

6 Cunha, 'The Cause of the Plague of Athens'.

7 Retief and Cilliers, 'The Epidemic of Athens, 430–426 BC'; Cunha, 'The Cause of the Plague of Athens'; Littman, 'The Plague of Athens'.

8 M. J. Papagrigorakis et al., 'DNA Examination of Ancient Dental Pulp Incriminates Typhoid Fever as a Probable Cause of the Plague of Athens', *International Journal of Infectious Diseases*, 10 (2006), pp. 206–14.

9 B. Shapiro, A. Rambaut and M.T.P. Gilbert, 'No Proof that Typhoid Caused the Plague of Athens (a reply to Papagrigorakis et al.)', *International Journal of Infectious Diseases*, 10 (2006), pp. 334–40.

10 Cunha and Cunha, 'Great Plagues of the Past and Remaining Questions'.

11 K. Harper, *The Fate of Rome* (Princeton, NJ, 2017).

12 Ibid.

13 Ibid.

14 R. J. Littman and M. L. Littman, 'Galen and the Antonine Plague', *American Journal of Philology*, 94 (1973), pp. 243–55.

15 Harper, *The Fate of Rome*; Cunha and Cunha, 'Great Plagues of the Past and Remaining Questions'.

16 J. F. Gilliam, 'The Plague under Marcus Aurelius', *American Journal of Philology*, 82 (1961), pp. 225–51; Littman and Littman, 'Galen and the Antonine Plague'.

17 Harper, *The Fate of Rome*.

18 Ibid.

19 F. McLynn, *Marcus Aurelius: Warrior, Philosopher, Emperor* (London, 2010).

20 J. N. Hays, *Epidemics and Pandemics: Their Impacts on Human History* (Santa Barbara, CA, 2005).

21 Harper, *The Fate of Rome*.

22 J. Horgan, 'Plague of Cyprian, 250–270 CE', *World History Encyclopedia*, 13 December 2016, www.ancient.eu.

23 Harper, *The Fate of Rome*.

24 Horgan, 'Plague of Cyprian, 250–270 CE'.

25 Harper, *The Fate of Rome*.

26 R. Stark, 'Epidemics, Networks, and the Rise of Christianity', *Semeia*, 56 (1992), pp. 159–75.

27 A. L. Rowse, *Bosworth Field and the Wars of the Roses* (London, 1998).

28 E. Bridson, 'The English "Sweate" (*Sudor Anglicus*) and Hantavirus Pulmonary Syndrome', *British Journal of Biomedical Science*, 58 (2001), pp. 1–6; P. Heyman, L. Simons and C. Cochez, 'Were the English Sweating

Sickness and the Picardy Sweat Caused by Hantaviruses?', *Viruses*, 6 (2014), pp. 151–71.

29 Bridson, 'The English "Sweate" (*Sudor Anglicus*)'; Heyman, Simons and Cochez, 'Were the English Sweating Sickness and the Picardy Sweat Caused by Hantaviruses?'

30 P. R. Hunter, 'The English Sweating Sickness, with Particular Reference to the 1551 Outbreak in Chester', *Reviews of Infectious Diseases*, 13 (1991), pp. 303–6.

31 Bridson, 'The English "Sweate" (*Sudor Anglicus*)'.

32 J.A.H. Wylie and L. H. Collier, 'The English Sweating Sickness (*Sudor Anglicus*): A Reappraisal', *Journal of the History of Medicine and Allied Sciences*, 36 (1981), pp. 425–45.

33 J. R. Carlson and P. W. Hammond, 'The English Sweating Sickness (1485–*c.* 1551): A New Perspective on Disease Etiology', *Journal of the History of Medicine*, 54 (1999), pp. 23–54.

34 Bridson, 'The English "Sweate" (*Sudor Anglicus*)'; Hunter, 'The English Sweating Sickness'.

35 Bridson, 'The English "Sweate" (*Sudor Anglicus*)'; Heyman, Simons and Cochez, 'Were the English Sweating Sickness and the Picardy Sweat Caused by Hantaviruses?'

36 Bridson, 'The English "Sweate" (*Sudor Anglicus*)'.

37 Wylie and Collier, 'The English Sweating Sickness (*Sudor Anglicus*): A Reappraisal'.

38 Heyman, Simons and Cochez, 'Were the English Sweating Sickness and the Picardy Sweat Caused by Hantaviruses?'

39 Bridson, 'The English "Sweate" (*Sudor Anglicus*)'; Wylie and Collier, 'The English Sweating Sickness (*Sudor Anglicus*): A Reappraisal'.

40 W. Boeck, 'La Radesyge', in C. W. Boeck and D. C. Danielssen, *Samling af Iakttagelser om hudens sygdomme*, vol. II (Christiania, 1860).

41 B. Bjorvatn and A. Danielsen, 'Radesyken: en Norsk Tragedie', *Tidsskrift for den Norske Legeforening*, 123 (2003), pp. 3557–8; F. Grøn, 'Tidsrummet, 1500–1800', in *Medisinens historie i Norge*, ed. I. Reichborn-Kjennerud, F. Grøn and I. Kobro (Oslo, 1936), pp. 101–207.

42 A. K. Lie, 'Tanker om radesyken i Norge: "den hentærer sine Offere langsomt"', *Tidsskrift for den Norske Legeforening*, 123 (2003), pp. 3562–4; Bjorvatn and Danielsen, 'Radesyken: en Norsk Tragedie'.

43 Lie, 'Tanker om radesyken i Norge'.

44 Ibid.

45 Grøn, 'Tidsrummet, 1500–1800'.

46 Bjorvatn and Danielsen, 'Radesyken: en Norsk Tragedie'.

47 Grøn, 'Tidsrummet, 1500–1800'.

SIX **The Contribution Made by Epidemics to the Fall of Empires**

1 W. H. McNeill, *Plagues and Peoples* (New York, 1976).

2 L. Schofield, *The Mycenaeans* (Los Angeles, CA, 2007).

3 L. Walløe, 'Was the Disruption of the Mycenaean World Caused by Repeated Epidemics of Bubonic Plague?', *Opuscula Atheniensa*, 24 (1999), pp. 121–6.

4 M. A. Spyrou et al., 'Analysis of 3800-year-old *Yersinia pestis* Genomes Suggests Bronze Age Origin for Bubonic Plague', *Nature Communications*, 9 (2018).

5 G. R. Schlug et al., 'Infection, Disease, and Biosocial Processes at the End of the Indus Civilization', *PLoS Neglected Tropical Diseases*, 8 (2013), e84814.

6 M. R. Mughal, 'The Decline of the Indus Civilization and the Late Harappan Period in the Indus Valley', *Lahore Museum Bulletin*, 3 (1990), pp. 1–17; A. Lawler, 'Climate Spurred Later Indus Decline', *Science*, 316 (2007), pp. 978–9.

7 Schlug et al., 'Infection, Disease, and Biosocial Processes at the End of the Indus Civilization'.

8 P. W. Ewald, *Evolution of Infectious Disease* (Oxford, 1994).

9 M. A. Soupios, 'Impact of the Plague in Ancient Greece', *Infectious Disease Clinics of North America*, 18 (2004), pp. 45–51.

10 Ibid.

11 J. N. Hays, *Epidemics and Pandemics: Their Impacts on Human History* (Santa Barbara, CA, 2005).

12 A. Demandt, *Der Fall Roms: Die Auflösung des Römisches Reiches im Urteil der Nachwelt* (Munich, 1984).

13 C. Wald, 'The Secret History of Ancient Toilets', *Nature*, 533 (2016), pp. 456–8.

14 K. Harper, *The Fate of Rome* (Princeton, NJ, 2017).

15 R. J. Littman and M. L. Littman, 'Galen and the Antonine Plague', *American Journal of Philology*, 94 (1973), pp. 243–55; J. F. Gilliam, 'The Plague under Marcus Aurelius', *American Journal of Philology*, 82 (1961), pp. 225–51.

16 Harper, *The Fate of Rome*.

17 Ibid.

18 Ibid.

19 W. Rosen, *Justinian's Flea: Plague, Empire and the Birth of Europe* (London, 2008); L. K. Little, ed., *Plague and the End of Antiquity. The Pandemic of 541–750* (Cambridge, 2007).

20 Ibid.

21 A. W. Crosby, *The Columbian Exchange: Biological and Cultural Consequences of 1492* (Westport, CT, 1972).

22 McNeill, *Plagues and Peoples*.

23 D. R. Hopkins, *Princes and Peasants: Smallpox in History* (Chicago, IL, 1983).

24 McNeill, *Plagues and Peoples*; Crosby, *The Columbian Exchange*.

25 V. W. von Hagen, *The Ancient Sun Kingdoms of the Americas* (St Albans, 1977).

26 Hopkins, *Princes and Peasants*.

SEVEN **New Infections, New Challenges**

1 A. S. Fauci, 'Infectious Diseases: Considerations for the 21st Century', *Clinical Infectious Diseases*, 32 (2001), pp. 675–85.

2 F. M. Burnet, *Natural History of Infectious Disease*, 4th edn (Cambridge, 1972).

3 K. E. Jones et al., 'Global Trends in Emerging Infectious Diseases', *Nature*, 451 (2008), pp. 990–93.

4 M. S. Smolinski, M. A. Hamburg and J. Lederberg, *Microbial Threats to Health: Emergence, Detection, and Response* (Washington, DC, 2003).

5 L. Garrett, *The Coming Plague: Newly Emerging Diseases in a World out of Balance* (New York, 1994); R. Preston, *The Hot Zone* (New York, 1995).

6 L. K. Dropulic and H. M. Lederman, 'Overview of Infections in the Immunocompromised Host', *Microbiology Spectrum*, 4 (2016), pp. 1–43; L. H. Kahn, 'The Growing Number of Immunocompromised', *Bulletin of the Atomic Scientists*, 6 January 2008, https://thebulletin.org.

7 Dropulic and Lederman, 'Overview of Infections in the Immunocompromised Host'; Kahn, 'The Growing Number of Immunocompromised'.

8 Dropulic and Lederman, 'Overview of Infections in the Immunocompromised Host'; Kahn, 'The Growing Number of Immunocompromised'.

9 S. Fox et al., *Infections in the Immune Compromised Host* (Oxford, 2018).

10 F. A. Murphy and C. J. Peters, 'Ebola Virus: Where Does It Come from and Where Is It Going?', in *Emerging Infections*, ed. R. M. Krause (New York, 1998), pp. 375–410.

11 D. Malvy et al., 'Ebola Virus Disease', *The Lancet*, 393 (2019), pp. 936–48.

12 Ibid.

13 Murphy and Peters, 'Ebola Virus: Where Does It Come from and Where Is It Going?'; Malvy al., 'Ebola Virus Disease'.

14 A. Caron et al., 'Ebola Virus Maintenance: If Not (Only) Bats, What Else?', *Viruses*, 10 (2018), p. 549.

15 J. Olivero et al., 'Recent Loss of Closed Forests Is Associated with Ebola Virus Disease Outbreaks', *Scientific Reports*, 7 (2017), article 14291.

16 Malvy et al., 'Ebola Virus Disease'.

17 J. D. Quick with B. Fryer, *The End of Epidemics. The Looming Threat to Humanity and How to Stop It* (London, 2018).

18 B. A. Cunha et al., 'Legionnaires' Disease', *The Lancet*, 387 (2016), pp. 376–85; Garrett, *The Coming Plague*.

19 Cunha et al., 'Legionnaires' Disease'; Garrett, *The Coming Plague*.

20 Cunha et al., 'Legionnaires' Disease'; Garrett, *The Coming Plague*.

21 L. A. Herwaldt and A. R. Marra, '*Legionella*: A Reemerging Pathogen', *Current Opinion in Infectious Diseases*, 31 (2018), pp. 325–33.

22 D. D. Richman, ed., *Human Immunodeficiency Virus* (London, 2003).

23 Ibid.

24 M. Crichton, *The Andromeda Strain* (New York, 1969).

25 Richman, ed., *Human Immunodeficiency Virus*.

26 Ibid.

27 C. Zimmer, *A Planet of Viruses* (Chicago, IL, and London, 2011).

28 J. Pépin, *The Origins of* AIDS (Cambridge, 2011).

29 Richman, ed., *Human Immunodeficiency Virus*.

30 Pépin, *The Origins of* AIDS.

31 S. S. Frøland et al. 'HIV-1 Infection in Norwegian Family before 1970', *The Lancet*, 331 (1988), pp. 1344–5.

32 T. Ø. Jonassen et al., 'Sequence Analysis of HIV-1 Group O from Norwegian Patients Infected in the 1960s', *Virology*, 231 (1997), pp. 43–7.

33 Pépin, *The Origins of* AIDS.

34 S. S. Frøland et al., 'Acquired Immunodeficiency Syndrome (AIDS): Clinical, Immunological, Pathological, and Microbiological Studies of the First Case Diagnosed in Norway', *Scandinavian Journal of Gastroenterology, Supplement*, 107 (1985), pp. 82–93.

35 H.-J. Han et al., 'Bats as Reservoirs of Severe Emerging Infectious Diseases', *Virus Research*, 205 (2015), pp. 1–6.

36 R. Shipley et al., 'Bats and Viruses: Emergence of Novel Lyssaviruses and Association of Bats with Viral Zoonoses in the EU', *Tropical Medicine and Infectious Disease*, 4 (2019), p. 31.

37 Han et al., 'Bats as Reservoirs of Severe Emerging Infectious Diseases'.

38 T. Schountz, 'Immunology of Bats and Their Viruses: Challenges and Opportunities', *Viruses*, 6 (2014), pp. 4880–901.

39 D. Quammen, *Spillover: Animal Infections and the Next Human Pandemic* (New York, 2012); Han et al., 'Bats as Reservoirs of Severe Emerging Infectious Diseases'.

40 B.S.P. Ang, T.C.C. Lim and L. Wang, 'Nipah Virus Infection', *Journal of Clinical Microbiology*, 56 (2018), e01875–7.

41 E. S. Gurley et al., 'Convergence of Humans, Bats, Trees, and Culture in Nipah Virus Transmission, Bangladesh', *Emerging Infectious Diseases*, 23 (2017), pp. 1446–53.

42 Ang, Lim and Wang, 'Nipah Virus Infection'.

43 Quick with Fryer, *The End of Epidemics*.

44 E. de Wit et al., 'SARS and MERS: Recent Insights into Emerging Coronaviruses', *Nature Reviews Microbiology*, 14 (2016), pp. 523–34; Quick with Fryer, *The End of Epidemics*.

45 Ibid.

46 L. Hawryluck, S. E. Lapinsky and T. E. Stewart, 'Clinical Review: SARS – Lessons in Disaster Management', *Critical Care*, 9 (2005), pp. 384–9.

47 Z. Shi and Z. Hu, 'A Review of Studies on Animal Reservoirs of the SARS Corona Virus', *Virus Research*, 133 (2008), pp. 74–87.

48 De Wit et al., 'SARS and MERS: Recent Insights into Emerging Coronaviruses'.

49 J.-E. Park et al., 'MERS Transmission and Risk Factors: A Systematic Review', BMC *Public Health*, 18 (2018), p. 574; De Wit et al., 'SARS and MERS: Recent Insights into Emerging Coronaviruses'.

50 C. Poletto et al., 'Risk of MERS Importation and Onward Transmission: A Systematic Review and Analysis of Cases Reported to WHO', BMC *Infectious Diseases*, 16 (2016), p. 448; Park et al., 'MERS Transmission and Risk Factors'.

51 Poletto et al., 'Risk of MERS Importation and Onward Transmission'.

52 G. Lu et al., 'Bat-to-Human: Spike Features Determining "Host Jump" of Coronaviruses SARS-Cov. MERS-Cov., and Beyond', *Trends in Microbiology*, 23 (2015), pp. 468–78.

53 Garrett, *The Coming Plague*.

54 W. G. Downs, 'Lassa Fever', in *The Cambridge Historical Dictionary of Disease*, ed. K. F. Kiple (Cambridge, 2003), pp. 184–5; T. Newman, 'Everything You Need to Know about Lassa Fever', *Medical News Today*, 28 June 2018, www.medicalnewstoday.com.

55 'Lassa Fever and Global Health Security', *The Lancet*, 18 (2018), p. 357.

56 Downs, 'Lassa Fever'; Newman, 'Everything You Need to Know about Lassa Fever'.

57 S. S. Morse, ed., *Emerging Viruses* (Oxford, 2003).

58 V. Saxena, B. G. Bolling and T. Wang, 'West Nile Virus', *Clinics in Laboratory Medicine*, 37 (2017), pp. 243–52; L. H. Gould and E. Fikrig, 'West Nile Virus: A Growing Concern?', *Journal of Clinical Investigation*, 113 (2004), pp. 1102–7.

59 Saxena, Bolling and Wang, 'West Nile Virus'.

60 S. Paz and J. C. Semenza, 'Environmental Drivers of West Nile Fever Epidemiology in Europe and Western Asia: A Review', *International Journal of Environmental Research and Public Health*, 10 (2013), pp. 3543–62.

61 Saxena, Bolling and Wang, 'West Nile Virus'; Gould and Fikrig, 'West Nile Virus: A Growing Concern?'

62 Ibid.

63 Paz and Semenza, 'Environmental Drivers of West Nile Fever Epidemiology'.

64 J. Vasudevan et al., 'Zika Virus', *Reviews in Medical Microbiology*, 29 (2018), pp. 43–50.

65 Ibid.

66 J. Cohen, 'Are Wild Monkeys Becoming a Reservoir for Zika Virus in the Americas?', *Science*, 31 October 2018, www.sciencemag.org, accessed 16 March 2021.

67 Vasudevan et al., 'Zika Virus'.

68 Z.-Y. Liu et al., 'The Evolution of Zika Virus from Asia to the Americas', *Nature Reviews Microbiology*, 17 (2019), pp. 131–9.

69 K. S. Maclea, 'What Makes A Prion: Infectious Proteins from Animals to Yeast', *International Review of Cell and Molecular Biology*, 329 (2016), pp. 227–76.

70 M. Howell and P. Ford, *The Ghost Disease and Twelve Other Stories of Detective Work in the Medical Field* (Harmondsworth, 1986); S. Lindenbaum, 'Kuru, Prions, and Human Affairs: Thinking about Epidemics', *Annual Review of Anthropology*, 30 (2001), pp. 363–85.

71 Howell and Ford, *The Ghost Disease*.

72 Lindenbaum, 'Kuru, Prions, and Human Affairs'.

73 S. B. Prusiner, 'Novel Proteinaceous Infectious Particles Cause Scrapie', *Science*, 216 (1982), pp. 136–44.

74 Maclea, 'What Makes A Prion'; Lindenbaum, 'Kuru, Prions, and Human Affairs'.

75 G. Mackenzie and R. Will, 'Creutzfeldt-Jakob Disease: Recent Developments', *F1000research*, 6 (2017), p. 2053.

76 M. T. Osterholm et al., 'Chronic Wasting Disease in Cervids: Implications for Prion Transmission to Humans and Other Animal Species', *mBio*, 10 (2019), e01091–19.

77 Z. Allam, 'The First 50 Days of COVID-19: A Detailed Chronological Timeline and Extensive Review of Literature Documenting the Pandemic', *Elsevier Public Health Emergency Collection*, 24 July 2020, DOI: 10.1016/B978-0-12-824313-8.00001-2; E. Garcia de Jesus, 'Here's What We Learned in Six Months of COVID-19 – and What We Still Don't Know', *Science News*, 30 June 2020, www.sciencenews.org.

78 Visual and Data Journalism Team, 'COVID-19: The Global Crisis – in Data', *Financial Times*, 18 October 2020; Visual and Data Journalism Team, 'COVID-19 Pandemic: Tracking the Global Coronavirus Outbreak', BBC *News*, 11 December 2020.

79 W. J. Wiersinga et al., 'Pathophysiology, Transmission, Diagnosis, and Treatment of Coronavirus Disease 2019 (COVID-19)', *Journal of the American Medical Association*, 324 (2020), pp. 782–93.

80 N. Wilson et al., 'Airborne Transmission of COVID-19', *British Medical Journal*, 370 (2020), M3206.

81 Wiersinga et al., 'Pathophysiology, Transmission, Diagnosis, and Treatment of Coronavirus Disease 2019 (COVID-19)'.

82 W. Ni et al., 'Role of Angiotensin-converting Enzyme 2 (ACE2) in COVID-19', *Critical Care*, 24 (2020), p. 424; Wiersinga et al., 'Pathophysiology, Transmission, Diagnosis, and Treatment of Coronavirus Disease 2019 (COVID-19)'.

83 Ibid.

84 C. del Rio, L. F. Collins and P. Malani, 'Long-term Health Consequences of COVID-19', *Journal of the American Medical Association*, 324 (2020), pp. 1723–4.

85 Garcia de Jesus, 'Here's What We Learned in Six Months of COVID-19'; Wiersinga et al., 'Pathophysiology, Transmission, Diagnosis, and Treatment of Coronavirus Disease 2019 (COVID-19)'.

86 E. J. Williamson et al., 'Factors Associated with COVID-19-related Death Using OpenSAFELY', *Nature*, 584 (2020), pp. 430–36.

87 J. E. Weatherhead et al., 'Inflammatory Syndromes Associated with SARS-CoV-2 Infection: Dysregulation of the Immune Response across the Age Spectrum', *Journal of Clinical Investigation*, 130 (2020), pp. 6194–7.

88 H. Zeberg and S. Pääbo, 'The Major Genetic Risk Factor for Severe COVID-19 Is Inherited from Neanderthals', *Nature*, 587 (2020), pp. 610–12.

89 S. Perlman, 'COVID-19 Poses a Riddle for the Immune System', *Nature*, 584 (2020), pp. 345–6.

90 J. S. Faust et al., 'Mortality among Adults Ages 25–44 in the United States during the COVID-19 Pandemic', *medRxiv*, 25 October 2020, www.medrxiv.org, accessed 16 March 2021.

91 L. Piroth et al., 'Comparison of the Characteristics, Morbidity, and Mortality of COVID-19 and Seasonal Influenza: A Nationwide,

Population-based Cohort Study', *Lancet Respiratory Medicine*, 9 (2021), pp. 251–9; N. F. Brazeau et al., 'Report 34: COVID-19 Infection Fatality Ratio Estimates from Seroprevalence', MRC *Centre for Global Infectious Disease Analysis*, 29 October 2020, www.imperial.ac.uk.

92 D. A. Relman, 'Opinion: To Stop the Next Pandemic, We Need to Unravel the Origins of COVID-19', *Proceedings of the National Academy of Sciences*, 117 (2020), pp. 29246–8.

93 Ibid.

94 G. Readfearn, 'How Did Coronavirus Start and Where Did It Come From? Was It Really Wuhan's Animal Market?', *The Guardian*, 28 April 2020.

95 Ibid.

96 Visual and Data Journalism Team, 'COVID-19: The Global Crisis – in Data'; Visual and Data Journalism Team, 'COVID-19 Pandemic'.

97 A. Green, 'Li Wenliang', *The Lancet*, 395 (2020), p. 682.

98 Visual and Data Journalism Team, 'COVID-19: The Global Crisis – in Data'.

99 Ibid.

100 Ibid.; Visual and Data Journalism Team, 'COVID-19 Pandemic: Tracking the Global Coronavirus Outbreak'.

101 C. Aschwanden, 'The False Promise of Herd Immunity', *Nature*, 587 (2020), pp. 26–8.

102 Visual and Data Journalism Team, 'COVID-19 Pandemic: Tracking the Global Coronavirus Outbreak'.

103 Ibid.

104 Visual and Data Journalism Team, 'COVID-19: The Global Crisis – in Data'.

105 S. Blecker et al., 'Hospitalizations for Chronic Disease and Acute Conditions in the Time of COVID-19', JAMA *Internal Medicine*, 181 (2020), pp. 269–71.

106 M. Kulldorff et al., 'Great Barrington Declaration', https://gbdeclaration. org, accessed 16 March 2021.

107 Aschwanden, 'The False Promise of Herd Immunity'.

108 European Centre for Disease Prevention and Control, 'Rapid Risk Assessment: Outbreak of Plague in Madagascar, 2017', 9 October 2017, www.ecdc.europa.eu.

109 D. Lantagne et al., 'The Cholera Outbreak in Haiti: Where and How Did It Begin?', *Current Topics in Microbiology and Immunology*, 379 (2014), pp. 145–64.

110 D. J. Gubler, 'Resurgent Vector-borne Diseases as a Global Health Problem', *Emerging Infectious Diseases*, 4 (1998), pp. 442–50.

EIGHT **When Microbes Are Used as Weapons**

1 V. Barras and G. Greub, 'History of Biological Warfare and Bioterrorism', *Clinical Microbiology and Infection*, 20 (2014), pp. 497–502.

2 G. W. Christopher et al., 'Biological Warfare', *Journal of the American Medical Association*, 278 (1997), pp. 412–17.

3 Barras and Greub, 'History of Biological Warfare and Bioterrorism'; Christopher et al., 'Biological Warfare'.

4 W. Barnaby, *The Plague Makers: The Secret World of Biological Warfare* (London, 1997); Barras and Greub, 'History of Biological Warfare and Bioterrorism'.

5 Barnaby, *The Plague Makers*.

6 Christopher et al., 'Biological Warfare'; Barnaby, *The Plague Makers*.

7 Barras and Greub, 'History of Biological Warfare and Bioterrorism'; Christopher et al., 'Biological Warfare'; Barnaby, *The Plague Makers*.

8 Ibid.

9 E. M. Spiers, *A History of Chemical and Biological Weapons* (London, 2010).

10 Ibid.

11 Ibid.

NINE *Homo sapiens* Strikes Back

1 R. J. Stevenson et al., 'Proactive Strategies to Avoid Infectious Disease', *Philosophical Transactions of the Royal Society of London: Biological Sciences*, 366 (2011), pp. 3361–3.

2 V. A. Curtis, 'Dirt, Disgust and Disease: A Natural History of Hygiene', *Journal of Epidemiology and Community Health*, 61 (2007), pp. 660–64; C. Sarabian et al., 'Evolution of Pathogen and Parasite Avoidance Behaviours', *Philosophical Transactions of the Royal Society of London: Biological Sciences*, 373 (2018), 20170256.

3 M. Schaller, 'The Behavioural Immune System and the Psychology of Human Sociality', *Philosophical Transactions of the Royal Society of London: Biological Sciences*, 366 (2011), pp. 3418–26.

4 Curtis, 'Dirt, Disgust and Disease: A Natural History of Hygiene'.

5 Ibid.

6 E. Tognotti, 'Lessons from the History of Quarantine from Plague to Influenza A', *Emerging Infectious Diseases*, 19 (2013), pp. 254–9; G. F. Gensini et al., 'The Concept of Quarantine in History: From Plague to SARS', *Journal of Infection*, 49 (2004), pp. 257–61.

7 M. Harrison, *Contagion: How Commerce Has Spread Disease* (New Haven, CT, 2012); E. H. Ackerknecht, 'Anticontagionism between 1821 and 1867', *International Journal of Epidemiology*, 38 (February 2009), pp. 7–21.

8 D. R. Hopkins, *Princes and Peasants: Smallpox in History* (Chicago, IL, 1983).

9 A. Allen, *Vaccine: The Controversial Story of Medicine's Greatest Life Saver* (New York, 2007); Hopkins, *Princes and Peasants*.

10 G. Miller, 'Putting Lady Mary in Her Place: A Discussion of Historical Causation', *Bulletin of the History of Medicine*, 55 (1981), pp. 2–16.

11 P. Sköld, *The Two Faces of Smallpox: A Disease and Its Prevention in Eighteenth- and Nineteenth-century Sweden*, Report No. 12 from the Demographic Data Base, Umeå University (Umeå, 1996).

12 Allen, *Vaccine: The Controversial Story of Medicine's Greatest Life Saver*.

13 Hopkins, *Princes and Peasants*.

14 I. Glynn and J. Glynn, *The Life and Death of Smallpox* (London, 2004); Hopkins, *Princes and Peasants*; Allen, *Vaccine: The Controversial Story of Medicine's Greatest Life Saver*.

15 A. Boylston, 'The Origins of Vaccination: Myths and Reality', *Journal of the Royal Society of Medicine*, 106 (2013), pp. 351–4.

16 Hopkins, *Princes and Peasants*.

17 Allen, *Vaccine: The Controversial Story of Medicine's Greatest Life Saver*; Hopkins, *Princes and Peasants*.

18 Hopkins, *Princes and Peasants*.

19 Allen, *Vaccine: The Controversial Story of Medicine's Greatest Life Saver*.

20 C. R. Damaso, 'Revisiting Jenner's Mysteries: The Role of the Beaugency Lymph in the Evolutionary Path of Ancient Smallpox Vaccines', *Lancet Infectious Diseases*, 18 (2018), pp. e55–63.

21 R. P. Gaynes, *Germ Theory: Medical Pioneers in Infectious Diseases* (Washington, DC, 2011); J. Waller, *The Discovery of the Germ: Twenty Years that Transformed the Way We Think about Disease* (New York, 2002).

22 Gaynes, *Germ Theory*.

23 G. L. Geison, *The Private Science of Louis Pasteur* (Princeton, NJ, 1995).

24 Gaynes, *Germ Theory*.

25 E. Bendiner, 'From Rabies to AIDS: 100 Years at Pasteur', *Hospital Practice*, 22 (1987), pp. 119–24.

26 S. Plotkin, 'History of Vaccination', *Proceedings of the National Academy of Sciences*, 111 (2014), pp. 12283–7.

27 B. S. Graham et al. 'Novel Vaccine Technologies: Essential Components of an Adequate Response to Emerging Viral Diseases', *Journal of the American Medical Association*, 319 (2018), pp. 1431–2; J. Abbasi, 'COVID-19 and MRNA Vaccines: First Large Test for a New Approach', *Journal of the American Medical Association*, 324 (2020), pp. 1125–7.

28 A. Allen, *The Fantastic Laboratory of Dr Weigl: How Two Brave Scientists Battled Typhus and Sabotaged the Nazis* (New York, 2015).

29 Ibid.

30 Plotkin, 'History of Vaccination'.

31 M. Harrison, *Medicine and Victory: British Military Medicine in the Second World War* (Oxford, 2004).

32 L. Trogstad et al., 'Narcolepsy and Hypersomnia in Norwegian Children and Young Adults Following the Influenza A(H1N1) 2009 Pandemic', *Vaccine*, 35 (2017), pp. 1879–85.

33 M. M. Eibl, 'Vaccination in Patients with Primary Immune Deficiency, Secondary Immune Deficiency and Autoimmunity with Immune Regulatory Abnormalities', *Immunotherapy*, 7 (2015), pp. 1273–92.

34 L. R. Platt, 'Vaccine-associated Paralytic Poliomyelitis: A Review of the Epidemiology and Estimation of the Global Burden', *Journal of Infectious Diseases*, 210 (2014), suppl. 1, pp. s380–89.

35 R. Rappuoli et al., 'Vaccines for the Twenty-first Century Society', *Nature Reviews Immunology*, 11 (2011), pp. 865–72.

36 B. S. Graham et al., 'Novel Vaccine Technologies: Essential Components of an Adequate Response to Emerging Viral Diseases', *Journal of the American Medical Association*, 319 (2018), pp. 1431–2.

37 P. Piot et al., 'Immunization: Vital Progress, Unfinished Agenda', *Nature*, 575 (2019), pp. 119–29.

38 D. R. Burton, 'Advancing an HIV Vaccine: Advancing Vaccinology', *Nature Reviews Immunology*, 19 (2019), pp. 77–8.

39 P. Andersen and T. J. Scriba, 'Moving Tuberculosis Vaccine from Theory to Practice', *Nature Reviews Immunology*, 19 (2019), pp. 550–62.

40 M. Eisenstein, 'Towards a Universal Flu Vaccine', *Nature*, 573 (2019), pp. S50–52.

41 J. S. Tregoning et al., 'Vaccine for COVID-19', *Clinical and Experimental Immunology*, 202 (2020), pp. 162–92.

42 Graham et al., 'Novel Vaccine Technologies: Essential Components'; Abbasi, 'COVID-19 and MRNA Vaccines: First Large Test for a New Approach'.

43 C. Aschwanden, 'The False Promise of Herd Immunity', *Nature*, 587 (2020), pp. 26–8.

44 H. Schmidt, 'COVID-19: How to Prioritize Worse-off Populations in Allocating Safe and Effective Vaccines', *British Medical Journal*, 37 (5 October 2020), M3795.

45 Rappuoli et al., 'Vaccines for the Twenty-first Century Society'.

46 B. M. Tebeje et al., 'Schistosomiasis Vaccines: Where Do We Stand?', *Parasites and Vectors*, 9 (2016), article 528.

47 S.H.E. Kaufmann, 'Remembering Emil von Behring: From Tetanus Treatment to Antibody Cooperation with Phagocytes', *mBio*, 8 (2017), e00117–17.

48 F. Winau and R. Winau, 'Emil von Behring and Serum Therapy', *Microbes and Infection*, 4 (2002), pp. 185–8.

49 Gaynes, *Germ Theory*.

50 Ibid.

51 S.H.E. Kaufmann, 'Emil von Behring: Translational Medicine at the Dawn of Immunology', *Nature Reviews Immunology*, 17 (2017), pp. 341–3; Gaynes, *Germ Theory*.

52 A. Casadevall and M. D. Scharff, 'Serum Therapy Revisited: Animal Models of Infection and Development of Passive Antibody Therapy', *Antimicrobial Agents and Chemotherapy*, 38 (1994), pp. 1695–702.

53 C. J. Tsay, 'Julius Wagner-Jauregg and the Legacy of Malarial Therapy for the Treatment of General Paresis of the Insane', *Yale Journal of Biological Medicine*, 86 (2013), pp. 245–54.

54 Gaynes, *Germ Theory*.

55 A. C. Hüntelmann, 'Paul Ehrlich: His Passion for Staining, and his Role for Microbiology', *Reviews in Medical Microbiology*, 28 (2017), pp. 79–87.

56 Gaynes, *Germ Theory*.

57 P. de Kruif, *Microbe Hunters* (New York, 2002).

58 W. Rosen, *Miracle Cure: The Creation of Antibiotics and the Birth of Modern Medicine* (New York, 2018); Gaynes, *Germ Theory*.

59 Rosen, *Miracle Cure*; Gaynes, *Germ Theory*.

60 J. M. Fenster, *Mavericks, Miracles, and Medicine* (New York, 2003).

61 F. Ryan, *The Forgotten Plague: How the Battle against Tuberculosis Was Won – and Lost* (Boston, MA, 1992); Rosen, *Miracle Cure*.

62 Ryan, *The Forgotten Plague*; Rosen, *Miracle Cure*.

63 Ibid.

64 E. Bendiner, 'Alexander Fleming: Player with Microbes', *Hospital Practice*, 24 (1989), pp. 283–316.

65 E. Lax, *The Mould in Dr Florey's Coat: The Remarkable True Story of the Penicillin Miracle* (London and New York, 2004).

66 Gaynes, *Germ Theory*.

67 Bendiner, 'Alexander Fleming: Player with Microbes'; Lax, *The Mould in Dr Florey's Coat*.

68 B. L. Ligon, 'Sir Howard Walter Florey: The Force behind the Development of Penicillin', *Seminars in Pediatric Infectious Diseases*, 15 (2004), pp. 109–14.

69 Lax, *The Mould in Dr Florey's Coat*.

70 Gaynes, *Germ Theory*.

71 Ligon, 'Sir Howard Walter Florey'.

72 Bendiner, 'Alexander Fleming: Player with Microbes'.

73 G. Greene, *The Third Man and Other Stories* (London, 2017).

74 P. N. Newton and B. Timmerman, 'Fake Penicillin, *The Third Man*, and Operation Claptrap', *British Medical Journal*, 355 (2016), i6494.

75 Ryan, *The Forgotten Plague*.

76 Ibid.

77 T. M. Daniel, *Captain of Death: The Story of Tuberculosis* (Rochester, NY, 1997).

78 Ryan, *The Forgotten Plague*; Rosen, *Miracle Cure*.

79 S. Keshavjee and P. E. Farmer, 'Tuberculosis, Drug Resistance, and the History of Modern Medicine', *New England Journal of Medicine*, 367 (2012), pp. 931–6.

80 S. Tibur et al., 'Tuberculosis: Progress and Advances in Development of New Drugs, Treatment Regimens, and Host Directed Therapies', *Lancet Infectious Diseases*, 18 (2018), e183–98.

81 K. Gould, 'Antibiotics: From Prehistory to the Present Day', *Journal of Antimicrobial Chemotherapy*, 71 (2016), pp. 572–5.

82 R. Aminov, 'History of Antimicrobial Drug Discovery: Major Classes and Health Impact', *Biochemical Pharmacology*, 133 (2017), pp. 4–19.

83 E. De Clercq, 'Looking Back in 2009 at the Dawning of Antiviral Therapy Now 50 Years Ago: An Historical Perspective', *Advances in Virus Research*, 73 (2009), pp. 1–53.

84 G. Antonelli and O. Turriziani, 'Antiviral Therapy: Old and Current Issues', *International Journal of Antimicrobial Agents*, 40 (2012), pp. 95–102.

85 E. De Clercq, 'Fifty Years in Search of Selective Antiviral Drugs', *Journal of Medicinal Chemistry*, 62 (2019), pp. 7322–39; D. D. Richman, ed., *Human Immunodeficiency Virus* (London, 2003).

86 P. Chigwedere et al., 'Estimating the Lost Benefits of Antiretroviral Drug Use in South Africa', *Journal of Acquired Immune Deficiency Syndromes*, 49 (2008), pp. 410–15.

87 T. Ndung'u, J. M. McCune and S. G. Deeks, 'Why and Where an HIV Cure Is Needed and How It Might Be Achieved', *Nature*, 576 (2019), pp. 397–405.

88 S. Pol and S. Lagaye, 'The Remarkable History of the Hepatitis C Virus', *Genes and Immunity*, 20 (2019), pp. 436–46.

89 A. Pedrana et al., 'Global Hepatitis C Elimination: An Investment Framework', *Lancet Gastroenterology and Hepatology*, 5 (2020), pp. 927–39.

90 J. Cohen, 'Forgotten No More', *Science*, 362 (2018), pp. 984–7.

91 N. Principi et al., 'Drugs for Influenza Treatment: Is There Significant News?', *Frontiers in Medicine*, 6 (2019), p. 109.

92 K.A.O. Tikkinen et al., 'COVID-19 Clinical Trials: Learning from Exceptions in the Research Chaos', *Nature Medicine*, 26 (2020), pp. 1671–2.

93 M. A. Martinez, 'Clinical Trials of Repurposed Antivirals for SARS-CoV-2', *Antimicrobial Agents and Chemotherapy*, 64 (2020), e01101–20.

94 The RECOVERY Collaborative Group, 'Effect of Hydroxychloroquine in Hospitalized Patients with Covid-19', *New England Journal of Medicine*, 383 (2020), pp. 2030–40; WHO Solidarity Trial Consortium, 'Repurposed Antiviral Drugs for Covid-19: Interim WHO Solidarity Trial Results', *New England Journal of Medicine*, 384 (2021), pp. 497–511.

95 Ibid.

96 J. H. Beigel et al., 'Remdesivir for the Treatment of Covid-19: Final Report', *New England Journal of Medicine*, 383 (2020), pp. 1813–26.

97 A. Casadevall et al., 'Passive Antibody Therapy for Infectious Diseases', *Nature Reviews Microbiology*, 2 (2004), pp. 695–703.

98 V. A. Simonovich et al., 'A Randomized Trial of Convalescent Plasma in Covid-19 Severe Pneumonia', *New England Journal of Medicine*, 384 (2021), pp. 619–29.

99 The RECOVERY Collaborative Group, 'Dexamethasone in Hospitalized Patients with Covid-19: Preliminary Report', *New England Journal of Medicine*, 384 (2021), pp. 693–74.

100 J. B. Parr, 'Time to Reassess Tocilizumab's Role in COVID-19 Pneumonia', *Journal of the American Medical Association Internal Medicine*, 181 (2021), pp. 12–15.

101 J. R. Perfect, 'The Antifungal Pipeline: A Reality Check', *Nature Reviews Drug Discovery*, 16 (2017), pp. 603–16.

102 Ibid.

103 J. Utzinger et al., 'Neglected Tropical Diseases: Diagnosis, Clinical Management, Treatment and Control', *Swiss Medical Weekly*, 142 (2012), w13727.

104 M. De Rycker et al., 'Challenges and Recent Progress in Drug Discovery for Tropical Diseases', *Nature*, 559 (2018), pp. 498–506.

105 F. Mueller-Langer, 'Neglected Infectious Diseases: Are Push and Pull Incentive Mechanisms Suitable for Promoting Drug Development Research?', *Health Economics, Policy and Law*, 8 (2013), pp. 185–208.

TEN **New Challenges from the Microbes – and Possible Countermeasures**

1 S. S. Morse et al., 'Prediction and Prevention of the Next Pandemic Zoonosis', *The Lancet*, 380 (2012), pp. 1956–65.

2 T. Allen et al., 'Global Hotspots and Correlates of Emerging Zoonotic Diseases', *Nature Communications*, 8 (2017), article 1124; Morse et al., 'Prediction and Prevention of the Next Pandemic Zoonosis'.

3   D. M. Morens and J. K. Taubenberger, 'Pandemic Influenza: Certain
    Uncertainties', *Reviews in Medical Virology*, 21 (2011), pp. 262–84.

4   J.S.M. Peiris et al., 'Interventions to Reduce Zoonotic and Pandemic Risks
    from Avian Influenza in Asia', *Lancet Infectious Diseases*, 16 (2016),
    pp. 252–8.

5   L.-F. Wang and D. E. Anderson, 'Viruses in Bats and Spillover to Animals
    and Humans', *Current Opinion in Virology*, 34 (2019), pp. 79–89.

6   D. S. Hui and M. Peiris, 'Severe Acute Respiratory Syndrome and Other
    Emerging Severe Respiratory Viral Infections', *Respirology*, 24 (2019),
    pp. 410–12.

7   C. Castillo-Chavez et al., 'Beyond Ebola: Lessons to Mitigate Future
    Pandemics', *Lancet Global Health*, 3 (2015), pp. E354–5.

8   A. T. Price-Smith, *Contagion and Chaos* (Cambridge, MA, 2009).

9   S. K. Cohn, 'Pandemics: Waves of Disease, Waves of Hate from the Plague
    of Athens to AIDS', *Historical Research*, 85 (2012), pp. 535–55; Price-Smith,
    Contagion and Chaos.

10 A. Maxmen, 'Battling Ebola in a War Zone', *Nature*, 570 (2019), pp. 426–7.

11 J. D. Quick with B. Fryer, *The End of Epidemics. The Looming Threat to
    Humanity and How to Stop It* (London, 2018).

12 P. Sands et al., 'Assessment of Economic Vulnerability to Infectious Disease
    Crises', *The Lancet*, 388 (2016), pp. 2443–8.

13 Price-Smith, *Contagion and Chaos*.

14 Quick with Fryer, *The End of Epidemics*.

15 B. Bennett and T. Carney, 'Planning for Pandemics: Lessons from the Past
    Decade', *Bioethical Inquiry*, 12 (2015), pp. 418–28.

16 B. Jester et al., 'Readiness for Responding to a Severe Pandemic 100 Years
    after 1918', *American Journal of Epidemiology*, 187 (2018), pp. 2596–602.

17 T. Pang, 'Is the Global Health Community Prepared for Future
    Pandemics? A Need for Solidarity, Resources and Strong Governance',
    EMBO Molecular Medicine, 8 (2016), pp. 587–8.

18 J. T. Ladner et al., 'Precision Epidemiology for Infectious Disease Control',
    Nature Medicine, 25 (2019), pp. 206–11.

19 E. C. Holmes, A. Rambaut and K. G. Andersen, 'Pandemics: Spend on
    Surveillance, Not Prediction', *Nature*, 558 (2018), pp. 180–81.

20 J. A. Røttingen et al., 'New Vaccines against Epidemic Infectious Diseases',
    New England Journal of Medicine, 376 (2017), pp. 610–13.

21 H. D. Marston, C. I. Paules and A. S. Fauci, 'The Critical Role of
    Biomedical Research in Pandemic Preparedness', *Journal of the American
    Medical Association*, 318 (2017), pp. 1757–8.

22 D. Carroll et al., 'The Global Virome Project', *Science*, 359 (2018),
    pp. 872–4.

23 Bennett and Carney, 'Planning for Pandemics'.

24 Maxmen, 'Battling Ebola in a War Zone'.

25 M. Enserink, 'Risk of Exposure', *Science*, 347 (2015), pp. 498–500.

26 Quick with Fryer, *The End of Epidemics*.

27 H. D. Marston et al., 'Antimicrobial Resistance', *Journal of the American
    Medical Association*, 316 (2016), pp. 1193–204.

28 Ibid.

29 J. Perry, N. Waglechner and G. Wright, 'The Prehistory of Antibiotic Resistance', *Cold Spring Harbor Perspectives in Medicine*, 6 (2016), a025197.

30 S. B. Levy, *The Antibiotic Paradox: How the Misuse of Antibiotics Destroys their Curative Powers*, 2nd edn (Cambridge, MA, 2002).

31 J. Davies and D. Davies, 'Origins and Evolution of Antibiotic Resistance', *Microbiology and Molecular Biology Reviews*, 74 (2010), pp. 417–33.

32 Marston et al., 'Antimicrobial Resistance'; Levy, *The Antibiotic Paradox*.

33 Ibid.

34 M. T. Osterholm and M. Olshaker, *Deadliest Enemy: Our War against Killer Germs* (New York, 2017); Marston et al., 'Antimicrobial Resistance'; Davies and Davies, 'Origins and Evolution of Antibiotic Resistance'.

35 J. Wilkinson and A. Boxall, 'The First Global Study of Pharmaceutical Contamination in Riverine Environments', SETAC Europe 29th Annual Meeting, Helsinki, 28 May 2019; see also C. Wilke, 'Antibiotics Pollute Many of the World's Rivers', *Science News for Students*, 2 July 2019, www.sciencenewsforstudents.org.

36 M. Dolejska and J. Literak, 'Wildlife Is Overlooked in the Epidemiology of Medically Important Antibiotic-resistant Bacteria', *Antimicrobial Agents and Chemotherapy*, 63 (2019), e01167–19.

37 U. Theuretzbacher et al., 'Analysis of the Clinical Antibacterial and Antituberculosis Pipeline', *Lancet Infectious Diseases*, 19 (2019), e40–50.

38 H. Naci, A. W. Carter and E. Mossialos, 'Why the Drug Development Pipeline Is Not Delivering Better Medicines', *British Medical Journal*, 351 (2015), h5542.

39 Interagency Coordination Group on Antimicrobial Resistance, 'No Time to Wait: Securing the Future from Drug-resistant Infections', Report to the Secretary-General of the United Nations, April 2019.

40 W. Hall, A. McDonnell and J. O'Neill, *Superbugs: An Arms Race against Bacteria* (Cambridge, MA, 2018).

41 B. Spellberg, 'The New Antibiotic Mantra: "Shorter Is Better"', *J ournal of the American Medical Association*, 176 (2016), pp. 1254–5.

42 K. U. Jansen et al., 'The Role of Vaccines in Preventing Bacterial Antimicrobial Resistance', *Nature Medicine*, 24 (2018), pp. 10–19.

43 Marston et al., 'Antimicrobial Resistance'; Naci, Carter and Mossialos, 'Why the Drug Development Pipeline Is Not Delivering Better Medicines'.

44 D. M. Shlaes and P. A. Bradford, 'Antibiotics – from There to Where?: How the Antibiotic Miracle Is Threatened by Resistance and a Broken Market and What We Can Do About It', *Pathogens and Immunity*, 13 (2018), pp. 19–43; L.J.V. Piddock, 'The Crisis of No New Antibiotics: What Is the Way Forward?', *Lancet Infectious Diseases*, 12 (2012), pp. 249–53.

45 K. Moelling, F. Broecker and C. Willy, 'A Wake-up Call: We Need Phage Therapy Now', *Viruses*, 10 (2018), p. 688.

46 O. Bergh et al., 'High Abundance of Viruses Found in Aquatic Environments', *Nature*, 340 (1989), pp. 467–8.

47 Moelling, Broecker and Willy, 'A Wake-up Call: We Need Phage Therapy Now'.

48 D. M. Lin, B. Koskella and H. C. Lin, 'Phage-therapy: An Alternative to Antibiotics in the Age of Multi-drug Resistance', *World Journal of Gastrointestinal Pharmacology and Therapeutics*, 6 (2017), pp. 162–73.

49 Moelling, Broecker and Willy, 'A Wake-up Call: We Need Phage Therapy Now'.

50 F. L. Gordillo Altamirano and J. J. Barr, 'Phage Therapy in the Postantibiotic Era', *Clinical Microbiology Reviews*, 32 (2019), e00066–18.

51 A. Kakasis and G. Panitsa, 'Bacteriophage Therapy as an Alternative Treatment for Human Infections: A Comprehensive Review', *International Journal of Antimicrobial Agents*, 53 (2019), pp. 16–21; K. Abdelkader et al., 'The Preclinical and Clinical Progress of Bacteriophages and their Lytic Enzymes: The Parts Are Easier than the Whole', *Viruses*, 11 (2019), p. 96.

52 R. M. Dedrick et al., 'Engineered Bacteriophages for Treatment of a Patient with a Disseminated Drug-resistant *Mycobacterium Abscessus*', *Nature Medicine*, 25 (2019), pp. 730–33.

53 A. Zumla et al., 'Host-directed Therapies for Infectious Diseases: Current Status, Recent Progress, and Future Prospects', *Lancet Infectious Diseases*, 16 (2016), pp. e47–63.

54 J. Rhodes and M. C. Fisher, 'Global Epidemiology of Emerging *Candida Auris*', *Current Opinion in Microbiology*, 52 (2019), pp. 84–9.

55 J. M. Rybak, J. R. Fortwendel and P. D. Rogers, 'Emerging Threat of Triazole-resistant *Aspergillus Fumigatus*', *Journal of Antimicrobial Chemotherapy*, 74 (2019), pp. 835–42.

56 E. Rodriguez Mega, 'Alarming Surge in Drug-resistant HIV Uncovered', *Nature Briefing*, 30 July 2019.

57 N. Slivinski, 'Are We Headed for a New Era of Malaria Drug Resistance?', *The Scientist*, 20 March 2019.

58 A. Allen, *Vaccine: The Controversial Story of Medicine's Greatest Life Saver* (New York, 2007).

59 J.-F. Bach, 'The Hygiene Hypothesis in Autoimmunity: The Role of Pathogens and Commensals', *Nature Reviews Immunology*, 18 (2018), pp. 105–20.

60 The Editors of *The Lancet*, 'Retraction: Ileal-lymphoid-nodular Hyperplasia, Non-specific Colitis, and Pervasive Developmental Disorder in Children', *The Lancet*, 375 (2010), pp. 1302–4.

61 Allen, *Vaccine: The Controversial Story of Medicine's Greatest Life Saver*.

62 M. J. Mina et al., 'Long-term Measles-induced Immunomodulation Increases Overall Childhood Infectious Disease Mortality', *Science*, 348 (2015), pp. 694–9.

63 M. J. Mina et al., 'Measles Virus Infection Diminishes Preexisting Antibodies that Offer Protection from Other Pathogens', *Science*, 366 (2019), pp. 599–606.

64 P. Hotez, 'The Physician-scientist: Defending Vaccines and Combating Antiscience', *Journal of Clinical Investigation*, 129 (2019), pp. 2169–71.

65 M. E. Sundaram, L. B. Guterman and S. B. Omer, 'The True Cost of Measles Outbreaks during the Postelimination Era', *Journal of the American Medical Association*, 321 (2019), pp. 1155–6.

66 S. B. Omer, C. Betsch and J. Leask, 'Mandate Vaccination with Care', *Nature*, 571 (2019), pp. 469–72.

67 H. J. Larson, 'The Biggest Pandemic Risk? Viral Misinformation', *Nature*, 562 (2018), p. 309.

68 Hotez, 'The Physician-scientist: Defending Vaccines and Combating Antiscience'.

69 Quick with Fryer, *The End of Epidemics*.

70 M. S. Green et al., 'Confronting the Threat of Bioterrorism: Realities, Challenges, and Defensive Strategies', *Lancet Infectious Diseases*, 19 (2019), pp. e2–13.

71 Quick with Fryer, *The End of Epidemics*.

72 H. W. Cohen et al., 'The Pitfalls of Bioterrorism Preparedness: The Anthrax and Smallpox Experience', *American Journal of Public Health*, 94 (2004), pp. 1667–71.

73 Green et al., 'Confronting the Threat of Bioterrorism'.

74 N. Khardori, 'Bioterrorism and Bioterrorism Preparedness: Historical Perspective and Overview', *Infectious Disease Clinics of North America*, 20 (2006), pp. 179–211.

75 B. Lorber, 'Are All Diseases Infectious?', *Annals of Internal Medicine*, 125 (1996), pp. 844–51.

76 P. W. Ewald, *Plague Time. How Stealth Infections Cause Cancers, Heart Disease, and Other Deadly Ailments* (New York, 2000).

77 G. K. Hansson, 'Inflammation, Atherosclerosis, and Coronary Artery Disease', *New England Journal of Medicine*, 352 (2005), pp. 1685–95.

78 Ewald, *Plague Time*.

79 M. S. Rezaee-Zavareh, M. Tohidi and A. Saburi, 'Infectious and Coronary Artery Disease', ARYA *Atherosclerosis*, 12 (2016), pp. 41–9.

80 G. Aarabi et al., 'Roles of Oral Infections in the Pathomechanism of Atherosclerosis', *International Journal of Molecular Sciences*, 19 (2018), p. 1978.

81 O. Patrakka et al., 'Oral Bacterial Signatures in Cerebral Thrombi of Patients with Acute Ischemic Stroke Treated with Thrombectomy', *Journal of the American Heart Association*, 8 (2019), p. e012330.

82 Ewald, *Plague Time*.

83 P. E. Castle and M. Maza, 'Prophylactic HPV Vaccination: Past, Present, and Future', *Epidemiology and Infection*, 144 (2016), pp. 449–68; Ewald, *Plague Time*.

84 R. F. Itzhaka, 'Corroboration of a Major Role for Herpes Simplex Virus Type 1 in Alzheimer's Disease', *Frontiers in Aging Neuroscience*, 10 (2018), p. 324.

85 M. C. Norton et al., 'Greater Risk of Dementia When Spouse has Dementia? The Cache County Study', *Journal of the American Geriatrics Society*, 58 (2010), pp. 895–900.

86 S. S. Lollis et al., 'Cause-specific Mortality among Neurosurgeons', *Journal of Neurosurgery*, 113 (2010), pp. 474–8.

87 G. Morris et al., 'Myalgic Encephalomyelitis and Chronic Fatigue Syndrome: How Could the Illness Develop?', *Metabolic Brain Disease*, 34 (2019), pp. 385–415.

88 F. Khan and M. Ali, 'The Last Case of Smallpox', *Lancet Infectious Diseases*, 18 (2018), p. 1318.

89 L. Klotz, 'Human Error in High-biocontainment Labs: A Likely Pandemic Threat', *Bulletin of Atomic Scientists*, 25 February 2019, www.thebulletin. org.

90 A. Casadevall and M. J. Imperiale, 'Risks and Benefits of Gain-of-function Experiments with Pathogens of Pandemic Potential, such as Influenza Virus: A Call for a Science-based Discussion', *mBio*, 5 (2014), e01730-14.

91 J. Kaiser, 'Controversial Flu Studies Can Resume, U.S. Panel Says', *Science*, 363 (2019), pp. 676–7.

92 B. Ekser, P. Li and D.K.C. Cooper, 'Xenotransplantation: Past, Present, and Future', *Current Opinion in Organ Transplantation*, 22 (2017), pp. 513–21.

93 J. A. Fishman, 'Infectious Disease Risks in Xenotransplantation', *American Journal of Transplantation*, 18 (2018), pp. 1856–64.

94 X. Wu et al., 'Impact of Climate Change on Human Infectious Diseases: Empirical Evidence and Human Adaptation', *Environment International*, 86 (2016), pp. 14–23; P. R. Epstein, 'Climate and Emerging Infectious Diseases', *Microbes and Infection*, 3 (2001), pp. 747–54.

95 K. D. Lafferty and E. A. Mordecai, 'The Rise and Fall of Infectious Disease in a Warmer World', *F1000research*, 5 (2016).

96 K. L. Gage et al., 'Climate and Vectorborne Diseases', *American Journal of Preventive Medicine*, 35 (2008), pp. 436–50.

97 D. Sumilo et al., 'Climate Change Cannot Explain the Upsurge of Tick-borne Encephalitis in the Baltics', *PLoS One*, 2 (2007), e500.

98 C. Baker-Austin and J. D. Oliver, '*Vibrio vulnificus*: New Insights into a Deadly Opportunistic Pathogen', *Environmental Microbiology*, 20 (2018), pp. 423–30.

99 A. Casadevall, D. P. Kontoyiannis and V. Robert, 'On the Emergence of *Candida auris*: Climate Change, Azoles, Swamps, and Birds', *mBio*, 10 (2019), e01397–19.

100 D. R. MacFadden et al., 'Antibiotic Resistance Increases with Local Temperature', *Nature Climate Change*, 8 (2018), pp. 510–14.

101 J. K. Jansson and N. Tas, 'The Microbial Ecology of Permafrost', *Nature Reviews Microbiology*, 12 (2014), pp. 414–25.

102 'What Lies Beneath', *Scientific American*, 315 (2016), pp. 11–12; repr. as 'As Earth Warms, the Diseases that May Lie within Permafrost Become a Bigger Worry', *Scientific American*, 1 November 2016, www.scientificamerican.com.

103 R. Meyer, 'The Zombie Diseases of Climate Change', *The Atlantic*, 16 November 2017.

104 C. Abergel and J.-M. Claverie, '*Pithovirus sibericum*: Réveil d'un virus géant de plus de 30,000 ans', *Médecine/Sciences*, 30 (2014), pp. 329–31; M. Legendre et al., 'In-depth Study of *Mollivirus sibericum*, a New 30,000-y-old Giant Virus Infecting *Acanthamoeba*', *Proceedings of the National Academy of Sciences*, 112 (2015), pp. e5327–35.

105 C. Wickramasinghe, 'Panspermia According to Hoyle', *Astrophysics and Space Science*, 285 (2003), pp. 535–8.

106 E. J. Steele et al., 'Cause of Cambrian Explosion: Terrestrial or Cosmic?', *Progress in Biophysics and Molecular Biology*, 136 (2018), pp. 3–23.

107 I. Gyollai et al., 'Mineralized Biosignatures in ALH-77005 Shergottite: Clues to Martian Life?', *Open Astronomy*, 28 (2019), pp. 32–9.

108 A. C. Sielaff et al., 'Characterization of the Total and Viable Bacterial and Fungal Communities Associated with the International Space Station Surfaces', *Microbiome*, 7 (2019), article 50.

109 C. Urbaniak et al., 'Detection of Antimicrobial Resistance Genes Associated with the International Space Station Environmental Surfaces', *Scientific Reports*, 8 (2018), p. 814.

110 N. Guéginou et al., 'Could Spaceflight-associated Immune System Weakening Preclude the Expansion of Human Presence Beyond Earth's Orbit?', *Journal of Leukocyte Biology*, 86 (2009), pp. 1027–38.

111 B. V. Rooney et al., 'Herpes Virus Reactivation in Astronauts during Spaceflight and its Application on Earth', *Frontiers in Microbiology*, 7 February 2019, www.frontiersin.org.

112 B. E. Crucian et al., 'Immune System Dysregulation during Spaceflight: Potential Countermeasures for Deep Space Exploration Missions', *Frontiers in Immunology*, 28 June 2018.

113 Ibid.

114 A. C. Clarke, *Tales of Ten Worlds* (New York, 1973).

Epilogue: The Never-ending Duel

1 D. Durack and S. V. Lynch, 'The Gut Microbiome: Relationships with Disease and Opportunities for Therapy', *Journal of Experimental Medicine*, 216 (2018), pp. 20–40.

2 B. Pulendran, 'Immunology Taught by Vaccines', *Science*, 366 (2019), pp. 1074–5.

3 S. Gupta, E. Allen-Vercoe and E. O. Petrof, 'Fecal Microbiota Transplantation: In Perspective', *Therapeutic Advances in Gastroenterology*, 9 (2016), pp. 229–39.

4 M. Cully, 'Microbiome Therapeutics Go Small Molecule', *Nature Reviews Drug Discovery*, 18 (2019), pp. 569–72.

5 M. Jimenez, R. Langer and G. Traverso, 'Microbial Therapeutics: New Opportunities for Drug Delivery', *Journal of Experimental Medicine*, 216 (2019), pp. 1005–9.

SELECT BIBLIOGRAPHY

Allen, A., Vaccine: *The Controversial Story of Medicine's Greatest Life Saver*
(New York, 2007)

Barnaby, W., *The Plague Makers: The Secret World of Biological Warfare*
(London, 1997)

Barrett, R., and G. J. Armelagos, *An Unnatural History of Emerging Infections*
(Oxford, 2013)

Barry, J. M., *The Great Influenza: The Epic Story of the Deadliest Plague in
History* (New York, 2004)

Benedictow, O. J., *The Black Death, 1346–1353: The Complete History*
(Woodbridge, 2004)

Bray, R. S., *Armies of Pestilence: The Impact of Disease on History*
(Cambridge, 1996)

Bruce-Chwatt, L. J., and J. Zulueta, *The Rise and Fall of Malaria in Europe*
(Oxford, 1980)

Cartwright, F. F., *Disease and History* (New York, 1972)

Cohen, M. N., *Health and the Rise of Civilization* (New Haven, CT, 1989)

Crosby, A. W., *The Columbian Exchange: Biological and Cultural Consequences
of 1492* (Westport, CT, 1972)

Daniel, T. M., *Captain of Death: The Story of Tuberculosis* (Rochester,
NY, 1997)

De Kruif, P., *Microbe Hunters* [1926] (New York, 2002)

Diamond, J., Guns, *Germs, and Steel: The Fates of Human Societies*
(New York, 1999)

Ewald, P. W., *Evolution of Infectious Disease* (Oxford, 1994)

Gaynes, R. P., *Germ Theory: Medical Pioneers in Infectious Diseases*
(Washington, DC, 2011)

Geison, G. L., *The Private Science of Louis Pasteur* (Princeton, NJ, 1995)

Gradmann, C., *Laboratory Disease* (Baltimore, MD, 2009)

Harper, K., *The Fate of Rome* (Princeton, NJ, 2017)

Hays, J. N., *Epidemics and Pandemics: Their Impacts on Human History*
(Santa Barbara, CA, 2005)

Hopkins, D. R., *Princes and Peasants: Smallpox in History* (Chicago, IL, 1983)

Jouanna, J., *Hippocrates* (Baltimore, MD, 1999)

Kiple, K. F., ed., *The Cambridge World History of Human Disease*
(Cambridge, 1994)

Levy, S. B., *The Antibiotic Paradox: How the Misuse of Antibiotics Destroys
their Curative Powers*, 2nd edn (Cambridge, MA, 2002)

Little, L. K., ed., *Plague and the End of Antiquity: The Pandemic of 541–750* (Cambridge, 2007)

McNeill, W. H., *Plagues and Peoples* (New York, 1976)

Mattern, S. P., *The Prince of Medicine: Galen in the Roman Empire* (Oxford, 2013)

Morse, S. S., ed., *Emerging Viruses* (Oxford, 2003)

Nutton, V., *Ancient Medicine* (London, 2004)

Oldstone, M.B.A., *Viruses, Plagues and History* (Oxford, 1998)

Osterholm, M. T., and M. Olshaker, *Deadliest Enemy: Our War against Killer Germs* (New York, 2017)

Paul, J. R., *A History of Poliomyelitis* (New Haven, CT, 1971)

Pepin, J., *The Origins of AIDS* (Cambridge, 2011)

Playfair, J., and G. Bancroft, *Infection and Immunity*, 2nd edn (Oxford, 2004)

Porter, R., *The Greatest Benefit to Mankind: A Medical History of Humanity from Antiquity to the Present* (London, 1999)

Price-Smith, A. T., *Contagion and Chaos* (Cambridge, MA, 2009)

Quétel, C., *History of Syphilis* (Cambridge, 1990)

Rosen, W., *Justinian's Flea: Plague, Empire and the Birth of Europe* (London, 2008)

—, *Miracle Cure: The Creation of Antibiotics and the Birth of Modern Medicine* (New York, 2018)

Sherman, I. W., *The Power of Plagues* (Washington, DC, 2006)

Spiers, E. M., *A History of Chemical and Biological Weapons* (London, 2010)

Thucydides, *The Peloponnesian War*, trans. Martin Hammond (Oxford, 2009)

Waller, J., *The Discovery of the Germ: Twenty Years that Transformed the Way We Think about Disease* (New York, 2002)

Winslow, C.-E. A., *The Conquest of Epidemic Disease: A Chapter in the History of Ideas* (Madison, WI, 1980)

Ziegler, P., *The Black Death* (London, 1997)

Zinsser, H., *Rats, Lice and History* (Boston, MA, 1934)

PHOTO ACKNOWLEDGEMENTS

The author and publishers wish to express their thanks to the below sources of illustrative material and/or permission to reproduce it. Some locations of artworks are also given below, in the interest of brevity:

Accademia di belle arti G. Carrara, Bergamo: p. 246; photo AFP Photo/Egyptian Ministry of Antiquities: p. 363; Bibliothèque royale de Belgique (KBR), Brussels (MS 13077, fol. 16v)/© KIK-IRPA, Brussels: p. 145; photo Andrea Booher/FEMA: p. 97; Château de Versailles: pp. 182, 231; Creutzfeldt-Jakob Disease (CJD) Foundation Inc, Akron, OH: p. 45; photo courtesy Dallas Museum of Art, TX: p. 367; De Agostini Picture Library/Getty Images: p. 143; Deutsches Historisches Museum, Berlin: p. 157; from Gustave Doré and Blanchard Jerrold, *London: A Pilgrimage* (London, 1872): p. 83; courtesy Ellen Finsberg: p. 55; photo Stig S. Frøland: p. 395 (*left*); photo D. Carleton Gajdusek: p. 432; Gallerie degli Uffizi, Florence: p. 281; Glinka State Central Museum of Musical Culture, Moscow: p. 87; from the collections of The Henry Ford, Dearborn, MI: p. 335 (*top*); iStock.com: pp. 48 (ChrisChrisW), 164 (Yevgeniy Drobotenko), 526 (Marcin Klapczynski/ Alpha Tauri 3D), 570 (Adrian Wojcik), 574 (3000ad); photo Carol A. Kauffman, MD: p. 396; courtesy David Keeping: p. 211; photo George E. Koronaios: p. 374; from Atichat Kuadkitkan, Nitwara Wikan, Wannapa Sornjai and Duncan R. Smith, 'Zika virus and microcephaly in Southeast Asia: A cause for concern?', *Journal of Infection and Public Health*, XIII/1 (January 2020): p. 429; Kunsthistorisches Museum, Vienna: p. 261; Kupferstichkabinett, Staatliche Museen zu Berlin (MS 78 E 1, fol. 80v): p. 140; from Pierre Lalouette, *Nouvelle méthode de traiter les maladies vénériennes, par la fumigation: avec les procès-verbaux des guérisons opérés* (Paris, 1776), photo Wellcome Library, London: p. 249; Landesbibliothek Mecklenburg-Vorpommern Günther Uecker, Schwerin (MS 376, fol. 103v): p. 146; from Geoffroy de La Tour-Landry and Marquart von Stein, trans., *Der Ritter vom Turn von den Exempeln der Gotsforcht und Erberkeit* (Augsburg, 1498), photo Library of Congress, Lessing J. Rosenwald Collection, Washington, DC: p. 248; Library of Congress, Prints and Photographs Division, Washington, DC: pp. 183, 265; from James D. McCabe Jr, *Great Fortunes, and How They Were Made: Or, the Struggles and Triumphs of our Self-Made Men* (Philadelphia, New York and Boston, 1871): p. 233; Philippe Maillard/akg-images: p. 132; from Shauna Milne-Price, Kerri L. Miazgowicz and Vincent J. Munster, 'The emergence of the Middle East Respiratory Syndrome coronavirus', *Pathogens and Disease*, LXXI/2 (March 2014): p. 423; Munch-museet, Oslo: p. 242; Musée Alexandre Dumas,

Villers-Cotterêts: p. 283; Musée du Louvre, Paris: p. 90; Musée d'Orsay, Paris: p. 30; Museu de Belles Arts de València: p. 148; Narodowe Archiwum Cyfrowe, Warsaw: p. 486; Nasjonalbiblioteket, Oslo: pp. 29, 370; Nasjonalmuseet, Oslo: pp. 152 (photo Morten Thorkildsen), 153 (photo Dag Andre Ivarsøy), 251 (photo Jacques Lathion), 277 and 340 (photos Børre Høstland); The National Gallery, London: p. 20; National Library of Medicine, Bethesda, MD: p. 497 (*top*); National Museum of Health and Medicine, Silver Spring, MD: pp. 335 (Otis Historical Archives, NCP 1603; *bottom*), 485; National Portrait Gallery, London: pp. 282, 285, 365; NTB scanpix: pp. 26 (Mary Evans Picture Library), 100 (Luis Montanya/ Marta Montanya/Science Photo Library), 116 (Science Photo Library), 141 (Album/ Fine Art Images), 150 (AB Svensk Filmindustri/Album), 169, 175 (Heritage Art/ Heritage Images), 179 (akg/North Wind Picture Archive), 180 (Barbara Cushing/ Everett Collection), 181 (Historia/REX/Shutterstock), 205 (Dennis Kunkel Microscopy/Science Photo Library), 210 (The Granger Collection, New York), 299 (photo © Tore Wuttudal/NN/Samfoto; *bottom*), 301 (© 20thCentFox/Everett Collection), 402 (*top*), 404 (photo Abbas Dulleh; *top*), 404 (photo Florian Plaucheur; *bottom*), 410 (Kateryna Kon/Science Photo Library), 411 (WSPA/ K. Ammann/REX/Shutterstock), 415 (imageBROKER/Ivan Kuzmin), 449 (SOPA Images/SIPA USA), 497 (*bottom*), 508 (St Mary's Hospital Medical School/Science Photo Library), 511 (AP), 563 (Universal Pictures/Album); Ny Carlsberg Glyptotek, Copenhagen: p. 345; Oslo Museum: p. 253; private collection: p. 286; Public Health Image Library (PHIL), Centers for Disease Control and Prevention, U.S. Department of Health and Human Services (HHS): pp. 133, 158 (Rocky Mountain Laboratories, NIAID, NIH), 161 (photo Dr Pratt; *top*), 172 (photo James Hicks), 185 and 312 (photos James Gathany), 401 (Dr Frederick A. Murphy), 403, 422 (Alissa Eckert, MSMI, and Dan Higgins, MAMS), 433 (Teresa Hammett); from Marcus Rainsford, *An Historical Account of the Black Empire of Hayti* (London, 1805), photo John Carter Brown Library, Brown University, Providence, RI: p. 232; from Kamleshun Ramphul, Stephanie G. Mejias, Vivian C. Agumadu, et al., 'The Killer Virus Called Nipah: A Review,' *Cureus*, x/8 (August 2018): p. 418; from *Review of Reviews*, II/12 (December 1890): p. 33; Royal Collection Trust/© Her Majesty Queen Elizabeth II 2022: p. 368; Shutterstock.com: pp. 320 (VectorMine), 407 (Alila Medical Media); from G. Elliot Smith, *Catalogue général des antiquités égyptiennes du Musée du Caire* (Cairo, 1912): p. 176; Special Collections and University Archives, Rutgers University Libraries, New Brunswick, NJ: p. 515; The State Tretyakov Gallery, Moscow: pp. 196, 257; StudioCanal/REX/Shutterstock: p. 513; from Norman Walker, *An Introduction to Dermatology*, 7th edn (Edinburgh, 1922), photo Wellcome Library, London: p. 294; Yale Center for British Art, Paul Mellon Collection, New Haven, CT: p. 473.

CDC Global Health, the copyright holder of the image on p. 203, and Matt-80, the copyright holder of the image on p. 84, have published them online under conditions imposed by a Creative Commons Attribution 2.0 Generic License. El Bingle/ Sean Robinson (University of Sunderland), the copyright holders of the image on p. 144, have published it online under conditions imposed by a Creative Commons Attribution-NonCommercial 2.0 Generic License. J. G. Collomb/ World Resources Institute (WRI), the copyright holders of the image on p. 402 (*bottom*), have published it online under conditions imposed by a Creative

INDEX OF NAMES

Illustration page numbers are in *italics*